Hematology and Oncology

Hematology and Oncology

Editor: Wedge Burton

FOSTER
ACADEMICS
www.fosteracademics.com

www.fosteracademics.com

FOSTER ACADEMICS

Cataloging-in-Publication Data

Hematology and oncology / edited by Wedge Burton.
p. cm.
Includes bibliographical references and index.
ISBN 978-1-63242-737-3
1. Hematology. 2. Oncology. 3. Hematological oncology. 4. Blood--Diseases. I. Burton, Wedge.
RC280.H47 H46 2019
616.994 18--dc23

Foster Academics,
118-35 Queens Blvd., Suite 400,
Forest Hills, NY 11375, USA

ISBN 978-1-63242-737-3 (Hardback)

Printed and bound in China.

Contents

Preface

Hematology is a branch of medicine that is concerned with the study of the cause, treatment, prognosis and prevention of diseases related to blood. The treatment of diseases affecting the production of blood and its components like hemoglobin, bone marrow, blood cells, blood proteins, platelets, blood vessels, etc. is under the scope of this field. Some of these diseases are leukemia, lymphoma and multiple myeloma. These are all cancers of the blood. The treatment of blood cancer is also under the scope of oncology. When there is a suspicion of a hematological malignancy, various analyses such as a blood film and a complete blood count are conducted. In case of a lymphadenopathy, a biopsy of a lymph node or a bone marrow biopsy are generally done. Imaging techniques of positron emission tomography (PET CT) and computerized tomography (CT) are also used for diagnosis. This book brings forth some of the most innovative concepts and elucidates the unexplored aspects of hematology and oncology. The topics covered in this extensive book deal with the core aspects of the care and management of blood cancer. It aims to equip students and experts with the advanced topics and upcoming concepts in this area.

This book is a result of research of several months to collate the most relevant data in the field.

When I was approached with the idea of this book and the proposal to edit it, I was overwhelmed. It gave me an opportunity to reach out to all those who share a common interest with me in this field. I had 3 main parameters for editing this text:

- Accuracy – The data and information provided in this book should be up-to-date and valuable to the readers.
- Structure – The data must be presented in a structured format for easy understanding and better grasping of the readers.
- Universal Approach – This book not only targets students but also experts and innovators in the field, thus my aim was to present topics which are of use to all.

Thus, it took me a couple of months to finish the editing of this book.

I would like to make a special mention of my publisher who considered me worthy of this opportunity and also supported me throughout the editing process. I would also like to thank the editing team at the back-end who extended their help whenever required.

Editor

1

Glabridin Mediate Caspases Activation and Induces Apoptosis through JNK1/2 and p38 MAPK Pathway in Human Promyelocytic Leukemia Cells

Hsin-Lien Huang[1]❡, Ming-Ju Hsieh[1,2,3]❡, Ming-Hsien Chien[4,5], Hui-Yu Chen[1], Shun-Fa Yang[1,6], Pei-Ching Hsiao[7,8]*

1 Institute of Medicine, Chung Shan Medical University, Taichung, Taiwan, **2** Cancer Research Center, Changhua Christian Hospital, Changhua, Taiwan, **3** School of Optometry, Chung Shan Medical University, Taichung, Taiwan, **4** Graduate Institute of Clinical Medicine, College of Medicine, Taipei Medical University, Taipei, Taiwan, **5** Wan Fang Hospital, Taipei Medical University, Taipei, Taiwan, **6** Department of Medical Research, Chung Shan Medical University Hospital, Taichung, Taiwan, **7** School of Medicine, Chung Shan Medical University, Taichung, Taiwan, **8** Department of Internal Medicine, Chung Shan Medical University Hospital, Taichung, Taiwan

Abstract

Background: Glabridin, a prenylated isoflavonoid of *G. glabra L.* roots, has been associated with a wide range of biological properties such as regulation of energy metabolism, estrogenic, neuroprotective, anti-osteoporotic, and skin-whitening in previous studies. However, the effect of glabridin on tumor cells metastasis has not been clearly clarified. Here, the molecular mechanism by which glabridin anticancer effects in human promyelocytic leukemia cells was investigated.

Methodology and Principal Findings: The results showed that glabridin significantly inhibited cell proliferation of four AML cell lines (HL-60, MV4-11, U937, and THP-1). Furthermore, glabridin induced apoptosis of HL-60 cells through caspases-3, -8, and -9 activations and PARP cleavage in dose- and time-dependent manner. Moreover, western blot analysis also showed that glabridin increase phosphorylation of ERK1/2, p38 MAPK and JNK1/2 in dose- and time-dependent manner. Inhibition of p38 MAPK and JNK1/2 by specific inhibitors significantly abolished the glabridin-induced activation of the caspase-3, -8 and -9.

Conclusion: Taken together, our results suggest that glabridin induced HL-60 cell apoptosis through p38 MAPK and JNK1/2 pathways and could serve as a potential additional chemotherapeutic agent for treating AML.

Editor: Yuan-Soon Ho, Taipei Medical University, Taiwan

Funding: This study was supported by a grant (CSH-2014-C-020) from Chung Shan Medical University Hospital, Taiwan. The funders had no role in the study design, data collection and analysis, decision to publish, or preparation of the manuscript.

Competing Interests: The authors have declared that no competing interests exist.

* E-mail: cshy046@csh.org.tw

❡ These authors contributed equally to this work.

Introduction

Naturally occurring plant products have gained increasing attention for potential use in intervention against malignant invasive progression in late stage neoplastic diseases [1,2]. There is increasing focus on providing a scientific basis for use of these agents as a preventive strategy for people with high risk of cancers. Glabridin as a key chemical and biological marker of G. glabra and have significant impact on food, dietary supplements (DSs) and cosmetic markets. Glabridin is an isoflavane, a type of isoflavonoid. This product is part of a larger family of plant-derived molecules, the natural phenols. The group's previous study showed that glabridin can inhibit lung and breast cancer metastasis [3,4]. Glabridin have shown positive effects in fields like LDL protection against oxidation and anti-obesity could potentially provide benefits to human health [5–7]. However, the effects of glabridin on human promyelocytic leukemia have yet to be evaluated.

Acute myeloid leukemia (AML), is a cancer of the myeloid line of blood cells, characterized by the rapid growth of abnormal white blood cells that accumulate in the bone marrow and interfere with the production of normal blood cells [8,9]. Exposure to anticancer chemotherapy can increase the risk of subsequently developing AML. The risk is highest about three to five years after chemotherapy [10]. Conventional chemotherapy of AML combination treatment with cytarabine or daunorubicin induces complete remission in more than 50% of patients, only 20–30% of patients enjoy long-term disease-free survival and these chemo drugs can also affect normal cells causing unpleasant side effects such as anemia, bleeding, and infection. Thus, there is a need for new agents to treat AML. In recent years, some natural products have been used as alternative treatments for cancers including AML. Icariside II, a flavonoid compound derived from Epimedium koreanum, was suggested as an antileukemic agent for AML therapy [11]. Moreover, matrine, an alkaloid extracted from Sophora flavescens Aif, targets mitochondrial apoptotic pathways in HL-60 [12]. Wogonin, an active compound in Scutellaria baicalensis, induces apoptosis by inhibiting telomerase activity in HL-60 [13]. In the present study, we investigated the cytotoxic effects of glabridin on HL-60 and its underlying mechanisms in vitro.

Materials and Methods

Chemicals

Glabridin, ≥98% (HPLC), powder was purchased from Sigma Chemical Co. (St. Louis, MO, USA). Stock solution of Glabridin was made at 10, 20 and 40 μM concentration in DMSO and stored at −20°C. The final concentration of DMSO for all treatments was consistently less than 0.1%. 3-(4,5-dimethylthiazol-2-yl)-2,5-diphenyltetrazolium bromide (MTT) was obtained from Sigma Chemical Co. (St. Louis, MO, USA). Specific inhibitors for ERK1/2 (U0126), JNK1/2 (SP600125) or p38 (SB202190) were purchased from Calbiochem (San Diego, CA). Antibodies, specifically of Bax, Bad, Bid, Bcl-2, cleaved caspase-3, caspase-8, caspase-9, poly (ADP-ribose) polymerase (PARP), p-extracellularly regulated kinase (ERK)1/2, p-p38, p-c-Jun N-terminal kinase (JNK), ERK1/2, p38, JNK1/2, α-tubulin and β-actin (for the Western blot analysis), were purchased from Santa Cruz Biotechnology.

Cell Culture

Human AML cell lines of MV4-11 were kindly provided by Dr. L.-I. Lin (National Taiwan University, Taipei, Taiwan), while the HL-60, U937, and THP-1 cell lines were purchased from the American Type Culture Collection (ATCC) (Manassas, VA). Human normal cells of WI-38 (lung fibroblast) and HOK (human oral keratinocyte cell) were purchased from ATCC. All cells were cultured in the recommended conditions, supplemented with 10% fetal bovine serum (FBS), 0.1 mM nonessential amino acids, 1 mM glutamine, 1% penicillin/streptomycin, 1.5 g/L sodium bicarbonate, and 1 mM sodium pyruvate (Sigma, St. Louis, Mo, USA) and maintained at 37°C in a humidified atmosphere of 5% CO2.

In vitro Cytotoxicity Assay

The effect of glabridin on cell growth was assayed by the MTT (3- (4,5-cimethylthiazol-2-yl)-2,5-diphenyl tetrazolium bromide) method, as previously described [14]. Briefly, cells were cultured in 24-well plates (5×10^4/well) and stimulated with different concentrations of glabridin (0, 10, 20, 40, 80 μM) in culture media. After 24 hours of glabridin stimulation, MTT was added to each well (0.5 mg/ml final concentration) with a further incubation for 4 h. The viable cell number was directly proportional to the production of frmazan following the solubilization with isopropanol. The color intensity was measured at 570 nm [15]. Each condition was performed in triplicate and data were obtained from at least 3 separate experiments.

Cell Cycle Analysis

To determine the effect of glabridin on cell cycle, cells (1×10^6/ml) were first cultured in serum-free medium for starvation at 18 hours and then exposed to glabridin for 24 hours. After cells were washed, fixed with 70% ethanol, and incubated for 30 minutes in the dark at room temperature with propidium iodide (PI) buffer (4 μg/ml PI, 1% Triton X-100, 0.5 mg/ml RNase A in PBS) and then filtered through a 40-μm nylon filter (Falcon, USA) [16]. The cell cycle distribution was analyzed for 5,000 collected cells by a FACS Vantage flow cytometer that uses the CellQuest acquisition and analysis program (Becton Dickinson FACSCalibur).

Annexin V/PI Double Staining

To detect apoptosis in HL-60 cell line after exposure to glabridin, an FITC Annexin V Apoptosis Detection Kit I (BD Biosciences, USA) was used to quantify cell number in different stages of cell death [17]. Briefly, 1×10^5 cells were resuspended in 100 μl 1× binding buffer (0.01 M Hepes/NaOH (pH 7.4), 0.14 M NaCl, 2.5 mM CaCl2). After the addition of FITC Annexin V and PI (5 μl each), the cell suspension was gently vortexed and incubated for 15 minutes at room temperature in the dark. Add 400 μl of 1 × binding buffer to each tube and analyze by flow cytometry within 1 h [18].

Western Blot Analysis

Cell lysates were separated in a 10% or 15% polyacrylamide gel and transferred onto a PVDF membrane (Millipore Corporation, Milford, MA, USA) [19]. The blot was subsequently incubated with 5% non-fat milk in PBS for 1 h to block non-specific binding, and probed with a corresponding antibody against a specific protein for 37°C at 2 h or overnight at 4°C, and then with an appropriate peroxidase conjugated secondary antibody for 1 h. After the final washing, signal was developed by ECL detection system and relative photographic density was quantitated by a gel documentation and analysis (AlphaImager 2000, Alpha Innotech Corporation, San Lean 189 dro, CA, USA) [20].

Statistical Analysis

Values represent the means ± standard deviation and the experiments were repeated three times (n = 3). Statistical analyses were performed using the one-way analysis of variance (ANOVA) followed by Tukey's posthoc test was used when more than three groups were analyzed. Data comparisons were performed with Student's t test (Sigma-Stat 2.0, Jandel Scientific, San Rafael, CA, USA) when two groups were compared. A p value <0.05 was considered to be statistically significant.

Results

Cytotoxic Effects of Glabridin-treated AML Cell Lines

The chemical structure of glabridin was shown in Figure 1A. To determine the cytotoxicity and the effect on cell proliferation of glabridin on four AML cell lines (HL-60, MV4-11, U937, and THP-1), cells were treated with different concentrations of glabridin (0–80 μM) for 24 h. As shown in Figure 1B, after treatment for 24 h, glabridin significantly reduced the cell viability in a concentration-dependent manner for the four AML cell lines. Moreover, glabridin did not alter the cell viability of normal lung fibroblast cells (WI-38) and human oral keratinocyte cell (HOK) (Figure 1C).

Glabridin-induced Cell Apoptosis in HL-60 and MV4-11 Cells

To determine whether the inhibitory effect of cell viability of glabridin is associated with induction of cell apoptosis, HL-60 and MV4-11 cells were treated with different concentrations (0–40 μM) of glabridin for 24 h. Cell cycle analysis by flow cytometry was showed a dose-dependent increased accumulation of cell population in sub-G1 phase after a 24-hour treatment with glabridin (Figure 2A). Meanwhile, Annexin-V and PI double-staining displayed an increased percentage of apoptotic cells after a 24 h treatment of glabridin (Figure 2B), respectively.

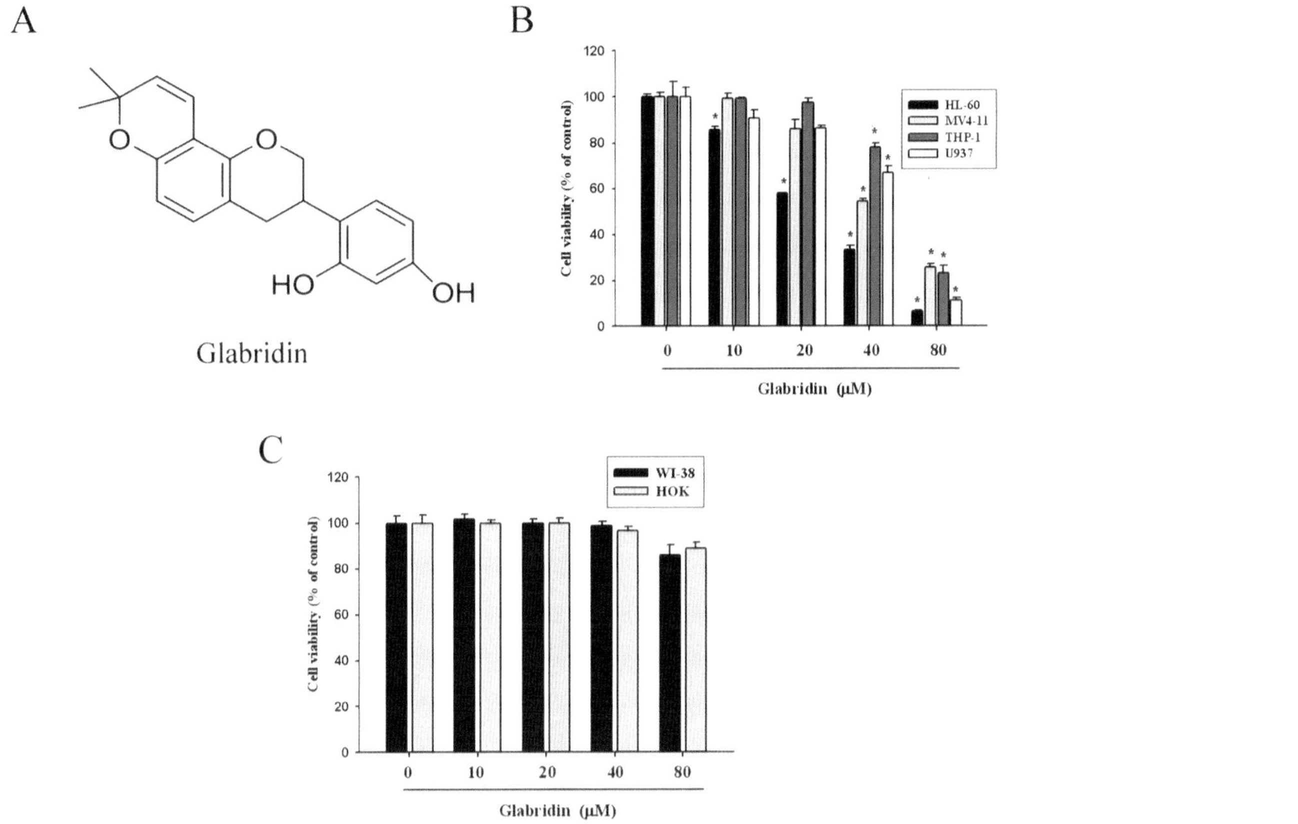

Figure 1. Cytotoxic effect of glabridin in four AML cell lines (HL-60, MV4-11, U937, and THP-1) and two human normal cells (WI-38 and HOK). (A) Structure of glabridin. (B) Cell viability analysis of four AML cell lines (HL-60, MV4-11, U937, and THP-1) cultured in presence of glabridin for 24 h by MTT assay. (C) Cell viability analysis of two normal cells (WI-38 and HOK) cultured in presence of glabridin for 24 h by MTT assay. Data represent mean of 3 determinations per condition repeated 3 times. Results are shown as mean ± SE.

Glabridin Induced Activation of Caspase-3, -8 and -9 in HL-60 Cells

To further confirm the involvement of caspase activation in glabridin-induced apoptosis, activation of caspases-3, -8, and -9 and cleavage of PARP were detected. Figure 3A shows that exposure of HL-60 cells to glabridin (0–40 μM) for 24 h, caused concentration-dependent increased of the cleaved fragments of caspases-9, -8, and -3. Furthermore, cleaved PARP was also significantly increased in glabridin treated HL-60 cells. Glabridin treatment at 40 μM for 24 h significantly increased expression levels of cleaved caspases-3, -8, -9 and PARP by 4.1-, 2.37-, 5.37 and 3.87-fold, respectively, compared to the control (Figure 3B). Moreover, treatment of HL-60 cells with glabridin (40 μM) also resulted in a time-dependent increase in activated caspases-3, -8, and -9 (Figure 3C). Glabridin treatment at 40 μM for 24 h significantly increased expression levels of cleaved caspases-3, -8 and -9 by 2.12-, 2.11- and 1.5-fold, respectively, compared to the control (Figure 3D). Glabridin caused concentration-dependent decreases in the truncate Bid and Bcl-2, in addition, the expression levels of Bax and Bad were increases in glabridin-treated HL-60 cells (Figure 3E). Glabridin treatment at 40 μM for 24 h significantly increased expression levels of Bad and Bax by 1.3 and 1.48-fold, it also decreased expression levels of truncate Bid and Bcl-2 by 29% and 31%, respectively, compared to the control (Figure 3F).

The Apoptosis Induction by Glabridin is Dependent on the Regulation of JNK and P38 MAPK Signaling Pathways in HL-60 Cells

Several signaling pathways have been implicated MAPK signaling pathway plays an important role in the action of chemotherapeutic drugs in the regulation of apoptosis [21]. In a further investigation for the underlying molecular mechanisms, we determined whether MAPKs were activated in glabridin-treated HL-60 cells by a Western blot analysis. Results showed that the phosphorylation of ERK1/2, JNK1/2 and p38 MAPK were increased in cells treated with glabridin in a dose-dependent manner (Figure 4A, 4B and 4C). Moreover, treatment of HL-60 cells with glabridin (40 μM) also resulted in a time-dependent increase in phosphorylation of ERK1/2, JNK1/2 and p38 MAPK (Figure 4D and 4E). Next, we further investigated relationships among glabridin induced activation of caspases-9, -8, and -3 and MAPKs. HL-60 cells were pretreated with 20 μM U0126 (an ERK inhibitor), SP600125 (a JNK inhibitor), or SB202190 (a p38 inhibitor) for 1 h, treated with 40 μM glabridin for another 24 h, and then analyzed by Western blotting. As shown in Figure 5, treatment SB202190 and SP600125 significantly attenuated glabridin-induced caspase-9, -8, and -3 activation. These findings suggest that activation of JNK1/2 and p38 MAPK might play a critical upstream role in glabridin-mediated caspase activation in HL-60 cells.

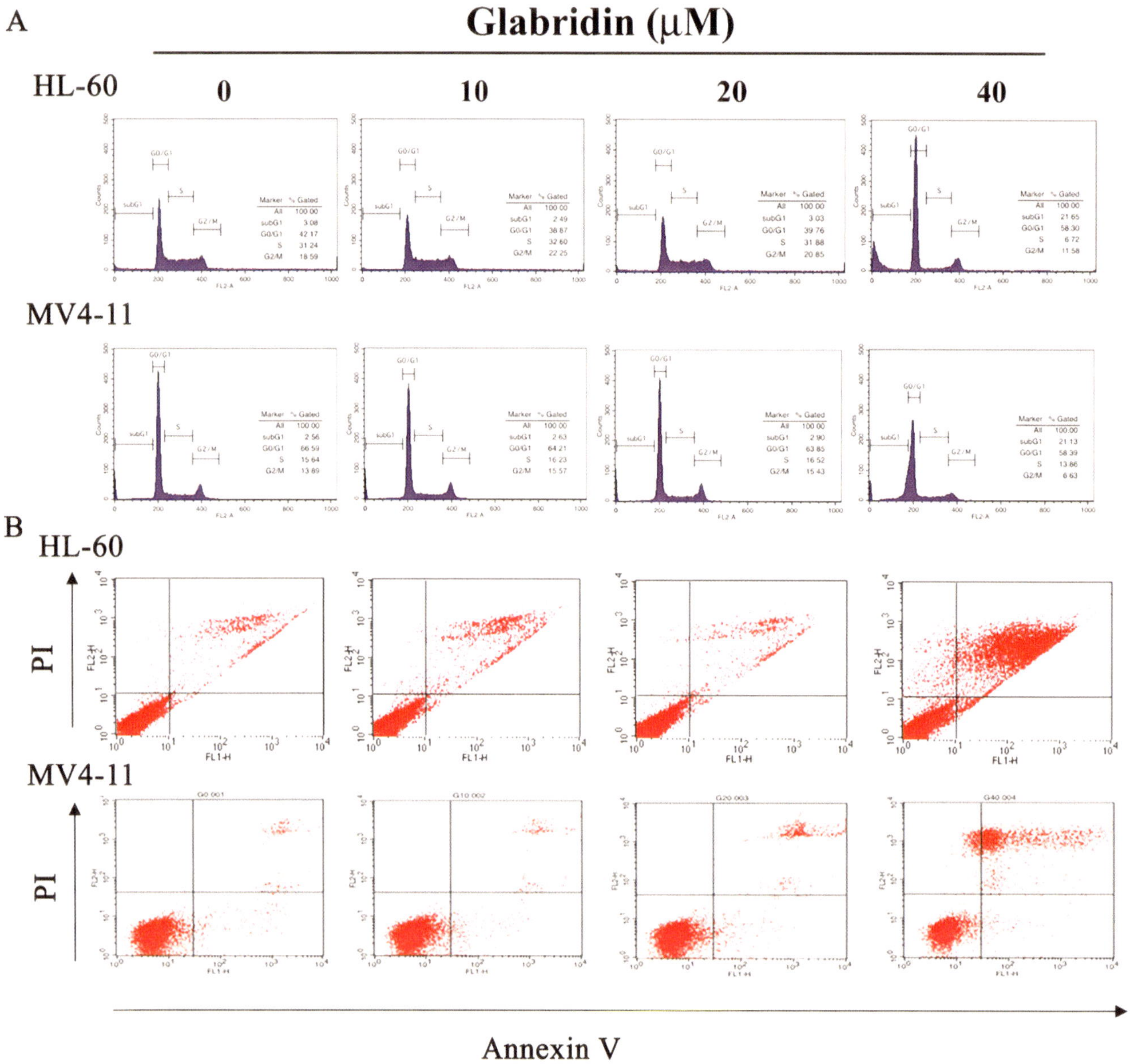

Figure 2. Glabridin induced cell apoptosis in HL-60 and MV4-11 cells. (A) HL-60 and MV4-11 cells were incubated for 18 h in the absence of serum and then treated with indicated concentrations of glabridin for 24 h, after which the cells were stained with PI, and analyzed for DNA content by flow cytometry. Furthermore, after being treated with different concentration of glabridin for 24 h, cells were harvested and then subjected to quantitative analysis of cell apoptosis by Annexin-V and PI double-stained flow cytometry (B).

Discussion

Acute myeloid leukemia (AML) is a fatal hematological malignancy which is resistant to a variety of chemotherapy drugs. Natural herbal products have a promising and potential role in developing novel chemotherapeutics for various cancers [22–24]. Various ethnic societies worldwide have traditionally used herbal products in the prevention and/or treatment of several chronic diseases [25–27]. Glabridin is a polyphenolic flavonoid, a main constituent in the roots of *Glycyrrhiza glabra* possesses various biological activities, has reported protection against oxidation, anti-obesity and inhibit lung and breast cancer metastasis [4,28,29]. Glabridin being a natural product and with known safety in human is a suitable candidate for drug development [30]. The present study demonstrates, for the first time, that glabridin induced apoptosis of HL-60 cells.

Apoptosis, is a form of programmed cell death that occurs naturally in cells and can be beneficial to cancer therapy as previously reported [31,32]. Natural herbal products have been extensively studied for its antitumor effect including antiproliferative activities, cell cycle arrest and apoptosis induction via the mitochondrial and some other pathways [33,34]. Recently, targeted elimination of AML cells by inducing apoptosis has emerged as a valuable strategy for combating AML [12,35]. Moreover, several naturally occurring drugs such as homoharringtonine and etoposide are used in the clinic for treating AML [36]. In this study, several hallmarks of apoptosis such as significant increases in sub-G1 content, and Annexin V-positive

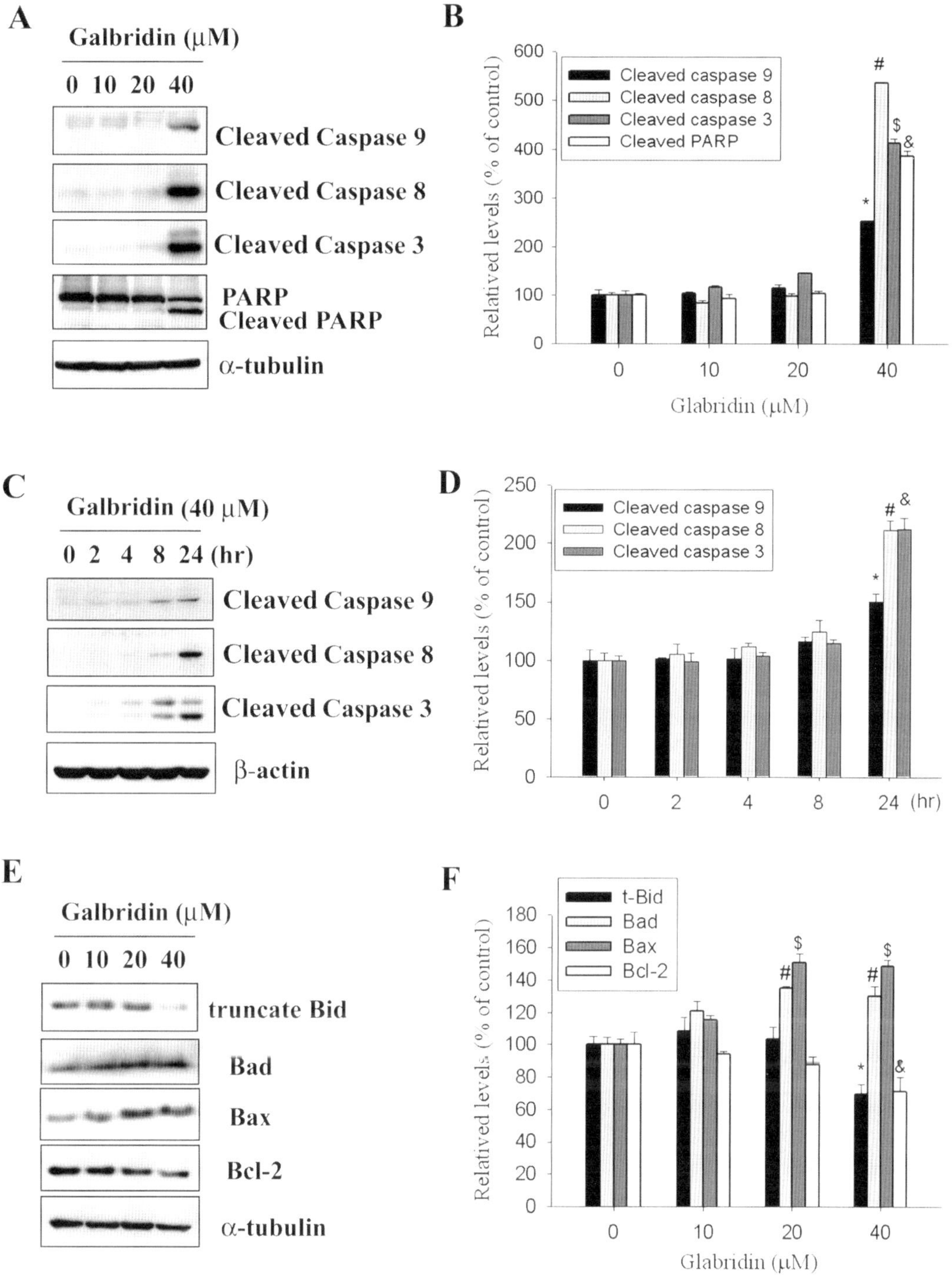

Figure 3. Activation of caspase 3, -8, -9 and PARP were increased in Glabridin-treated HL-60 cells. (A) HL-60 cells were treated with 10, 20 and 40 μM glabridin for 24 h and subjected to western blotting with an antibody against PARP or caspase-3, -8 and -9 antibody. (B) The values under each lane indicate relative density of the band normalized to α-tubulin using a densitometer. Values represent the mean ± SE of three independent experiments. (*, #, &, $) $p<0.05$ compared to the vehicle control groups. (C) HL-60 cells were treated with 40 μM glabridin for 2, 4, 8 and 24 h, subjected to western blotting with an antibody against caspase-3, -8 and -9 antibody. (D) The values under each lane indicate relative density of the band normalized to β-actin using a densitometer. Values represent the mean ± SE of three independent experiments. (*, #, &) $p<0.05$ compared to the vehicle control groups. (E) HL-60 cells were treated with 10, 20 and 40 μM glabridin for 24 h and subjected to western blotting with an antibody against Bid, Bax, Bad and Bcl-2 antibody. (F) The values under each lane indicate relative density of the band normalized to α-tubulin using a densitometer. Values represent the mean ± SE of three independent experiments. (*, #, &, $) $p<0.05$ compared to the vehicle control groups.

cells were observed in HL-60 cells after glabridin treatment for 24 h. Glabridin (40 μM) can induce increases of sub-G1 content and Annexin V-positive cells by 6.7- and 8.2-fold, respectively.

Apoptosis is mediated by proteolytic enzymes called caspases, which trigger cell death by cleaving specific proteins in the cytoplasm and nucleus. The activation process is initiated by either

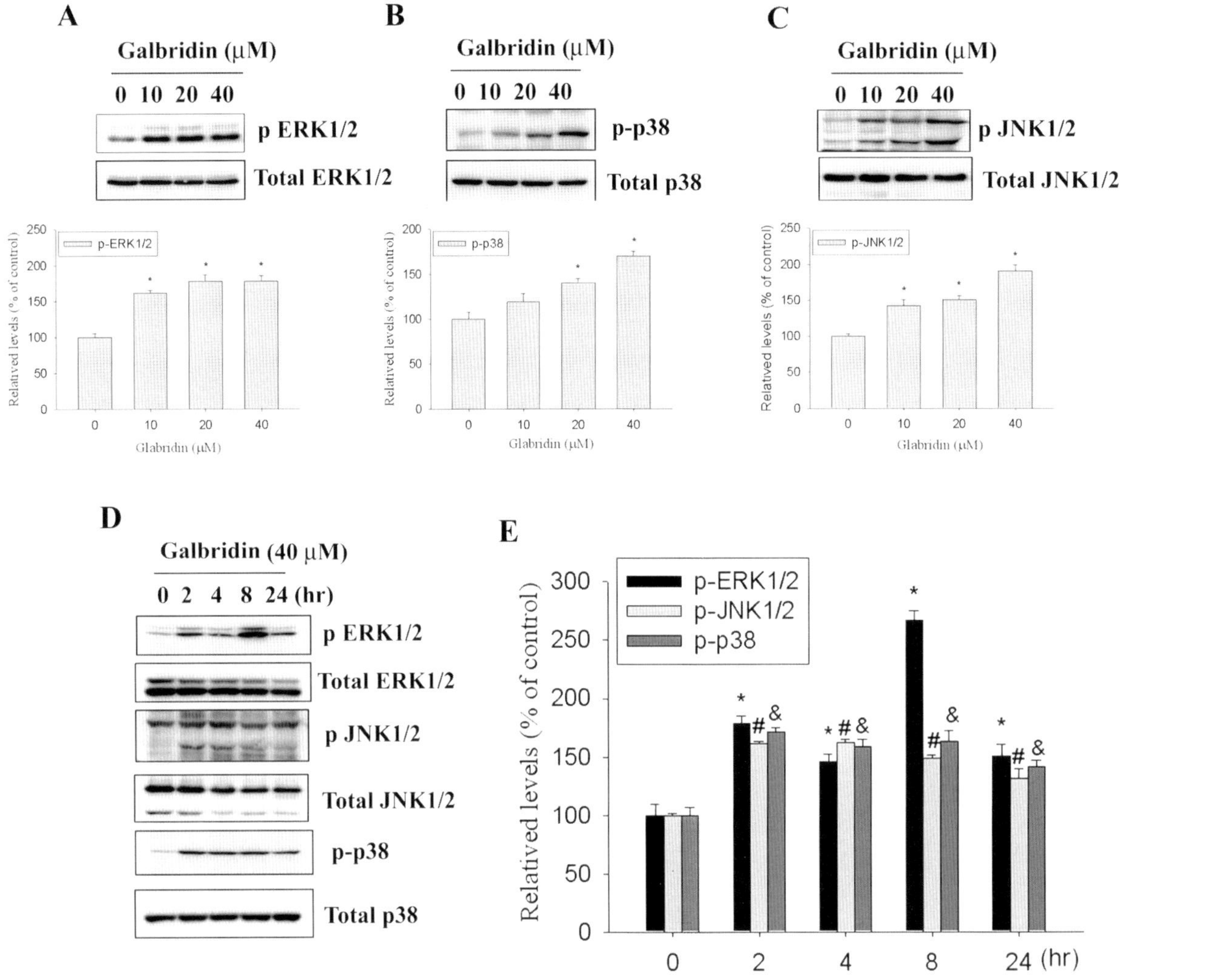

Figure 4. Glabridin activates the phosphorylation of ERK1/2, p38 MAPK and JNK1/2 in HL-60 cells. (A–C, upper panel)) Cells were treated with different concentrations of glabridin (0–40 μM) for 24 h and then subjected to western blotting with an antibody against ERK1/2, JNK1/2, and p38 MAPK. (A–C, lower panel) Quantitative results of p-ERK1/2, p-p38, and p-JNK1/2 protein levels, which were adjusted with the total ERK1/2, p38, and JNK1/2 protein levels and expressed as multiples of induction beyond each respective control. Values represent the mean ± SE of three independent experiments. (*) $p<0.05$ compared to the vehicle control group. (D) HL-60 cells were treated with 40 μM glabridin for 2, 4, 8 and 24 h, subjected to western blotting with an antibody against ERK1/2, JNK1/2, and p38 MAPK antibody. (E) The values under each lane indicate relative density of the band normalized to β-actin using a densitometer. Values represent the mean ± SE of three independent experiments. (*, #, &, $) $p<0.05$ compared to the vehicle control groups.

extracellular or intracellular death signals, which cause intracellular adaptor molecules to aggregate and activate procaspases [37]. The present results suggest that glabridin may partially act through the initiator caspase-8 and then the executioner caspase-3 to increase the cleavage form of PARP to induce AML cell apoptosis. Moreover, many papers pointed out that the ability of anticancer agents to induce apoptosis of tumor cells was correlated with the ability to decrease expression of Bcl-2 [38]. Meanwhile, we found that expression of the antiapoptotic proteins Bcl-2 also was decreased in HL-60 cells after glabridin treatment for 24 h. Other members of the Bcl-2 family are not death inhibitors, but instead promote procaspase activation and cell death. Some of these apoptosis promoters, such as Bad, function by binding to and inactivating the death-inhibiting members of the family, whereas others, like Bax and Bak, stimulate the release of cytochrome *c* from mitochondria. Bax and Bak are themselves activated by other apoptosis-promoting members of the Bcl-2 family such as Bid [39]. In the present study, an increase in the Bad and Bax protein expression levels, a decrease in the expression of Bid, and activation of caspases-3/−9 occurred after treatment with glabridin, suggesting that glabridin inducing apoptosis in HL-60 cells might partly occur through a mitochondrion-mediated pathway.

Previous studies have suggested that MAPKs can be induced by various compounds and involved in cell death or cytoprotection in AML cells [40–42]. On the basis of previous reports, we further investigated activation of MAPK family proteins in glabridin treated HL-60 cells. The results showed that the phosphorylation of ERK1/2, JNK1/2, and p38 MAPK were increased in glabridin-treatment HL-60 cells and glabridin (40 μM) induced activation of ERK1/2, JNK1/2, and p38 MAPK in a time-dependent manner. However, treatment with JNK specific inhibitor (SP600125) or p38 MAPK specific inhibitor (SB202190) effectively inhibit activation of caspases-3, -8, and -9

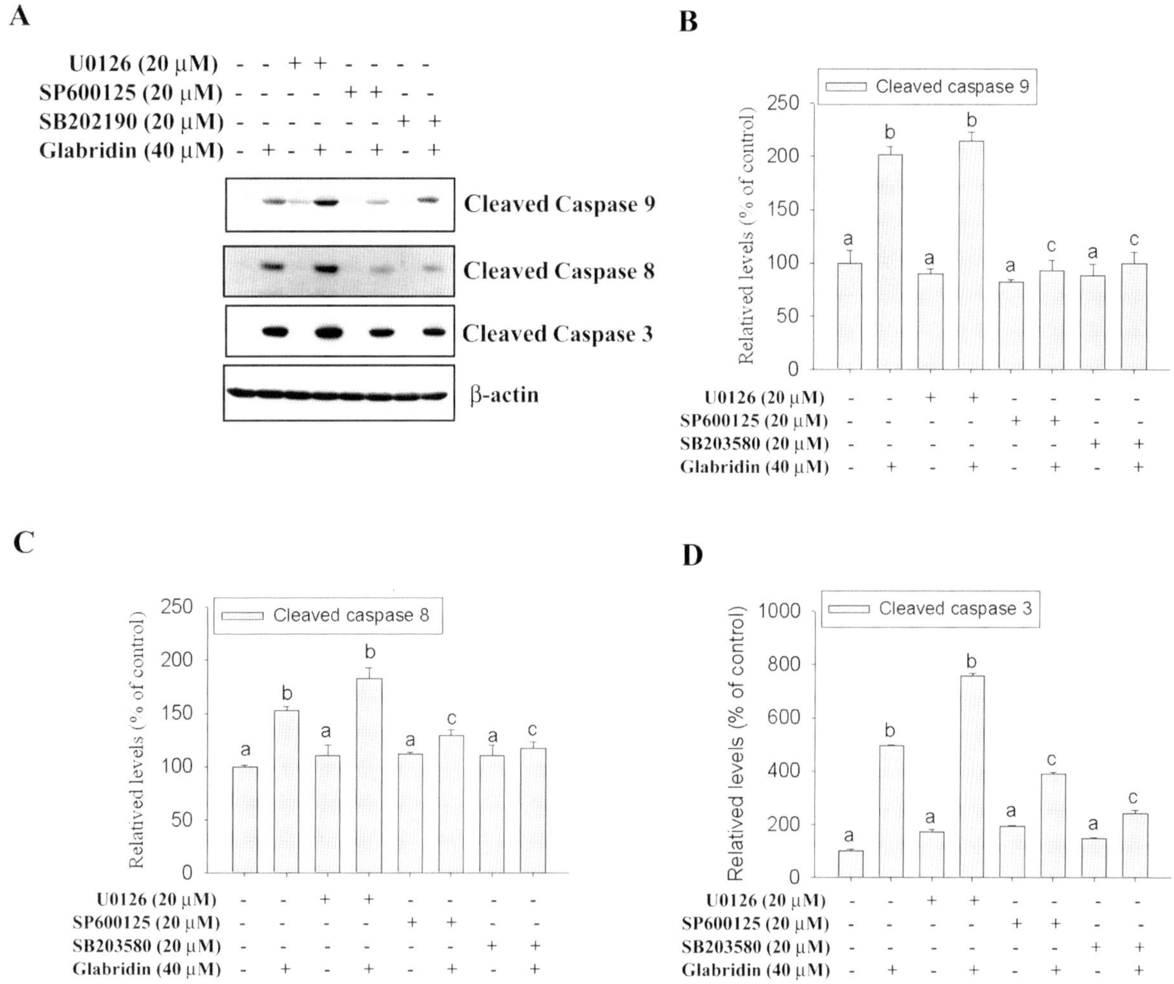

Figure 5. JNK1/2 and p38 MAPK are essential for caspase activation induced by glabridin. (A) HL-60 cells were treated for 24 hours with 40 μM glabridin with or without a 1-hour pretreatment of 20 μM U0126, SP600125, or SB202190. The expression of cleaved caspase-9, -8 and -3 were detected by western blotting. (B–D) Quantitative results of cleaved caspase-9, -8, and -3 protein levels, which were adjusted to the β-actin protein level and expressed as multiples of induction beyond each respective control. Values represent the mean ± SE of three independen experiments. Data were analyzed using a one-way ANOVA with Tukey's posthoc tests at 95% confidence intervals; different letters represent different levels of significance.

induced by glabridin, whereas U0126 (an ERK1/2 inhibitor) had no effect on glabridin-induced caspase activation. Taken together, these results suggest that activation of JNK1/2 and p38 MAPK plays an important role in glabridin-induced apoptosis.

In conclusion, we first demonstrated that glabridin could induce the phosphorylation of JNK1/2, and p38 MAPK, inhibit the expressions of Bcl-2 and Bid, subsequent stimulate the activation of caspase-3, -8, and -9, which eventually result in the cleaved of PARP and inhibition of proliferation and apoptosis induction of HL-60 cells. Our findings revealed that glabridin may be a useful candidate as a chemotherapeutic agent for AML therapy.

Author Contributions

Conceived and designed the experiments: HLH PCH. Performed the experiments: MJH SFY MHC. Analyzed the data: HYC SFY. Contributed reagents/materials/analysis tools: SFY MHC. Contributed to the writing of the manuscript: HLH PCH.

References

1. Ravindranath MH, Ramasamy V, Moon S, Ruiz C, Muthugounder S (2009) Differential growth suppression of human melanoma cells by tea (Camellia sinensis) epicatechins (ECG, EGC and EGCG). Evid Based Complement Alternat Med 6: 523–530.
2. Shankar S, Ganapathy S, Hingorani SR, Srivastava RK (2008) EGCG inhibits growth, invasion, angiogenesis and metastasis of pancreatic cancer. Front Biosci 13: 440–452.
3. Tsai YM, Yang CJ, Hsu YL, Wu LY, Tsai YC, et al. (2011) Glabridin inhibits migration, invasion, and angiogenesis of human non-small cell lung cancer A549 cells by inhibiting the FAK/rho signaling pathway. Integr Cancer Ther 10: 341–349.
4. Hsu YL, Wu LY, Hou MF, Tsai EM, Lee JN, et al. (2011) Glabridin, an isoflavan from licorice root, inhibits migration, invasion and angiogenesis of MDA-MB-231 human breast adenocarcinoma cells by inhibiting focal adhesion kinase/Rho signaling pathway. Mol Nutr Food Res 55: 318–327.
5. Carmeli E, Fogelman Y (2009) Antioxidant effect of polyphenolic glabridin on LDL oxidation. Toxicol Ind Health 25: 321–324.
6. Belinky PA, Aviram M, Mahmood S, Vaya J (1998) Structural aspects of the inhibitory effect of glabridin on LDL oxidation. Free Radic Biol Med 24: 1419–1429.

7. Ahn J, Lee H, Jang J, Kim S, Ha T (2013) Anti-obesity effects of glabridin-rich supercritical carbon dioxide extract of licorice in high-fat-fed obese mice. Food Chem Toxicol 51: 439-445.
8. Jemal A, Thomas A, Murray T, Thun M (2002) Cancer statistics, 2002. CA Cancer J Clin 52: 23-47.
9. Tallman MS, Gilliland DG, Rowe JM (2005) Drug therapy for acute myeloid leukemia. Blood 106: 1154-1163.
10. Bishop JF (1997) The treatment of adult acute myeloid leukemia. Semin Oncol 24: 57-69.
11. Kang SH, Jeong SJ, Kim SH, Kim JH, Jung JH, et al. (2012) Icariside II induces apoptosis in U937 acute myeloid leukemia cells: role of inactivation of STAT3-related signaling. PLoS One 7: e28706.
12. Zhang S, Zhang Y, Zhuang Y, Wang J, Ye J, et al. (2012) Matrine induces apoptosis in human acute myeloid leukemia cells via the mitochondrial pathway and Akt inactivation. PLoS One 7: e46853.
13. Huang ST, Wang CY, Yang RC, Chu CJ, Wu HT, et al. (2010) Wogonin, an active compound in Scutellaria baicalensis, induces apoptosis and reduces telomerase activity in the HL-60 leukemia cells. Phytomedicine 17: 47-54.
14. Yang SF, Chen MK, Hsieh YS, Yang JS, Zavras AI, et al. (2010) Antimetastatic effects of Terminalia catappa L. on oral cancer via a down-regulation of metastasis-associated proteases. Food Chem Toxicol 48: 1052-1058.
15. Yu YL, Su KJ, Chen CJ, Wei CW, Lin CJ, et al. (2012) Synergistic anti-tumor activity of isochaihulactone and paclitaxel on human lung cancer cells. J Cell Physiol 227: 213-222.
16. Huang SM, Cheung CW, Chang CS, Tang CH, Liu JF, et al. (2011) Phloroglucinol derivative MCPP induces cell apoptosis in human colon cancer. J Cell Biochem 112: 643-652.
17. Tsai CF, Yeh WL, Huang SM, Tan TW, Lu DY (2012) Wogonin induces reactive oxygen species production and cell apoptosis in human glioma cancer cells. Int J Mol Sci 13: 9877-9892.
18. Casciola-Rosen L, Nicholson DW, Chong T, Rowan KR, Thornberry NA, et al. (1996) Apopain/CPP32 cleaves proteins that are essential for cellular repair: a fundamental principle of apoptotic death. J Exp Med 183: 1957-1964.
19. Lu DY, Yeh WL, Huang SM, Tang CH, Lin HY, et al. (2012) Osteopontin increases heme oxygenase-1 expression and subsequently induces cell migration and invasion in glioma cells. Neuro Oncol 14: 1367-1378.
20. Wu CS, Yen CJ, Chou RH, Li ST, Huang WC, et al. (2012) Cancer-associated carbohydrate antigens as potential biomarkers for hepatocellular carcinoma. PLoS One 7: e39466.
21. Chen T, Wong YS (2008) Selenocystine induces S-phase arrest and apoptosis in human breast adenocarcinoma MCF-7 cells by modulating ERK and Akt phosphorylation. J Agric Food Chem 56: 10574-10581.
22. Casciola-Rosen L, Rosen A, Petri M, Schlissel M (1996) Surface blebs on apoptotic cells are sites of enhanced procoagulant activity: implications for coagulation events and antigenic spread in systemic lupus erythematosus. Proc Natl Acad Sci U S A 93: 1624-1629.
23. Lee YR, Lei HY, Liu MT, Wang JR, Chen SH, et al. (2008) Autophagic machinery activated by dengue virus enhances virus replication. Virology 374: 240-248.
24. Jia W, Gao W, Tang L (2003) Antidiabetic herbal drugs officially approved in China. Phytother Res 17: 1127-1131.
25. Li X, Wang H (2005) Chinese herbal medicine in the treatment of chronic kidney disease. Adv Chronic Kidney Dis 12: 276-281.
26. Wang J, Xiong X, Xing Y, Liu Z, Jiang W, et al. (2013) Chinese Herbal Medicine for Acute Mountain Sickness: A Systematic Review of Randomized Controlled Trials. Evid Based Complement Alternat Med 2013: 732562.
27. Zhou F, Hao YF, Chen Y, Wang T (2013) Chinese herbal medicine in treatment of polyhydramnios:a meta-analysis and systematic review. Chin Med Sci J 28: 72-81.
28. Wu F, Jin Z, Jin J (2013) Hypoglycemic effects of glabridin, a polyphenolic flavonoid from licorice, in an animal model of diabetes mellitus. Mol Med Rep 7: 1278-1282.
29. Kim HS, Suh KS, Ko A, Sul D, Choi D, et al. (2013) The flavonoid glabridin attenuates 2-deoxy-D-ribose-induced oxidative damage and cellular dysfunction in MC3T3-E1 osteoblastic cells. Int J Mol Med 31: 243-251.
30. Aoki F, Nakagawa K, Kitano M, Ikematsu H, Nakamura K, et al. (2007) Clinical safety of licorice flavonoid oil (LFO) and pharmacokinetics of glabridin in healthy humans. J Am Coll Nutr 26: 209-218.
31. Chinkwo KA (2005) Sutherlandia frutescens extracts can induce apoptosis in cultured carcinoma cells. J Ethnopharmacol 98: 163-170.
32. Kroemer G, Martin SJ (2005) Caspase-independent cell death. Nat Med 11: 725-730.
33. Cai J, Liu M, Wang Z, Ju Y (2002) Apoptosis induced by dioscin in Hela cells. Biol Pharm Bull 25: 193-196.
34. Wang Y, Che CM, Chiu JF, He QY (2007) Dioscin (saponin)-induced generation of reactive oxygen species through mitochondria dysfunction: a proteomic-based study. J Proteome Res 6: 4703-4710.
35. Carter BZ, Mak DH, Shi Y, Fidler JM, Chen R, et al. (2012) MRx102, a triptolide derivative, has potent antileukemic activity in vitro and in a murine model of AML. Leukemia 26: 443-450.
36. Efferth T, Li PC, Konkimalla VS, Kaina B (2007) From traditional Chinese medicine to rational cancer therapy. Trends Mol Med 13: 353-361.
37. Spencer SL, Sorger PK (2011) Measuring and modeling apoptosis in single cells. Cell 144: 926-939.
38. Vermes I, Haanen C, Steffens-Nakken H, Reutelingsperger C (1995) A novel assay for apoptosis. Flow cytometric detection of phosphatidylserine expression on early apoptotic cells using fluorescein labelled Annexin V. J Immunol Methods 184: 39-51.
39. Cotter TG (2009) Apoptosis and cancer: the genesis of a research field. Nat Rev Cancer 9: 501-507.
40. Li Q, Huai L, Zhang C, Wang C, Jia Y, et al. (2013) Icaritin induces AML cell apoptosis via the MAPK/ERK and PI3K/AKT signal pathways. Int J Hematol 97: 617-623.
41. Repicky A, Jantova S, Cipak L (2009) Apoptosis induced by 2-acetyl-3-(6-methoxybenzothiazo)-2-yl-amino-acrylonitrile in human leukemia cells involves ROS-mitochondrial mediated death signaling and activation of p38 MAPK. Cancer Lett 277: 55-63.
42. Sanchez Y, Amran D, Fernandez C, de Blas E, Aller P (2008) Genistein selectively potentiates arsenic trioxide-induced apoptosis in human leukemia cells via reactive oxygen species generation and activation of reactive oxygen species-inducible protein kinases (p38-MAPK, AMPK). Int J Cancer 123: 1205-1214.

2

Renal Involvement in Non-Hodgkin Lymphoma: Proven by Renal Biopsy

Shi-Jun Li, Hui-Ping Chen, Ying-Hua Chen, Li-hua Zhang, Yuan-Mao Tu, Zhi-hong Liu*

National Clinical Research Center of Kidney Diseases, Jinling Hospital, Nanjing University of Medcine, Nanjing, China

Abstract

Aims: To determine the spectrum of renal lesions in patients with kidney involvement in non-Hodgkin's lymphoma (NHL) by renal biopsy.

Methods: The clinical features and histological findings at the time of the renal biopsy were assessed for each patient.

Results: We identified 20 patients with NHL and renal involvement, and the diagnosis of NHL was established following the kidney biopsy in 18 (90%) patients. The types of NHL include the following: chronic lymphocytic leukemia/small lymphocytic lymphoma (n = 8), diffuse large B-cell lymphoma (n = 4), T/NK cell lymphoma (n = 3), lymphoplasmacytic lymphoma (n = 2), cutaneous T-cell lymphoma (n = 1), mucosa-associated lymphoid tissue lymphoma (n = 1) and mantle cell lymphoma (n = 1). All presented with proteinuria, and 15 patients had impaired renal function. The pathological findings included (1) membranoproliferative glomerulonephritis-like pattern in seven patients; (2) crescent glomerulonephritis in four; (3) minimal-change disease in three, and glomeruli without specific pathological abnormalities in three; (4) intraglomerular large B-cell lymphoma in one; (5) intracapillary monoclonal IgM deposits in one; (6) primary diffuse large B-cell lymphoma of the kidneys in one; and (7) lymphoma infiltration of the kidney in eight patients.

Conclusion: A wide spectrum of renal lesions can be observed in patients with NHL, and NHL may be first proven by renal biopsies for evaluation of kidney injury or proteinuria. Renal biopsy is necessary to establish the underlying cause of renal involvement in NHL.

Editor: Maria Pia Rastaldi, Fondazione IRCCS Ospedale Maggiore Policlinico & Fondazione D'Amico per la Ricerca sulle Malattie Renali, Italy

Funding: The authors have no support or funding to report.

Competing Interests: The authors have declared that no competing interests exist.

* E-mail: zhihong—liu@hotmail.com

Introduction

Renal involvement in non-Hodgkin lymphoma (NHL) has been reported previously, including glomerulonephritis, acute kidney injury (AKI), and lymphoma infiltrating the kidney parenchyma [1–4]. Previous studies have shown that up to 10% of patients with NHL and lymphocytic leukemia may have kidney injury [5]. However, a limited number of cases of GN have been described in patients with NHL demonstrated by renal biopsy in the literature to date [6–8]. Considering that the morphology of glomerular injury in patients with lymphoma are often heterogeneous, the myriad of etiologies of renal injury due to NHL often present a diagnostic challenge to clinician. Here, we retrospectively analyzed the spectrum of renal lesions proven by renal biopsy in patients with NHL in single center, to better establish the relationship between renal injury and NHL.

Materials and Methods

Patient selection

We reviewed the renal pathology archives of the Research Institute of Nephrology at Nanjing University of Medicine from 2001 through 2012 and identified 20 patients with NHL and renal dysfunction of sufficient severity and/or proteinuria that a renal biopsy was obtained. The diagnosis of NHL was based on the 2008 WHO classification system [9]. This study was approved by the Ethical Committee of Nanjing University. According to the ethics committee recommendation, written consent was not required for this non interventional study. Patients or surrogates provided verbal informed consent prior to study inclusion. Verbal consent was obtained through a session of patient or family information explaining the study, its aims and the non interventional design. The consent was recorded in the medical chart of each patient. Patients or relatives had the opportunity to decline study participation at any time.

Data collection

Baseline data at the time of renal biopsy were obtained from the medical records for all cases. The following data were collected: sex, age, clinical presentation, ultrasound of kidneys, extra renal presentations and relevant clinical history.

Clinical and laboratory data at the time of kidney biopsy were assessed for each patient. Cryoglobulinemia was detected by cold precipitation of serum samples from blood that had been collected and processed at 37°C. Proteinuria was defined as a urine protein level >0.4 g/24 h, and hematuria, assessed using light microscopy, was defined as a red blood cell count >10,000/ml in the urinary sediment. Nephrotic syndrome was defined as a urinary protein excretion >3.5 g/d and a serum albumin level <30 g/L. Impaired renal function was defined as a GFR<60 ml/min per 1.73 m^2according to the Modification of Diet in Renal Disease (MDRD) formula. Acute kidney injury was defined according to the KIDIGO criteria.

Renal biopsy studies

All patients underwent a percutaneous renal biopsy. No symptom perirenal haematoma and macroscopic haematuria have been observed in these patients. Each renal sample contained more than 10 glomeruli. The renal biopsy procedure was as follows: the samples were embedded in paraffin and sectioned at 2 μm, followed by hematoxylin-eosin, Masson, periodic acid-Schiff or periodic acid-silver methenamine (PASM) staining. For immunofluorescence (IF), the samples were sectioned at 3 μm using a cryostat, followed by use of a panel of FITC-conjugated rabbit anti-human antibodies to IgG, IgM, IgA, C3, C1q, and κ and λ light chains (polyclonal, Dako Corporation). These samples were also stained with Congo red. The intensity of the immunofluorescence staining was semiquantitatively scored on a scale of 0 to 2+. Immunophenotyping of the lymphomas was performed on frozen sections using the immunoperoxidase and avidin-biotin techniques. The phenotype of the cellular infiltrate was studied using biotinylated anti-CD4, -CD8, -CD20 and -CD68 antibodies (Dako) and visualized using a peroxidase-streptavidin conjugate. Electron microscopy was performed using a Hitachi 7500 electron microscope after routine sections were prepared from renal tissues, followed by double staining with uranyl acetate and lead citrate. Renal biopsies from all patients were reviewed by two renal pathologists.

Results

Clinical findings

The clinical characteristics of all 20 patients are summarized in Table 1. There were 17 men and 3 women aged 16 to 68 years at the time of renal biopsy (mean age 53 years). At the time of the renal biopsy, only 2 (10%) of 20 patients had an established diagnosis of NHL, the remaining 18 patients had renal biopsies performed before the diagnosis of the lymphoma. Six patients (30%) presented with recurring fever of unknown origin. Enlargement of the inguinal, axillary, submaxillary or supraclavicular lymph nodes were found in eight patients (40%). Computed tomography (CT) scans revealed numerous intumesced lymph nodes in the neck, mediastinal septum and retroperitoneal space in five patients (25%). CT revealed markedly enlarged kidneys bilaterally in nine (45%) patients, enlargement of the spleen in three patients. (See Table 1). The anatomic sites of sampling used for the primary diagnosis of the lymphoid neoplasm were the lymph nodes (n = 7), bone marrow (n = 6), gastrointestinal tract (n = 2), nasal cavity/sinus (n = 2), kidney (n = 2) and skin (n = 1).

Of the 20 patients with NHL, 16 (80%) had B-cell neoplasms, including chronic lymphocytic leukemia/small lymphocytic lymphoma (CLL/SLL, n = 8), diffuse large B-cell lymphoma (DLBCL, n = 4), lymphoplasmacytic lymphoma (LPL, n = 2), mucosa-associated lymphoid tissue lymphoma (MALT, n = 1) and mantle cell lymphoma (MCL, n = 1). Four patients (20%) had mature T/NK-cell neoplasms, including extra nodal NK/T-cell lymphoma, nasal type T/NK cell lymphoma (n = 2), cutaneous T-cell lymphoma (n = 1) and adult T-cell lymphoma (n = 1).

All patients presented with proteinuria, and 15 patients (75%) had impaired renal function(eGFR<60 ml/min). The mean serum creatinine level was 228±181 μmol/l (range 50 to 752 μmol/L). Microscopic hematuria was found in 15 patients (75%), and gross hematuria in 4 patients (20%). Renal symptoms included nephrotic syndrome in 6 patients, while accompanied by AKI in 4 patients; rapidly progressive glomerulonephritis (RPGN) in 5 patients; AKI in 5 patients and mild proteinuria/microscopic hematuria in the remaining 4 patients (see Table 2).

Eighteen patients (90%) had anemia (5.9 to 11.3 g/dl), five had leukocytosis, three had leucopenia and three had thrombopenia. Two patients were positive for ANA, two were positive for cytoplasmic antineutrophil cytoplasmic antibodies (C-ANCA) and anti-proteinase 3 ANCA (PR3-ANCA) and one was positive for anti-glomerular basement membrane antibody (anti-GBM). IgM (kappa) monoclonal protein was detected in five patients by immunofixation electrophoresis. Cryoglobulinemia was also identified in three patients (see Table 2).

Histological findings

The histological findings of 20 patients are summarized in Table 3. Membranoproliferative glomerulonephritis -like patterns was found in seven patients with B-cell lymphoma. Light microscopy showed increased cellularity in all glomeruli and accentuation of the lobular architecture (Fig. 1 A). Silver staining showed double contours within the capillary loops. Capillary loops contained infiltrating leucocytes (more than 10 cells). Immunofluorescence studies revealed granular staining in a lobular pattern for IgG, IgM or C3 in five patients (Fig. 1 B). IgG was undetectable, and only IgM and C3 were present in mesangial area in case 6 and 18. The interstitium was diffusely or focally infiltrated by mononuclear cells. Electron microscopy showed fine subendothelial and mesangial electron-dense deposits together with frequent double-contoured appearance (Fig. 1 C).

Crescent glomerulonephritis was demonstrated in 4 patients, two patients had T/NK cell lymphoma, and the remaining two had CLL/SLL. No evidence of immune complex deposition was found in case1, 2; and serum PR3-ANCA was positive in case 2. IgG line deposits along the GBM and anti-GBM antibody was positive in case 7. Cellular crescents and focal necrotizing capillary by LM and IgG, IgM, IgA and C3 deposits in the mesangial and capillary were confirmed in case 8. In addition to the glomerular lesions, mononuclear cell infiltration was observed in the peritubular capillaries (PTCs) in all 4 patients.

Three patients (case 4,10,11) had minimal change in the glomeruli observed by light microscopy and no immune complex deposition by IF assay, but ultrastructural examination of these glomeruli revealed extensive effacement of the foot processes characteristic of minimal-change disease (MCD). The other three patients(case 3,5,17) revealed glomeruli without specific pathological abnormalities, ultrastructural examination revealed only segmental effacement of the foot processes, and the IF assay showed staining for IgG and IgM deposits in the glomeruli in two patients(case 3,5). Mononuclear cell infiltration was also observed in the PTCs in five patients (Fig. 1 E, F).

Primary diffuse large B-cell lymphoma of the kidney was found in case 13. Severe cell infiltration throughout the cortex and marked destruction of both the glomeruli and the tubular structure, with only two ruined glomeruli were observed. The accumulation of large atypical lymphoid cells with hyperchromatic nuclei was observed in renal specimens under high-power magnification (Fig. 2A). IF did not reveal any glomerular immune deposits. The lymphoid cell were positive for CD20 (+++) (Fig. 2B) and CD79a (+) but negative for CD3, CD43 and CD138.

Intraglomerular large B-cell lymphoma was identified in case 14. Lymphoid cells were present only within the lumina of the

Table 1. Clinical features of patients with NHL and renal involvement

Patient	Sex	Age	Type of lymphoma	Biopsy site	Clinical symptoms of lymphoma	Renal symptoms	Treatment	Patient outcome	Renal Outcome (Scr μmol/l)
1	M	16	T/NK	Nasal mucosa	Anemia, fever, nasal discharge	RPGN	EPOCH	Died (1 yr)	NA
2	F	38	T/NK	Nasal mucosa	Fever, nasal discharge	NS	Steroids	Died (2 mo)	NA
3	F	39	TCL	Lymph node	Fever, lymphadenectasis	proteinuria	CHOP	Died (2 mo)	NA
4	M	40	TCL	Skin	Skin rash	NS	Steroids	NA	NA
5	M	61	CLL/SLL	Bone marrow	Anemia, weakness	AKI	Chlorambucil	Died (2 mo)	NA
6	F	57	CLL/SLL	Lymph node	Anemia, lymphadenectasis	RPGN	Chlorambucil	NA	NA
7	M	64	CLL/SLL	Lymph node	Lymphadenectasis	RPGN	FC	Died (3 mo)	NA
8	M	55	CLL/SLL	Lymph node	Lymphadenectasis	RPGN	FC	Alive (3 yr)	dialysis
9	M	59	CLL/SLL	Bone marrow	Leucocytosis	RPGN	Steroids	Alive (6 yr)	126
10	M	61	CLL/SLL	Bone marrow	Anemia, weakness	NS+AKI	FC	Alive (3 yr)	137
11	M	68	CLL/SLL	Bone marrow	Anemia, lymphadenectasis	NS+AKI	Steroids	Died (4 mo)	NA
12	M	62	CLL/SLL	Bone marrow	Anemia, leucopenia	AKI	CTX	Alive (1 yr)	350
13	M	47	DLBCL	Kidney	Fever, weakness	AKI	CHOP	Alive (1 yr)	109
14	M	56	DLBCL	Kidney	Anemia	AKI	CHOP	Died (2 yr)	NA
15	M	62	DLBCL	Lymph node	Anemia, lymphadenectasis	AKI	Steroids	Alive (8 yr)	156
16	M	37	DLBCL	Ileum	Fever, diarrhea	proteinuria	CHOP	Died (2 yr)	NA
17	M	53	LPL	Lymph node	Anemia, lymphadenectasis	proteinuria	Steroids	Alive (2 yr)	89
18	M	68	LPL	Bone marrow	Fever, Anemia, skin rash	proteinuria	CTX	Died (1 yr)	NA
19	M	65	MCL	Lymph node	Anemia, lymphadenectasis	NS+AKI	CHOP	Alive (1 yr)	101
20	M	52	MALT	Stoma mucosa	Anemia, stomachache	NS+AKI	R+Steroids	Alive (1 yr)	249

CLL/SLL: chronic lymphocytic leukemia/small lymphocytic lymphoma, DLBCL: diffuse larger B-cell lymphoma, T/NK:T/NK cell lymphoma, TCL: T-cell lymphoma, MALT: mucosa-associated lymphoid tissue lymphoma, MCL: mantle cell lymphoma, LPL: lymphoplasmacytic lymphoma, NS: nephritic syndrome,
AKI: acute kidney injury, RPGN: rapidly progressive glomerulonephritis, R: radiotherapy, NA: not available.
CHOP: cyclophosphamide, hydroxydaunomycin, oncovin, prednisone. CTX: cyclophosphamide.
EPOCH:Etoposide, prednisone, oncovin, cyclophosphamide, hydroxydaunomycin, FC: fludarabine, cyclophosphamide

glomerular capillaries and not within the interstitium (Fig 2C). Large pleomorphic lymphoid cells often occluded the glomerular capillaries. The lymphoid cells had large vesicular nuclei. In the IF analysis of frozen sections, the lymphoid cells were $CD45^+$, $CD3^-$ and $CD20^{3+}$ (Fig 2D).

Intracapillary monoclonal IgM deposits (ICMDD) was observed in case 12. The most striking glomerular lesions consisted of periodic acid Schiff-positive intracapillary deposits that were variable in size and distribution (Fig. 3A). In the IF assay, all of the deposits were strongly stained for IgM and the κ light chain (Fig. 3B, C). EM revealed large intracapillary deposits that dilated the capillary lumen. No organized structure was observed (Fig. 3D).

The monomorphic lymphocytes infiltrates were patchy in 7 cases, diffuse in case 13 (Table 3), renal tubules were separated and atrophic or destroyed as a result of interstitial infiltrates. Staining with various immunohistochemical markers revealed that the infiltrating lymphocyte cells were positive for predominance of CD20, while $CD68^+$ cells within the infiltration (Table 3), which is consistent with B-cell lymphoma.

Outcome

During follow-up, two patients were lost, nine patients died. Among those who died, three patients with T/NK cell lymphoma died of infection after they received specific chemotherapy; the remaining six patients died as a direct or indirect result of the lymphoma during the first 2 years after NHL diagnosis. In these nine patients, four patients had AKI, four patients had CKD in last record. At the end of the follow-up period (6-96 months, average 35 months), three patients had normal serum creatinine, five patients had renal function stable or improved after chemotherapy, and one patient required permanent hemodialysis. (See Table 1).

Discussion

In this study, we confirmed that a wide spectrum of NHL is associated with renal injury, particularly with B-cell lymphocytic type NHL. CLL/SLL was the most common type of lymphoma associated with renal involvement (40%), followed by DLBCL and NK/T-cell lymphoma (20%). The profile of the NHL reported in the literature is similar to that observed our study. Kowalewska et al. [6] found a similar pattern of distribution; among 18 patients with neoplasms and kidney injury, the most common type of lymphoma was CLL/SLL, followed by DLBCL. However, Sun et al. [10] showed that the most common subtype of lymphoma was DLBCL (36.2%) in China, followed by extranodal NK/T-cell lymphoma, nasal type (11.0%); CLL/SLL accounted for only 3.7% of all lymphoid neoplasm. This finding suggests that renal involvement may be commonly associated with CLL/SLL. The pathogenesis of CLL/SLL-associated glomerulonephritis is not well understood. Notably, four of eight patients with CLL/SLL had serum positive for ANA or ANCA, three had M-component and two had cryoglobulinemia in their sera. Therefore, glomerulonephritis may also be related to the production of cryoglobulins

Table 2. Summary of clinical data in patients with NHL and renal involvement

Patient	Hb (g/L)	WBC (*10^9/L)	Scr (μmol/l)	eGFR (ml/min)	albumin (g/L)	globulin (g/L)	Urine protein (g/d)	Urine RBC (10^4/ml)	Urine NAG (U/g·cr)	Urine RBP (mg/L)	Renal size (mm/mm)	Antibody or Cryo	SIFE
1	70	6.6	187	44.8	33	31.3	2.72	2500	40.7	65.5	115/109	N	N
2	90	4.1	61	105	28.2	35.3	3.5	95	31.2	1.51	103/101	ANA PR3-ANCA	N
3	65	4.5	100	52.7	32.6	28.8	1.58	N	47.6	1.32	104/100	N	N
4	147	5.2	95	85.9	20.4	16.4	5.37	15	39.4	1.13	109/105	N	N
5	59	2.8	543	13	38.4	38.7	1.3	2000	40.2	7.78	106/102	PR3-ANCA	N
6	66	4.0	151	32.8	36.4	29.9	3.02	1850	94	1.88	99/98	ANA	N
7	91	5.1	338	15.6	36.5	26.3	1.41	1250	26.9	10.2	107/103	A-GBM	N
8	99	10.1	477	12.6	31.6	45.7	2.75	3000	35.5	10.2	127/122	Cryo	N
9	87	25.3	188	32.9	38.9	27.8	4.24	750	83.2	0.43	100/98	N	N
10	99	11.4	320	18.3	23.6	29.9	10.2	15	48.2	31.7	97/96	N	IgM, k
11	111	7.3	235	25.6	17.1	29.1	14.9	570	75.4	53.4	94/96	N	IgM, k
12	89	3.3	392	17.8	27.7	17.7	0.71	N	25.2	4.5	123/120	Cryo	IgM, k
13	135	8.8	158	46.3	44.2	29.7	0.39	N	20.2	10	167/146	N	N
14	98	5.6	166	37.2	40.6	27.4	0.84	N	32.4	3.44	114/110	N	N
15	113	4.2	168	34.2	38.3	15.5	1.24	47	21.1	0.13	103/101	N	N
16	107	10.6	77	103	36	18	0.68	50	25.7	0.1	106/101	N	N
17	109	4.5	74	103	34	40.3	0.41	N	26.2	0.93	129/120	N	IgM, k
18	78	9.4	50	95.8	27.2	18.8	0.7	230	82.3	0.84	111/110	Cryo	N
19	80	13.8	164	34.8	28.4	28.6	6.92	260	25	15.5	112/115	N	N
20	106	3.7	263	36.5	32.3	18.7	7.96	1100	119	11.9	112/106	N	IgM, k

Hb, hemoglobin; WBC, white blood count; BUN, blood urea nitrogen; SCr, serum creatinine; eGFR: estimated Glomerular Filtration Rate
NAG, N-acetyl-pD glucosaminidase enzyme, RBP: retinol-binding protein (RBP). ANA: antinuclear antibody, C-ANCA: antineutrophil cytoplasmic antibody, PR3-ANCA: anti-proteinase 3 ANCA, A-GBM: anti-glomerular basement membrane antibody, Cryo: cryoglobulinemia; SIFE: serum immunofixation electrophoresis, N negative

Table 3. Renal biopsy findings

	Glomerular Disease	Infiltrating cells		Immunofluorescence							Immunoperoxidase	
		Glomerular	PTC	IgG	IgA	IgM	C3	C1q	κ	λ	CD20(n/mm²)	CD68(n/mm²)
1	Crescent GN	>5	Y	-	-	-	-	-	-	-	NA	192
2	Crescent GN	2–3	Y	-	-	-	-	-	-	-	NA	NA
3	NSPA	2–3	No	+	-	+	-	-	-	-	96	NA
4	MCD	2–3	Y	-	-	-	-	-	-	-	Multifocal	152
5	NSPA	>3	Y	++	-	-	++	++	-	+	NA	624
6	MPGN	>10	Y	-	-	+	+	+	-	-	Diffuse	548
7	Crescent GN	>5	Y	++	-	-	-	-	-	+	Multifocal	Diffuse
8	Crescent GN	>5	Y	++	+	+	++	++	+	+	Multifocal	592
9	MPGN	>10	Y	++	+	++	++	+	++	+	Multifocal	152
10	MCD	3–5	Y	-	-	-	-	-	-	-	184	872
11	MCD	3–5	Y	-	-	-	-	-	-	-	72	356
12	ICMDD	3–5	Y	-	-	++	-	-	++	-	Diffuse	140
13	No glomerular	ND	Y	-	-	-	-	-	-	-	192	1192
14	Lymphoma	ND	Y	-	+	+	-	-	-	-	16	848
15	MPGN	>10	Y	++	+	++	+	++	+	++	NA	NA
16	MPGN	>10	No	++	++	-	++	-	+	+	144	NA
17	NSPA	3–5	Y	-	-	-	-	-	-	-	Multifocal	312
18	MPGN	>5	Y	-	++	-	++	-	+	-	Focal	268
19	MPGN	>10	No	++	-	-	++	++	-	+	180	420
20	MPGN	>10	No	++	++	-	++	-	++	+	NA	312

MPGN: Membranoproliferative glomerulonephritis. FSNGN: Focal segmental necrotizing glomerulonephritis. PTC: ICMDD: Intracapillary monoclonal IgM deposits. Lymphoma: Intraglomerular lymphoma. MCD: Minimal-change disease NSPA:No specific pathologic abnormalities; NA: not available. Immunofluorescence: -, negative; +, mild; ++, intense. λ: λ light chain; κ: κ light chain.

and/or immunoglobulins (paraprotein production) by secretory B-cell clones in patients with CLL/SLL.

In our series, the most common presentations of renal involvement in NHL patients were renal impairment and proteinuria. All patients presented with proteinuria, and 75% had impaired renal function; 30% had nephrotic syndrome and 25% had RPGN. It is difficult to distinguish lymphoma-associated glomerulonephritis from primary kidney disease in the clinic. Interestingly, at the time of the renal biopsy, only 10% patients in our series had an established diagnosis of current NHL. Therefore, renal biopsy may be suggested as the diagnostic method of choice.

The most common pattern of glomerular involvement in our series was glomerulonephritis with MPGN-like patterns. All seven cases of MPGN-like patterns were associated with B-cell neoplasm. Among these patients, three were positive for serum ANA, M-component or cryoglobulinemia. IgG deposition was not observed in two patients, which is different from typical MPGN. Moulin et al. [11] retrospectively analyzed 13 patients with glomerulonephritis and chronic lymphocytic leukemia (CLL) or B-cell lymphoma; MPGN was observed in eight patients, five patients had cryoglobulinemia and two patients had circulating M-component. Therefore, MPGN- like patterns associated with NHL may directly result from the lymphoma through a paraprotein deposition process that results in cryoglobulinemia or monoclonal immunoglobulin deposition disease, or it may be induced indirectly through immune-mediated mechanisms.

Four patients had crescent glomerulonephritis in our series; one patient with PR3-ANCA, one with anti-GBM antibody. Pauci-immune crescentic glomerulonephritis associated with NHL and ANCA has also been reported by Henriksen and Dussol [12–13]. However, we describe a previously unreported unique case of anti-GBM glomerulonephritis in a patient with CLL/SLL. Given that NHL patients have defective T-cell colony-forming capacity and T-cell regulatory function, the simultaneous presence of NHL, anti-GBM and crescentic glomerulonephritis may not be a coincidence.

Minimal-change nephrotic syndrome is described as a paraneoplastic manifestation of classical Hodgkin's lymphoma (HL) that occurs in 0.4% of Hodgkin's lymphoma patients but is a rare complication of NHL [14 15]. In our series, three patients presented with nephritic syndrome, and showed MCD by EM. Increased cytokine levels caused by T- or B-cell lymphoma cytokine-induced altered glomerular permeability and podocyte injury may be responsible for nephrotic syndrome [15]. In these patients, mononuclear cell infiltration into the PTC and lymphocytic infiltration of the tubule interstitium were also observed. It is not clear why patients with NHL associated renal injury have mononuclear cell infiltration into the PTC. One possibility would be that NHL induces the release of proinflammatory molecules, which induce infiltrating cells infiltration. These results suggest that the immune processes involved in the pathogenesis of NHL-associated MCD are different from those of idiopathic MCD.

ICMDD was defined as PAS-positive intracapillary thrombi in glomeruli that were sufficiently voluminous to occlude the capillary lumens and thrombi positive for IgM and either κ or λ LC by IF. This type of renal lesion was first reported in

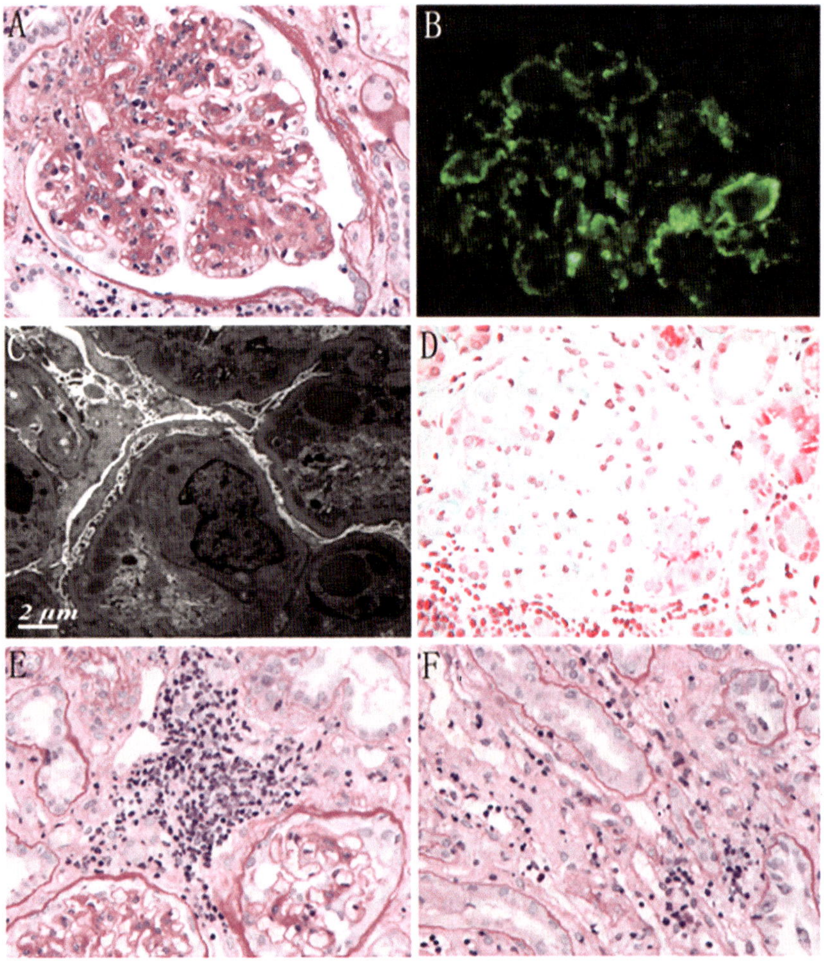

Figure 1. Representative renal histological change in patients with NHL. A Light microscopy showed increased cellularity in glomeruli and the accentuation of the lobular architecture (patient 9 PAS×400). B Immunofluorescence showed granular staining in a lobular pattern for IgG (patient 9 IF×400). C Electron microscopy showed fine subendothelial electron-dense deposits (patient 9 EM). D Glomeruli with focal segmental necrosis and lymphoid cell infiltration around glomeruli (patient 8 Masson×400). E Glomeruli without pathological abnormalities visualized by LM with lymphocyte-like cell infiltration in the interstitial tissue (patient 5 PAS×200). F Mononuclear cell infiltration in the peritubular capillaries (patient 5 PAS×400).

Waldenstrom macroglobulinemia (WM). However, Audard et al. [16] reported that only three of five patients with ICMDD had WM, whereas the two other patients had an IgM-related disorder and a B-cell lymphoma. In our study, patients with intraglomerular thrombi were found to have circulating monoclonal IgM and κ LC. Cellular proliferation in the glomeruli was absent or mild; no organized microtubular structures were visualized by EM, which suggests a diagnosis of ICMDD rather than cryoglobulinemic glomerulonephritis. Therefore, ICMDD may be applied to IgM-secreting B-cell lymphoma. In addition, κ and/or λ light chain staining was positive by immunofluorescence in 10 patients in our study. However, no linear deposits of κ or λ light chain staining within GBM and TBM was observed, which was the characteristic for light chain deposition disease (LCDD).

Renal involvement is rare in patients with diffuse large B-cell lymphoma (DLBCL). Villa et al. [17] identified renal involvement in only 2% (55/2656) of patients with DLBCL at the time of diagnosis. In the present study, computed tomography (CT) revealed markedly enlarged kidneys bilaterally in case 13, and the renal parenchyma was massively infiltrated by $CD20^{+}$ lymphoid cells; the lymphoma was classified as diffuse large B-cell lymphoma. Intravascular large B-cell lymphoma (IVLBCL) is a very rare subtype of NHL lymphoma. To the best of our knowledge, no more than 20 cases have been published in the literature [18–19]. The patients with intraglomerular large B-cell lymphoma may present with proteinuria, renal dysfunction, which may clinically mimic primary glomerulonephritis. The glomerular lesion may appear confusingly like endocapillary proliferative glomerulonephritis; only immunocytochemical characteristics can reveal the true lymphoid cells [20]. In such cases, kidney biopsy is the only way to establish the correct diagnosis.

In our study, 40% patients showed lymphomatous infiltration of the interstitium. All of these patients had B-cell lymphoma, and seven of eight presented with AKI. Lymphocytic infiltrations of the renal tubulointerstitium and AKI have been reported previously [2,6]. The mechanism of AKI due to lymphomatous infiltration of the kidneys is unknown; infiltrate may destruct of the normal renal architecture and cause intrarenal obstruction. The aggregates of inflammatory cells such as CD68+ cells can also be seen in these patients, which suggest to inflammatory response to lymphomatous infiltration. A monotonous appearance and aggregates of infiltrative pattern of the lymphomatous cell population in kidney

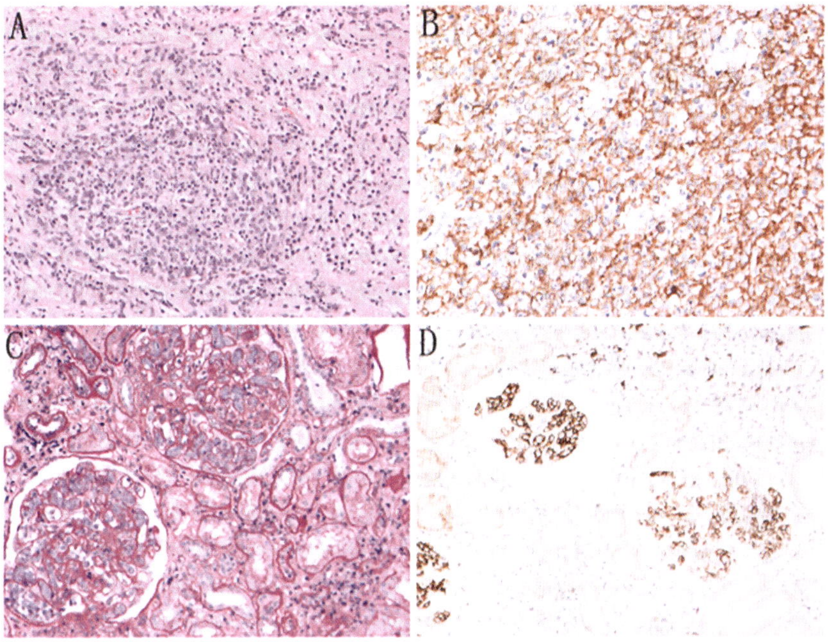

Figure 2. Diffuse infiltration into the renal parenchyma and intraglomerular lymphoma in DLBCL. A. Accumulation of large atypical lymphoid cells was observed in renal specimens (patient 13 PAS×400). B. Immunohistochemical staining showing strong staining for CD20 in the lymphoid cells (patient 13 IH×400). C. Glomerular capillary lumina containing atypical large cells in the enlarged glomeruli (patient 14 PAS ×400). D Immunohistochemistry showing strong staining for CD20 in lymphoid cells localized within the glomerular capillary lumina (patient 14 IH×400).

should prompt the examiner to perform an additional workup to rule out or confirm lymphoma.

The differentiation between a primary glomerular disease and lymphoma-associated glomerulonephritis is difficult. Therefore, we need to implement screening for the underlying hematological malignancy if a patient presents with (1) severe anemia, leukocytosis and/or thrombopenia; (2) enlarged lymph nodes and/or enlarged kidneys; (3) mononuclear cells in the PTC or

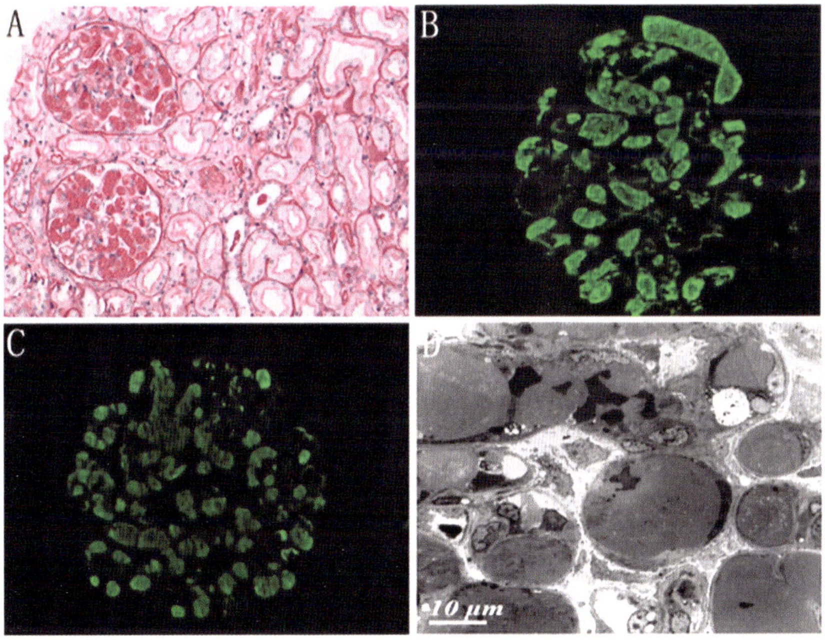

Figure 3. Intracapillary monoclonal deposition disease in an NHL patient (patient 12). A PAS-positive intracapillary thrombi in glomerulus (PAS, ×200). B Immunofluorescence showed bright staining of the intraglomerular thrombi for IgM. C Immunofluorescence showed bright staining of the intraglomerular thrombi for κ LC.D Electron microscopy showed that the glomerular capillary lumen was filled with granular electron-dense material. No organized structure was observed.

monomorphic lymphoid cells infiltration in renal parenchyma. If a patient has one or more of the above conditions, it is imperative that the patient undergo a full workup for lymphoma, which should include lymph node biopsy, bone marrow aspiration and biopsy, serum immunofixation studies and cryoglobulinemia detection. If these tests are positive, then a series of immunohistochemical staining studies is warranted to determine whether the kidney injury is caused by underlying lymphoma.

In conclusion, we confirmed that a wide spectrum of renal pathological findings can be observed in patients with NHL, and NHL may be first diagnosed by renal biopsies for evaluation of kidney injury or proteinuria. CLL/SLL were the most common types of NHL associated with renal injury, and the most common pattern of glomerular lesion was MPGN-like pattern. Renal biopsy is necessary to establish the underlying cause of renal involvement in NHL.

Author Contributions

Conceived and designed the experiments: S-JL Z-hL. Analyzed the data: Y-HC L-hZ Y-MT. Wrote the paper: S-JL H-PC.

References

1. Ronco PM. (1999) Paraneoplastic glomerulopathies: new insights into an old entity. Kidney Int 56:355 377.
2. Cohen LJ, Rennke HG, Laubach JP, Humphreys BD. (2010) The spectrum of kidney involvement in lymphoma: a case report and review of the literature. Am J Kidney Dis 56:1191 1196.
3. Rault R, Holley JL, Banner BF, el-Shahawy M.(1992) Glomerulonephritis and non-Hodgkin's lymphoma: a report of two cases and review of the literature. Am J Kidney Dis. 20:84 89.
4. Stokes MB, Wood B, Alpers CE. (2002) Membranoproliferative glomerulonephritis associated with low-grade B cell lymphoma presenting in the kidney. Clin Nephrol 57:303 309.
5. Da'as N, Polliack A, Cohen Y, Amir G, Darmon D, et al. (2001) Kidney involvement and renal manifestations in non-Hodgkin's lymphoma and lymphocytic leukemia: a retrospective study in 700 patients. Eur J Haematol 67:158 164.
6. Kowalewska J, Nicosia RF, Smith KD, Kats A, Alpers CE. (2011) Patterns of glomerular injury in kidneys infiltrated by lymphoplasmacytic neoplasms. Hum Pathol. 42:896 903.
7. Shi SF, Zhou FD, Zou WZ, Wang HY. (2012) Acute kidney injury and bilateral symmetrical enlargement of the kidneys as first presentation of B-cell lymphoblastic lymphoma. Am J Kidney Dis 60:1044 1048.
8. Yeo SC, Chuah KL, Lee HY, Liew A. (2013) An unusual case of glomerulonephritis in a patient with non-Hodgkin mucosal associated lymphoid tissue (MALT) B-cell lymphoma. BMC Nephrol 22;14:158
9. Swerdlow SH, Campo E, Harris NL, et al. (2008) WHO Classification of Tumours of Haematopoietic and Lymphoid Tissues. 4th ed. Lyon, France: IARC Press.
10. Sun J, Yang Q, Lu Z, He M, Gao L, et al. (2012) Distribution of lymphoid neoplasms in China: analysis of 4,638 cases according to the World Health Organization classification. Am J Clin Pathol 138:429 434.
11. Moulin B, Ronco PM, Mougenot B, Francois A, Fillastre JP, et al. (1992) Glomerulonephritis in chronic lymphocytic leukemia and related B-cell lymphomas. Kidney Int 42:127 135.
12. Dussol B, Brunet P, Vacher-Coponat H, Bouabdallah R, Chetaille P, et al. (1997) Crescentic glomerulonephritis with antineutrophil cytoplasmic antibodies associated with chronic lymphocytic leukaemia. Nephrol Dial Transplant 12:785 786.
13. Henriksen KJ, Hong RB, Sobrero MI, Chang A. (2011) Rare association of chronic lymphocytic leukemia/small lymphocytic lymphoma, ANCAs, and pauci-immune crescentic glomerulonephritis. Am J Kidney Dis 57:170 174.
14. Harper L, Adu D. (1997) Glomerulonephritis and non-Hodgkin lymphoma: Nephrol Dial Transplant 12:1520 1525.
15. Audard V, Larousserie F, Grimbert P,Abtahi M, Sotto JJ, et al. (2006) Minimal change nephrotic syndrome and classical Hodgkin's lymphoma: report of 21 cases and review of the literature. Kidney Int. 69:2251 2260.
16. Audard V, Georges B, Vanhille P, Toly C, Deroure B, et al. (2008) Renal Lesions Associated with IgM-Secreting Monoclonal Proliferations: Revisiting the Disease Spectrum. Clin J Am Soc Nephrol 3:1339 1349.
17. Villa D, Connors JM, Sehn LH, Gascoyne RD, Savage KJ. (2011) Diffuse large B-cell lymphoma with involvement of the kidney: outcome and risk of central nervous system relapse. Haematologica 96:1002 1007.
18. Bai X, Li X, Wan L, Wang G, Jia N, et al. (2011) Intravascular large B-cell lymphoma of the kidney: a case report. Diagn Pathol 6:86.
19. Kameoka Y, Takahashi N, Komatsuda A. (2009) Kidney-limited intravascular large B cell lymphoma: a distinct variant of IVLBCL? Int J Hematol 89:533 537.
20. Wood SM, Boyd SM, Taylor JE, Savill J. (1996) A case of non-Hodgkin lymphoma presenting primarily with renal failure. Nephrol Dial Transplant 11:535 536

3

Antileukemic Activity of Sulforaphane in Primary Blasts from Patients Affected by Myelo- and Lympho-Proliferative Disorders and in Hypoxic Conditions

Carmela Fimognari[1]*, Eleonora Turrini[1], Piero Sestili[2], Cinzia Calcabrini[2], Giovanni Carulli[3], Giulia Fontanelli[3], Martina Rousseau[3], Giorgio Cantelli-Forti[1], Patrizia Hrelia[4]

1 Department for Life Quality Studies, Alma Mater Studiorum-University of Bologna, Rimini, Italy, **2** Department of Biomolecular Sciences, University of Urbino "Carlo Bo", Urbino, Italy, **3** Division of Hematology, Department of Clinical and Experimental Medicine, University of Pisa, Pisa, Italy, **4** Department of Pharmacy and BioTechnology, Alma Mater Studiorum-University of Bologna, Bologna, Italy

Abstract

Sulforaphane is a dietary isothiocyanate found in cruciferous vegetables showing antileukemic activity. With the purpose of extending the potential clinical impact of sulforaphane in the oncological field, we investigated the antileukemic effect of sulforaphane on blasts from patients affected by different types of leukemia and, taking into account the intrinsically hypoxic nature of bone marrow, on a leukemia cell line (REH) maintained in hypoxic conditions. In particular, we tested sulforaphane on patients with chronic lymphocytic leukemia, acute myeloid leukemia, T-cell acute lymphoblastic leukemia, B-cell acute lymphoblastic leukemia, and blastic NK cell leukemia. Sulforaphane caused a dose-dependent induction of apoptosis in blasts from patients diagnosed with acute lymphoblastic or myeloid leukemia. Moreover, it was able to cause apoptosis and to inhibit proliferation in hypoxic conditions on REH cells. As to its cytotoxic mechanism, we found that sulforaphane creates an oxidative cellular environment that induces DNA damage and Bax and p53 gene activation, which in turn helps trigger apoptosis. On the whole, our results raise hopes that sulforaphane might set the stage for a novel therapeutic principle complementing our growing armature against malignancies and advocate the exploration of sulforaphane in a broader population of leukemic patients.

Editor: Persio Dello Sbarba, Università degli Studi di Firenze, Italy

Funding: This work was supported by Fondazione Cassa di Risparmio di Imola (Italy) and by Fondazione del Monte di Bologna e Ravenna (Italy). The funders had no role in study design, data collection and analysis, decision to publish, or preparation of the manuscript.

Competing Interests: The authors have declared that no competing interests exist.

* Email: carmela.fimognari@unibo.it

Introduction

Sulforaphane (SR) is a dietary isothiocyanate found in cruciferous vegetables able to provide protection against multistep carcinogenesis [1]. Epidemiological studies evidenced an inverse correlation between the consumption of a diet rich in cruciferous vegetables (i.e., broccoli and cabbage) and the incidence of breast, lung, prostate, colon, and bladder cancer [2–7], largely attributed to the activity of isothiocyanates derived from the metabolism of glucosinolates that accumulate in cruciferous vegetables [8]. SR is a highly reactive and hydrophobic compound that can alter many cellular processes. Inhibition of cell proliferation, increased apoptosis, anti-inflammatory and antioxidant activities, induction of phase-II detoxification enzymes, inhibition of cyclooxygenase 2, and various other mechanisms have been proposed to explain the anticancer effects of SR [9].

SR induces apoptosis in several cancer cell lines, such as T-cell leukemia, breast, colon, and prostate cancer, by targeting different molecules, such as caspases, PARP, p21, p53 and Bax [10–14]. SR also blocks cell cycle through the modulation of G1/S and G2/M phases and alters the levels of cyclin A, cyclin B1, cyclin D1, p21cip1/waf1, and KLF4 [12,15–19]. The antileukemic effect of SR was demonstrated in many different cell lines and, recently, also in blasts from pediatric patients with acute lymphoblastic leukemia (ALL) [20].

Leukemias are malignant neoplasms involving cells originally derived from hematopoietic precursor cells that include many diverse and biologically distinct subgroups. All leukemias start in the bone marrow, that is diffusely replaced by abnormally proliferating neoplastic cells. The neoplastic cells may spill out of the bone marrow and reach the blood, where they may be present in large numbers, resulting in the clinical presentations of the disease. Generally, the leukaemias can be divided into acute myeloid leukemia (AML) and related disorders, B-lymphoblastic leukemias, T-lymphoblastic leukemias, leukemias of ambiguous lineage [21].

Although leukemia is the most common malignancy among children and adolescents, the majority of cases of leukemia occur in older people [22].

The treatment of leukemia still largely revolves around chemotherapy to induce a complete remission and to consolidate this with further cycles of chemotherapy. For example, the standard therapy of AML is based on the association of an anthracycline and ARA-C and the efficacy of such therapy still is unsatisfactory, since the rate of complete remission ranges 30–60%, depending on age, and the survival rate has not changed significantly in years [23].

Table 1. Clinical features of patients.

Patients	Age	Sex	Diagnosis	Timing	Previous therapy
1	67	F	CLL	Stable disease	None
2	76	F	CLL	Stable disease	None
3	38	M	AML	Studied at diagnosis	None
4	39	M	AML	Non-responder	3+7[a]
5	31	F	AML	Non-responder	3+7
6	19	F	AML	Studied at diagnosis	None
7	30	F	AML	Studied at diagnosis	None
8	60	F	AML	Relapse	3+7, allogeneic HSCT[b]
9	47	F	AML	Studied at diagnosis	None
10	24	M	T-ALL	Studied at diagnosis	None
11	24	F	T-ALL	Studied at diagnosis	None
12	48	M	B-ALL	Studied at diagnosis	None
13	55	F	AML	Studied at diagnosis	None
14	31	F	BNKAL	Studied at diagnosis	None

[a]a combination drug protocol used as induction chemotherapy and consisting of three days of anthracyclines and seven days of cytarabine;
[b]allogeneic HSCT: transplantation of allogeneic hematopoietic stem cells.

Several new therapeutic approaches are under investigation, alone or in combination with conventional chemotherapy. Despite the development of multiple new agents, the development of chemoresistance frequently hampers the successful treatment of acute and chronic leukemias either at the initial presentation or (more frequently) following primary or subsequent relapses [24], and relapse continues to be the most common cause of death [25]. Those therapeutic issues can also be imputable to tumor microenvironment, which is characterized not only by marked gradients in drug concentration, but also by regions of hypoxia, which can influence tumor cell sensitivity to drug treatment. Taking into account the intrinsically hypoxic nature of bone marrow, hypoxia is also an important environmental factor in leukemia [26].

Thus, leukemias remain a formidable therapeutic challenge that requires the identification and the development of novel agents for the treatment of this disease.

Based on these considerations and with the aim to extend the potential clinical impact of SR in the oncological field, we investigated whether purified SR is effective against hematological malignancies. To this end, we explored the antileukemic effect of SR on blasts from patients affected by different types of leukemia. In particular, we tested SR on patients with chronic lymphocytic leukemia (CLL), AML, T-cell ALL (T-ALL), B-cell ALL (B-ALL), and blastic NK cell leukemia (BNKAL). Since SR activity was marked on samples from acute leukemias, we next analyzed the proapoptotic activity of SR in two acute leukemia cell lines. To better understand whether the level of oxygen is relevant for the therapeutic efficacy of SR, we treated a leukemia cell line with SR in hypoxic conditions and analyzed the formation of ROS and the induction of apoptosis.

Materials and Methods

Chemicals

Ethidium bromide, NaOH, 2′,7′-dichlorofluorescein-diacetate (DCFH-DA), chloroform, phenol, NaH_2PO_4 were purchased from Sigma (USA). Synthetic DL- SR was dissolved in dimethyl sulfoxide (DMSO) to generate a 40 mM stock concentration and stored at −20°C. Cells were treated with different concentrations of SR (0.0–30.0 μM), selected on the basis of previous studies performed on leukemia cells [15].

Leukemic cell lines

REH (acute lymphocytic leukemia) and HL-60 (acute promyelocytic leukemia) cell lines were bought from ATCC-LGC, grown in suspension and propagated in RPMI 1640 supplemented with 10% (REH) or 20% (HL-60) heat-inactivated bovine serum, 1% antibiotics (all obtained from Sigma). To maintain exponential growth, the cultures were divided every third day by dilution to a concentration of 1×10^5 cells/mL. Cells were treated with different concentrations of SR for different times at 37°C in both normoxic (20% O_2) and hypoxic conditions.

Hypoxic conditions

Leukemic cells were cultivated in an INVIVO$_2$ 200 hypoxia workstation (Ruskinn Technology LTD, England) at <1% O_2. Treatments and all cell manipulations were performed in the workstation, thus ensuring a full maintenance of hypoxia for the entire duration of the experiments.

Ethics statement

The described study was approved (Comitato Etico e Sperimentazione del Farmaco dell'Azienda Ospedaliero-Universitaria Pisana) and written informed consent was obtained from the patients. All clinical investigation was conducted according to the principles expressed in the Declaration of Helsinki.

Hematologic patients

Patients include cases of CLL (n = 2), AML (n = 8), B-cell ALL (n = 1), T-cell ALL (n = 2), BNKAL (n = 1). The general characteristics of patients are shown in Table 1. Diagnosis of leukemia was established according to the 2008 WHO classification [21] and by the combination of morphological, immunological, cytogenetic and molecular methods, which were applied to peripheral blood samples. The immunological assays were made by fluorochrome-conjugated monoclonal antibodies and analysis

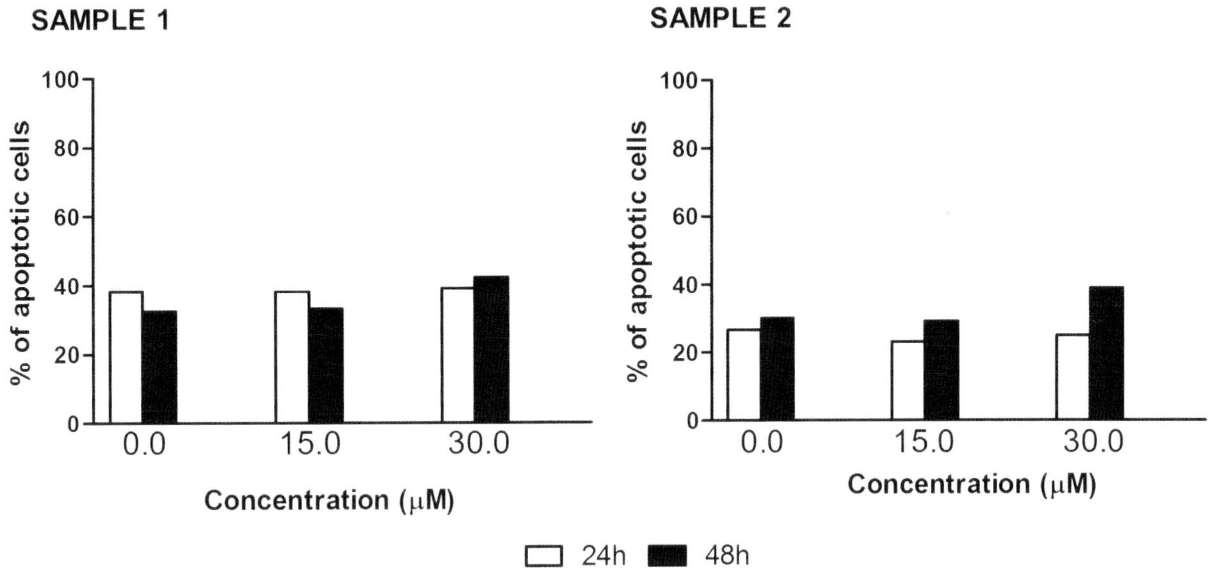

Figure 1. Fraction of apoptotic cells induced by SR on mononuclear cells isolated from CLL patients. Cells were treated with 0 to 30 μM SR for 24 or 48 h.

by a three-laser (488, 633, 405 nm)-equipped flow cytometer (FacsCanto II, Becton Dickinson, USA). A six-color method was applied; therefore the following fluorochrome combination was used: fluorescein isothiocyanate, phycoerythrin, peridinin chlorophyll protein complex, phycoerythrin-cyanine 7, allophycocyanin, allophycocyanin-cyanine 7. Diagnosis of acute leukemia was established by means of a wide panel of monoclonal antibodies, which included: CD45, CD13, CD33, CD34, CD117, HLA-DR, CD4, CD14, CD64, CD38, MPO, CD11b, CD16, CD15, CD56, CD7, CD19, CD3, CD2, CD5, CD4, CD8, CD10, CD20, CD58, TdT (from Becton Dickinson) and rabbit polyclonal F(ab′)2 antibodies directed to cyIgM and surface immunoglobulin K and lambda chains (from Dako, USA). CLL samples were subjected to an antibody panel which included CD45, CD3, CD4, CD8, CD16-56, CD5, CD19, CD20, CD23, CD22, CD79b, CD200, CD38, CD25, CD11c, surface immunoglobulin K and lambda chains. Patients were studied at the time of diagnosis; one patient was studied during his first relapse and two patients in a phase of resistant disease.

Preparation of leukemic cells

Peripheral blood samples of patients were collected in tubes containing preservative-free heparin. Leukemic cells were obtained by Ficoll-Histopaque density gradient centrifugation. 3 mL of Histopaque 1.077 g mL^{-1} were placed into a 10 mL plastic centrifuge tube, overlaid with 3 mL anticoagulated blood diluted 1:1 with phosphate-buffered saline (PBS), and centrifuged at 400×g for 30 min at room temperature. Interphase mononuclear cells banded at the interface between the plasma and the Histopaque were recovered, washed twice with PBS and then resuspended in RPMI 1640 medium (Sigma) containing 15% heat-inactivated bovine serum. The samples always contained > 95% blasts.

Flow cytometry

All flow cytometric analyses were performed by using the easyCyte 5HT flow cytometer (Millipore Guava Technologies, USA).

Detection of apoptosis

After 24, 48 or 72 h of treatment with different concentrations of SR, aliquots of 2.0×10^4 cells were stained with 100 μL of Guava Nexin Reagent containing ANNEXIN-V-phycoerythrin and 7-amino-actinomycin D. During apoptosis, the cells react to annexin V once chromatin condenses but before the plasma membrane loses its ability to exclude 7-amino-actinomycin D. Hence, by staining cells with a combination of phycoerythrin annexin V and 7-amino-actinomycin D it is possible to detect non apoptotic live cells, early apoptotic cells and late apoptotic or necrotic cells. Cells were incubated for 20 min at room temperature in the dark and then analyzed by flow cytometry.

Fast halo assay (FHA)

The assay has been carried out as previously described [27,28]. Briefly, after the treatments, the cells were resuspended at 4.0×10^4/mL in ice-cold PBS containing 5 mM EDTA: 25 μL of this cell suspension was diluted with an equal volume of 2% low melting agarose in PBS and immediately sandwiched between an agarose-coated slide and a coverslip. After complete gelling on ice, the coverslips were removed and the slides were immersed in NaOH 300 mM for 15 min at room temperature. Ethidium bromide (10 μg/mL) was directly added to NaOH during the last 5 min of incubation. The slides were then washed and destained for 5 min in distilled water. The ethidium bromide-labelled DNA was visualized using a Leica DMLB/DFC300F fluorescence microscope (Leica Microsystems, Germany) equipped with an Olympus Colorview IIIU CCD camera (Olympus Italia Srl, Italy) and the resulting images were digitally recorded on a PC and processed with an image analysis software (Scion Image, Scion Corporation, USA). The amount of fragmented DNA diffusing out of the nuclear cage, i.e. the extent of strand scission, was quantified by calculating the nuclear diffusion factor (NSF), which represents the ratio between the total area of the halo and nucleus and that of the nucleus. To allow the detection and recognition of DNA double strand breaks (DSBs) FHA was carried out at non-denaturing pH conditions as follows: the slides were submersed in a lysis solution (0.15 M NaOH, 0.1 M NaH_2PO_4, 1 mM EDTA,

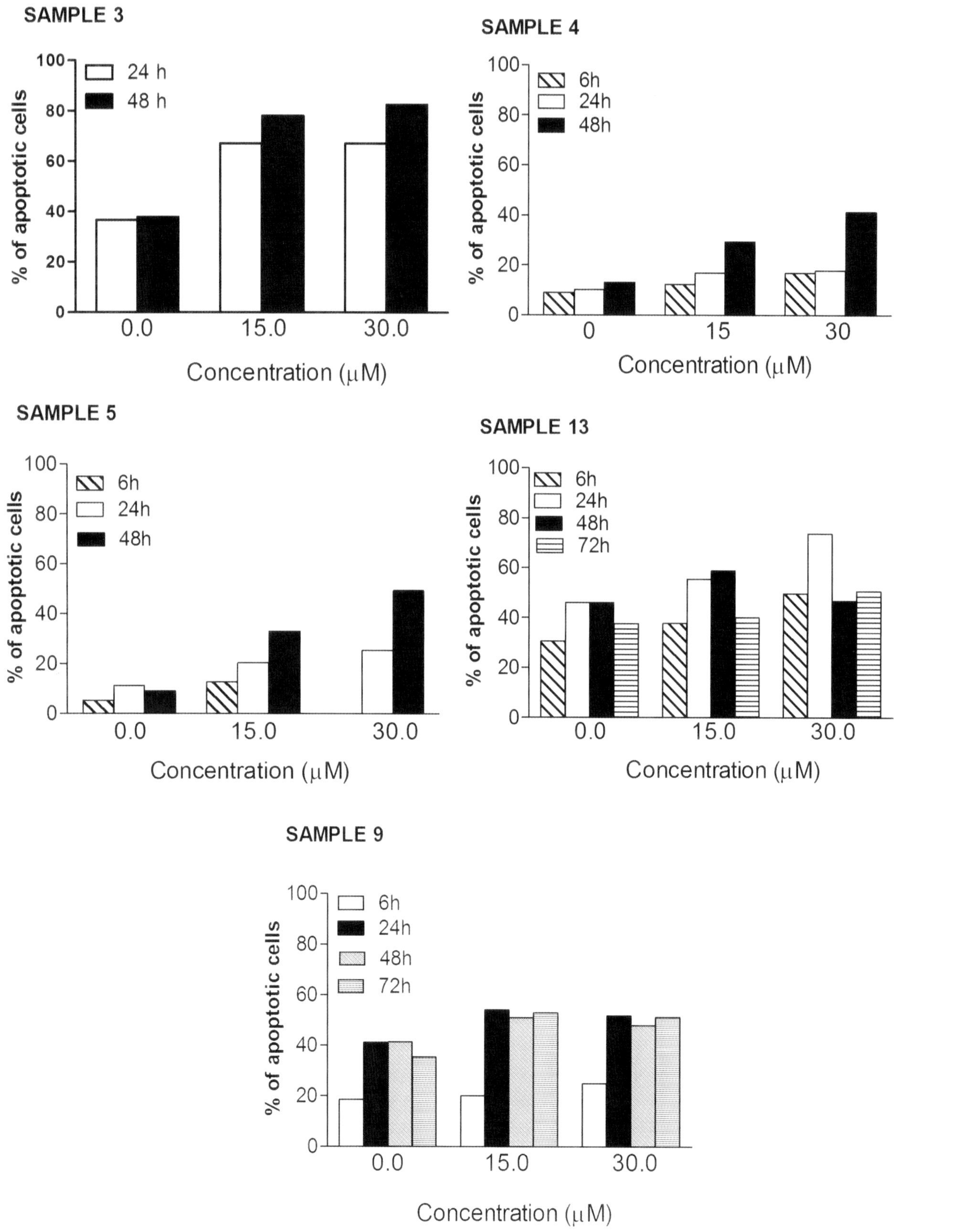

Figure 2. Fraction of apoptotic cells induced by SR on mononuclear cells isolated from AML patients. Cells were treated with 0 to 30 μM SR for 6, 24, 48 or 72 h.

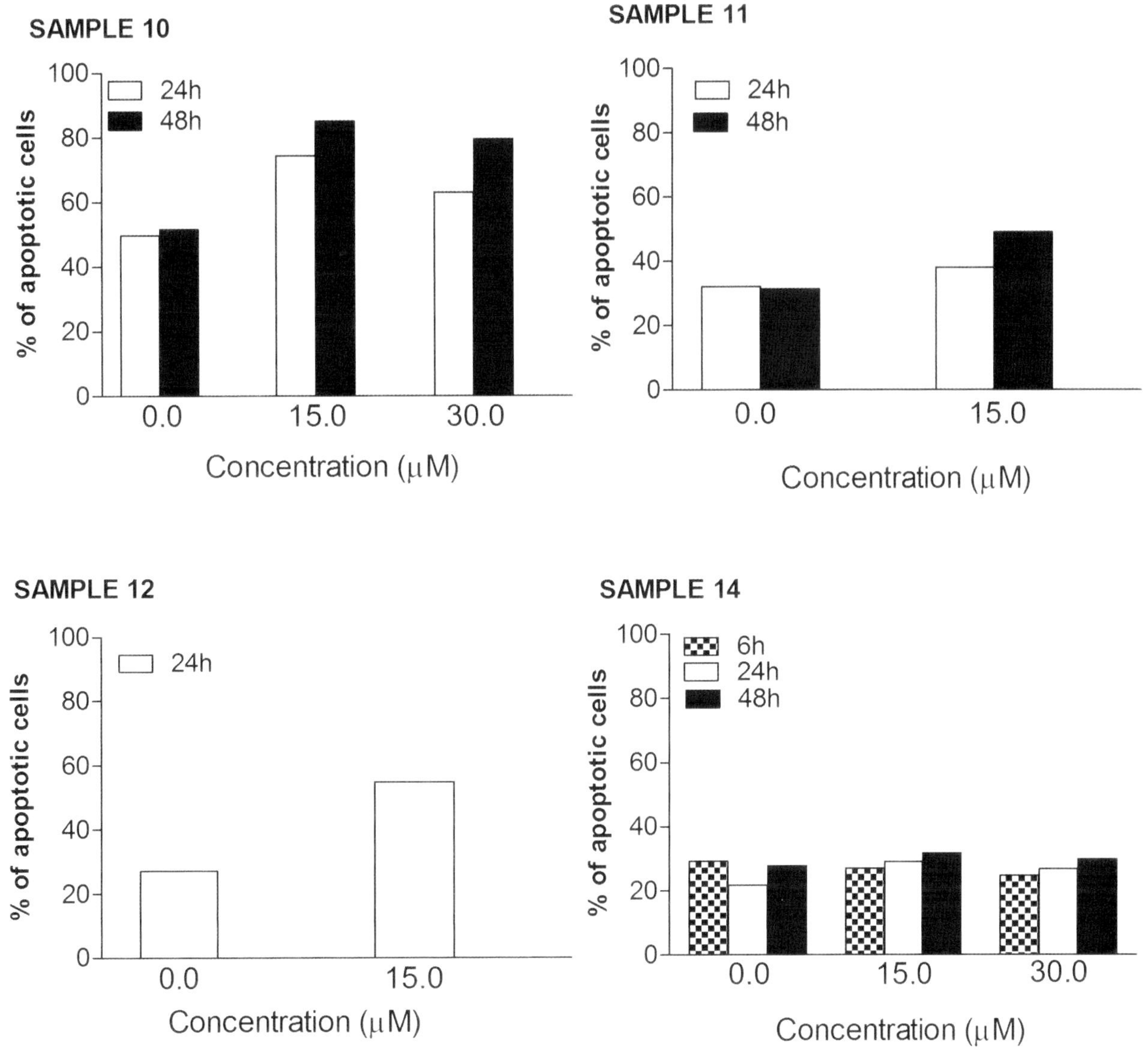

Figure 3. Fraction of apoptotic cells induced by SR on mononuclear cells isolated from ALL and BNKAL patients. Cells were treated with 0 to 30 μM SR for 6, 24 or 48 h.

Triton ×100 1% v/v, pH 10.1) for 10 min, incubated for further 15 min in PBS (pH 7.4) containing 0.1 mg/mL RNase (bovine pancreas Type IA); ethidium bromide was directly added to this solution during the last 5 min of incubation. The slides were then washed and destained for 5 min in distilled water and analyzed as described above.

ROS detection

DCFH-DA was used for ROS detection. DCFH-DA is cleaved intracellularly by nonspecific esterases to form 2′,7′-dichlorodihydrofluorescein (DCFH), which is further oxidized by ROS to form the highly fluorescent compound 2′,7′-dichlorodihydrofluorescein (DCF). Briefly, 1×10^6 cells were pre-treated with 15 or 30 μM SR for 30, 60, 180 or 360 min. Then, samples were washed and 1×10^6 cells were stained with 10 μM DCHF-DA. After 20 min of incubation at 37°C, fluorescence intensity was monitored by flow cytometry. Data were expressed as percentage of the control (untreated cells).

Analysis of apoptotic proteins

After treatment with SR, 1×10^6 cells were fixed and permeabilized by 2% of paraformaldehyde in PBS 1× and 90% of cold methanol. They were then incubated with Bax (1:100, Santa Cruz Biotechnology, Santa Cruz, CA, USA), Bcl-2 (1:100, Santa Cruz Biotechnology), p53 (1:100, Invitrogen), or isotype-matched negative control (1:100, e-Bioscience, San Diego, CA, USA) antibodies. The cells were washed and incubated with fluorescein isothiocyanate-labeled secondary antibody (1:100, Sigma). The cells were then analyzed to quantify fluorescein isothiocyanate binding by flow cytometry. Mean fluorescence intensity values were calculated. Non-specific binding was excluded by gating around those cells which were labeled by the fluorescein isothiocyanate-conjugate isotype control.

Analysis of cell cycle

Cell were treated with different concentrations of SR for 8, 24 and 48 h, and then fixed with ice-cold ethanol. Samples were then

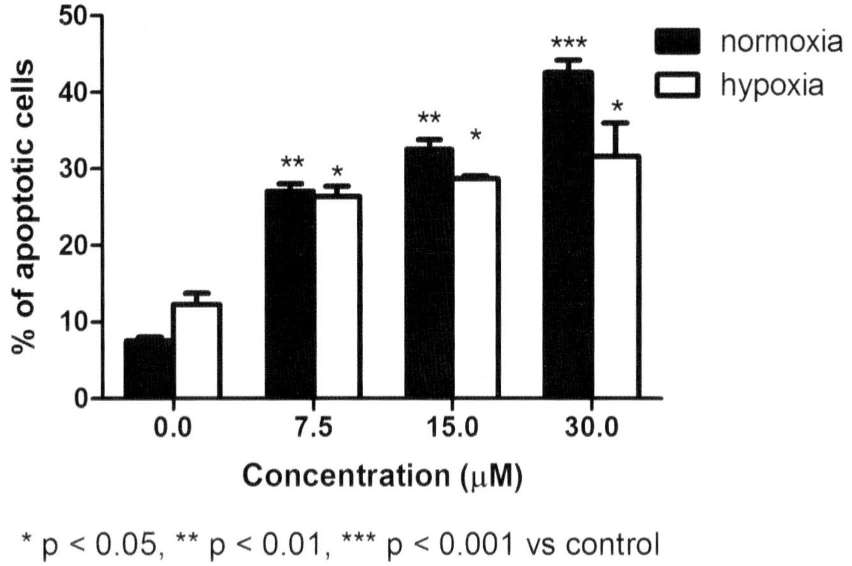

Figure 4. Induction of apoptosis by SR in normoxic and hypoxic conditions on REH cells. Cells were treated with 0 to 30 μM SR for 24 h. The % of apoptotic cells recorded in the untreated cultures was subtracted from that observed in cultures treated with SR. Data are presented as mean ± SEM of at least four different experiments.

stained with 200 μL of Guava Cell Cycle Reagent, containing propidium iodide that allows evaluating cellular DNA content. During the S phase of cell cycle, cells duplicate their content of DNA that will be double in the G_2/M phase compared to the G_0/G_1 phase. Cells were incubated at room temperature for 30 min in the dark, and analyzed via flow cytometry.

mRNA expression

After 6, 24 or 48 h of treatment in normoxic or in hypoxic conditions, total RNA was isolated using miRVana™ miRNA Isolation kit (Life Technologies, CA, USA), according to manufacturer's instructions. Briefly, cells were treated with lysis buffer, then subjected to acid - phenol: chloroform extraction. Ethanol was added to samples and they were passed through a filter cartridge containing a glass-fiber filter which immobilizes the RNA. The filter was washed and RNA was eluted with a low ionic strength solution. Total collected RNA was used for reversed transcription by High Capacity cDNA Reverse Transcription kit (Life Technologies). Briefly, 200 ng total RNA were added to 10 μL reaction kit mixture with RNase inhibitor according to manufacturer's instructions as well as the thermal cycler conditions. The obtained cDNA was stored at −20°C. Quantification of Bax, Bcl-2, TP53 and 18 S, as endogenous control, was performed in triplicate by real-time PCR (ABI Prism 7900HT, Life Technologies), using Universal Master Mix and TaqMan assays Hs00180269_m1 (Bax), Hs00608023_m1 (Bcl-2), Hs01034249_m1 (p53) and Hs99999901_s1 (18S) (Life Technologies). Each measurement was conducted in triplicate.

Statistical analysis

All results are expressed as the mean ± SEM of at least four different experiments. Differences in mRNA expression are reported as value ± SEM and represent the relative expression calculated through the $2^{-\Delta\Delta C}$t method [29]. One way ANOVA, followed by Dunnett or Bonferroni as post test was used to evaluate differences between treatments. GraphPad InStat version 5.0 (GraphPad Prism, San Diego, CA, USA) was used for all statistical analyses. $P<0.05$ was considered significant.

Results

Firstly, we examined the effects of different concentrations of SR on primary blasts collected from leukemic patients. Three samples (patients n. 6, 7 and 8) were excluded because they had a % of viable cells lower than 10% when untreated. SR seems not to have any activity on samples from patients with CLL. Even high concentrations (30 μM) and long times (48 h) of treatment only slightly increased the % of apoptotic cells compared to the control (42.3% vs. 32.4%, sample n. 1) (Fig. 1).

The pro-apoptotic effect of SR was recorded, however, in samples from patients with AML, where the % of apoptotic cells induced following treatment reached 49% (sample n. 5) (Fig. 2). Both samples 3 (about 45% apoptosis increase vs. control at 30 μM after 48 h incubation) and 5 (about 40% apoptosis increase vs. control at 30 μM after 48 h incubation) were highly sensitive to SR treatment (Fig. 2). In contrast, samples 4 (about 28% apoptosis increase vs. control at 30 μM after 48 h incubation), 13 (about 28% apoptosis increase vs. control at 30 μM after 24 h incubation), and 9 (about 13% apoptosis increase vs. control at 15 and 30 μM after 24 h incubation) were less sensitive (Fig. 2). Of note, the effect of SR was marked also on samples from non-responder patients. In the sample n. 5, for example, the fraction of apoptotic cells recorded after 48 h of treatment with 30 μM SR is more than 5 times higher than that recorded in untreated cultures (Fig. 2).

The activity of the isothiocyanate on samples from patients with ALL did not differ between T- or B- cell leukemia. The most marked effect was definitely observed on the sample from patient suffering from T-ALL, where the % of apoptotic cells reached 55% (vs. 27% in the control cultures) (sample n. 10) (Fig. 3). The effect on the other sample of T-ALL was milder (sample n. 11) (about 20% apoptosis increase vs. control at 15 μM after 48 h incubation) (Fig. 3). A 28% increase in the apoptotic effect was reached in the B-ALL sample at 15 μM after 24 h incubation (sample n. 12) (Fig. 3).

SR has not been shown to have any activity on the sample from BNKAL (sample n. 14) (Fig. 3).

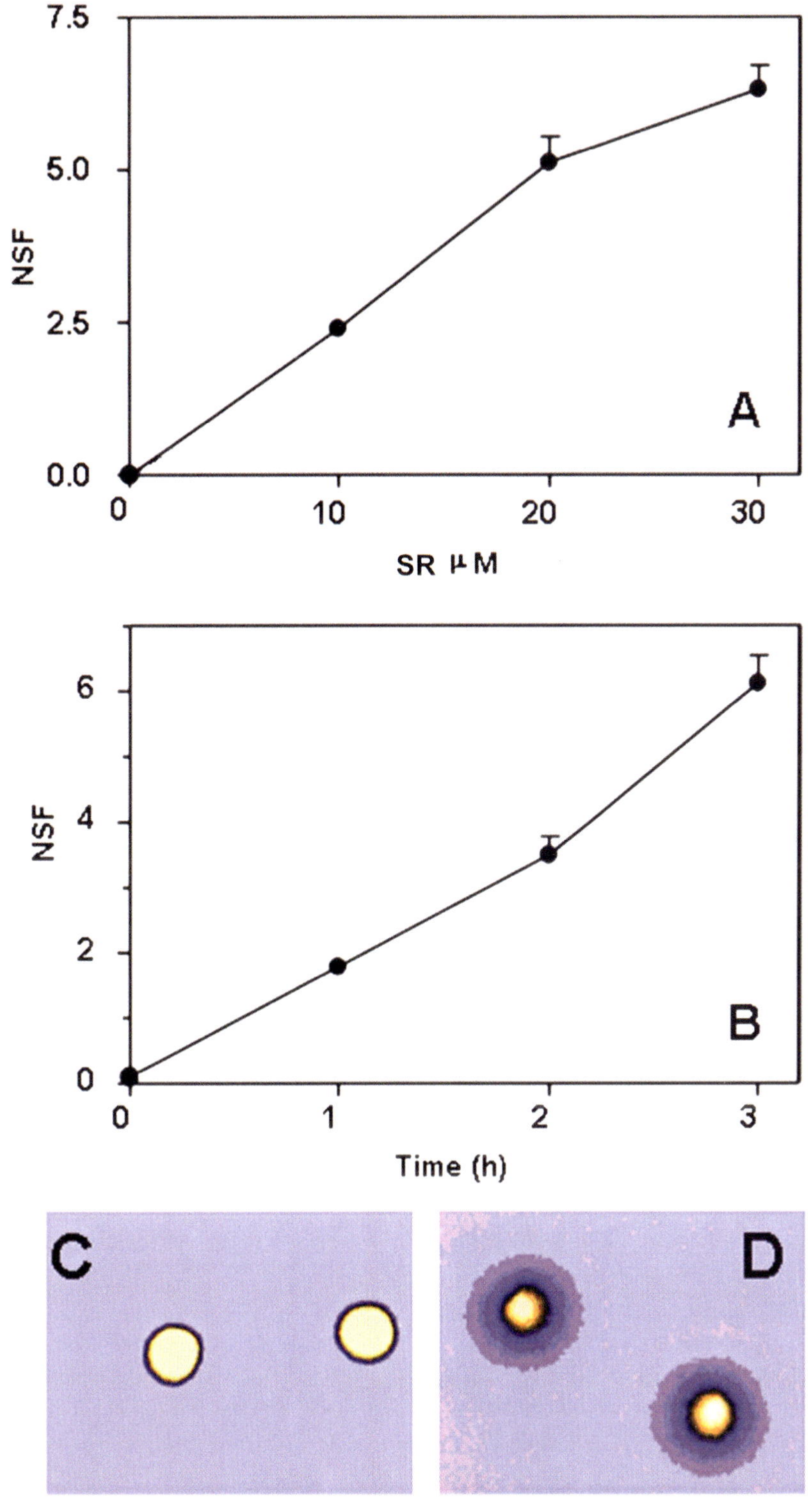

Figure 5. SR induces DNA damage in REH cells. Cells were treated with increasing concentrations of, or for increasing time intervals with, SR and immediately assayed for DNA breakage with FHA. A) DNA single strand breakage induced by 3 h SR treatment in REH cells. B) DNA single strand breakage induced by 30 μM SR in REH cells as a function of incubation time. Data are presented as mean ± SEM of three different experiments. C) and D) Representative, digitally pseudocolored (ICA look up table of the Image J software) micrographs of FHA-processed control (C) or 30 μM SR-treated (D) REH cells are also shown: note the wide halos in D as compared to C. Also shown (panel A, inset) the extent of DNA double strand breakage caused by SR (30 μM for 3 h) or etoposide (1 μg/mL for 3 h) in REH cells. Data are expressed as NSF (nuclear diffusion factor), which represents the ratio between the total area of the halo and nucleus and that of the nucleus.

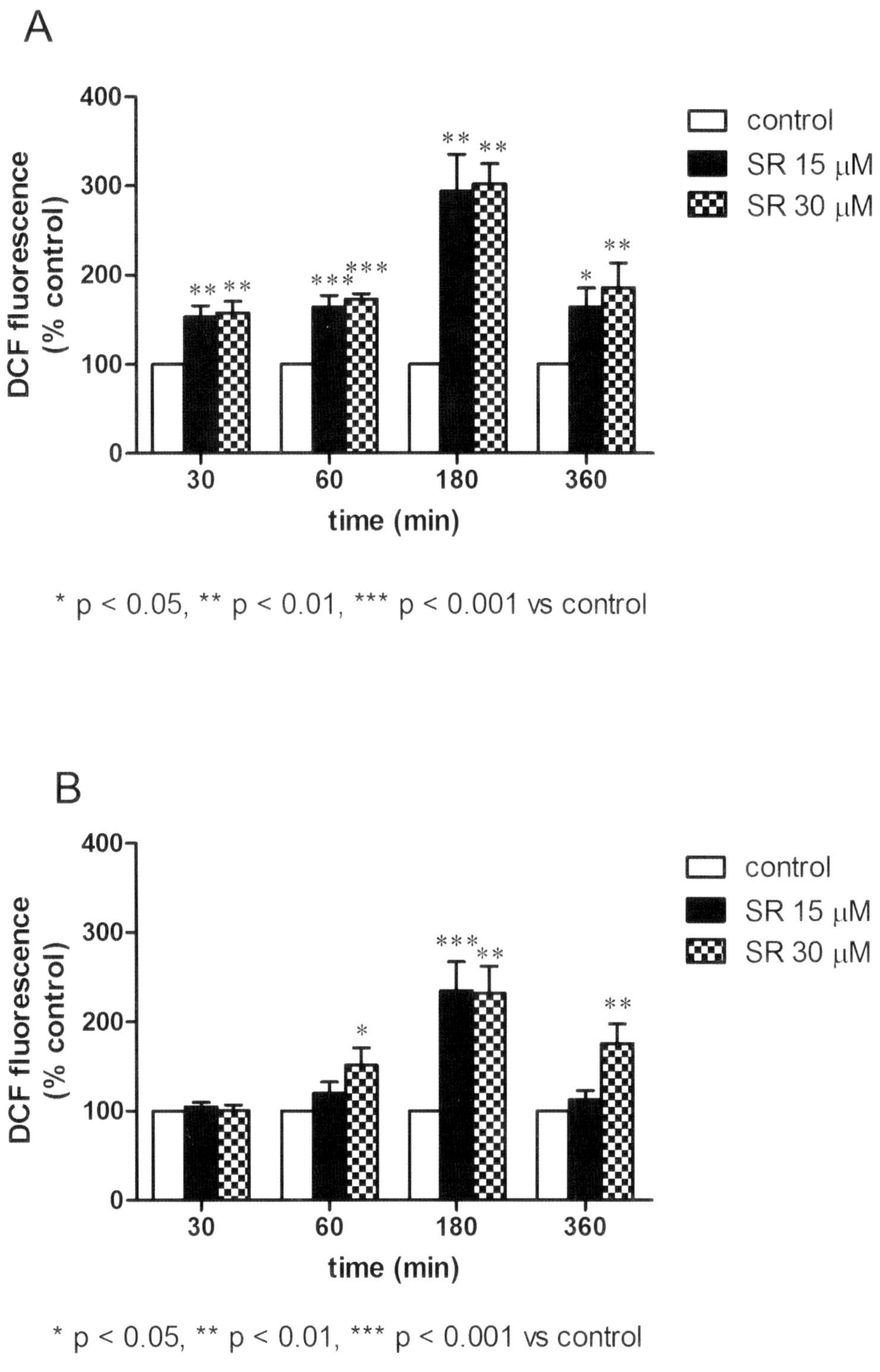

Figure 6. Effect of SR on ROS levels determined in normoxic (A) and hypoxic (B) conditions on REH cells. Cells were treated for 30–360 min with SR to analyze the oxidation state of the cell by using DCFH-DA as fluorogenic probe. Results are expressed as DCF (2′,7′-dichlorodihydrofluorescein) fluorescence (% of control) and are means ± SEM of four independent experiments.

We next analyzed the proapoptotic activity of SR and initially determined the induction of apoptosis after treating two acute leukemia cell lines with different doses of SR for 24 h. In REH cells, we observed a clear increase in the fraction of apoptotic cells under all conditions (Fig. 4). Similar results were observed in HL-60 cells, where we recorded a two-fold increase with respect to controls after 48 h of treatment.

Genomic DNA breaks represent an important trigger of apoptosis. Thus, we investigated the effect of SR on REH cells. REH cells were exposed to SR (10, 20 and 30 μM) for 3 h, and analyzed immediately for direct DNA strand scission using the

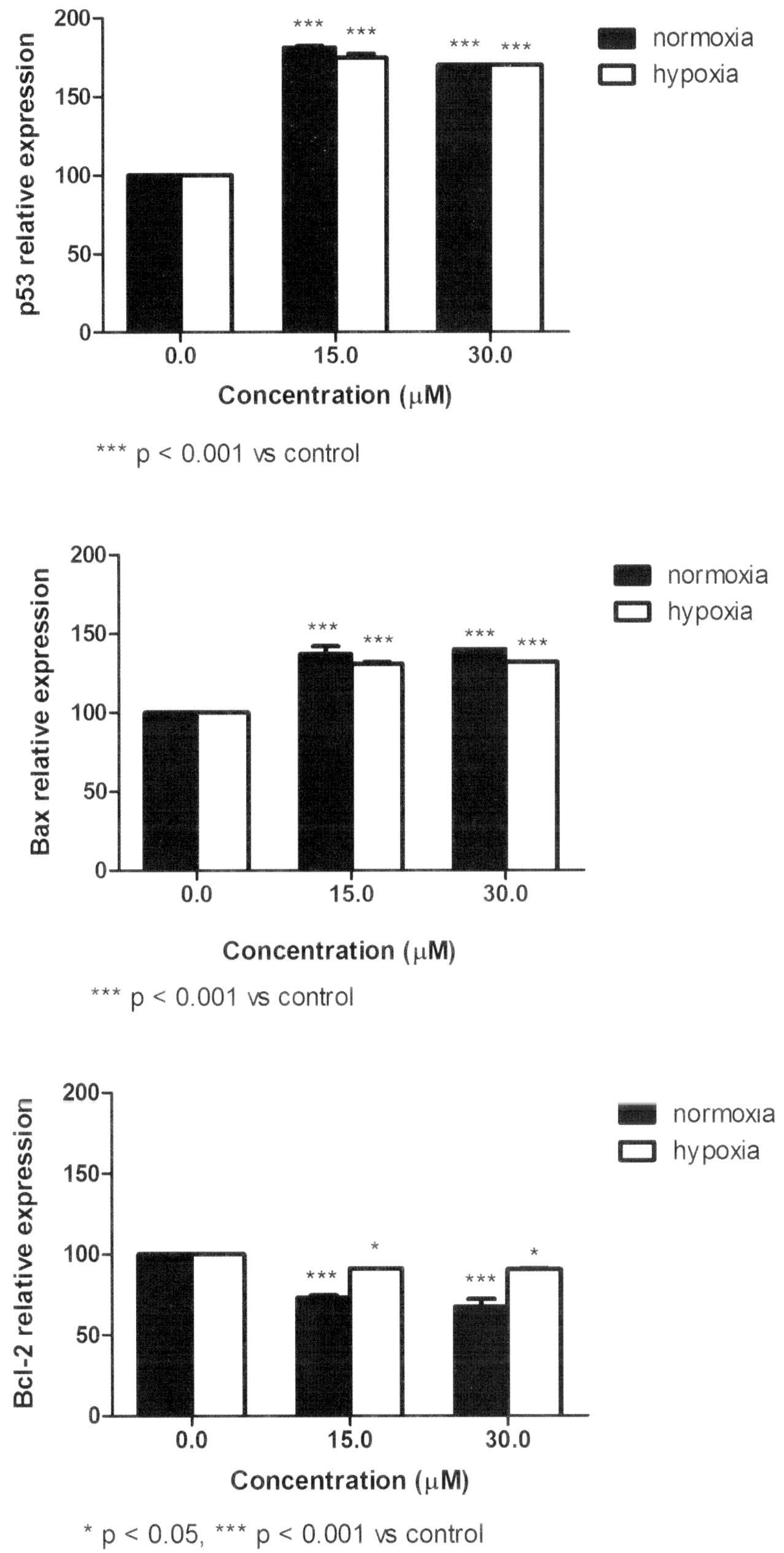

Figure 7. Effect of SR on p53, Bax and Bcl-2 protein expression determined in normoxic and hypoxic conditions on REH cells. Cells were treated with 0 to 30 μM SR for 24 h. Data are presented as mean ± SEM of at least four different experiments.

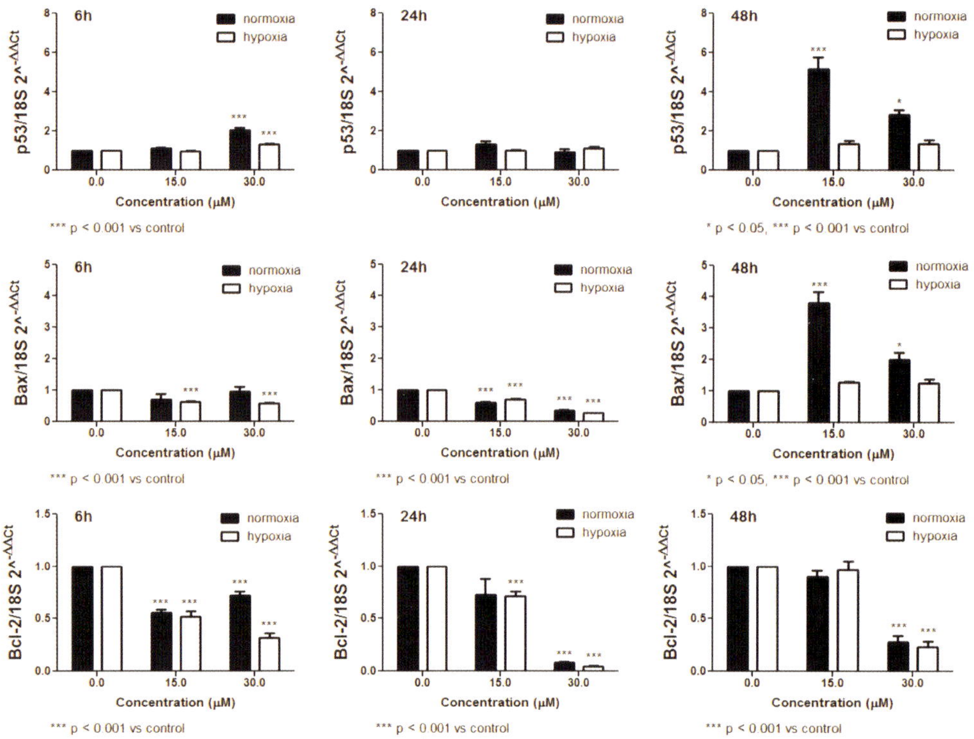

Figure 8. Effect of SR on p53, Bax and Bcl-2 mRNA relative expression calculated through the $2^{-\Delta\Delta C}t$ method and determined in normoxic and hypoxic conditions on REH cells. Cells were treated with 0 to 30 μM SR for 6, 24 or 48 h. Data are presented as mean ± SEM of at least four different experiments.

sensitive FHA. With this technique, DNA fragments resulting from the cleavage of DNA itself diffuse out of the nuclear cage as an inverse function of their size, thus producing a concentric halo whose radius reflects the extent of DNA damage. Halo formation was monitored at the single cell level with fluorescence microscopy, as seen in the representative micrographs shown in Fig. 5C–D. The results obtained indicate that SR promotes the formation of DNA breaks in a dose-dependent fashion (Fig. 5A). Formation of DNA breaks as a function of treatment time with 30 μM SR is linear over time (Fig. 5B).

We then explored the nature of SR-induced DNA lesions by analyzing the nuclear DNA of treated cells at lower -non denaturing conditions- lysis pH values, i.e. 9.3. Indeed, while operating at pH 13.00 does not allow to distinguish DNA single strand breaks (SSBs) from DSBs, at pH 9.3 nuclear DNA is not hydrolyzed into the two chains and only the DNA fragments resulting from double strand cleavage can be detected. Under these latter conditions (i.e. pH 9.3), no difference in terms of DNA fragmentation could be observed between treated (30 μM SFN for 3 h) and untreated REH cells (Fig. 5A, inset), thus suggesting that the lesions caused by SFN observed at pH 13.00 are frank SSBs. On the contrary, treatment of REH cells with etoposide (1 μg/ml for 3 h), included as a representative inducer of DNA DSBs, resulted in extensive DNA double strand breakage (Fig. 5A, inset).

As to the mechanism responsible for the induction of DNA damage in SR-treated cells, we previously reported that SR promotes the mitochondrial formation of ROS [30], which are the ultimate species mediating DNA cleavage. We then investigated the formation of ROS in REH cells. After 3 h of treatment with SR 30 μM, we recorded a significant induction of ROS. Results depicted in Fig. 6 indicate that SR caused the conversion of DCFH into its fluorescent by-product, a process which reflects the formation of ROS. Treatment of cells with SR greatly increased the formation of ROS. The effect was evident after just 30 min of treatment.

Chelation of iron ions blocks the Fenton reaction and thus the production and the propagation of oxygen radicals - i.e. the species responsible for DNA and cellular damages - within the cells [31]. The presence of the iron chelator *o*-phenanthroline prevented the formation of DNA breaks and reduced DCFH oxidation (data not shown). Thus, as to nuclear DNA, the data described so far indicate that REH, according to previous data obtained in Jurkat cells [30], are prone to the DNA damaging action caused by SR, and that ROS are the species mediating this effect in both cell lines.

In the second part of our work, we treated REH cells with different concentration of SR in hypoxic conditions and analyzed the formation of ROS and the induction of apoptosis.

Fig. 6 shows the formation of ROS in normoxic and hypoxic treatment protocols. ROS formation was also observed in hypoxic conditions. The trend is similar in both conditions, although the formation of ROS is higher in normoxia (Fig. 6A). Of note, DNA damage was observed also in hypoxic conditions after treatment with SR (data not shown).

The proapoptotic effect of SR in hypoxia was lower than that observed in normoxia (Fig. 4). As an example, after treatment with SR 7.5 μM, we observed a four-fold increase with respect to controls in normoxia and a two-fold increase in hypoxia. At the highest concentration tested, we recorded a six-fold and about a three-fold increase with respect to controls in normoxia and hypoxia, respectively. After longer time of treatment (i.e. 48 h) in hypoxic conditions, SR mainly induced necrotic events. As an example, at SR 30 μM we recorded 30% of necrotic cells (vs. 10% in the control) and 20% of apoptotic cells (vs. 15% in the control).

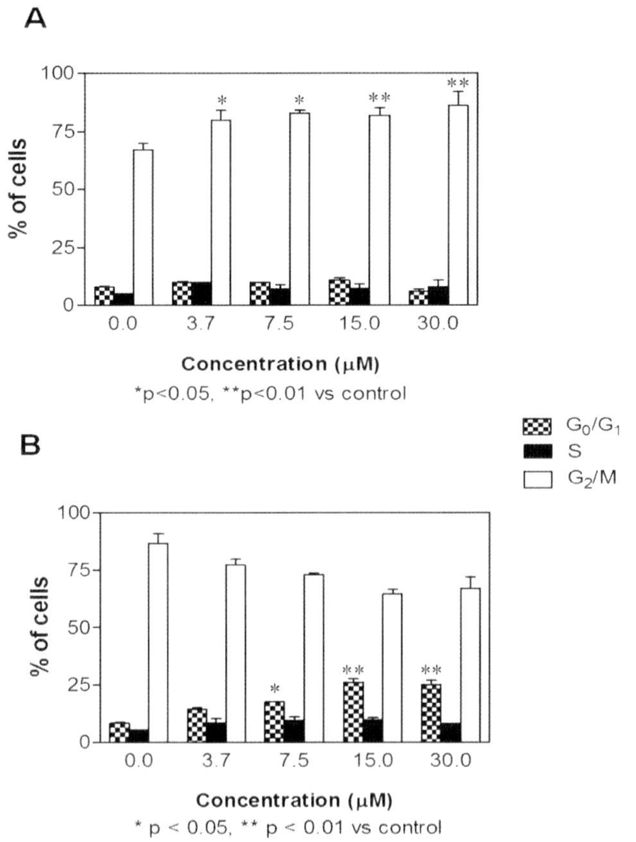

Figure 9. Cell-cycle distribution following 24 h culture in the absence or presence of SR in normoxic (A) and hypoxic (B) conditions on REH cells. Data are means ± SEM of four independent experiments.

This trend was not observed in normoxic conditions, where at SR 30 μM the % of necrotic cells was 25% (vs. 8% in the control) and 44% of apoptotic cells (vs. 10% in the control).

Survival of cancer cells is influenced by the interactions between pro- and anti-apoptotic proteins. We then analyzed the expression at mRNA and protein levels of some genes involved in the regulation of apoptosis. Following 48 h-treatment in normoxic conditions, SR induced a significant up-regulation of p53 and Bax protein expression (Fig. 7). However, the expression of the same genes at mRNA level seems more complex. After treatment with SR for 6, 24 or 48 h, we mainly observed an up-regulation of p53 expression (Fig. 8), while a down-regulation of Bax expression was recorded after 6 and 24 h of treatment. After 48 h, SR up-regulated Bax expression (Fig. 8). The expression of Bcl-2 was down-regulated at both mRNA and protein expression level and following 6, 24 or 48 h of exposure to SR (Figs. 7 and 8).

In hypoxic conditions, we observed a similar trend. However, the effects on p53 and Bax mRNA expression and the ratio of Bax/Bcl-2 proteins were less marked than in normoxia (Figs. 7 and 8).

The antileukemic effect of SR is strengthened by the inhibition of cell proliferation (Fig. 9) in both normoxic and hypoxic exposure to SR. In both conditions, the effect was recordable starting from the lowest concentration tested. However, the mechanism by which SR inhibits cell-cycle progression is different in the two treatment protocols. In normoxia, a block in G_2/M phase was recorded, while an increase in G_1 phase was observed in hypoxia.

Discussion

The main goal of this study was to test the antileukemic properties of SR in hematological cancers. We found that synthesized SR caused a dose-dependent induction of apoptosis in acute leukemia cell lines and primary lymphoblasts from patients diagnosed with B-ALL, T-ALL, and AML.

Due to the possibility to easily obtain blast samples from leukemic patients, SR was tested on an *ex vivo* leukemia model. *Ex vivo* samples represent a quite good surrogate for determining the cellular response of the patient to the treatment and predicting the clinical outcome [32–34]. This can not be realized by using cell lines, which markedly differ from blasts directly taken from leukemic patients in terms of growth kinetics and pharmacological determinants [35]. By the *ex vivo* model and in accordance with previous data [20,30], we confirmed that SR controlled the expansion of leukemic cells. However, our results show that SR can not be defined generically an antileukemic, as apparently it acts only on patients with particular types of leukemia. Indeed, we did not record any activity of SR on samples from CLL patients. CLL is generally described as a disease of failed apoptosis. Apoptosis resistance may stem from a combination of microenvironmental survival signals as well as from intrinsic alterations in the apoptotic machinery and deregulation of components of the DNA-damage response and repair pathways within the CLL cell [36]. Moreover, CD40 signaling has been recognized as a strong antiapoptotic pathway mediating drug resistance *in vitro*. All CLL cells express CD40, and *in vitro* resistance can be induced in 100% of patients [37]. The strong dependence on cellular and cytokine components of the microenvironment makes the *ex vivo* manipulation of CLL cells complex and resulting in biased findings [38]. Taking into account the absence of a cellular model for different types of CLL [39], further research might explore the effects of SR on blasts from CLL patients through the partial re-creation *in vitro* of the CLL microenvironment, including in particular leukemic cell survival signals.

One of the greatest problems for anticancer chemotherapy is chemoresistance, which is less frequent *ab initio* and has a major clinical impact during relapse. SR was tested also on non-responder patients. Although the number of patients was limited, it is interesting to note that SR retains its activity on this type of patients.

One of the more significant findings to emerge from this study is that SR exerts proapoptotic and antiproliferative effects in hypoxic conditions. Reduced oxygen tension affects cellular metabolism and the microenvironment, including pH level. These and other modulations caused by hypoxia can affect the response to pharmacological treatment [40]. Therefore, with the aim of gaining further mechanistic insight into the antileukemic activities of SR as well as the effects of the local environment on the outcome of treatment, we investigated the effects of SR in hypoxic conditions, which better mimics the tumor microenvironment *in vivo*. Our findings demonstrate that, despite hypoxic culture conditions, the antileukemic activity of SR is relatively preserved. We indeed recorded induction of apoptosis and production of ROS after treatment of leukemia cells with SR in both normoxic and hypoxic conditions. As to the mechanism through which SR induces apoptosis, an important trigger is likely to reside in its ability of damaging nuclear DNA. Indeed DNA damage is known as an event causally linked to the apoptotic commitment of target cells. The mechanism whereby DNA breaks are produced clearly involves the intracellular generation of ROS. Paradoxically, exposure of cells to low oxygen (hypoxia) leads to an increase in mitochondrial production of ROS, that are central upstream regulators of many of the cellular responses to hypoxia. Low levels of ROS are required for cellular processes such as proliferation and differentiation, while additional amounts of ROS above a certain threshold may cause cell-cycle arrest and/or apoptosis. The equilibrium of ROS concentration will thus be reached at the point where maximal signaling is permitted without causing irreversible damage to cellular components. Indeed, irreversible damage to cellular proteins, DNA, or lipids seems to be the case as compounds that raise ROS levels can effectively kill a variety of tumor cell lines [41]. Increasing ROS levels may indeed represent a therapeutic strategy to increase killing of cancer cells. Accordingly with those observations, in our experimental setting SR creates an oxidative cellular environment that induces DNA damage and Bax and p53 gene activation, which in turn helps trigger apoptosis. Indeed, the % of apoptotic cells and the up-regulation of p53 and Bax are particularly marked in normoxic conditions, where the production of ROS is higher than in hypoxia. However, the effect of SR on the mRNA expression of p53 and Bax is different, particularly for Bax, for which a down-regulation was observed after short times of treatment with SR. The quantification of both of these expression levels is not an exercise in redundancy. Indeed, analyses of mRNA and protein levels are complementary and both are necessary for a complete understanding of how the cell works. The different modulation of a gene at mRNA and protein levels caused by a xenobiotic can be due to different reasons, such as the poor definition of the complicated and varied post-transcriptional mechanisms involved in turning mRNA into protein, or the different half lives of proteins [42]. The differential effect of SR at mRNA and protein level seems not be imputable to an inhibition of proteasome. Instead, SR appears to stimulate proteasome [43,44]. Alternately, a further study could assess the modulation by SR of microRNAs that moderate the p53 and Bax transcriptional program.

The results of this investigation show that SR is also able to inhibit cell-cycle progression through a block in the G_2/M phase in normoxia and in the G_1 phase in hypoxia. The G_2/M block induced by SR in normoxia was reported in many cell lines [1]. The differential effect in hypoxic conditions is not surprising. As a matter of fact, cells subject to severe hypoxia will arrest in G_1 or early S phase and cells in late S, G_2 or M phase will finish cell division and arrest in G_1, unless the hypoxia is severe [45].

As to the concentrations of SR used in this study, they could be not achievable from food supply. However, after a single oral dose of SR at 150 µmol/kg in rat, plasma concentrations of SR equivalents increase to 15.2 µM [46]. Furthermore, the potential development of SR in clinical practice could lead to the application of a drug delivery system to improve drug absorption.

In conclusion, *in vitro* and *ex vivo* experiments performed in the present study suggest that SR could represent an interesting therapeutic approach for patients affected by acute proliferative disorders and might set the stage for a novel therapeutic principle complementing our growing armature against malignancies. Large clinical trials will be necessary to confirm this attractive perspective *in vivo*.

Author Contributions

Conceived and designed the experiments: CF. Performed the experiments: ET CC GF MR. Analyzed the data: CF ET PS. Wrote the paper: CF PS GC GCF PH.

References

1. Fimognari C, Hrelia P (2007) Sulforaphane as a promising molecule for fighting cancer. Mutat Res 635: 90 104.
2. Ambrosone CB, McCann SE, Freudenheim JL, Marshall JR, Zhang Y, et al. (2004) Breast cancer risk in premenopausal women is inversely associated with consumption of broccoli, a source of isothiocyanates, but is not modified by GST genotype. J Nutr 134: 1134 8.
3. Joseph MA, Moysich KB, Freudenheim JL, Shields PG, Bowman ED, et al. (2004) Cruciferous vegetables, genetic polymorphisms in glutathione S-transferases M1 and T1, and prostate cancer risk. Nutr Cancer 50: 206 13.
4. Probst-Hensch NM, Tannenbaum SR, Chan KK, Coetzee GA, Ross RK, et al. (1998) Absence of the glutathione S-transferase M1 gene increases cytochrome P4501A2 activity among frequent consumers of cruciferous vegetables in a Caucasian population. Cancer Epidemiol Biomarkers 7: 635–8.
5. Spitz MR, Duphorne CM, Detry MA, Pillow PC, Amos CI, et al. (2000) Dietary intake of isothiocyanates: evidence of a joint effect with glutathione S-transferase polymorphisms in lung cancer risk. Cancer Epidemiol Biomarkers Prev 9: 1017 20.
6. Traka M, Gasper AV, Melchini A, Bacon JR, Needs PW, et al. (2008) Broccoli consumption interacts with GSTM1 to perturb oncogenic signalling pathways in the prostate. PLoS One 3: e2568.
7. Tang L, Zirpoli GR, Guru K, Moysich KB, Zhang Y, et al. (2008) Consumption of raw cruciferous vegetables is inversely associated with bladder cancer risk. Cancer Epidemiol Biomarkers Prev 17: 938 44.
8. Fimognari C, Turrini E, Ferruzzi L, Lenzi M, Hrelia P (2012) Natural isothiocyanates: genotoxic potential versus chemoprevention. Mutat Res 750: 107 31.
9. Hsu YC, Chang SJ, Wang MY, Chen YL, Huang TY (2013) Growth inhibition and apoptosis of neuroblastoma cells through ROS-independent MEK/ERK activation by sulforaphane. Cell Biochem Biophys 66: 765–74.
10. Fimognari C, Lenzi M, Hrelia P (2009) Apoptosis induction by sulfur-containing compounds in malignant and nonmalignant human cells. Environ Mol Mutagen 50: 171–89.
11. Parnaud G, Li P, Cassar G, Rouimi P, Tulliez J, et al. (2004) Mechanism of sulforaphane-induced cell cycle arrest and apoptosis in human colon cancer cells. Nutr Cancer 48: 198 206.
12. Jackson SJ, Singletary KW (2004) Sulforaphane inhibits human MCF-7 mammary cancer cell mitotic progression and tubulin polymerization. J Nutr 134: 2229 36.
13. Singh AV, Xiao D, Lew KL, Dhir R, Singh SV (2004) Sulforaphane induces caspase-mediated apoptosis in cultured PC-3 human prostate cancer cells and retards growth of PC-3 xenografts in vivo. Carcinogenesis 25: 83 90.
14. Myzak MC, Dashwood WM, Orner GA, Ho E, Dashwood RH (2006) Sulforaphane inhibits histone deacetylase in vivo and suppresses tumorigenesis in Apc-minus mice. FASEB J 20: 506 8.
15. Fimognari C, Nüsse M, Berti F, Iori R, Cantelli-Forti G, et al. (2003) Sulforaphane modulates cell cycle and apoptosis in transformed and non-transformed human T lymphocytes. Ann N Y Acad Sci 1010: 393 8.
16. Pham NA, Jacobberger JW, Schimmer AD, Cao P, Gronda M, et al. (2004) The dietary isothiocyanate sulforaphane targets pathways of apoptosis, cell cycle arrest, and oxidative stress in human pancreatic cancer cells and inhibits tumor growth in severe combined immunodeficient mice. Mol Cancer Ther 3: 1239 48.
17. Gamet-Payrastre L, Li P, Lumeau S, Cassar G, Dupont MA, et al. (2000) Sulforaphane, a naturally occurring isothiocyanate, induces cell cycle arrest and apoptosis in HT29 human colon cancer cells. Cancer Res 60: 1426 33.
18. Singh SV, Herman-Antosiewicz A, Singh AV, Lew KL, Srivastava SK, et al. (2004) Sulforaphane-induced G2/M phase cell cycle arrest involves checkpoint kinase 2-mediated phosphorylation of cell division cycle 25C. J Biol Chem 279: 25813 22.
19. Traka M, Gasper AV, Smith JA, Hawkey CJ, Bao Y, et al. (2005) Transcriptome analysis of human colon Caco-2 cells exposed to sulforaphane. J Nutr 135: 1865 72.
20. Suppipat K, Park CS, Shen Y, Zhu X, Lacorazza HD (2012) Sulforaphane induces cell cycle arrest and apoptosis in acute lymphoblastic leukemia cells. PLoS One 7: e51251.
21. Vardiman JW, Thiele J, Arber DA, Brunning RD, Borowitz MJ, et al. (2009) The 2008 revision of the World Health Organization (WHO) classification of myeloid neoplasms and acute leukemia: rationale and important changes. Blood 114: 937 51.
22. Jemal A, Siegel R, Xu J, Ward E (2010) Cancer statistics, 2010. CA Cancer J Clin 60: 277 300.
23. Fathi AT, Karp JE (2009) New agents in acute myeloid leukemia: beyond cytarabine and anthracyclines. Curr Oncol Rep 11: 346 52.
24. Arcangeli A, Pillozzi S, Becchetti A (2012) Targeting ion channels in leukemias: a new challenge for treatment. Curr Med Chem 19: 683 96.

25. Karp JE, Ross DD, Yang W, Tidwell ML, Wei Y, et al. (2003) Timed sequential therapy of acute leukemia with flavopiridol: in vitro model for a phase I clinical trial. Clin Cancer Res 9: 307 15.
26. Filippi I, Naldini A, Carraro F (2011) Role of the hypoxic microenvironment in the antitumor activity of tyrosine kinase inhibitors. Curr Med Chem 18: 2885 92.
27. Sestili P, Martinelli C, Stocchi V (2006) The fast halo assay: an improved method to quantify genomic DNA strand breakage at the single-cell level. Mutat Res 607: 205 14.
28. Sestili P (2009) The fast-halo assay for the assessment of DNA damage at the single-cell level. Methods Mol Biol 521: 517 33.
29. Livak KJ, Schmittgen TD (2001) Analysis of relative gene expression data using real-time quantitative PCR and the 2(-Delta Delta C(T)) method. Methods 25: 402 8.
30. Sestili P, Paolillo M, Lenzi M, Colombo E, Vallorani L, et al. (2010) Sulforaphane induces DNA single strand breaks in cultured human cells. Mutat Res 689: 65 73.
31. Sestili P, Diamantini G, Bedini A, Cerioni L, Tommasini I, et al. (2002) Plant-derived phenolic compounds prevent the DNA single-strand breakage and cytotoxicity induced by tert-butylhydroperoxide via an iron-chelating mechanism. Biochem J 364: 121 8.
32. Bromidge TJ, Turner DL, Howe DJ, Johnson SA, Rule SA (1998) In vitro chemosensitivity of chronic lymphocytic leukaemia to purine analogues correlation with clinical course. Leukemia 12: 1230 5.
33. Morabito F, Stelitano C, Callea I, Dattola A, Console G, et al. (1998) In vitro drug-induced cytotoxicity predicts clinical response to fludarabine in B-cell chronic lymphocytic leukaemia. Br J Haematol 102: 528 31.
34. Bosanquet AG, Burlton AR, Bell PB (2002) Parameters affecting the ex vivo cytotoxic drug sensitivity of human hematopoietic cells. J Exp Ther Oncol 2: 53 63.
35. O'Connor R, Cesano A, Lange B, Finan J, Nowell PC, et al. (1991) Growth factor requirements of childhood acute T-lymphoblastic leukemia: correlation between presence of chromosomal abnormalities and ability to grow permanently in vitro. Blood 77: 1534 45.
36. Mohr J, Helfrich H, Fuge M, Eldering E, Bühler A, et al. (2011) DNA damage-induced transcriptional program in CLL: biological and diagnostic implications for functional p53 testing. Blood 117: 1622 32.
37. Dietrich S, Krämer OH, Hahn E, Schäfer C, Giese T, et al. (2012) Leflunomide induces apoptosis in fludarabine-resistant and clinically refractory CLL cells. Clin Cancer Res 18: 417 31.
38. Ghia P, Chiorazzi N, Stamatopoulos K (2008) Microenvironmental influences in chronic lymphocytic leukaemia: the role of antigen stimulation. J Intern Med 264: 549 62.
39. Ghamlouch H, Ouled-Haddou H, Damaj G, Royer B, Gubler B, et al. (2013) A combination of cytokines rescues highly purified leukemic CLL B-cells from spontaneous apoptosis in vitro. PLoS One 8: e60370.
40. Lodi A, Tiziani S, Khanim FL, Drayson MT, Günther UL, et al. (2011) Hypoxia triggers major metabolic changes in AML cells without altering indomethacin-induced TCA cycle deregulation. ACS Chem Biol 6: 169 75.
41. Hamanaka RB, Chandel NS (2010) Mitochondrial reactive oxygen species regulate cellular signaling and dictate biological outcomes. Trends Biochem Sci 35: 505 13.
42. Greenbaum D, Colangelo C, Williams K, Gerstein M (2003) Comparing protein abundance and mRNA expression levels on a genomic scale. Genome Biol 4: 117.
43. Balasubramanian S, Chew YC, Eckert RL (2011) Sulforaphane suppresses polycomb group protein level via a proteasome-dependent mechanism in skin cancer cells. Mol Pharmacol 80: 870 8.
44. Liu Y, Hettinger CL, Zhang D, Rezvani K, Wang X, et al. (2014) Sulforaphane enhances proteasomal and autophagic activities in mice and is a potential therapeutic reagent for Huntington's disease. J Neurochem doi: 10.1111/jnc.12647
45. Box AH, Demetrick DJ (2004) Cell cycle kinase inhibitor expression and hypoxia-induced cell cycle arrest in human cancer cell lines. Carcinogenesis 25: 2325 35.
46. Veeranki OL, Bhattacharya A, Marshall JR, Zhang Y (2013) Organ-specific exposure and response to sulforaphane, a key chemopreventive ingredient in broccoli: implications for cancer prevention. Br J Nutr 109: 25 32.

Epigenetic Silencing of TFPI-2 in Canine Diffuse Large B-Cell Lymphoma

Serena Ferraresso[1]*, Silvia Bresolin[2], Arianna Aricò[1], Stefano Comazzi[3], Maria Elena Gelain[1], Fulvio Riondato[4], Luca Bargelloni[1], Laura Marconato[5], Geertruy te Kronnie[2], Luca Aresu[1]

1 Department of Comparative Biomedicine and Food Science, University of Padova, Padova, Italy, **2** Department of Women's and Children's Health, University of Padova, Padova, Italy, **3** Department of Animal Pathology Hygiene and Veterinary Public Health, University of Milano, Milano, Italy, **4** Department Veterinary Science, University of Torino, Torino, Italy, **5** Centro Oncologico Veterinario, Sasso Marconi, Italia

Abstract

Epigenetic modifications are important early events during carcinogenesis. In particular, hypermethylation of CpG islands in the promoter region of tumor suppressor genes is a well-known mechanism of gene silencing that contributes to cancer development and progression. Tissue factor pathway inhibitor 2 (TFPI-2) is a tumor suppressor involved in invasiveness inhibition. Although TFPI-2 transcriptional silencing, through promoter hypermethylation, has been widely reported in several human malignancies, it has never been explored in lymphoma. In the present study TFPI-2 methylation and gene expression have been investigated in canine Diffuse Large B-cell lymphomas (cDLBCL). The methylation level of 23 CpGs located within the TFPI-2 promoter was investigated by bisulfite-specific PCR and next generation amplicon deep sequencing (GS Junior 454, Roche) in 22 cDLBCLs and 9 controls. For the same specimens, TFPI-2 gene expression was assessed by means of Real-time RT-PCR. Sequence analysis clearly demonstrated that TFPI2 is frequently hypermethylated in cDLBCL. Hypermethylation of the TFPI-2 promoter was found in 77% of DLBCLs (17 out of 22) and in one normal lymph node. Globally, dogs with DLBCL showed a mean methylation level significantly increased compared to controls ($p<0.01$) and analysis of hypermethylation by site identified 19 loci out of 23 (82%) with mean methylation levels from 2- to 120-fold higher in cDLBCL. Gene expression analysis confirmed a significant down-regulation of TFPI-2 ($p<0.05$) in DLBCLs compared with normal lymph nodes, suggesting that TFPI-2 hypermethylation negatively regulates its transcription. In addition, a significant positive correlation ($p<0.01$) was found between TFPI-2 methylation levels and age providing the first indication of age-associated epigenetic modifications in canine DLBCL. To conclude, our findings demonstrated that epigenetic dysregulation of TFPI-2, leading to its reduced expression, is frequently detected in canine DLBCL. In the next future, the aberrant TFPI-2 promoter hypermethylation may be considered in association with prognosis and therapy.

Editor: Ken Mills, Queen's University Belfast, United Kingdom

Funding: This work was founded by a grant from Ministry of Health (PRIN). The funders had no role in study design, data collection and analysis, decision to publish, or preparation of the manuscript.

Competing Interests: The authors have declared that no competing interests exist.

* E-mail: serena.ferraresso@unipd.it

Introduction

Canine diffuse large B-cell lymphoma (DLBCL) is an aggressive malignancy of the mature B-lymphocytes showing significant overlaps with the human disease and it is considered curable in less than 10% of dogs. Although advances in treatment have improved outcome, survival time is quite variable, ranging from months to years [1]. This incomplete success indicates the need for further studies to elucidate the pathogenesis through the identification of altered gene expression and cellular pathways, thereby influencing the aggressive behavior of DLBCL, and representing a target for novel therapeutic strategies.

In human DLBCL, gene-expression profiling has identified two biologically and clinically distinct molecular subtypes, which consistently correlate with treatment response, regardless of the regimen used ([2] for a review). Nevertheless, paucity remains in the understanding of the molecular events underlying the development and progression of DLBCL, especially in terms of activation of oncogenes or inactivation of tumor suppressor genes (TSG). Recently, it has become clear that, in addition to genetic changes (i.e. mutations, rearrangements), epigenetic modifications represent an important step in the pathogenesis of lymphoma, and such changes may be of interest in the definition of prognosis and delineation of specific therapy [3]. A common epigenetic event is DNA methylation at cytosine residues of CpG islands [4]. CpG islands are short CpG-rich regions, often mapping at the promoter and exonic regions of the gene. Increased methylation of CpG islands within gene promoters is associated with transcriptional gene silencing. In particular, hypermethylation of CpG islands in the promoter region of TSGs is a well-known mechanism of gene silencing that contributes to cancer development and progression [5]. Identifying aberrant methylated genes may provide better understanding of the pathogenesis of lymphoma, thereby paving the way for the development of novel tumor markers and therapeutic targets.

A candidate gene for epigenetic regulation of lymphomagenesis is Tissue Factor Pathway Inhibitor-2 (TFPI-2), a Kunitz-type serine proteinase inhibitor that directly regulates the activation of matrix metallo-proteinases (MMPs) and plays a significant role in the regulation of ECM degradation, which is an essential step for cell remodeling, as well as tumor invasiveness and metastasis. In humans, TFPI-2 is inactivated or absent during tumor progression, conferring an important role for this gene in the pathogenesis of malignancies [6]. Aberrant methylation has been suggested as a possible mechanism for loss of TFPI-2 expression in several human cancers [7–11].

We recently characterized the transcriptome profiles of twenty-one dogs with DLBCL and five normal lymph nodes by using an array–based approach [12]. Statistical analyses identified two molecular subtypes similarly to human DLBCL. These two clusters revealed distinct signatures with NFKB2 and other genes related to proliferation having increased expression in the main subgroup. Two probe sets revealed a significant down-regulation of TFPI-2 mRNA levels in both DLBCL groups compared to healthy controls.

The role of TFPI-2 in hematopoietic malignancies is scarcely documented. Epigenetic dysregulation of TFPI-2, leading to its reduced expression, has been observed in pediatric acute myeloid leukemia [13], while no information is available for lymphoma. Major improvements in sequencing technologies have now provided an unprecedented opportunity to examine the cancer-associated genomic alterations even in non-model species.

The aim of the present study was to investigate the TFPI-2 epigenetic status in lymph nodes from dogs with DLBCL and healthy controls. TFPI-2 methylation levels were quantified by means of bisulfite-specific PCR and next generation amplicon deep sequencing. Additionally, the methylation status of TFPI-2 promoter has been correlated to gene expression levels in order to evaluate whether abnormal methylation of the promoter region might be responsible for TFPI-2 transcription silencing.

Materials and Methods

Samples and Nucleic Acid Extraction

All lymphoma samples were taken as part of normal diagnostic procedures from dogs with newly diagnosed, previously untreated lymphoma. Only dogs with confirmed DLBCL after histopathological and immunohistochemical analysis (CD20/CD79 marker analysis) were enrolled (Table 1). The study was approved by the

Table 1. Samples included in the study.

	ID	Breed	Age	Gender	Stage	Substage
Healthy ctrls	Ctrl1	German shepherd	5	M		
	Ctrl2	Cane Corso	5	F		
	Ctrl3	Mixed breed	6	M		
	Ctrl4	Mixed breed	4	M		
	Ctrl5	Siberian husky	9	F		
	Ctrl6	Mixed breed	10	F		
	Ctrl7	Mixed breed	9	F		
	Ctrl8	American Pittbul	7	M		
	Ctrl9	Mixed breed	2	F		
DLBCL	DLBCL1	Mixed breed	14	F	5	a
	DLBCL2	Scottish terrier	10	F	4	a
	DLBCL3	Pyrenean sheepdog	12	M	3	a
	DLBCL4	English setter	12	F	3	a
	DLBCL5	Labrabor retriever	5	M	4	a
	DLBCL6	Labrador retriever	6	F	4	a
	DLBCL7	Mixed breed	7	F	3	a
	DLBCL8	German shepherd	8	M	3	a
	DLBCL9	Tibetian terrier	8	F	4	a
	DLBCL10	Mixed breed	3	F	3	a
	DLBCL11	Mixed breed	9	M	4	a
	DLBCL12	Epagneul Breton	7	F	5	b
	DLBCL13	Yorkshire terrier	6	M	5	b
	DLBCL14	Mixed breed	12	F	5	a
	DLBCL15	Cocker spaniel	5	F	3	a
	DLBCL16	Mixed breed	4	F	3	a
	DLBCL17	Mixed breed	6	F	4	a
	DLBCL18	German shepherd	8	F	3	a
	DLBCL19	Mixed breed	8	M	5	a
	DLBCL20	Mixed breed	5	F	4	a
	DLBCL21	Mixed breed	5	M	4	a
	DLBCL22	Mixed breed	11	F	5	b

Table 2. Primer pairs employed for PCR amplification and amplicon library preparation.

	Primer	Primer sequence	Amplicon (bp)
First-round PCR	TFPI2_2F	GGGGAGGTAGGTTTAATTTGG	493
	TFPI2_Rd	TCCTAAACRCCCTATACAACTAAAA	
Amplicon library preparation	TFPI2_LF	GTGTGGGGTATGAATTAGTTAGG	212
	TFPI2_LR	AACCAACRAAATCCATAC	

University Committee (protocol 20085MSFH2) and a mandatory written consent from patient owners was also requested. Portion of the tumour was obtained under sterile conditions. Normal lymph node samples were obtained from healthy dogs.

Samples were preserved in RNA-later and stored at minus 80°C prior to RNA and DNA extraction. For all samples, DNA extraction was conducted using the DNeasy Blood & Tissue Kit (Qiagen, Hilden, Germany) according to the manufacturer's specifications. Total RNA was extracted using the RNAeasy Mini Kit (Qiagen) according to manufacturer's specifications. For each sample, RNA integrity and quality were estimated on the Agilent 2100 Bioanalyzer (Agilent Technologies, Palo Alto, CA). DNA and RNA concentrations were determined with a NanoDrop ND-1000 UV-Vis spectrophotometer (NanoDrop Technologies, Wilmington, USA).

In silico Prediction of TFPI-2 CpG Island and Primer Design

In order to identify putative CpG island on promoter region, TFPI-2 genomic sequence (ENSCAFG00000002040), as stored on Ensembl genome browser (http://www.ensembl.org/index.html), including 1000 bp upstream the ATG site was employed as query sequence. Two different softwares, CpGPlot software (http://www.ebi.ac.uk/Tools/seqstats/emboss_cpgplot/) and MethylPrimer Express v1.0 (Applied Biosystem) were applied. Parameters set for CpG island identification were: 1) minimun length of 200 nt, 2) CG content ≥50% and, 3) CpG observed/CpG expected ratio ≥ 0.6.

On the CpG island identified, Bisulfite-specific primers (BSPs) were then designed by means of Methyl Primer Express software to amplify a region of 493 bp (see Table 2). In the same way, a second primer pair was designed as "template specific portion" of Fusion primers (see below) employed for 454 amplicon library preparation (see Table 2).

Bisulfite Treatment and PCR Amplification

For each sample, a total of 400 ng of genomic DNA was bisulfite treated using the MethylCode Bisulfite Conversion Kit (Invitrogen, Carlsbad, California) following manufacturer's specifications. A total of 10 ng of bisulfite-converted DNA was then employed as template for first-round PCR using TFPI2_2F and

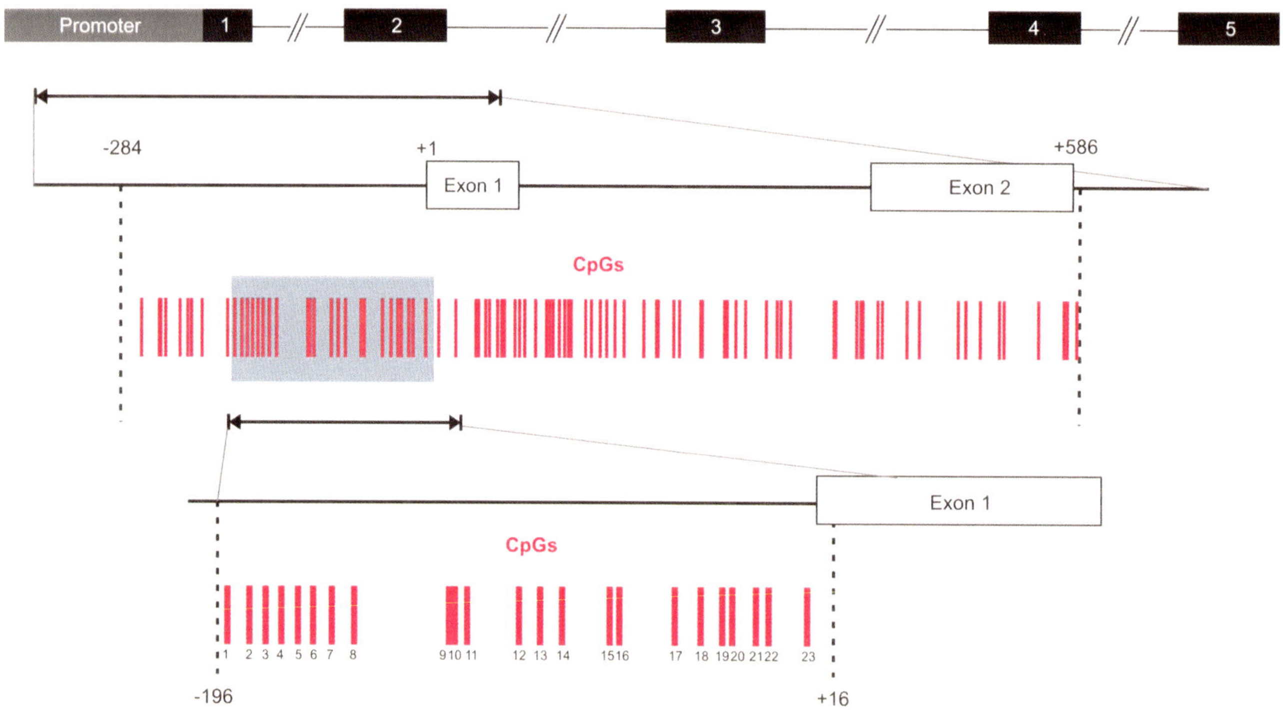

Figure 1. Schematic representation of of the TFPI-2 gene and CpG island. The black boxes indicate exons, +1 indicates the translation start site. Each vertical bar represents a CpG dinucleotide. From −284 to +586 is the location of the CpG island, the grey box (from −196 to +16) indicates the region analyzed by Bis-seq.

Table 3. TFPI-2 mean methylation level and total number of reads for each sample. Gene expression levels measured by means of qPCR are also reported.

	Sample	qPCR	Reads	Methylation level	Mean methylation
Healthy ctrls	Ctrl1	11.990	490	**0.093**	**0.141 (±0.08)**
	Ctrl2	1.336	459	**0.135**	
	Ctrl3	na	337	**0.121**	
	Ctrl4	na	273	**0.033**	
	Ctrl5	0.862	469	**0.308**	
	Ctrl6	1.290	349	**0.076**	
	Ctrl7	0.711	480	**0.158**	
	Ctrl8	1.563	427	**0.216**	
	Ctrl9	2.703	384	**0.128**	
DLBCLs	DLBCL1	0.030	410	**0.671**	**0.448 (±0.26)**
	DLBCL2	1.563	337	**0.931**	
	DLBCL3	4.636	364	**0.692**	
	DLBCL4	na	385	**0.863**	
	DLBCL5	0.184	485	**0.007**	
	DLBCL6	0.055	435	**0.133**	
	DLBCL7	0.031	441	**0.481**	
	DLBCL8	0.052	489	**0.395**	
	DLBCL9	1.441	331	**0.361**	
	DLBCL10	0.666	461	**0.082**	
	DLBCL11	1.324	236	**0.696**	
	DLBCL12	0.01	534	**0.552**	
	DLBCL13	0.000	402	**0.147**	
	DLBCL14	1.200	338	**0.889**	
	DLBCL15	0.114	352	**0.129**	
	DLBCL16	0.140	453	**0.324**	
	DLBCL17	na	374	**0.414**	
	DLBCL18	na	393	**0.382**	
	DLBCL19	2.264	457	**0.549**	
	DLBCL20	na	869	**0.306**	
	DLBCL21	1.546	397	**0.526**	
	DLBCL22	0.859	372	**0.316**	

TFPI2_Rd primers (see Table 2) in order to amplify a portion of 493 bp of TFPI-2 promoter. Cycling conditions were: initial incubation at 94°C for 2 min followed by 35 cycles at 94°C for 20 s, 61.7°C for 30 s and 72°C for 1 min. A final extension step at 72°C for 5 min was added at the end of the last cycle. Amplification products for each sample were then employed as template for amplicon library preparation.

Amplicon Library Preparation and GS Junior 454 Sequencing

The amplicon library was purified using Agencourt AMPure XP beads (Beckman Coulter, Krefeld, Germany), quantified using the Quant-iT PicoGreen dsDNA kit (Invitrogen, Carlsbad, CA, USA) and equimolar pooled together for the emPCR (library at 1×10^7 molecules/ul). All data were generated using GS Junior Sequencer Instrument software version 2.7 (Roche Applied Science, Mannheim, Germany). Image processing and amplicon pipeline analysis was performed using default settings of the GS RunBrowser software version 2.7 (Roche Applied Science).

Gene Expression Analysis of TFPI-2

TFPI-2 expression levels were tested on 25 samples (7 healthy controls and 18 DLBCLs) by means of real-time RT-PCR. A total of 100 ng of RNA for each sample was reverse transcribed to cDNA using High Capacity cDNA Reverse Transcription Kit (Life Technologies). An aliquot (2.5 µl) of diluted (1:50) cDNA template was amplified in a final volume of 10 µl, containing 5 µl Platinum SYBR Green qPCR SuperMix-UDG 2× (Invitrogen) and 0.25 µl of each gene-specific primer (10 µM). The amplification protocol consisted of an initial step of 2 min at 50°C and 2 min at 95° followed by 45 cycles of 10 s at 95°C and 30 s at 60°C. All experiments were carried out in a *LightCycler 480* thermocycler (Roche Diagnostics).

Each measurement was made in triplicate, and normalized to the reference gene, transmembrane BAX inhibitor motif containing 4 (TMBIM4), which was also measured in triplicate. TMBIM4

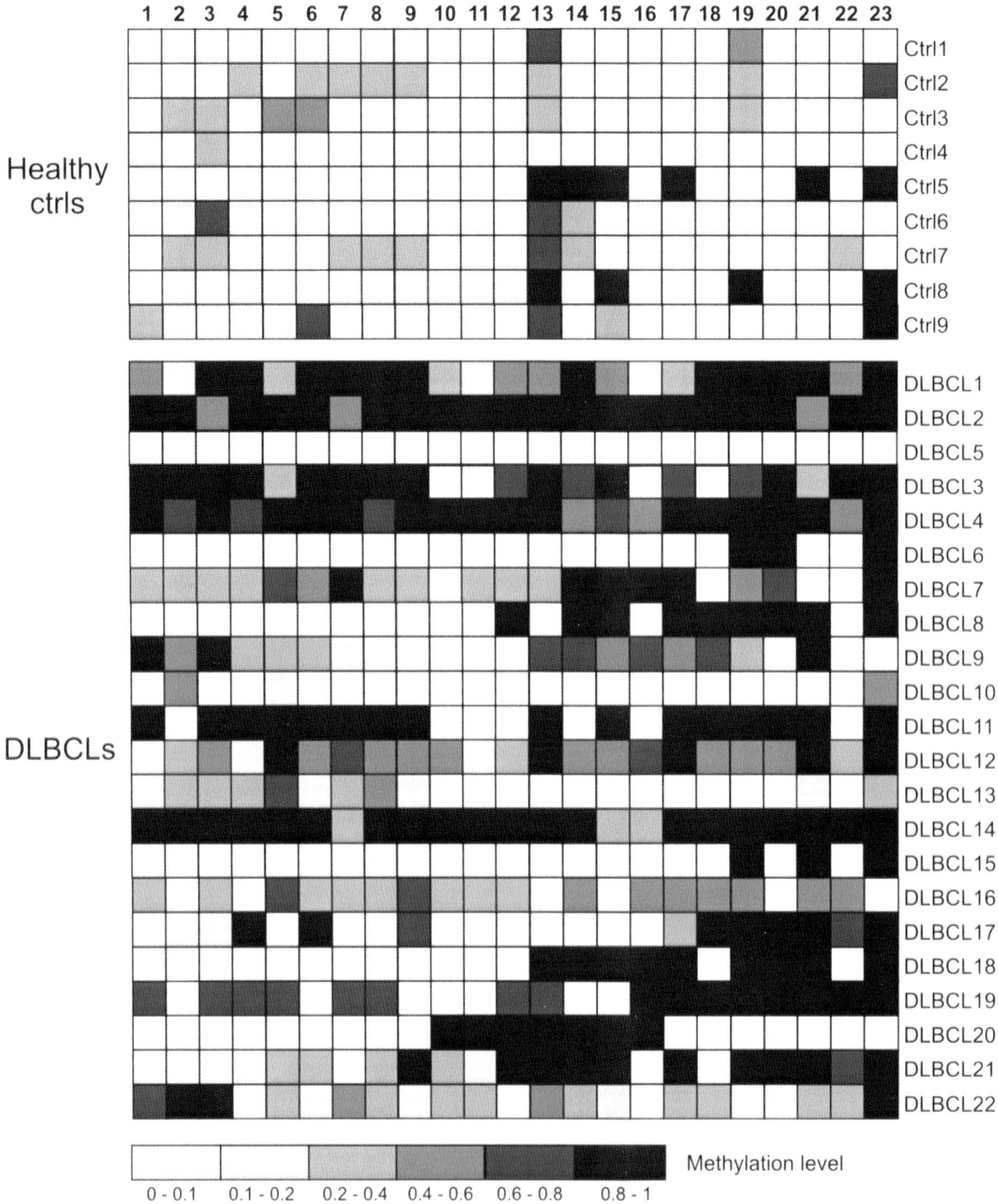

Figure 2. Bisulfite sequencing of the TFPI-2 CpG island. Each box indicates a CpG dinucleotide and each line of boxes represents analysis of a single dog. Color gradation indicated the methylation level of each CpG site (0–1); 0, totally unmethylated; 1 totally methylated.

was chosen as reference in qRT-PCR assays since it was already tested in canine lymphomas by Aricò et al. [14] and did not show differences in its expression profile between healthy and pathologic samples.

To evaluate the efficiency of each assay (TFPI-2 and TMBIM4), standard curves were constructed amplifying two-fold serial dilutions (from 1:20 up to 1:640) of the same cDNA, which was used as calibrator. For both transcripts, efficiency of primer pairs was within the range 95 - 105%. For each sample, the Cp (Crossing point) was used to determine the relative amount of target gene.

Data Analysis

The sets of reads from each sample, together with a "reference" genomic (not bisulfite converted) sequence, were analyzed by BiQ Analyzer HT software [15]. The methylation status of each read

Table 4. Kolmogorov-Smirnov test on 23 individuals TFPI-2 promoter CpG sites.

Site	p-value DLBCL n22	p-value DLBCL n17[(a)]
CpG1	0.082	0.014*
CpG2	0.517	0.410
CpG3	0.438	0.137
CpG4	0.143	0.034*
CpG5	0.016*	0.005**
CpG6	0.537	0.224
CpG7	0.17	0.058
CpG8	0.18	0.068
CpG9	0.143	0.034*
CpG10	0.138	0.031*
CpG11	0.622	0.239
CpG12	0.045*	0.006**
CpG13	0.537	0.410
CpG14	0.106	0.013*
CpG15	0.35	0.063
CpG16	0.143	0.031*
CpG17	0.016*	0.001**
CpG18	0.011*	0.002**
CpG19	0.042*	0.012*
CpG20	0.011*	0.002**
CpG21	0.007**	0.002**
CpG22	0.235	0.068
CpG23	0.031*	0.013*

[(a)]DLBCL5, DLBCL6, DLBCL10, DLBCL13 and DLBCL15 excluded from the analysis.
*$p<0.05$, **$p<0.01$.

sequence was then determined based on a C to T conversion at each CpG. For each analyzed sample-reference combination, the software provides information about the methylation pattern *per* read and the mean methylation level calculated for the amplicon. In addition, a Pearl-Necklace diagram summarizes methylation information for the whole set of filtered reads, by CpG loci. For each site, distribution of the "methylated", "unmethylated" and "unrecognized" states in the given set of bisulfite reads is also provided by the software.

The percentage of methylation (methylation level) at each CpG site within each amplicon was calculated based on the number of sequences containing methylated CpG sites versus the total number of sequences analyzed, assigned values range between 0 (0%, site unmethylated) and 1 (100%, site totally methylated).

Statistical analyses were performed using a commercially available statistical software program (SPSS v20.0). Data were analysed using non-parametric statistical methods because of the limited number of cases. Sample mean methylation levels, as well as methylation percentage of individual CpG sites, were evaluated for significant differences between healthy dogs and dogs with DLBCL using the Kolmogorov-Smirnov test.

Mann-Whitney test was performed on qPCR data to test for significant difference in TFPI-2 expression levels between controls and DLBCLs. Spearman's rank test was used to estimate the correlation between mean methylation levels and TFPI-2 gene expression values measured for the same individuals. A p-value $<$ 0.05 was selected as the level of significance.

Results

Twenty-two dogs with DLBCL were enrolled (Table 1). These were 15 females and 7 males, and the median age was 7,5 years (range, 3 to 14 years). Regarding breed, there were 11 mixed-breed, 2 German shepherds, 2 Labrador retrievers, and one each of Scottish terrier, Tibetan terrier, Pyrenean Sheepdog, Epagneul Breton, Yorkshire terrier, Cocker spaniel and English setter.

Nine healthy dogs were enrolled (Table 1): 5 mixed-breeds, 1 Siberian husky, 1 American Pit Bull terrier, 1 German shepherd, and 1 Cane Corso. Median age was 6 years (range, 2 to 10 years). There were 5 females and 4 males.

TFPI-2 Amplicon Sequencing

A region encompassing 870 nucleotides (−284 to +586) and containing 87 CG dinucleotides was identified as CpG island by means of CpG Plot software (Figure 1). A fragment of 212 nt, encompassing 23 CpG sites, was then chosen for ultradeep bisulfite sequencing analysis (see Methods).

A total of 14,755 sequences was obtained in a single 454 sequencing run with average read length of 229.97 bp. After quality filtering a total of 14,508 sequences (98.3%) was used for computing the mean methylation level for each sample. On average, 418 sequence reads (range of reads 236 869, including both forward and reverse strands) were obtained for each dog (see Table 3).

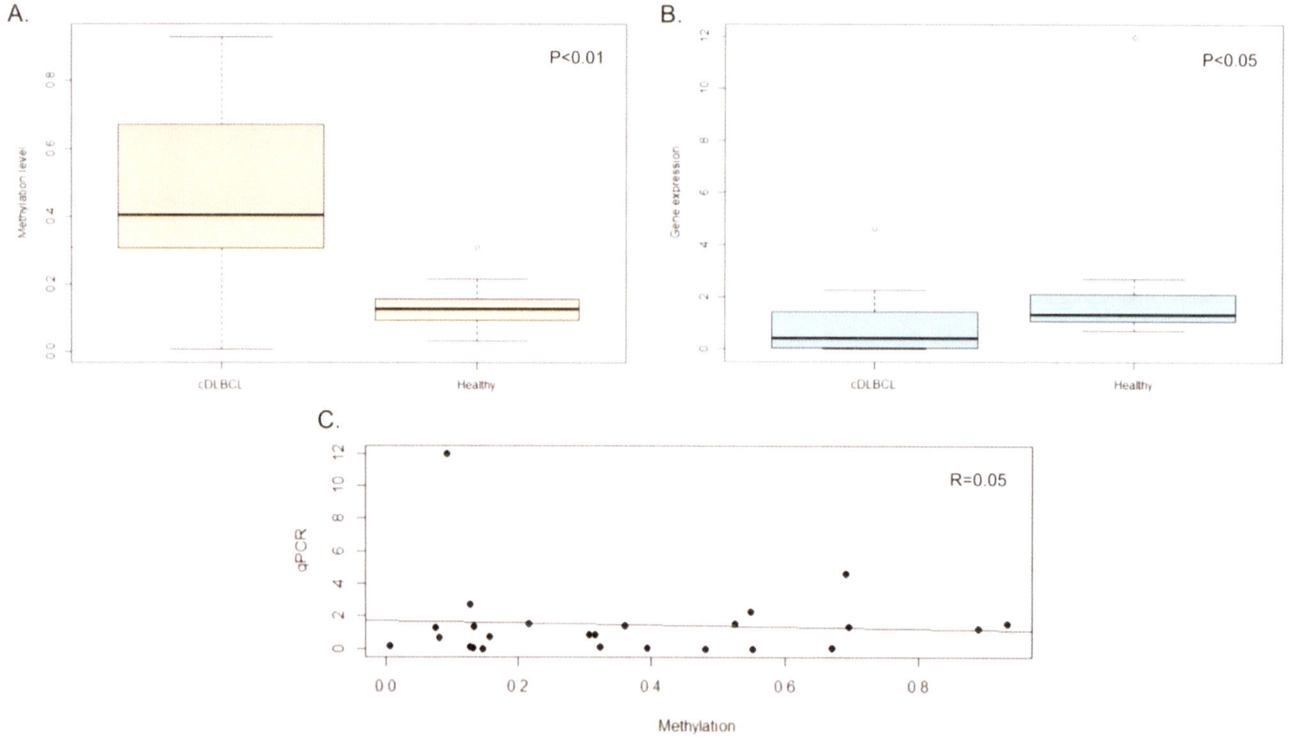

Figure 3. Relationship between TFPI-2 methylation and gene expression levels. A. Boxplot of TFPI-2 methylation levels measured in DLBCL and Healthy control group. **B.** Boxplot of TFPI-2 gene expression levels measured in the same samples and **C.** Correlation between TFPI-2 methylation and its gene expression values.

Quantitative DNA Methylation Analysis

For each sample, the mean methylation level (see Table 3) and the percentage of methylation for each CpG locus (reported in File S1) were calculated by means of BiQ Analyzer HT. Seventeen out of 22 DLBCLs (77.3%) exhibited a mean methylation ≥0.3, with 9 samples (40.9%) with level of methylation greater than 0.5. Control lymph nodes showed a mean methylation ≤0.3. Only one sample had a mean methylation of 0.31. Kolmogorov-Smirnov test was performed in order to compare methylation levels between controls and DLBCLs. A significant 3.2-fold increase of mean methylation levels in DLBCL dogs was observed compared to control lymph nodes ($p<0.01$). Five DLBCLs (i.e. DLBCL5, DLBCL6, DLBCL10, DLBCL13 and DLBCL15) did not show hypermethylation in TFPI-2 promoter, with mean methylation levels significantly reduced ($p<0.01$) compared to all other DLBCL samples.

DNA Methylation Patterns on Individual CpG Sites

When considering each CpG site individually (Figure 2), only one locus out of 23 showed a mean methylation percentage higher than 50% in healthy controls compared with 7 loci (30.4%) found in DLBCL samples (see File S1). The difference between the two groups was more evident if the threshold of the mean methylation percentage was lowered to 40% (0.4) with two loci (8.6%) and 15 loci (65.2%) for controls and DLBCL dogs, respectively. Statistical analysis for each CpG site identified eight loci with significant difference ($p<0.05$) in methylation level between DLBCL and control group (see Table 4). Excluding DLBCL5, DLBCL6, DLBCL10, DLBCL13 and DLBCL15 from the analysis, the number of loci found differentially methylated between the two groups increased up to 14 out of 23 (see Table 3).

Relationship between TFPI-2 Methylation Status and Gene Expression Levels

For a subset of samples including 7 controls and 18 DLBCLs (see Table 3), the association between TFPI-2 methylation levels and gene expression values was assessed by means of real-time RT-PCR (Figure 3). Gene expression analysis identified a significant down-regulation of TFPI-2 in DLBCL ($p<0.05$), with normal lymph nodes having 3-fold increased expression levels. Pearson correlation analysis between TFPI-2 methylation levels and gene expression, however, revealed a rho coefficient = 0.05 indicating that there is no linear correlation between the two variables (Figure 3).

Expression values obtained with qPCR were also correlated with those previously obtained using Canine genome 2.0 array (Affymetrix) [12] for the same specimens (n 19). Comparative analysis of microarray and qPCR expression data are reported in File S2. Statistical analysis identified a positive and highly significant correlation between qPCR and two microarray probes (Spearman's $0.68 \leq$ rho ≤ 0.78, $p<0.01$), thus validating microarray results.

The two oligonucleotide probes, Cfa.13994.1.S1_at and CfaAffx.3983.1.S1_at, showed a significant down-regulation of TFPI-2 in DLBCLs compared to control lymph nodes ($p<0.05$). However, as for qPCR, no linear correlation was documented between mean methylation levels and gene expression values.

Relationship between TFPI-2 Methylation Status and Clinical Data

The Spearman's correlations between TFPI-2 methylation levels, age, clinical signs, stage and substage were also assessed for all samples. Statistical analysis identified a significant positive correlation (Spearman's rho 0.745, $p<0.01$) between methylation levels and age of DLBCL dogs. The number of dogs older than 8 years in healthy control group was too low for properly assessing the correlation age/methylation in this group.

No correlation was observed between TFPI-2 methylation levels and staging of the disease (data not shown). The same analysis was conducted considering TFPI-2 mRNA levels and no correlation was found between TFPI-2 expression and age or staging.

Discussion

DLBCL is the most common subtype of canine lymphoma [14,16] and it shares many features with the human counterpart, including clinical presentation, biological behavior, tumor genetics and treatment response [1]. A genome-wide hypomethylation associated with a simultaneous promoter-associated CpG island hypermethylation is now considered a hallmark of cancer [17]. Recently, genome-scale studies reported that aberrant DNA methylation occurs at specific genomic locations [18,19]. It is widely reported that TSGs are frequently hypermethylated in neoplastic cells. This epigenetic modification contributes to the suppression of their expression ([20] and references therein) and makes cancer cells acquire growth advantages. However, the role of the single gene aberrant DNA methylation in controlling gene expression and tumor progression is still under debate.

TFPI-2 has been recently proposed as TSG since it plays a significant role in the maintenance of the stability of the tumor microenvironment and in the prevention of cancer progression by inhibiting tumor-related angiogenesis and members of ECM.

In particular, TFPI-2 has been reported to inhibit MMP-1, MMP-2, MMP3 and MMP-9 [21–23], proteolytic ECM enzymes whose increased expression has been demonstrated to be strongly associated with prognosis in canine lymphoma [14,24].

The transcriptional silencing of TFPI-2 by hypermethylation in the promoter region has been recently demonstrated in many human cancers, including nasopharyngeal, colorectal and gastric carcinoma [9–11,25]. No studies report TFPI-2 methylation in human lymphoma, although this phenomenon is described in pediatric acute myeloid leukemia [13].

In the present study, bisulfite conversion and 454 amplicon sequencing (Bis-seq) provided an accurate quantification of TFPI-2 methylation levels with a single base resolution, allowing the identification of CpG sites aberrantly methylated in canine DLBCLs. Sequence analysis clearly demonstrated that TFPI2 is frequently hypermethylated in canine DLBCL. Globally, dogs with DLBCL showed a mean methylation level over three-fold higher than controls and hypermethylation of the TFPI-2 promoter was found in 77% of DLBCLs (17 out of 22) against only one normal lymph node (~11%). The analysis of hypermethylation by site identified 19 loci out of 23 (82%) with mean methylation levels from 2- to 120-fold increased in DLBCL (File S1) and 8 CpG loci were significantly ($p<0.05$) hypermethylated in DLBCL dogs compared to controls.

One of the proposed regulatory mechanisms ascribed to DNA methylation is to prevent the binding of transcription factors [26]. In dogs, TFPI-2 gene is located in chromosome 14 and, similarly to humans, *in silico* analysis of its promoter region identified the binding sites for several transcription factors, including SP1, activating enhancer-binding protein-1 (AP-1), nuclear factor kappa B (NF-kB), lymphoid transcription factor-1 (Lyf-1) and Myeloid zinc finger 1 (MZF-1).

Here, bisulfite sequencing results provided a partial representation of the potential control apparatus of TFPI-2. However, the region analyzed in the present study included both AP-1 and NF-kB putative binding sites. No CpG dinucleotides were located in close proximity to the AP-1 consensus sequence, while the region with the highest density of hypermethylated CpG sites (Sites 17–21, see Table 4) encompassed the NF-kB binding motif. It is well known that the transcription factor NF-κB controls a wide range of genes that are involved in multiple cellular processes, from apoptosis to proliferation and inflammation. In particular, Rel/NF-kB families of transcription factors are key regulators of B-cell development, proliferation and survival [27]. Human and canine DLBCLs are characterized by constitutive canonical NF-kB activity [28,29] that promotes lymphomagenesis and chemotherapy resistance via overexpression of anti-apoptotic NF-kB target genes (i.e. Cyclin D1 and D2, Bcl-2). Very recently Mudaliar and co-workers [29], through the analysis of differentially expressed probe sets in canine and human DLBCL, found molecular signatures shared between dog and human. In particular, they reported the enrichment of the NF-kB signalling pathway in both species, with potential therapeutic implications, and further underscoring the dog as a translation model for human DLBCL.

In humans, mutations at either AP-1 or SP1 sites resulted in reduced TFPI-2 activity while NF-kB has not been demonstrated to directly control TFPI-2 transcription [30]. Whether TFPI-2 in dogs is controlled by the same mechanisms as in humans has not been assessed yet. However, the location of NF-kB binding motif in canine TFPI-2 promoter (i.e. immediately upstream of the ATG site) is different from humans, and it is unknown whether NF-kB exerts a role in regulating the transcription of this gene in dogs. In this context, it cannot be excluded that the hypermethylation of the NF-kB binding motif may exert a role in preventing the binding of this transcription factor.

The second aim of the present study was to assess the relationship between TFPI-2 methylation status and its gene expression levels measured by means of qRT-PCR. TFPI-2 showed a significant down-regulation in DLBCL compared with normal lymph nodes, suggesting that TFPI-2 hypermethylation negatively regulates its transcription.

In comparison with previous "semi-quantitative" approaches that mainly relied on the sequencing of 5–10 clones for measuring gene methylation levels, NGS allowed for a proper quantification of each CpG status. We decided then to verify whether a linear correlation between methylation levels and gene expression values could be determined.

No linear correlation was found between mean methylation levels and gene expression values. This was not unexpected, since a certain level of discordance between methylation and gene expression has been reported in both humans and dogs [31,32]. In these cases, gene promoters showed mixed methylation patterns with regions completely methylated and regions unmethylated, the latter being responsible for the continued gene expression.

In the present study, the extremely high GC content of TFPI-2 promoter, and the approach chosen for amplicon sequencing (i.e. sequencing only one amplicon in favor of a greater number of sequences), limited bisulfite evaluation to one forth (212/870 nt) of the entire CpG island thus giving only partial information on the methylation levels of the promoter. Although a good indication of the relationship between TFPI-2 methylation and gene transcription has been achieved, the analysis of the entire promoter region is needed in order to properly investigate the correlation between methylation level and gene expression, as well as to identify potential critical, hypomethylated, regions that allow transcription in spite of global promoter hypermethylation or *vice versa*.

In this context, of particular interest are five DLBCL cases (DLBCL5, DLBCL6, DLBCL10, DLBCL13 and DLBCL15) that showed TFPI-2 transcription silencing even if the promoter regions appeared to be unmethylated (Table 3). In addition to the binding of transcription factors, other mechanisms, known to regulate gene transcription at different levels (i.e. recruitment of other members of the "transcription machinery", interplay of enhancer molecules or small non-coding RNAs) may participate in controlling TFPI-2 mRNA levels thus leading to its silencing in DLBCL samples in spite of lower methylation levels.

Multiple changes such as decreased telomere length and altered gene expression have been linked to cellular aging. Recently, genomic hypomethylation and accumulation of CpG island hypermethylation has been associated with increasing age in humans [33]. Several genome-wide studies have revealed strong links between age-associated epigenetic changes and disease ([17] for a review). In particular, the hematopoietic stem cell decline in aging individuals was described as being determined by age-dependent changes in DNA methylation. To our knowledge, a similar phenomenon of accumulated promoter hypermethylation has not been demonstrated in dogs. In the present study, a significant positive correlation (rho 0.74, $p<0.01$) was appreciated between TFPI-2 methylation levels and age of DLBCL dogs.

This finding is in accordance with the study by Hannum and colleagues [33] where, by using a newly developed aging model based on whole genome DNA methylation, tumor tissue appears to be 40% older than the matched normal tissue from the same individual.

Although a higher number of samples both from normal dogs and dogs with DLBCL are needed, this study provides the first indication of age-associated epigenetic modifications in dogs.

To conclude, our results demonstrated that TFPI-2 promoter hypermethylation occurs frequently in DLBCL. TFPI-2 is also expressed at lower levels in neoplastic lymphoid cells compared to normal lymphoid cells, thus demonstrating an association between methylation and silencing of TFPI-2 expression.

Identifying aberrant methylated genes may provide a better understanding of the pathogenesis of canine DLBCL. The present analysis is far from showing a prognostic utility of TFPI-2 in cases of DLBCL. Further analysis will consider a set of canine lymphoma cell lines to test the efficacy of hypomethylating agents and a larger number of cases to assess whether TFPI-2 promoter hypermethylation may be considered in association with prognosis and therapy. In this context, novel gene therapy tools, including recombinant adenoviral-mediated TFPI-2 delivery, are currently being developed to regulate tumor growth providing potential novel therapeutic approaches for the treatment of DLBCL in dogs [34].

Author Contributions

Conceived and designed the experiments: LA GTK SF LB LM. Performed the experiments: SF SB AA. Analyzed the data: SF LA SB. Contributed reagents/materials/analysis tools: LM GTK LB SC FR MEG. Wrote the paper: SF LA. Edited the paper: SB SF LA GTK.

References

1. Marconato L, Frayssinet P, Rouquet N, Comazzi S, Leone VF, et al (2014) Randomized, Placebo-Controlled, Double-Blinded Chemoimmunotherapy Clinical Trial in a Pet Dog Model of Diffuse Large B-cell Lymphoma. Clin Cancer Res 20(3): 668–677.
2. Rosenwald A, Staudt LM (2003) Gene expression profiling of diffuse large B-cell lymphoma. Leuk Lymphoma 44 Suppl 3: S41–47.
3. Clozel T, Yang S, Elstrom RL, Tam W, Martin P, et al (2013) Mechanism-based epigenetic chemosensitization therapy of diffuse large B-cell lymphoma. Cancer Discov 3(9): 1002–1019.
4. Galm O, Herman JG, Baylin SB (2006) The fundamental role of epigenetics in hematopoietic malignancies. Blood Rev 20(1): 1–13.
5. Jones PA, Baylin SB (2002) The fundamental role of epigenetic events in cancer. Nat Rev Genet 3(6): 415–428.
6. Wong CM, Ng YL, Lee JM, Wong CC, Cheung OF, et al (2007) Tissue factor pathway inhibitor-2 as a frequently silenced tumor suppressor gene in hepatocellular carcinoma. Hepatology 45(5): 1129–1138.
7. Hubé F, Reverdiau P, Iochmann S, Rollin J, Cherpi-Antar C, Gruel Y (2003) Transcriptional silencing of the TFPI-2 gene by promoter hypermethylation in choriocarcinoma cells. Biol Chem 384(7): 1029–1034.
8. Guo H, Lin Y, Zhang H, Liu J, Zhang N, et al (2007) Tissue factor pathway inhibitor-2 was repressed by CpG hypermethylation through inhibition of KLF6 binding in highly invasive breast cancer cells. BMC Mol Biol 8: 110.
9. Wang S, Xiao X, Zhou X, Huang T, Du C, et al (2010) TFPI-2 is a putative tumor suppressor gene frequently inactivated by promoter hypermethylation in nasopharyngeal carcinoma. BMC Cancer 10: 617.
10. Hibi K, Goto T, Kitamura YH, Sakuraba K, Shirahata A, et al (2010) Methylation of the TFPI2 gene is frequently detected in advanced gastric carcinoma. Anticancer Res 30(10): 4131–4133.
11. Takada H, Wakabayashi N, Dohi O, Yasui K, Sakakura C, et al (2010) Tissue factor pathway inhibitor 2 (TFPI2) is frequently silenced by aberrant promoter hypermethylation in gastric cancer. Cancer Genet Cytogenet 197(1): 16–24.
12. Bresolin S, Mahmoodi P, Gelain ME, Riondato F, Mortarino M, et al (2013) Distinct gene expression profiles in a canine model of human DLBCL. Haematologica 98(s1): 353.
13. Jian P, Yan WS, Chao SL, Liang P, Zhen L, et al (2012) Promoter of TFPI-2 is hypermethylated in Chinese pediatric acute myeloid leukemia. J Pediatr Hematol Oncol 34(1): 43–46.
14. Aricò A, Giantin M, Gelain ME, Riondato F, Comazzi S, et al (2013) The role of vascular endothelial growth factor and matrix metalloproteinases in canine lymphoma: in vivo and in vitro study. BMC Vet Res 9: 94.
15. Lutsik P, Feuerbach L, Arand J, Lengauer T, Walter J, Bock C (2011) BiQ Analyzer HT:locus-specific analysis of DNA methylation by high-throughput bisulfite sequencing. Nucleic Acids Res 39(Web Server issue): W551–556.
16. Ponce F, Marchal T, Magnol JP, Turinelli V, Ledieu D, et al (2010) A morphological study of 608 cases of canine malignant lymphoma in France with a focus on comparative similarities between canine and human lymphoma morphology. Vet Pathol 47(3): 414–33.
17. Schoofs T, Berdel WE, Müller-Tidow C (2013) Origins of aberrant DNA methylation in acute myeloid leukemia. Leukemia In press.
18. Hansen KD, Timp W, Bravo HC, Sabunciyan S, Langmead B, et al (2011) Increased methylation variation in epigenetic domains across cancer types. Nat Genet 43: 768–775.
19. Irizarry RA, Ladd-Acosta C, Wen B, Wu Z, Montano C, et al (2009) The human colon cancer methylome shows similar hypo- and hypermethylation at conserved tissue-specific CpG island shores. Nat Genet 41: 178–186.
20. Herman JG, Baylin SB (2003) Gene silencing in cancer in association with promoter hypermethylation. N Engl J Med 349(21): 2042–2054.
21. Herman MP, Sukhova GK, Kisiel W, Foster D, Kehry MR, et al (2001) Tissue factor pathway inhibitor-2 is a novel inhibitor of matrix metalloproteinases with implications for atherosclerosis. J Clin Invest 107: 1117–1126.
22. Gaud G, Iochmann S, Guillon-Munos A, Brillet B, Petiot S, et al (2011) TFPI-2 silencing increases tumour progression and promotes metalloproteinase 1 and 3 induction through tumour-stromal cell interactions. J Cell Mol Med 15(2): 196–208.
23. Lavergne M, Jourdan ML, Blechet C, Guyetant S, Pape AL, et al (2013) Beneficial role of overexpression of TFPI-2 on tumour progression in human small cell lung cancer. FEBS Open Bio 3: 291–301.
24. Aresu L, Aricò A, Comazzi S, Gelain ME, Riondato F, et al (2012) VEGF and MMP-9: biomarkers for canine lymphoma. Vet Comp Oncol. DOI: 10.1111/j.1476-5829.2012.00328.x.
25. Glöckner SC, Dhir M, Yi JM, McGarvey KE, Van Neste L, et al (2009) Methylation of TFPI2 in stool DNA: a potential novel biomarker for the detection of colorectal cancer. Cancer Res 69(11): 4691–4699.
26. Daniel FI, Cherubini K, Yurgel LS, de Figueiredo MA, Salum FG (2011) The role of epigenetic transcription repression and DNA methyltransferases in cancer. Cancer 117(4): 677–687.
27. Keller U, Nilsson JA, Maclean KH, Old JB, Cleveland JL (2005) Nfkb 1 is dispensable for Myc-induced lymphomagenesis. Oncogene 24(41): 6231–6240.
28. Gaurnier-Hausser A, Patel R, Baldwin AS, May MJ, Mason NJ (2011) NEMO-binding domain peptide inhibits constitutive NF-κB activity and reduces tumor

burden in a canine model of relapsed, refractory diffuse large B-cell lymphoma. Clin Cancer Res 17(14): 4661 4671.

29. Mudaliar MA, Haggart RD, Miele G, Sellar G, Tan KA, et al (2013) Comparative Gene Expression Profiling Identifies Common Molecular Signatures of NF-κB Activation in Canine and Human Diffuse Large B Cell Lymphoma (DLBCL). PLoS One 8(9): e72591.
30. Konduri SD, Yanamandra N, Dinh DH, Olivero WC, Gujrati M, et al (2003) Physiological and chemical inducers of tissue factor pathway inhibitor-2 in human glioma cells. Int J Oncol 22(6): 1277 83.
31. Zinn RL, Pruitt K, Eguchi S, Baylin SB, Herman JG (2007) hTERT is expressed in cancer cell lines despite promoter DNA methylation by preservation of unmethylated DNA and active chromatin around the transcription start site. Cancer Res 67: 194 201.
32. Bryan JN, Jabbes M, Berent LM, Arthur GL, Taylor KH, et al (2009) Hypermethylation of the DLC1 CpG island does not alter gene expression in canine lymphoma. BMC Genet 10: 73.
33. Hannum G, Guinney J, Zhao L, Zhang L, Hughes G, et al (2013) Genome-wide methylation profiles reveal quantitative views of human aging rates. Mol Cell 49(2): 359 367.
34. Sun Y, Xie M, Liu M, Jin D, Li P (2006) Growth suppression of human laryngeal squamous cell carcinoma by adenovirus-mediated tissue factor pathway inhibitor gene 2. Laryngoscope 116(4): 596 601.

5

Expression of Neuron-Specific Enolase in Multiple Myeloma and Implications for Clinical Diagnosis and Treatment

Haiping Yang[1,2], Ruihua Mi[1], Qian Wang[1], Xudong Wei[1]*, Qingsong Yin[1], Lin Chen[1], Xinghu Zhu[1], Yongping Song[1]

1 Department of Hematology, Tumor Hospital of Zhengzhou University, Zhengzhou City, China, **2** Department of Hematology, First Affiliated Hospital of Henan University of Science and Technology, Zhengzhou City, China

Abstract

Objective: To determine the expression of neuron-specific enolase (NSE) in patients with multiple myeloma (MM) and to evaluate its clinical value as a tumor marker and, an indicator of disease progression and treatment efficacy.

Methods: Using electrochemiluminescence immunoassay (ECLIA), we measured the serum levels of NSE in 47 healthy subjects (control group), 25 patients with small cell lung cancer (lung cancer group), and 52 patients with MM (MM group). For the MM group, serum NSE levels were measured and other disease indicators and related symptoms were monitored before and after chemotherapy. The relationship between NSE expression and other MM-related factors was analyzed. In addition, immunohistochemical staining was performed on bone marrow biopsy specimens from patients with MM.

Results: In the control group, serum NSE levels were within the normal range as previously reported, while the lung cancer group and the untreated MM group exhibited NSE levels that were significantly higher relative to the control group ($P<0.05$). The difference in NSE expression between the lung cancer group and untreated MM group was statistically significant ($P<0.05$). NSE levels were significantly decreased in MM patients after chemotherapy and were positively correlated with an MM disease index [beta-2 microglobulin (β_2-MG)]. Changes in NSE were not related to the response rate to chemotherapy but rather were correlated with progression-free survival.

Conclusions: Patients with MM may have increased serum NSE levels, and changes in NSE may provide insight into treatment efficacy of chemotherapy and disease progression. Perhaps NSE expression is a viable biomarker for MM and can be a useful reference for the design and adjustment of clinical MM treatment programs.

Editor: Maria Fiammetta Romano, Federico II University, Naples, Italy

Funding: This study was supported by the National Natural Science Foundation of China (NO. 81170520) and the Henan Department of Health Provincial-Departmental collaboration project (NO. 2011010014). The funders had no role in study design, data collection and analysis, decision to publish, or preparation of the manuscript.

Competing Interests: The authors have declared that no competing interests exist.

* E-mail: xudongwei@zzu.edu.cn

These authors contributed equally to this work.

Introduction

Multiple myeloma (MM) is a malignant plasma cell disease typified by clonal plasma cells in the bone marrow (plasma cell neoplasms) and is associated with end-organ damage, including bone damage, and the presence of monoclonal protein (M protein) in the serum or urine [1–4]. Treatment efficacy and recurrence can be monitored by measuring the proportion of plasma cells in bone marrow by puncture or biopsy, M protein levels in serum and urine, immune electrophoresis, and the range, number and progression of osteolytic lesions [5]. Also, the levels of blood beta-2 microglobulin (β_2-MG), albumin, and urine light chain are used to determine therapeutic efficacy and disease progression [6]. The natural disease course of MM ranges widely from a few months to more than 20 years, and the response to treatment is variable. Recently, functional imaging tools, such as F-18 fluorodeoxyglucose (FDG) positron emission tomography (PET), have been considered for the assessment of responses [7]. However, application of this technique is quite limited due to the high cost. Therefore, the key to treatment success is to offer patients with an accurate prognosis and to adopt the appropriate treatment strategy after diagnosis.

It is becoming increasingly apparent that the identification of tumor markers is valuable in the diagnosis and treatment of various diseases [1]. Indeed, some markers have become important inference indices for cancer patients. For instance, in lung cancer, tumor markers can aid in the diagnosis of pathological type, stage, metastasis, recurrence, and prognosis. Neuron-specific enolase (NSE) is one of these markers and its application in clinical practice has been gradually increasing in recent years with significant diagnostic value [2–4].

Enolase is an enzyme that catalyzes the decomposition of glycerol in the glycolytic pathway and consists of three subunits (α, β, γ) and five isozymes (αα, ββ γγ, αγ, βγ) [3]. The isozymes containing a γ subunit are found in neuronal and endocrine tissue, and thus are known as the neuron-specific enolases (NSE). NSE has been implicated in tumorigenesis with neuroendocrine origin. Japanese scholars Jimbo *et al.* [1] and Nakajima *et al.* [2] and British scholars Sharma *et al.* [3] each reported a case where a patient with MM exhibited increased levels of NSE. In China, there are very few reports evaluating NSE levels in MM patients. Zhang *et al.* [4] reported that patients with MM who had increased NSE levels had a poorer prognosis than those patients with normal NSE levels. Patients with elevated NSE levels exhibited shorter overall survival and decreased progression-free survival. Moreover, although there was no correlation between NSE expression level and age, gender, M protein type, hemoglobin, or serum creatinine, there was a significant correlation between NSE expression and the abundance of myeloma plasma cells and blood β_2-MG expression level [4]. COX analysis suggested that the levels of NSE and β_2-MG are two independent prognostic factors that affect the survival of MM. Gao *et al.* [8] reported that NSE expression was increased in the U266 myeloma cell line and in 67% of MM patients. In addition, NSE expression trended upward as disease severity progressed and the degree of bone destruction increased. In this study, we examined the level of NSE in 52 MM patients before and after chemotherapy. In addition, we monitored the disease condition and efficacy of therapeutic intervention. Taken together, we sought to determine the relationship between NSE and MM, and to evaluate the viability of NSE as a biomarker for the diagnosis, treatment evaluation, and prognosis of MM.

Patients and Methods

1 Subjects

1.1 Control group. Forty-seven healthy were included in the control group and underwent physical examination. The group consisted of 29 males and 18 females with a median age of 37 (28–59) years old. ECLIA was used to detect tumor biomarkers in the following systems: respiratory, digestive, genitourinary, endocrine systems, etc. The physical examination included imaging, blood test, biochemistry analysis, infectious disease, immunization, electrocardiogram, and other tests. Those individuals without abnormalities in these tests were enrolled in the healthy control group.

1.2 Small cell lung cancer group. Twenty-five patients with small cell lung cancer were included in this group. These patients were hospitalized in the Department of Medical Oncology of our hospital between March 2009 and August 2010. They had clear pathological diagnosis and were composed of 21 males and four females with a median age of 53 (36–80) years old.

1.3 MM group. All 52 patients in this group were hospitalized with MM in either our hospital or the First Affiliated Hospital of Henan University of Science and Technology between May 2010 and April 2013, including 26 males and 26 females with a median age of 53 (47–62) years old. Hospitalization examinations were performed to confirm the diagnosis of MM, according to the diagnostic criteria defined in references [5,6]. These included bone marrow biopsy, ECT whole body bone scan (or CT, PET-CT, or other imaging methods), blood count, blood chemistry, blood tumor marker testing, serum protein electrophoresis, and immunofixation electrophoresis.

1.4 MM treatment programs. All MM patients were treated with either TD (thalidomide and dexamethasone) or VD (Velcade plus dexamethasone)-based programs for three courses of chemotherapy, combined with or without mitoxantrone, THP topiramate Star, cyclophosphamide, and etoposide. In patients with elevated NSE levels, 28 adopted the TD-based program (NSE+/T) and six adopted the VD-based program (NSE+/V). In patients with normal NSE levels, 14 adopted the TD program (NSE-/T) and four adopted the VD program (NSE-/V). The difference in choosing either program between the NSE+ and NSE- patient groups was not statistically significant ($P = 0.723$).

2 Research Methods

Ethics statement. Informed consent was obtained from all the patients in writing prior to enrollment in the study. This study was performed in strict accordance with the ethical guidelines of the Declaration of Helsinki, and the protocol was approved by the institutional Ethics Committee of Henan Cancer Hospital.

2.1 Equipment. Roche Elecsys 2010 (Basel, Switzerland) was used for electrochemiluminescence detection. KDC-2046 low-speed refrigerated centrifuge (Henan, China) was purchased from Anhui Zhongjia Co., Ltd.

2.2 Reagents. Reagents specific for ECLIA detection on Roche Elecsys 2010 included NSE detection kit, cleaning fluid (ISE Cleaning Solution), system reagent (Procell), standard solution, and quality control reagent (PreciControl Tumor Marer).

2.3 NSE detection method. For ECLIA detection of NSE, four ml of fasting blood was taken from patients in the morning prior to eating and drinking. After coagulation, blood serum was separated at 3000 rpm, and NSE concentration was measured within two hours after separation in strict accordance with the user manual guidelines of the Roche Elecsys 2010 and the NSE electrochemical luminescence detection kit. NSE levels were read automatically on Elecsys 2010. As for detection value criteria, the normal detection range was set from zero to 15 ng/ml, and any values beyond the normal range were considered positive.

In addition, NSE levels were examined by immunohistochemistry in bone marrow biopsy specimens from patients with previously untreated MM. All tissues were fixed in 10% neutral formalin and paraffin-embedded after routine dehydration. Five to six serial sections were prepared with a thickness of four μm. Sections were dewaxed and treated with fresh 3% H_2O_2 to block endogenous peroxidase. After rinsing three times with PBS for three min, citric acid antigen retrieval was performed under high pressure. The slices were blocked with normal goat serum for 30 min at room temperature to eliminate nonspecific staining, followed by incubation with primary antibody solution (Abcam, Cambridge, UK) at 4°C overnight. After recovery for 40 min at room temperature, ready-to-use secondary antibody solution (rabbit anti-mouse secondary antibody, Zhongshan Golden Bridge, Beijing, China) was added dropwise to the slices and incubated at room temperature for 40 min followed by three PBS washes for 3 min. DAB reagent was added dropwise to the slices afterwards and developed at room temperature. Slices were observed under a microscope for three to five min to determine the optimal developing time, after which slices were rinsed with tap water, stained with hematoxylin for 90 seconds, differentiated with the hydrochloric acid solution, and treated with saturated aqueous lithium carbonate for blue nuclear staining. Slices were mounted with neutral gum after routine dehydration and observed under a microscope. A positive result was determined by evaluating both staining intensity and positive rates. If the positive rate was less than 10% with weak staining, it was labeled as negative; if the positive rate was greater or equal to 10% with strong brownish-yellow granules, it was labeled as positive.

Table 1. Correlation analysis of serum NSE levels and IHC results.

Patient No.	1	2	3	4	5	6	7	8	9	10	11	12	13
NSE (ng/ml)	14.34	11.89	14.34	23.43	25.64	33.43	80.34	32.54	13.46	38.54	25.43	50.32	28.65
IHC result	-	-	-	+	+	+	+	+	+	+	+	+	+
Patient No.	14	15	16	17	18	19	20	21	22	23	24	25	26
NSE (ng/ml)	22.43	12.43	14.75	24.86	24.3	38.3	9.643	14.2	12.64	40.4	26.79	49.17	29.6
IHC result	-	-	+	+	+	+	-	+	-	+	-	+	+
Patient No.	27	28	29	30	31	32	33	34	35	36	37	38	39
NSE (ng/ml)	23.77	21.48	13.64	28.96	12.54	11.65	13.87	13.26	16.88	7.23	22.76	20.21	27.82
IHC result	+	+	-	+	-	-	+	-	-	-	+	+	+
Patient No.	40	41	42	43	44	45	46	47	48	49	50	51	52
NSE (ng/ml)	25.12	30.54	12.53	33.05	21.16	33.98	79.27	13.68	20.04	8.65	21.12	30.78	25.38
IHC result	+	+	-	+	+	+	+	-	+	-	+	+	+

Note: +, IHC result positive; -, IHC result negative.
Spearman's statistical analysis shows rr = 0.692, $p<0.05$, indicating that NSE serum levels in MM patients were positively correlated with the IHC results.

Table 2. Comparison of serum NSE levels between small cell lung cancer group and control group.

Indicator(ng/ml)	Group	Cases(n)	Percentile 25th	Percentile 50th	Percentile 75th	Range	Z	P
NSE	Control	47	8.11	9.33	10.8	5.73–14.40	6.937	$P<0.05$
	Lung cancer	25	30.86	44.6	95.85	13.91–370.0		

Table 3. Comparison of serum NSE levels between MM group and control group.

Indicator(ng/ml)	Group	Cases(n)	Percentile			Range	Z	P
			25th	50th	75th			
NSE	Control	47	8.11	9.33	10.8	5.73–14.40	5.356	P<0.05
	Lung cancer	52	13.72	23.10	30.31	7.23–880.34		

Table 4. Comparison of serum NSE levels between small cell lung cancer group and MM group.

Indicator(ng/ml)	Group	Cases(n)	Percentile			Range	Z	P
			25th	50th	75th			
NSE	Lung cancer	25	30.86	44.6	95.85	13.91–370.0	2.739	P<0.05
	Lung cancer	52	13.72	23.10	30.31	7.23–880.34		

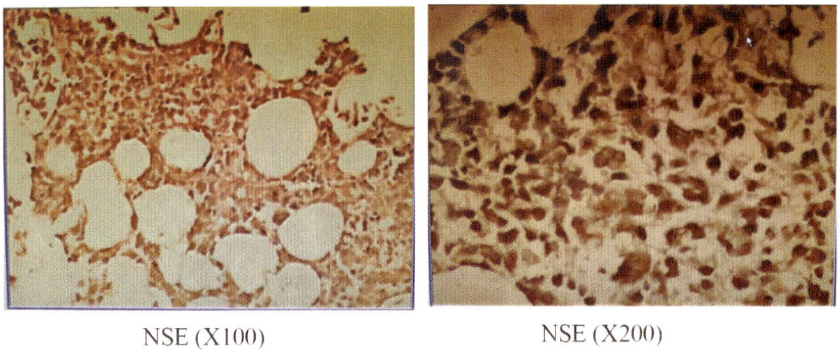

Figure 1. NSE immunohistochemical results of patients with previously untreated MM.

We also used reverse transcriptase polymerase chain reaction (RT-PCR) to detect NSE transcript levels in the bone marrow of patients. Two ml bone marrow samples were extracted by bone marrow biopsy from previously untreated MM patients and control healthy subjects. Mononuclear cells were enriched by density gradient centrifugation. Trizol extraction of total RNA was performed followed by PCR (Takara DRR002B). The upstream primer sequence for NSE: 5′-GACTGAGGACACATT-CATTGCTGAC-3′; downstream primer sequence: 5′-CAGCA-CACTGGGATTACGGAAG-3′. Eight μl reaction product together with 2 μl loading buffer was resolved on a 2% agarose ethidium bromide (EB)containing gel by electrophoresis. Results were documented under a UV transmission reflectometer.

3 Monitoring of patient condition indices

Prior to each course of chemotherapy, weekly routine preoperative examinations were performed on each patient. These included blood count, liver function, renal function, β_2-MG, serum NSE, serum protein electrophoresis, immunofixation electrophoresis, serum immunoglobulin (IgG, IgA and IgM) quantification, light chain (κ,λ) quantification, and bone marrow cell morphology. Meanwhile MM-associated symptoms, such as bone destruction, infection, high viscosity syndrome, anemia, hypercalcemia, and renal damage, were monitored and recorded.

4 Statistical analysis

SPSS16.0 software (Armonk, NY, USA) was used for statistical analysis. Because NSE level data in the control group, lung cancer group, and MM group exhibited a skewed distribution, percentiles were chosen for data presentation. Comparisons between the lung cancer group and control group, the MM group and control group, and the lung cancer group and the MM group were analyzed by rank-sum test. The correlation between NSE level in MM patients and the amount of the prognostic indicator β_2-MG was analyzed by Spearman's rank test.

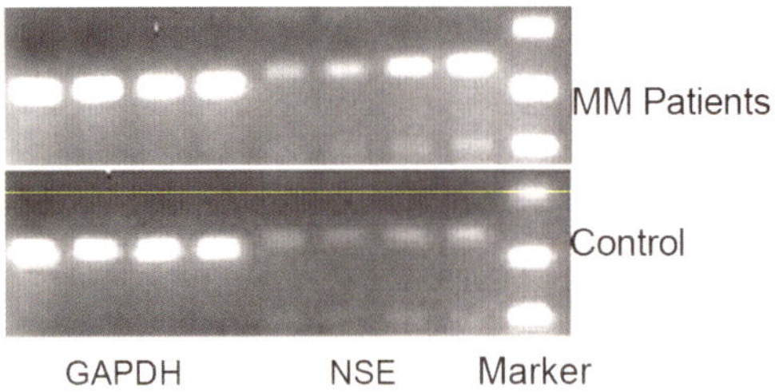

Figure 2. RT-PCR product electrophoresis for GAPDH (control and NSE) in previously untreated MM patients and controls.

Results

1

Among the 52 MM patients evaluated, 34 exhibited increased serum NSE levels, accounting for 65.4% of all patients with MM. Spearman's statistical analysis showed $r = 0.692$, $p<0.05$ (Table 1), indicating that NSE serum levels in MM patients were positively correlated with IHC results.

2 Comparison of serum NSE levels between the control and small cell lung cancer groups (Table 2)

As shown in Table 2, the serum NSE level in the control group all fell within the normal range, whereas the level in lung cancer group were significantly higher at the level of third percentile ($P< 0.05$).

3 Comparison of serum NSE levels between the control and MM groups (Table 3)

As shown in Table 3, NSE serum levels in 18 cases in the MM group were negative. However, at the level of third percentile, NSE levels of the MM group were significantly higher than those of the control group ($P<0.05$).

4 Comparison of serum NSE levels between the small cell lung cancer and MM groups (Table 4)

As shown in Table 4, at the level of third percentile, NSE levels in the small cell lung cancer group were significantly higher than those of the MM group ($P<0.05$).

5

Immunohistochemistry for NSE in patients with previously untreated MM (Figure 1) reveals clear brownish-yellow granules in cytoplasm with a positive rate of 45%.

6

RT-PCR was used to determine if RNA transcript levels of NSE were elevated in the bone marrow of untreated patients diagnosed with MM. Relative to healthy controls, MM patients exhibited elevated levels of NSE. GAPDH was used as an internal control, and its levels were unchanged between the two groups (Figure 2).

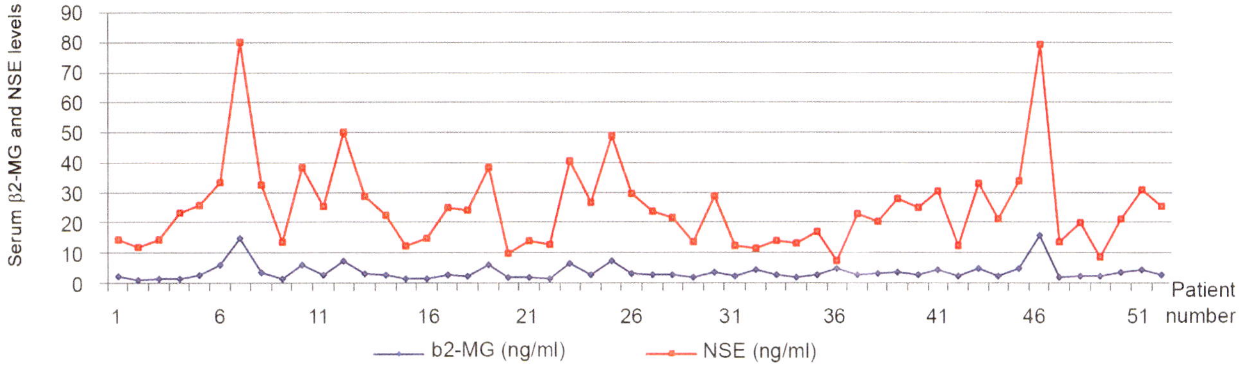

Figure 3. Correlation between NSE level in patients with previously untreated MM and the amount of the prognostic indicator β2-MG.

7 Correlation between NSE level in patients with previously untreated MM and the amount of the prognostic indicator β_2-MG (Figure 3)

According to Spearman's rank test, r = 0.749, P<0.01, there is a significant positive correlation between β_2-MG and NSE levels in MM patients.

8 Correlation between NSE level and the amount of prognostic indicator β_2-MG in MM patients after receiving three courses of chemotherapy (Figure 4)

According to Spearman's rank test, r = 0.618, P<0.01, there is even after chemotherapy a strong positive correlation between β_2-MG and NSE levels in MM patients.

9 Correlation between NSE level in MM patients and treatment response

After three courses of chemotherapy, the overall response rate (ORR) of the group with elevated NSE levels was 15/28 (53.6%), and three out of 28 patients (10.7%) achieved very good partial response (VGPR). In the group with normal NSE levels, the ORR was 10/14 (71.4%) and two patients (14.3%) achieved VGPR. In the group of patients with elevated NSE levels who adopted the TD-based program (NSE+/T group), the treatment was effective in 15 patients and the ORR was 53.6%. In the group of patients with elevated NSE levels who adopted the VD-based program (NSE+/V group), the treatment was effective in four patients and the ORR was 66.7%. In the group of patients with normal NSE levels who adopted the TD-based program (NSE-/T group), the treatment was effective in 10 patients and the ORR was 71.4%. In the group of patients with normal NSE levels who adopted the VD-based program (NSE-/V group), all four patients showed effective response. The difference in treatment efficiency between groups with elevated serum NSE levels and the ones with normal NSE levels was not statistically significant (P>0.05).

10 Correlation between NSE level in MM patients and progression-free survival (PFS)

The median PFS in patients with elevated and normal serum NSE levels was five months and 13 months, respectively. The difference in PFS was statistically significant (P<0.01) (Figure 5).

Discussion

To date, there are only a few published studies regarding elevated NSE levels in MM. Jimbo *et al.* [1] reported increased serum NSE level in a 53-year-old female patient diagnosed with IgG-λ type MM with a chest-wall plasmacytoma. Immunostaining of her bone marrow smears and left chest-wall tumor biopsy specimens revealed diffused cytoplasmic NSE staining in the abnormal plasma cells, confirming that myeloma cells can produce

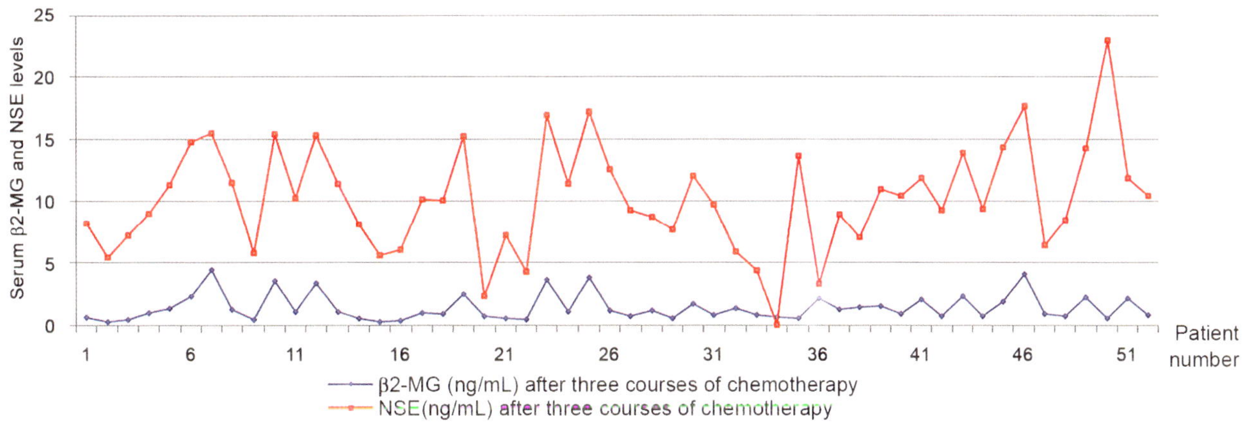

Figure 4. Correlation between NSE level and the amount of prognostic indicator β2-MG in MM patients after receiving three courses of chemotherapy.

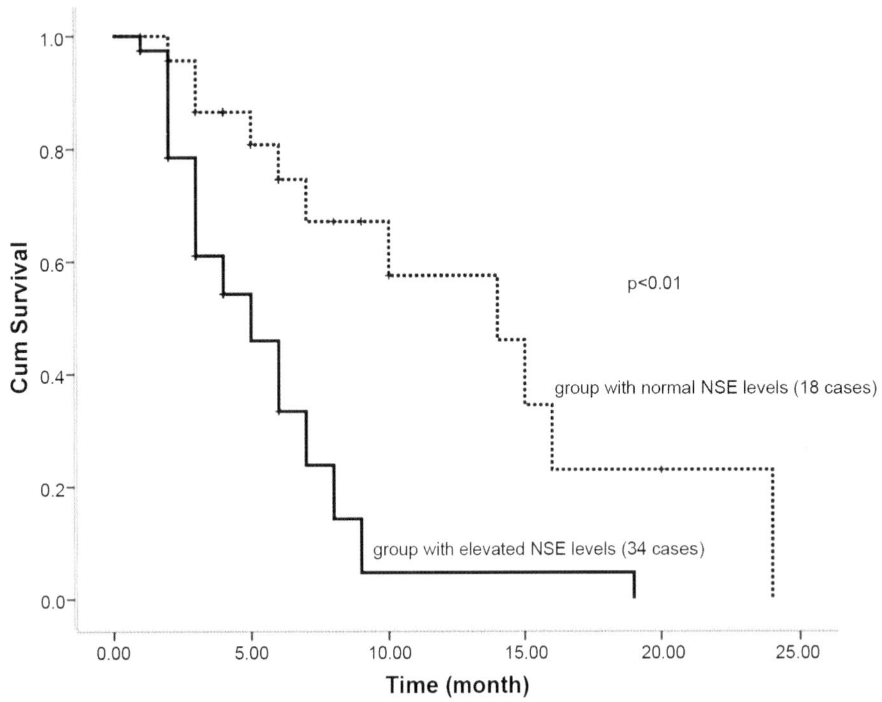

Figure 5. Correlation between NSE level in MM patients and progression-free survival (PFS).

NSE. After several cycles of chemotherapy, along with the disappearance of chest-wall plasmacytoma and plasma cells in the bone marrow, her serum NSE level returned to normal. Coincidentally, another Japanese group [2] reported a case of a 68-year-old patient with IgD-λ type MM exhibiting significantly elevated levels of serum NSE. Immunohistochemical staining confirmed NSE expression in myeloma cells. NSE level in this patient was reduced to normal after two cycles of combined interferon-α and vincristine, melphalan, cyclophosphamide, and prednisone (VMCP) chemotherapy. British scholars Sharma *et al.* [3] reported a case of a 75-year-old male patient who was initially hospitalized with sacral pain was diagnosed with prostate cancer. Following chemotherapy, the patient presented with multiple sites of bone pain, hypercalcemia, positive urine for B-J proteins, and elevated serum NSE. Bone marrow biopsy showed atypical plasma cells comprising 20–30% of the nucleated cells. In addition, immunohistochemical staining showed positive staining for CD138, κ light chain, and NSE. The patient was diagnosed with IgG-κ type MM and was treated with cyclophosphamide, thalidomide, and dexamethasone. Moreover, Japanese scholars reported detection of NSE expression in MM cell lines and primary cells by immunohistochemistry and PCR, further confirming the association of NSE expression with MM [9].

In the present study, 34 of the 52 MM patients examined showed elevated NSE levels in the initial detection of NSE. Following chemotherapy, NSE levels exhibited a downward trend. This was particularly true in patients treated with Velcade, a finding consistent with the downward trend of another MM monitoring indicator blood β_2-MG concentration. There was a significant positive correlation between NSE and β_2-MG levels. Although no significant correlation was detected, we observed that elevated NSE levels were often present in patients with severe bone pain symptoms or when the symptoms worsened. In contrast, NSE levels were not significantly related to other MM symptoms, such as anemia, hyperviscosity, and hypercalcemia. Consistent with previous reports, it is important to note that the PFS of patients with elevated NSE levels was significantly shorter than patients with normal levels of NSE. However, the overall survival data was not included for analysis since in all cases the observation time was less than three years, and the tumor burden in patients with disease progression had decreased to some extent after induction of remission therapy. These patients continue to be followed clinically, and the total sample size will continue to expand in order to study the correlation between NSE level and five year overall survival and the impact of different treatment programs on NSE level.

We also observed with the conduct of chemotherapy that MM indices such as proportion of plasma cells and M protein level declined. In parallel, individual NSE levels in each patient also decreased, suggesting that it can be used as an indicator for condition monitoring. The reason for the decline in NSE level with chemotherapy could be that during the process of tumor cell growth, the cell cycle is accelerated and glycolysis is strengthened. NSE is an acidic protease that is involved in glycolysis to catalyze the conversion of β-glycerophosphate into dihydroxy acetone phosphate. Therefore, the upregulation of intracellular NSE in tumor cells leads to increased release of NSE into the blood and results in increased level of serum NSE. Mature plasma cells are the dominant tumor cell type in the majority of myeloma, and the proportion of cells remaining in the cell division cycle is very small [10]. Plasma cell labeling index (PCLI) is a representative of plasma cell DNA synthesis and reflects the progression state of myeloma, and it is an important indicator of prognosis of patients with MM [11]. We speculate that, similar to PCLI, NSE does not primarily reflect the overall myeloma cell load but dynamically reflects the proliferation of myeloma cells. Therefore, NSE levels may become a new prognostic indicator. Importantly, since detection of NSE is simple and relatively inexpensive, NSE may be a more valuable clinical application than PCLI and can be incorporated into the routine examination of neoplastic diseases.

Consistent with previous studies, we found that the level of NSE was significantly higher in patients with untreated small cell lung cancer. It is widely agreed that the NSE level is a reliable indicator for the differential diagnosis of small cell lung cancer and a useful measure for the monitoring of the therapeutic efficacy of radiotherapy and chemotherapy [12–15]. For diagnosis of neuroblastoma, sensitivity of NSE measurements can be up to 90% and have also been used to monitor treatment efficacy and relapse [16]. Increased NSE expression has also been linked to a small number of tumor cell lines, including non-small cell lung cancers, medullary thyroid carcinoma, and pheochromocytoma [17]. Several studies have found that NSE can be used as a sensitive and specific indicator for brain damage, and increases in NSE reflect the size and severity of brain damage [18–19]. An increase in NSE has been found in cerebral ischemia and neuronal injury due to a variety of reasons, such as neonatal asphyxia, pediatric febrile seizures, brain infectious diseases, chronic obstructive pulmonary disease, cerebral infarction, cerebral hemorrhage, systemic lupus erythematosus, Wilson's degeneration, and depression. Bai *et al.* reported that the NSE levels in patients with lymphoma were significantly increased [20]. In addition, increased NSE was seen in patients with extramedullary hemolysis, such as autoimmune hemolytic anemia and paroxysmal nocturnal hemoglobinuria, and can be used as a diagnostic indicator to distinguish *in situ* and extramedullary hemolysis [21].

However, even though there was a multitude of research regarding NSE levels in numerous types of cancer and other disease, there was little data available in the Chinese literature regarding NSE levels in MM. One study by Zhang *et al.* [5] reported that MM patients with increased NSE levels had shorter overall survival, less progression-free survival, and a poorer prognosis than those with normal NSE levels. Consistent with this report, we observed in our study that the PFS of patients with elevated NSE levels was significantly shorter than patients with normal levels of NSE.

Given our data regarding the correlation between NSE level and MM condition changes and in consideration of the above-mentioned studies abroad, we propose that serum NSE levels in patients with multiple myeloma can be increased to varying degrees. NSE levels may not be useful for MM diagnosis or therapeutic evaluation but for the prognosis. However, due to the limited number of cases in this study, confirmation of our conclusions regarding the use of NSE as a prognostic indicator in multiple myeloma will require long-term, large-scale prospective clinical observation.

Author Contributions

Conceived and designed the experiments: YS XW. Performed the experiments: QW RM HY. Analyzed the data: RM QY LC. Contributed reagents/materials/analysis tools: XZ. Wrote the paper: RM HY.

References

1. Jimbo J, Sato K, Ikuta K, Inamura J, Hosoki T, et al (2006) A neuron specific enolase-producing multiple myeloma. Rinsho Ketsueki 10: 1381–1386.
2. Nakajima T, Noguchi T, Kumahara Y, Sugihara A, Yamazaki T, et al. (1995) Neuron specific enolase- producing IgD multiple myeloma with high serum amylase activity. Rinsho Ketsueki 36: 359–364.
3. Sharma RA, Wotherspoon AC, Cook G, Morgan GJ, Huddart RA (2006) Neuron-specific enolase expression in multiple myeloma. Lancet Oncol 7: 960.
4. Zhang Y, Hou J, Wei W, Guo Lieping, Shi Haotian, et al. (2012)Serum neuron-specific enolase activity on the prognosis of patients with multiple myeloma. Chinese Journal of Hematology 33:417–419.
5. Zhang Z, Shen T (2007) Diagnosis of blood diseases and treatment standards. 3rd edition, Beijing: Science Press. p232–235.
6. Multiple myeloma working group in China (2008) Multiple myeloma treatment guidelines. Chinese Journal of Internal Medicine 47: 869–872.
7. Bredella MA, Steinbach L, Caputo G, Segall G, Hawkins R (2005) Value of FDG PET in the assessment of patients with multiple myeloma. AJR Am J Roentgenol 184:1199–1204.
8. Gao W, Li H, Li X, Li Bin, He Di, et al. (2012)Expression of NSE in myeloma-related bone diseases. Journal of Chinese General Practice 10: 337–338.
9. Liu Sq, Otsuyama Ki, Ma Z, Abroun S, Shamsasenjan K, et al. (2007) Induction of Multilineage Markers in Human Myeloma Cells and Their Down-Regulation by Interleukin 6. Hematology 85: 49–58.
10. Song S, Chen Y (2004) Williams Hematology. Beijing: People's Health Publishing House. p1342–1368.
11. Zhang Z, Yang T, Hao Y (2003) Hematology. 1st edition. Beijing: People's Health Publishing House. 1341–1359.
12. Ebert W, Muley T, Drings P (1996)Does the assessment of serum markers in patients with lung cancer aid in the clinical decision making process? Anticancer Res 16:2161–2168.
13. Lamy PJ, Grenier J, Kramar A, Pujol JL (2000) Pro-gastrin-releasing peptide, neuron specific enolase and chromogranin A as serum markers of small cell lung cancer. Lung Cancer 29:197–203.
14. Jorgensen LG, Osterlind K, Genolla J, Gomm SA, Hernandez JR, et al. (1996)Serum neuron-specific enolase (S-NSE) and the prognosis in small-cell lung cancer (SCLC): a combined multivariable analysis on data from nine centres. Br J Cancer 74:463–467.
15. Pinson P, Joos G, Watripont P, Brusselle G, Pauwels R (1997) Serum neuron-specific enolase as a tumor marker in the diagnosis and follow-up of small-cell lung cancer. Respiration 64:102–107.
16. Riley RD, Heney D, Jones DR, Sutton AJ, Lambert PC (2004) A systematic review of molecular and biological tumor markers in neuroblastoma. Clin Cancer Res 10:4–12.
17. Zhang Q, Xu J, Wang Y (2005)Expression of human neuron-specific enolase expression in tumor cell lines and its significance. Chinese Journal of Laboratory Medicine 28: 728–731.
18. Bohmer AE, Oses JP, Schmidt AP, Peron CS, Krebs CL, et al. (2011) Neuron-specific enolase, S100B, and glial fibrillary acidic protein levels as outcome predictors in patients with severe traumatic brain injury. Neurosurgery 68:1624–1630.
19. Woertgen C, Rothoerl RD, Wiesmann M, Missler U, Brawanski A (2002) Glial and neuronal serum markers after controlled cortical impact injury in the rat. Acta Neurochir Suppl 81:205–207.
20. Bai Y, Wu D, Liu Y, et al. (2009) The value of serum neuron-specific enolase in the diagnosis of lymphoma. Clinical Hematology 22:379–380.
21. Chen K, Ding B, Zhu J, et al. (2010) NSE expression in the identification of in situ hemolysis and extramedullary hemolysis. Jiangsu Medicine 36:421–422.

6

The Choice of Regimens Based on Bortezomib for Patients with Newly Diagnosed Multiple Myeloma

Jingsong He[1], Li Yang[1], Xiaoyan Han[1], Gaofeng Zheng[1], Weiyan Zheng[1], Guoqing Wei[1], Wenjun Wu[1], Xiujin Ye[1], Jimin Shi[1], Wanzhuo Xie[1], Li Li[1], Jie Zhang[1], Weijia Huang[1], Yi Zhao[1], He Huang[1], Xuejin Zhang[2], Jiaping Fu[3], Zhen Cai[1]*

1 The Bone Marrow Transplantation center & Multiple Myeloma Treatment Center, The First Affiliated Hospital of Medical College, Zhejiang University, Hangzhou, Zhejiang, P. R. China, **2** Department of Hematology, Red Cross Hospital in Hangzhou, Zhejiang, P. R. China, **3** Department of Hematology, Shaoxing People's Hospital, Zhejiang, P. R. China

Abstract

Introduction: Bortezomib has significantly improved multiple myeloma (MM) response rates, but strategies for choosing bortezomib-based regimens for initial MM therapy are not standardized. Here, we describe four bortezomib-based therapies in Chinese MM patients to determine the optimal chemotherapeutic approach.

Methods: Newly diagnosed symptomatic MM patients at three hematological centers between February 1, 2006 and May 31, 2013 were treated with therapies including bortezomib plus dexamethasone (PD) or combinations of PD with either adriamycin (PAD), cyclophosphamide (PCD) or thalidomide (PTD) for every 28 days.

Results: The overall response rate of all the 215 eligible patients was 90.2%. The ORR for PCD, PAD, PTD and PD were 97.4%, 93.2%, 85.3% and 77.8% while the effects with VGPR or better were 63.7%, 62.7%, 44.2% and 37.8%, respectively. The effect of ORR, VGPR and CR/nCR for the PCD regimen was better than the PD protocol. Median PFS for all patients was 29.0 months with significant differences observed among treatment groups. Median OS of all the patients was not reached, but three-drug combinations were superior to PD alone. Frequently observed toxicities were neutropenia, thrombocytopenia, fatigue, infection, herpes zoster, and peripheral neuropathy. The incidence of peripheral neuropathy (PN) in PTD group was significantly higher than other three groups, especially grade 2–3 PN. Treatment with anti-viral agent acyclovir significantly reduced the incidence of herpes zoster.

Conclusions: Our experience indicated that bortezomib-based regimens were effective and well-tolerated in the Chinese population studied; three-drug combinations PCD, PAD were superior to PD, especially with respect to PCD.

Editor: John M. Koomen, Moffitt Cancer Center, United States of America

Funding: This work was supported by Major International (region) Co-elaboration Research Project of Chinese National Natural Science Foundation (Project No. 81120108018); National Natural Science Foundation of China (Project No. 91029740, 81071936, 30900533); Key project of the Ministry of Health of China (Project 2010-2012); Scientific Research Program for Public Interests from the Health Ministry of China (Project No. 201002024). The funders had no role in study design, data collection and analysis, decision to publish, or preparation of the manuscript.

Competing Interests: The authors have declared that no competing interests exist.

* E-mail: caiz@zju.edu.cn

These authors contributed equally to this work.

Introduction

Multiple myeloma (MM) is a malignant neoplasm of bone marrow plasma cells, representing the second most common hematologic malignancy worldwide [1]. Median survival for MM has historically been approximately 3–5 years with 5–8% of patients experiencing complete remission (CR) upon treatment with conventional therapy, such as melphalan and prednisone (MP) or vincristine, doxorubicin, dexamethasone (VAD), prior to the advent of novel therapies [1–3]. Bortezomib, a reversible inhibitor of the 26S proteasome, has anti-tumor activity conferred by multiple mechanisms. Clinical studies suggest that bortezomib is effective for the treatment of MM and offers improved remission and better survival [3–7]. At present there are bortezomib based combination chemotherapy with 2 or 3 drugs, but there is no clear strategy for choosing a regimen for different patients since few clinical trials are supported. Thus, we retrospectively analyzed the efficacy and adverse effects experienced by MM patients who received combination therapy based on bortezomib as the first-line therapy from three hematological centers in China and we report our findings here.

Materials and Methods

Patients

The study protocol was approved by the research ethics Committee of the First Affiliated Hospital, College of Medicine, Zhejiang University. All patients provided written informed consent and received bortezomib-based combination chemotherapy as first-line treatment. Patients with newly diagnosed symptomatic MM between February 1, 2006 and March 31, 2013 in three hematological centers who displayed either measurable blood or urine monoclonal protein (M protein) were included in this study. The diagnostic criteria were primarily derived from the World Health Organization (WHO) and we used both the International Staging System (ISS) and the Durie-Salmon (DS) staging for assessing patients.

Treatment

Patients received bortezomib-based combination chemotherapy in 28-day cycles as follows: bortezomib plus dexamethasone (PD) or three-drug combinations of PD with Adriamycin (PAD), cyclophosphamide (PCD) or thalidomide (PTD). Among the above regimens, bortezomib (1.3 mg/m^2) was given intravenously on days 1, 4, 8, 11, whereas dexamethasone (20 mg/day) was given intravenously on days 1–2, 4–5, 8–9, 11–12, adriamycin (10 mg/m^2) was given intravenously on days 1–4, cyclophosphamide (200 mg/m^2) was given intravenously on days 1–4 and thalidomide (100 mg) was administered orally each day.

Twenty patients received autologous stem cell transplantation (ASCT) after induction therapy including 3 cases who received PTD induction therapy, 4 cases who received PD, 5 cases who received PCD and 5 cases who received PAD. After induction therapy or ASCT, patients were given thalidomide (100 mg/d) for maintenance treatment until progression was observed or until they could not tolerate treatment due to adverse reactions.

Acyclovir was gived to 7 patients in the PTD group and to patients in the other groups. Routine anti-coagulation or anti-thrombotic agents were not used.

Response and Adverse Events Assessment

The International Melanoma Working Group (IMWG) uniform response criteria were used for the evaluation of response, including CR, very good partial response (VGPR), partial response (PR), stable disease (SD) and progressive disease [8]. Progression-free survival (PFS) was calculated from the time of first treatment to the time of progressive disease or until the time of the last follow-up or until a patient death. Overall survival (OS) was calculated from the time of start of therapy initiation until the date of death from any cause or to the time of the last follow-up. Adverse events were assessed at each visit and graded according to the National Cancer Institute's Common Terminology Criteria (version 3.0; NCI-CTC 3.0).

Statistical Analysis

All patients were followed-up until June 30, 2013, and patient assessment of patients began after one course of chemotherapy. Clinical characteristics, adverse effects rates and the 3-year OS and PFS rates were analyzed by the Pearson χ^2 test. Response rates were compared with multivariate logistic regression analysis, odds ratios (ORs) and 95% confidence intervals (CIs) were estimated by logistic regression. Kaplan-Meier methods were used to generate survival distribution graphs and differences in survival (e.g., PFS and OS) and statistically compared by the log-rank test. Multivariate analyses of prognostic factors were performed using Cox regression modeling. All probability values were two-sided and A P-value of 0.05 indicated statistical significance. All the data can be found in the Supporting Information files of the submission.

Results

Patient Characteristics

Two hundred and fifteen patients with MM were eligible for inclusion in this retrospective analysis, including a total of 135 male patients and 80 female patients, and the male-to-female ratio was 1.7:1. The median age at diagnosis was 60 years (range, 31–83 years). Of all the patients, 79.0% (170/215) were in stage III by DS staging while 76.3% (164/215) were in stage II and III by ISS staging. Baseline patient characteristics were well-balanced. The baseline demographic and disease characteristics of patients in deferent treatment groups were listed in Table 1.

Number of Cycles and Responses

A total of 215 patients received 1 to 8 cycles of treatment with median of 3 cycles, including 36 cases only receiving 1 cycle, 41 cases receiving 2 cycles, 55 cases receiving 3 cycles, 83 cases receiving 4 or more cycles of chemotherapy. Response rates were listed in Table 2.

Overall response rate (≥PR, ORR) of all the 215 eligible patients was 90.2% including 26.5% VGPR and 28.4% CR/nCR. Table 2 depicts details about ORR and treatment groups.

The patients received PCD or PAD demonstrated significant higher ORR compared to PD (97.4%, 93.2% vs 77.8%, $P=0.009$, 0.037). The response rate defined as VGPR or better in the all patients was 54.9%. Response rates defined as VGPR for PCD and PAD were significantly higher than PD (27.3%, 28.8%, vs 17.8%, $P=0.011$, 0.037). Rates of patients received CR/nCR in PCD and PAD were higher than PD (36.4%, 33.9%, vs 20.0%, $P=0.005$, 0.017). Patients receiving bortezomib-based therapies had a rapid treatment response with respect to ORR (77.2%) after one cycle, especially for the PCD group which performed better than other regimens and was superior to PD (especially for better than VGPR). Response for four regimens after every cycle are depicted in Table S1.

PFS and OS

The median duration of follow-up for the 215 patients from diagnosis was 22.5 months (range, 2.0–64.0 months). The median PFS of the 215 patients was 29.0 months (95% CI: 21.6–36.4 months). The median PFS was 27.0 months (95% CI: 15.9–38.1 months) for patients who received PDT, and 23.0 months (95% CI: 10.1–35.9 months) for those in the PD group and median PFS for PCD and PAD groups were not reached. There were significant differences among the groups and with respect to multivariate analysis (Fig. 1A, Table 3). Respective 3-year PFS was 71.4±6.1%, 70.3±7.1%, 50.2±9.7%, 46.1±9.8% in PCD, PAD, PTD and PD regimens. The 3-year PFS rate of PCD was significantly higher than PTD and PD ($\chi^2=4.752$, 7.414, $P=0.029$, 0.006), but without statistical significance compared to PAD ($\chi^2=0.060$, $P=0.806$). The 3-year PFS rate of PAD was significantly higher than PD ($\chi^2=5.524$, $P=0.019$), but without statistical significance compared to PTD ($\chi^2=3.491$, $P=0.062$). The 3-year PFS rate of PTD was not statistically higher than PD ($\chi^2=0.086$, $P=0.769$).

At the time of analysis, 33 (15.3%) patients had died, including 10 patients who had received PTD, and 14 patients in the PD groups, 7 patients in the PCD group and 2 in the PAD group died from treatment-related issues and MM. The median OS of the 215 patients was not reached at 64 months in either treatment arm and there were significant differences among groups ($P=0.005$; Fig. 1B). The median OS for the PD arm was 44.0 months (95% CI: 39.2–48.8 months) while other arms were not reached, but the median OS for PTD, PCD and PAD was significantly

Table 1. Patient characteristics and baseline demographics.

Variable	Total (n = 215)	PCD (n = 77)	PAD (n = 59)	PDT (n = 34)	PD (n = 45)
Age, n(%)					
<65	152(70.7)	53(68.8)	50(84.7)	24(70.6)	25(55.6)
≥65	63(29.3)	24(31.2)	9(15.3)	10(29.4)	20(44.4)
Gender, n(%)					
Male	135(62.8)	35(45.5)	45(76.3)	24(70.6)	31(68.9)
Female	80(37.2)	32(41.6)	24(40.7)	10(29.4)	14(31.1)
Type of myeloma, n(%)					
IgA	59(27.4)	23(29.8)	17(28.8)	7(20.6)	12(26.8)
IgG	101(47.0)	33(42.9)	26(44.1)	22(64.7)	20(44.4)
IgD	4(1.9)	0(0.0)	1(1.7)	1(2.9)	2(4.4)
Light chain	50(23.3)	21(27.3)	14(23.7)	4(11.8)	11(24.4)
Biphenotypic (IgG, IgA)	1(0.5)	0(0.0)	1(1.7)	0(0.0)	0(0.0)
Durie-Salmon Staging, n(%)					
1A	10(4.7)	2(2.6)	3(5.1)	2(5.9)	3(6.7)
2A	35(16.3)	10(13.0)	9(15.3)	5(14.7)	11(24.4)
3A	117(54.3)	47(61.0)	34(57.6)	17(50.0)	19(42.2)
3B	53(24.7)	18(23.4)	13(22.0)	10(29.4)	12(26.7)
International Staging System Staging, n(%)					
1	51(23.7)	20(26.0)	13(22.0)	4(11.8)	14(31.1)
2	79(36.7)	28(36.3)	23(39.0)	16(47.0)	12(26.7)
3	85(39.6)	29(37.7)	23(39.0)	14(41.2)	19(42.2)

longer than PD ($P = 0.015$, 0.013, 0.023). Respective 3-year OS was 86.3±5.3%, 75.1±11.0%, 75.5±8.1%, 65.3±8.8% with PCD, PAD, PTD and PD regimens. The 3-year OS rate of PCD was significantly higher than PD ($\chi^2 = 7.456$, $P = 0.006$), but this was not statistically significant compared to PAD and PTD ($\chi^2 = 2.680$, 1.421, $P = 0.102$, 0.233). The 3-year OS rate for PAD and PTD were not statistically higher than PD ($\chi^2 = 1.253$, 1.324, $P = 0.263$, 0.250). The 3-year OS rate of PAD was not statistically higher than PTD ($\chi^2 = 0.042$, $P = 0.838$). Comparing multivariate analysis of risk factors for PFS and OS, we found that patient's age at diagnosis, a higher D-S stage and the number of induction therapy cycles significantly affected patients' PFS and OS, certain cytogenetic abnormalities also affected OS, but these had little influence on PFS whereas ISS stage had no effect on PFS and OS (Table 3).

Adverse Events

Treatment-related deaths in the subgroups included 15 patients (7.0% of total recruited patients), for whom infection-related deaths accounted for most (N = 12) of the case. No significant difference in treatment-related deaths was observed between groups. Fequently observed hematologic toxicities (Grade 3/4) were: thrombocytopenia (15.9%), neutropenia (14.0%) and anemia (7.9%). Among the patients in every subgroup, there was no significant difference observed in grade 3 to 4 hematological toxicities. The most common non-hematologic toxicities included (all Grades) peripheral neuropathy (55.5%), fatigue (26.8%), infection (23.2%), constipation (20.7%), herpes zoster (15.9%) and diarrhea (14.0%) (Table 4).

The incidence of constipation for PTD arm was significantly higher than PCD, PAD, PD groups ($\chi^2 = 5.002$, 12.240, 9.876, $P = 0.025$, <0.001, 0.002). The incidence of diarrhea for PTD arm was significantly higher than PD groups ($\chi^2 = 5.577$, $P = 0.048$). The incidence of herpes zoster in the PTD was 40.0% which was significant higher than PCD (13.6%), PAD (8.6%) and PD (6.1%) group ($\chi^2 = 8.568$, 14.552, 12.641, $P = 0.003$, <0.001, <0.001), respectively). Peripheral neuropathy of all grades was more frequently reported in patients in the PTD group compared to the PD, PCD and PAD groups (83.3% vs 51.5%, 45.7%, 48.5%) ($\chi^2 = 4.819$, 18.848, 11.182, $P = 0.028$, <0.001, 0.001). The incidence of grade 2 to 3 peripheral neuropathy for PTD arm was significantly higher than PCD, PAD and PD groups ($\chi^2 = 7.562$, 14.190, 9.584, $P = 0.006$, <0.001, 0.002). There was no significant difference in other treatment-related adverse events among groups.

Discussion

MM is one of the most frequently observed hematologic cancers With an incidence in China of 1–2 per 100,000. Patients who can achieve CR are reported to be significantly improved with respect to PFS and OS whether in the patients received high-dose chemotherapy with ASCT or without ASCT, or relapse/refractory patients [7,9–13]. Recently years, many prospective randomized clinical trials have pushed forth advances in the treatment of MM with targeted drugs, such as bortezomib-, thalidomide-, and lenalidomie-based regimens, effects of which have been reported to be significantly better than traditional therapies [1–6]. However, few clinical trials have compared

Table 2. Overall response rates of regimens.

	ORR			PR			VGPR			nCR/CR		
	N (%)	OR, 95%CI	P	N (%)	OR, 95%CI	P	N (%)	OR, 95%CI	P	N,%	OR, 95%CI	P
PD	35(77.8)	1[a]		18(40.0)	1		8(17.8)	1[b]		9(20.0)	1[c]	
PCD	75(97.4)	9.11, 1.75–47.32	0.009	26(33.8)	6.79, 1.23–37.36	0.028	21 (27.3)	10.49, 1.70–64.78	0.011	28(36.4)	13.19, 2.20–79.22	0.005
PAD	55(93.2)	4.64, 1.10–19.60	0.037	18(30.5)	3.17, 0.69–14.55	0.139	17(28.8)	5.57, 1.11–29.86	0.037	20(33.9)	7.15, 1.41–36.16	0.017
PDT	29(85.3)	1.62, 0.44–5.96	0.466	14(41.2)	1.50, 0.38–6.03	0.566	11(32.4)	2.65, 0.56–12.44	0.218	4(11.8)	0.95, 0.17–5.25	0.950

[a]Patients received PCD or PAD demonstrated significant higher ORR compared to PD (97.4%, 93.2% vs 77.8%, $P = 0.009$, 0.037).
[b]Response rates defined as VGPR for PCD and PAD were significantly higher than PD (27.3%, 28.8%, vs 17.8%, $P = 0.011$, 0.037).
[c]Rates of patients received CR/nCR in PCD and PAD were higher than PD (36.4%, 33.9%, vs 20.0%, $P = 0.005$, 0.017).

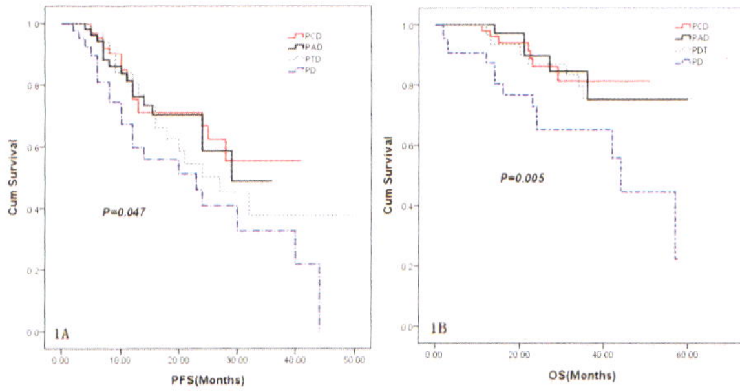

Figure 1. Kaplan-Meier survival curves for patients who received PCD, PAD, PTD and PD. 1A: Median PFS of the 215 patients was 29.0 months (95% CI: 21.6–36.4 months). Median PFS was 27.0 months (95% CI: 15.9–38.1 months) for patients who received PDT, and 23.0 months (95% CI: 10.1–35.9 months) in PD respectively whereas the median PFS for PCD and PAD were not reached but with significant differences were observed among the groups ($P = 0.047$). The respective 3-year PFS was 71.4±6.1%, 70.3±7.1%, 50.2±9.7%, 46.1±9.8% with PCD, PAD, PTD and PD regimens, respectively. **1B:** Median OS of the 215 patients was not reached at 64 months in either treatment arm and significant differences were observed among the groups ($P = 0.005$; Fig. 1B). Median OS for the PD arm was 44.0 months (95% CI: 39.2–48.8 months) and this was not reached in the other treatment arms. Median OS for PTD, PCD and PAD was significantly longer than the PD group ($P = 0.015$, 0.013, 0.023). The respective 3-year OS was 86.3±5.3%, 75.1±11.0%, 75.5±8.1%, 65.3±8.8% for the PCD, PAD, PTD and PD regimens.

regimens to develop a strategy to direct initial MM treatment, especially for the OS and patient quality of life [14].

At this time, regimens in China are mainly bortezomib-based therapies, including doublet regimens (PD), and triplet regimes such as PCD, PAD and PTD. Bortezomib, as a component of these protocols is given 1.3 mg/m^2 twice a week, or 1.5 mg/m^2 once a week. Dexamethasone is given at 160 mg for every course and sometimes as high as 480 mg every course. In our analysis, bortezomib was given twice a week and dexamethasone was administered at 160 mg for every course. ORRs reached 65–88% for the PD regimen, including at least 30–40% VGPR and about 20% CR/nCR [3,15–17]. A phase 3 clinical trial IFM 2005-01 reported that in newly diagnosed patients who were suitable for ASCT, the ORR, CR/nCR, and effects better than VGPR for PD was 78.5%, 14.8% and 37.7%, respectively. The same results were observed in patients with poor disease stage or with adverse chromosomal abnormalities [3]. However, PD offered slight advantages with respect to PFS and OS but these were not statistically significant. The ORR of patients who received PD in our study was 77.8%, including 20.0% with CR/nCR and 17.8% of VGPR as reported.

Adding another drug to the PD regimen, such as an immunomodulatory agent, thalidomide or a conventional chemotherapeutic such as adriamycin or cyclophosphamide can achieve ORR as high as 90% with at least 60–70% VGPR and 40–50% CR/nCR [7,18,19–22]. In our study patients received treatment with median cycles of three drugs and above 30% cases only received 1 or 2 cycles, among which the PCD regimen had the optimal efficacy. With ORR, VGPR and CR/nCR rates for PCD of 97.4%, 27.3%, and 36.4%, these treatment modalities were all superior to PD. The effect of PAD was similar to PCD but PTD was only slightly better than PD. Because Cyclophosphamide has fewer adverse effects and is less expensive, a PCD regimen should gain favorable attention over time. In a phase II clinical trial [18] ORR, VGPR or better and CR/nCR rates were better for patients who received total four courses of PCD (28 days with

Table 3. Multivariate Analysis of Risk Factors for PFS and OS.

	PFS			OS		
Risk Factor	**HR**	**95%CI**	***P***	**HR**	**95%CI**	***P***
Age	1.039	1.013–1.066	0.003	1.053	1.013–1.095	0.009
DS stage	1.735	1.166–2.582	0.007	1.914	1.012–3.621	0.046
ISS stage	0.992	0.685–1.437	0.967	0.726	0.387–1.364	0.320
FISH[a]	1.189	0.886–1.594	0.249	1.690	1.127–2.534	0.011
Regimens[b]	0.491	0.286–0.845	0.010	0.283	0.132–0.608	0.001
Cycles[c] (N)	0.811	0.662–0.994	0.043	0.603	0.438–0.831	0.002

Abbreviations: OS, overall survival; PFS, progression-free survival; HR, hazard ratio; CI, confidence intervals; DS, Durie-Salmon; ISS, International Staging System; FISH, interphase fluorescence in situ hybridization;
[a]Patients with abnormalities of 13q14, 1q21, 14q32 and 17p13 compared with no FISH abnormalities.
[b]Three-drug combinations compared with PD.
[c]Patients with 3 number of cycles or more compared with less than 3 cycles.

every course, bortezomib was used twice per week, CTX at 1,200 mg/m^2, dexamethasone at 480 mg every course). ORR, VGPR or better and CR/nCR rates were 88%, 61% and 39% respectively and the treatment onset of action was rapid. We observed similar effects with PCD. However, PCD with bortezomib once a week and less dexamethasone has similar effects with less adverse reaction [22].

Three-drug combinations were more effective than PD regimen, and for PFS, a three drug combination was better and OS was superior to PD. The median OS for the PD arm was 44.0 months while other arms were not reached, Respective 3-year OS was 86.3%, 75.1%, 75.5%, 65.3% with PCD, PAD, PTD and PD regimens, respectively. Because ours was only a retrospective study and the data can be affected by many factors although all the treatment center reach the consensus of MM. Therefore, further prospective randomized clinical trials are needed to confirm the induction treatment effect on PFS and OS.

At present, prognostic factors of patients with MM include host factors, such as age, abnormal cytogenetics, D-S stage and ISS stage [23]. ISS stage was derived from more than 11,000 patients and based on serum beta 2-microglobulin and albumin measurements and this criteria defines three risk groups with median survivals of 62, 44 and 29 months, respetcively [24]. In our study, ISS appears to be less helpful for predicting PFS and OS in

Table 4. Treatment-related adverse events.

	Total	PDT	PCD	PAD	PD
Adverse events, n(%)	**(n = 215)**	**(n = 34)**	**(n = 77)**	**(n = 59)**	**(n = 45)**
Hematologic events(3/4 grade)					
Neutropenia	23(14.0)	4(13.3)	11(16.7)	5(14.3)	3(9.1)
Thrombocytopenia	26(15.9)	6(20.0)	10(15.2)	6(17.1)	4(12.1)
Anemia	13(7.9)	3(10.0)	7(10.6)	2(5.7)	1(3.0)
Non-hematologic events (All grades)					
Fatigue	44(26.8)	10(33.3)	18(27.3)	9(25.7)	7(21.2)
Infection	38(23.2)	10(33.3)	15(22.7)	6(17.1)	7(21.2)
Constipation[a]	34(20.7)	13(43.3)	12(18.2)	5(14.3)	4(12.1)
Diarrhea[b]	23(14.0)	6(20.0)	12(18.2)	2(5.7)	3(9.1)
Pleural effusion and ascites	10(6.1)	4(13.3)	3(4.5)	1(2.9)	2(6.1)
Herpes zoster[c]	26(15.9)	12(40.0)	9(13.6)	3(8.6)	2(6.1)
Deep vein thrombosis	1(0.6)	1(3.3)	0(0.0)	0(0.0)	0(0.0)
Peripheral neuropathy[d]	91(55.5)	25(83.3)	34(51.5)	16(45.7)	16(48.5)
Grade 1	54(32.9)	11(36.7)	18(27.3)	13(37.1)	12(36.4)
Grade 2/3[e]	37(22.6)	14(46.7)	13(19.7)	5(14.3)	5(16.7)

[a]Incidence of constipation for the PTD arm was significantly higher than the PCD, PAD and PD groups (χ^2 = 5.002, 12.240, 9.876, P = 0.025, <0.001, 0.002).
[b]Incidence of diarrhea for the PTD arm was significantly higher than the PD group (χ^2 = 5.577, P = 0.048).
[c]Incidence of herpes zoster for the PTD arm was significantly higher than the PCD, PAD and PD groups (χ^2 = 8.568, 14.552, 12.641, P = 0.003, <0.001, <0.001).
[d]Peripheral neuropathy of all grades was more frequently reported in patients in the PTD group compared to the other groups which was obviously higher than that of the PCD, PAD and PD groups (χ^2 = 4.819, 18.848, 11.182, P = 0.028, <0.001, 0.001).
[e]Incidence of grade 2 to 3 peripheral neuropathy for the PTD arm was significantly higher than the PCD, PAD and PD groups (χ^2 = 7.562, 14.190, 9.584, P = 0.006, <0.001, 0.002). There was no significant difference in other treatment-related adverse events among groups.

Chinese populations [25], the results suggested that ISS had limitation when used for MM patients in China, but further randomized clinical trals are required to confirm this assertion.

Combination therapies based on bortezomib do not appear to cause serious adverse events [3–7,15–22], and we found this to be true as well. The most common non-hematologic toxicities included peripheral neuropathy, fatigue, infection, constipation, herpes zoster and diarrhea. Herpes zoster was documented in 5–13% of cases in the US and Europe [6,15,26], but this was higher in Asia [26–31]. In our study, the incidence of herpes zoster was 41.4% in patients of the PTD group without routine anti-viral therapy, but much more lower in other groups with anti-viral therapy. No serious adverse events emerged, so short-term treatment with a low dose may be safe and effective [26,32].

Peripheral neuropathy (PN) is another frequent adverse event of bortezomib but it is dose-limited and reversible [33–37]. However, how it occurs is not clear. The incidence of PN was higher in this study compared to reports from the US and Europe [15–19,33–36], and this was true in the PTD group but whether bortezomib combined with thalidomide increased the PN incidence and its severity remained uncertain [20,21,33–36]. In our study, PN of a grade 2 or higher was observed in nearly half of the patients who received the PTD regimen, a finding that was significantly higher than in other groups. And the discontinuation rate of thalidomide maintenance in PTD group was higher than PCD, PAD and PD. In fact, this may be a potential contributor to the reduced PFS in PTD group versus other triplet agent therapies. further prospective studies expanding the number of cases should be performed for a more reliable result. However, there were no significant differences among PAD, PCD and PD groups.

Deep vein thrombosis (DVT) is another common treatment-related adverse event with bortezomib and other agents and it is observed in 3–7% of patients in the US and Europe [18,38]. Patients who received PTD have a higher risk of DVT. In our study, routine anti-coagulation or anti-thrombosis agents were not used, and only one patient suffered from DVT/PE but did well with treatment. This frequency may be related to race and particulars of the local population and should be further studied to draw conclusions.

In conclusion, a three-drug combination is superior to bortezomib and dexamethasone, and PAD and PCD regimens are more efficacious with fewer adverse reactions, and the therapy is well-tolerated. In terms of the occurrence frequency and degree of PN, PAD and PCD are superior to PTD, especially the PCD. Considering drug toxicity, convenience and expense, we recommend a PCD scheme as a first-line therapy for MM for initial treatment.

Supporting Information

Table S1 Number of cycles and response rates. Response for four regimens after every cycle are depicted in the Table.

Data S1

Acknowledgments

We are grateful to the staff of Zhejiang University School of Medicine and professor Yunxian Yu for his guidance for the statistical analysis of the study data.

Author Contributions

Conceived and designed the experiments: ZC. Performed the experiments: XYH GFZ JMS WZX LL JZ WJH WYZ GQW WJW YZ XJZ JPF XJY HH. Analyzed the data: JSH LY. Wrote the paper: JSH LY.

References

1. Kyle RA, Rajkumar SV (2008) Multiple myeloma. Blood. 111(6): 2962–2972.
2. Cavo ME, Zamagni P, Tosi P, Tacchetti C, Cellini D, et al. (2005). "Superiority of thalidomide and dexamethasone over vincristine-doxorubicindexamethasone (VAD) as primary therapy in preparation for autologous transplantation for multiple myeloma." Blood 106(1): 35–39.
3. Harousseau JL, Attal M, Avet-Loiseau H, Marit G, Caillot D, et al. (2010) Bortezomib plus dexamethasone is superior to vincristine plus doxorubicin plus dexamethasone as induction treatment prior to autologous stem cell transplantation in newly diagnosed multiple myeloma: results of the IFM 2005-01 phase III trial. J Clin Oncol 28: 4621–4629.
4. Sonneveld P, Schmidt-Wolf IG, van der Holt B, El Jarari L, Bertsch U, et al. (2012) Bortezomib induction and maintenance treatment in patients with newly diagnosed multiple myeloma: results of the randomized phase III HOVON-65/GMMG-HD4 trial. J Clin Oncol 30: 2946–2955.
5. Wang L, Ran X, Wang B, Sheng Z, Liu L (2012) Novel agents-based regimens as induction treatment prior to autologous stem-cell transplantation in newly diagnosed multiple myeloma: a meta-analysis of randomized controlled trials. Hematol Oncol 30: 57–61.
6. Harousseau JL, Palumbo A, Richardson PG, Schlag R, Dimopoulos MA, et al. (2010) Superior outcomes associated with complete response in newly diagnosed multiple myeloma patients treated with nonintensive therapy: analysis of the phase 3 VISTA study of bortezomib plus melphalan-prednisone versus melphalan-prednisone. Blood 116: 3743–3750.
7. De la Rubia J, Roig M. (2011) Bortezomib for previously untreated multiple myeloma. Expert Rev Hematol. 4: 381–398.
8. Durie BG, Harousseau JL, Miguel JS, Blade J, Barlogie B, et al. (2006) International uniform response criteria for multiple myeloma. Leukemia 20: 1467–1473.
9. van de Velde HJ, Liu X, Chen G, Cakana A, Deraedt W, et al. (2007) Complete response correlates with long-term survival and progression-free survival in high-dose therapy in multiple myeloma. Haematologica 92: 1399–1406.
10. Niesvizky R, Richardson PG, Rajkumar SV, Coleman M, Rosinol L, et al. (2008) The relationship between quality of response and clinical benefit for patients treated on the bortezomib arm of the international, randomized, phase 3 APEX trial in relapsed multiple myeloma. Br J Haematol 143: 46–53.
11. Harousseau JL, Attal M, Avet-Loiseau H. (2009) The role of complete response in multiple myeloma. Blood. 114(15): 3139–3146.
12. Lahuerta JJ, Mateos MV, Martinez-Lopez J, Rosinol L, Sureda A, et al. (2008) Influence of pre- and post-transplantation responses on outcome of patients with multiple myeloma: sequential improvement of response and achievement of complete response are associated with longer survival. J Clin Oncol 26: 5775–5782.
13. Barlogie B, Anaissie E, Haessler J, van Rhee F, Pineda-Roman M, et al. (2008) Complete remission sustained 3 years from treatment initiation is a powerful surrogate for extended survival in multiple myeloma. Cancer 113: 355–359.
14. Rajkumar SV. (2012) Doublets, triplets, or quadruplets of novel agents in newly diagnosed myeloma? Hematology Am Soc Hematol Educ Program. 351–361.
15. Harousseau JL, Attal M, Leleu X, Troncy J, Pegourie B, et al. (2006) Bortezomib plus dexamethasone as induction treatment prior to autologous stem cell transplantation in patients with newly diagnosed multiple myeloma: results of an IFM phase II study. Haematologica 91: 1498–1505.
16. Rosinol L, Oriol A, Mateos MV, Sureda A, Garcia-Sanchez P, et al. (2007) Phase II PETHEMA trial of alternating bortezomib and dexamethasone as induction regimen before autologous stem-cell transplantation in younger patients with multiple myeloma: efficacy and clinical implications of tumor response kinetics. J Clin Oncol 25: 4452–4458.
17. Jagannath S, Durie BG, Wolf JL, Camacho ES, Irwin D, et al. (2009) Extended follow-up of a phase 2 trial of bortezomib alone and in combination with dexamethasone for the frontline treatment of multiple myeloma. Br J Haematol 146: 619–626.
18. Reeder CB, Reece DE, Kukreti V, Chen C, Trudel S, et al. (2009) Cyclophosphamide, bortezomib and dexamethasone induction for newly diagnosed multiple myeloma: high response rates in a phase II clinical trial. Leukemia 23: 1337–1341.
19. Palumbo A, Gay F, Falco P, Crippa C, Montefusco V, et al. (2010) Bortezomib as induction before autologous transplantation, followed by lenalidomide as consolidation-maintenance in untreated multiple myeloma patients. J Clin Oncol 28: 800–807.
20. Cavo M, Tacchetti P, Patriarca F, Petrucci MT, Pantani L, et al. (2010) Bortezomib with thalidomide plus dexamethasone compared with thalidomide plus dexamethasone as induction therapy before, and consolidation therapy after, double autologous stem-cell transplantation in newly diagnosed multiple myeloma: a randomised phase 3 study. Lancet 376: 2075–2085.

21. Mateos MV, Oriol A, Martinez-Lopez J, Gutierrez N, Teruel AI, et al. (2010) Bortezomib, melphalan, and prednisone versus bortezomib, thalidomide, and prednisone as induction therapy followed by maintenance treatment with bortezomib and thalidomide versus bortezomib and prednisone in elderly patients with untreated multiple myeloma: a randomised trial. Lancet Oncol 11: 934–941.
22. Reeder CB, Reece DE, Kukreti V, Chen C, Trudel S, et al. (2010) Once- versus twice-weekly bortezomib induction therapy with CyBorD in newly diagnosed multiple myeloma. Blood 115: 3416–3417.
23. Bladé J, Rosiñol L, Cibeira MT. (2008) Prognostic factors for multiple myeloma in the era of novel agents. Ann Oncol. 7: 117–120.
24. Greipp PR, San Miguel J, Durie BG, Crowley JJ, Barlogie B, et al. (2005) International staging system for multiple myeloma. J Clin Oncol 23: 3412–3420.
25. Tao ZF, Fu WJ, Yuan ZG, Wang DX, Chen YB, et al. (2007) Prognostic factors and staging systems of multiple myeloma. Chin Med J (Engl) 120: 1655–1658.
26. Chanan-Khan A, Sonneveld P, Schuster MW, Stadtmauer EA, Facon T, et al. (2008) Analysis of herpes zoster events among bortezomib-treated patients in the phase III APEX study. J Clin Oncol 26: 4784–4790.
27. Aoki T, Nishiyama T, Imahashi N, Kitamura K (2011) Efficacy of continuous, daily, oral, ultra-low-dose 200 mg acyclovir to prevent herpes zoster events among bortezomib-treated patients: a report from retrospective study. Jpn J Clin Oncol 41: 876–881.
28. Tong Y, Qian J, Li Y, Meng H, Jin J (2007) The high incidence of varicella herpes zoster with the use of bortezomib in 10 patients. Am J Hematol 82: 403–404.
29. Ohguchi H, Sugawara T, Ishikawa I, Okuda M, Tomiya Y, et al. (2009) A retrospective analysis of bortezomib therapy for Japanese patients with relapsed or refractory multiple myeloma: beta2-microglobulin associated with time to progression. Int J Hematol 89: 342–347.
30. Zheng W, Wei G, Ye X, He J, Li L, et al. (2009) Bortezomib in combination with dexamethasone and subsequent thalidomide for newly-diagnosed multiple myeloma: a Chinese experience. Leuk Res 33: 1615–1618.
31. Kim SJ, Kim K, Kim BS, Lee HJ, Kim H, et al. (2008) Bortezomib and the increased incidence of herpes zoster in patients with multiple myeloma. Clin Lymphoma Myeloma 8: 237–240.
32. Vickrey E, Allen S, Mehta J, Singhal S (2009) Acyclovir to prevent reactivation of varicella zoster virus (herpes zoster) in multiple myeloma patients receiving bortezomib therapy. Cancer 115: 229–232.
33. Chaudhry V, Cornblath DR, Polydefkis M, Ferguson A, Borrello I (2008) Characteristics of bortezomib- and thalidomide-induced peripheral neuropathy. J Peripher Nerv Syst 13: 275–282.
34. Badros A, Goloubeva O, Dalal JS, Can I, Thompson J, et al. (2007) Neurotoxicity of bortezomib therapy in multiple myeloma: a single-center experience and review of the literature. Cancer 110: 1042–1049.
35. Chaudhry V, Cornblath DR, Polydefkis M, Ferguson A, Borrello I (2008) Characteristics of bortezomib- and thalidomide-induced peripheral neuropathy. J Peripher Nerv Syst 13: 275–282.
36. Richardson PG, Sonneveld P, Schuster MW, Stadtmauer EA, Facon T, et al. (2009) Reversibility of symptomatic peripheral neuropathy with bortezomib in the phase III APEX trial in relapsed multiple myeloma: impact of a dose-modification guideline. Br J Haematol 144: 895–903.
37. Mohty B, El-Cheikh J, Yakoub-Agha I, Moreau P, Harousseau JL, et al. (2010) Peripheral neuropathy and new treatments for multiple myeloma: background and practical recommendations. Haematologica 95: 311–319.
38. Palumbo A, Gay F, Bringhen S, Falcone A, Pescosta N, et al. (2008) Bortezomib, doxorubicin and dexamethasone in advanced multiple myeloma. Ann Oncol 19: 1160–1165.

7

Isolation and Characterization of CD34+ Blast-Derived Exosomes in Acute Myeloid Leukemia

Chang Sook Hong[1], Laurent Muller[1,2], Michael Boyiadzis[1,3], Theresa L. Whiteside[1,4]*

1 University of Pittsburgh Cancer Institute, Pittsburgh, Pennsylvania, United States of America, **2** University Hospital, Department of Otolaryngology and Head & Neck Surgery, Basel, Switzerland, **3** University of Pittsburgh School of Medicine, Division of Hematology-Oncology, Pittsburgh, Pennsylvania, United States of America, **4** University of Pittsburgh School of Medicine, Departments of Pathology, Immunology and Otolaryngology, Pittsburgh, Pennsylvania, United States of America

Abstract

Exosomes are membrane-bound vesicles found in all biological fluids. AML patients' plasma collected at diagnosis contains elevated exosome levels relative to normal donor (ND) plasma. The molecular profile of AML exosomes changes in the course of therapy and may serve as a measure of disease progression or response to therapy. However, plasma contains a mix of exosomes derived from various cell types. To be able to utilize blast-derived exosomes as biomarkers for AML, we have developed an immunoaffinity-based capture method utilizing magnetic microbeads coated with anti-CD34 antibody (Ab). This Ab is specific for CD34, a unique marker of AML blasts. The capture procedure was developed using CD34+ exosomes derived from Kasumi-1 AML cell culture supernatants. The capture capacity of CD34microbeads was shown to linearly correlate with the input exosomes. A 10 uL aliquot of CD34 microbeads was able to capture all of CD34+ exosomes present in 100–1,000 uL of AML plasma. The levels of immunocaptured CD34+ exosomes correlated with the percentages of CD34+ blasts in the AML patients' peripheral blood. The immunocaptured exosomes had a typical cup-shaped morphology by transmission electron microscopy, and their molecular cargo was similar to that of parental blasts. These exosomes were biologically-active. Upon co-incubation with natural killer (NK) cells, captured blast-derived exosomes down-regulated surface NKG2D expression, while non-captured exosomes reduced expression levels of NKp46. Our data provide a proof-of-principle that blast-derived exosomes can be quantitatively recovered from AML patients' plasma, their molecular profile recapitulates that of autologous blasts and they retain the ability to mediate immune suppression. These data suggest that immunocaptured blast-derived exosomes might be useful in diagnosis and/or prognosis of AML in the future.

Editor: Zhuang Zuo, UT MD Anderson Cancer Center, United States of America

Funding: National Institutes of Health, USA grants PO1-CA109688 and R01-CA168628 to TLW (www.nih.gov). The funders had no role in study design, data collection and analysis, decision to publish, or preparation of the manuscript.

Competing Interests: The authors have declared that no competing interests exist.

* Email: whitesidetl@upmc.edu

Introduction

Although advances in acute myeloid leukemia (AML) therapy have considerably improved initial response rates and patients' quality of life, survival rates remain low, largely due to disease relapse [1,2]. The failure of conventional therapies to control leukemic relapse has stimulated the search for novel, more effective therapeutic approaches. Recently, tumor-derived exosomes (TEX) have emerged as one of the key modulators of immune evasion/suppression in cancer, including hematologic malignancies [3–6]. In view of emerging evidence for the critical role of the host immune system in cancer progression, evaluation of the impact TEX exert on the disease activity, severity and response to therapy in AML is of great interest.

Exosomes are 30 to 100 nm intraluminal vesicles (ILV) generated by inward budding of endosomal multivesicular bodies (MVB). MVB traffic to and fuse with the plasma membrane, releasing ILV into the extracellular space [7]. The exosomal cargo includes proteins/glycoproteins expressed on the cell membrane as well as molecules and soluble factors present in the cytosol of parental cells. Exosomes are found in all biological fluids, including urine, plasma or ascites. While exosome secretion occurs under physiologic conditions, and all cells are capable of their release, tumor cells are avid exosome producers. Importantly, exosome fractions obtained from plasma of cancer patients are enriched in molecules which play a role in tumor proliferation, immune escape and metastasis [8–12].

Plasma of newly-diagnosed AML patients contains higher levels of exosomal protein (in µg/mL plasma) than normal donors' (ND) plasma [13,14]. Also, AML exosomes have a distinct molecular profile. In addition to conventional exosome markers, such as tetraspanins, they contain membrane-associated TGF-β1, MICA/MICB, FasL and myeloid blast markers, CD33, CD34 and CD117 [13]. When tested *ex vivo*, AML exosomes decreased natural killer (NK)-cell cytotoxicity by down-regulating NKG2D expression levels in normal NK cells [13,14]. Antibody neutralization of TGF-β1 carried by AML exosomes partially restored NK-cell functions, suggesting that exosome-associated TGF-β1 is in part responsible for NK-cell dysfunction in AML. Thus, exosomes present in AML patients' plasma have a potential to modulate innate immune responses and could influence disease progression or response to therapy.

Exosomes are purified from biological fluids using differential centrifugation, ultrafiltration, size-exclusion chromatography and high-speed ultracentrifugation [13,14]. However, exosomes isolated from human plasma are largely derived from normal cells, such as e.g., platelets, which are known to be strong exosome producers [15]. TEX, if present in plasma, probably account for only a fraction of all isolated exosomes. We hypothesize that AML blast-derived exosomes are more biologically active than exosomes produced by normal cells and that they largely mediate immune suppression. To be able to perform molecular analyses of blast-derived exosomes, establish their clinical significance and determine their role as potential biomarkers of disease progression/relapse, it is first necessary to separate them from plasma exosomes derived from normal cells. Because AML blast-derived exosomes carry a unique set of membrane-associated molecules, which mimic those present in the membrane of AML blasts, they can be distinguished and separated from non-blast exosomes present in the same plasma. Based on this principle, we have developed an immunoaffinity-based capture method for AML blast-derived exosomes using microbeads coated with anti-CD34 antibody (Ab). Our data provide a proof-of- principle that blast-derived exosomes can be quantitatively recovered from AML patients' plasma and that their molecular profile recapitulates that of the blasts. These isolated exosomes are biologically-active, mediate immune suppression and might be useful in AML diagnosis and/or prognosis in the future.

Materials and Methods

Cell culture supernatants

A human CD34+ leukemic cell line (Kasumi-1) was purchased from American Type Culture Collection (Manassas, VA, USA) and cultured in RPMI supplemented with 2 mM/ml L-glutamine, 100 U/ml penicillin, 100 ug/ml streptomycin and 10% (v/v) fetal bovine serum (FBS). All reagents were purchased from Invitrogen (Grand Island, NY, USA). FBS was depleted of bovine exosomes by ultracentrifugation at 100,000×g for 3 hrs. Conditioned media (CM) were collected from 48–72 hr sub-confluent cell cultures after centrifugation at 10,000 g for 30 min and concentrated using a Vivacell 100 unit (Sartorius Corp, Bohemia, NY, USA). Concentrated CM was filtered using a 0.22 um syringe-filter unit and used for exosome isolation.

Plasma of AML patients and healthy donors

Samples of venous blood (20–50 mL) were obtained from newly-diagnosed AML patients prior to any treatment and from age-matched healthy volunteers. All subjects participating in this study signed an informed consent approved by the Institutional Review Board of the University of Pittsburgh (IRB #960279, IRB #0403105 and IRB #0506140). Peripheral blood was collected into heparinized vacutainer tubes, and the samples were hand-carried to the laboratory. Plasma was centrifuged at 1000×g for 10 min to remove blood cells and cell fragments. Clear plasma was collected and immediately used for exosome capture or aliquoted into vials, which were stored in liquid N_2. Frozen and thawed plasma was centrifuged at 10,000 g for 30 min and used for exosome isolation and for immunoaffinity capture as described below.

Exosome isolation from plasma or cell supernatants

Exosomes were isolated from CM of cultured cells or from clarified plasma of ND or AML patients as previously described [13,14] with minor modifications. Briefly, following centrifugation at 10,000×g for 30 min, aliquots of plasma (up to 9 mL) were passed through a 0.22 μm pore size filter and applied to Bio-Gel A50 m columns (Bio-Rad Laboratories, Hercules, CA, USA) packed with Sepharose 2B (Sigma-Aldrich, St. Louis, MO, USA). The column was eluted with phosphate buffered saline (PBS). Fractions between 10 and 28 mL (the void volume peak), which contained proteins of more than 50 million kDa, were collected into a Beckman Optiseal Centrifuge Tube and centrifuged in a Beckman Optima LE-80K Ultracentrifuge (Beckman Coulter, Atlanta, GA, USA) at 100,000×g for 2 h at 4°C. The pellet was resuspended in PBS (200 μL) and analyzed using a protein assay kit (Bio-Rad Laboratories, Hercules, CA, USA).

Immunoaffinity capture of exosomes from plasma

To isolate blast-derived exosomes from plasma of patients with $CD34^+$ blasts, the CD34 microbead kit (Miltenyi Biotec, Auburn, CA, USA) was used. From 0.1 to 1 mL of freshly-thawed plasma was used for immune capture. Exosomes captured on CD34 Ab-coated magnetic beads were recovered from the magnetic column by eluting with Tris Buffered Saline (TBS) as described by the manufacturer (MS column, Miltenyi Biotec, Auburn, CA, USA). Exosome-coated beads were pelleted by centrifugation at 10,000×g for 30 min. Captured exosomes were visualized by transmission electron microscopy (TEM), co-cultured with NK cells or lysed in 2x Laemmli sample buffer for Western blot analyses. In separate experiments, $CD61^+$ exosomes were also captured from patients' plasma using CD61 microbead kits (Miltenyi Biotec, Auburn, CA, USA) to capture and remove platelet-derived exosomes.

Transmission electron microscopy

TEM was performed at the Center for Biologic Imaging at the University of Pittsburgh. Freshly-isolated exosomes were put on a copper grid coated with 0.125% Formvar in chloroform. The grids were stained with 1% v/v uranyl acetate in ddH2O and the samples were examined immediately. A JEOL 1011 transmission electron microscope was used for imaging.

Western blots

Isolated or immunocaptured exosomes were tested for the presence of CD63, CD81, CD34, GAPDH, CD200, CD44 and CD105 using western blots as previously described [14]. Briefly, 10 μg of exosomes were lysed with Laemmli sample buffer (Bio-Rad Laboratories, Hercules, CA, USA), separated on 7–15% SDS/PAGE gels and transferred onto PVDF membrane (Millipore, Billerica, MA, USA) for western blot analysis. Membranes were incubated overnight at 4°C with antibodies specific for: CD63 (1:200, sc-15363, Santa Cruz, CA, USA), CD34 (1:2000, ab81289, Abcam, Cambridge, MA, USA), CD81 (1:200, PA5-13582, Thermo Fisher, Pittsburgh, PA, USA), GAPDH (1:500, FL-335, Santa Cruz, CA, USA), CD200 (1:2000, AF2724, R&D, Minneapolis, MN, USA), CD44 (1:1000, ab41478, Abcam, Cambridge, MA, USA), CD105 (1:1000, ab169545, Abcam, Cambridge, MA, USA), platelet IIb/IIIa (1:200, sc-73544, Santa Cruz, CA, USA). Next, the HRP-conjugated secondary antibody (1:5000, Pierce, Thermo Fisher, Pittsburgh, PA, USA) was added for 1 hr at room temperature (RT) and blots were developed with ECL detection reagents (GE Healthcare Biosciences, Pittsburgh, PA, USA). The intensities of the bands on exposed films were quantified using Image J software (NIH, USA).

Flow cytometry

Kasumi-1 cells (2×10^5) were labeled with phycoerythrin (PE)-conjugated anti-CD33, CD34, CD117 or CD81 antibodies (all from Beckman Coulter, Atlanta, GA, USA) for 20 minutes at 4°C and analyzed using a 4-color Beckman Coulter XL, and data were analyzed using the Expo32-Software.

Functional studies with captured CD34+ exosomes

Normal human NK cells were co-incubated with isolated exosomes to determine expression levels of the natural cytotoxicity receptor NKp46 and of NKG2D on the surface of these cells as previously described [13,14]. Briefly, NK cells (1×10^5) were co-incubated for 24 h with CD34+ exosomes captured directly from 1 mL AML plasma or unbound $CD34^{negative}$ exosomes. Then, flow cytometry for expression of NKG2D or NKp46 was performed and data expressed as mean fluorescence intensity (MFI). NK cells incubated in medium without exosomes were used as controls. Isolation of human NK cells from normal donor buffy coats using AutoMACS (Miltenyi Biotec, Auburn, CA, USA) was previously described [13,14]. PE-conjugated anti-NKG2D and anti-NKp46 antibodies or isotype controls were purchased from Beckman Coulter (Atlanta, GA, USA).

Results

Immunoaffinity exosome capture

The strategy used for exosome capture from patients' plasma is illustrated in Figure 1A. Freshly harvested or frozen/thawed plasma was processed as shown in Figure 1B, yielding the captured CD34+exosome fraction and non-captured CD34neg exosomes.

Characteristics of Kasumi-1 cell line-derived exosomes

Kasumi-1 cell line is a leukemic cell line established from peripheral blood of an AML patient with 8; 21 chromosome translocation. It originated from early myeloid stem cell [16,17] and expresses leukemic blast markers, including CD34, CD33, CD117 (Figure 2A). Exosomes present in supernatants of cultured Kasumi-1 cells were initially isolated by ultracentrifugation and used to implement the strategy shown in Figure 1A. Isolated Kasumi-1 exosomes floated at density of 1.10–1.14 on a continuous sucrose density gradient (Figure 2B) and were visualized by TEM as typical cup-shaped vesicles measuring 30–70 nM in diameter (Figure 2C). In Western blots, their protein profile included CD34, a blast marker, as well as CD81, the tetraspanin used as an exosomal marker (Figure 2D). Exosomes isolated from supernatants of Kasumi cells recapitulated the molecular profile of the Kasumi cell line (Figure 2D). In addition, Kasumi-1 exosomes also carried proteins known to be expressed in leukemia stem cells: CD44, CD200 and CD105 (Figure 2D). Exosomes isolated from ND plasma were not $CD34^+$ (Figure 2D).

Development of immunocapture using $CD34^+$ exosomes isolated from Kasumi-1 supernatants

Anti-CD34 Ab-coated microbeads were used to establish optimal conditions for capture of CD34+ exosomes from supernatants of Kasumi-1 cells. First, exosomes were isolated from Kasumi-1 supernatants by ultracentrifugation. The capture capacity of microbeads was calibrated using densitometric analysis of western blot bands reactive with anti-CD34 Ab. As shown in Figure 3A, pixel intensity of each CD34 band linearly correlated with the exosomal protein level loaded on the SDS/PAGE gel. A 5 to10 μL aliquot of CD34 Ab-coated microbeads was able to capture all $CD34^+$ exosomes from 20 μg of isolated Kasumi-1 exosomes (Figure 3B, *left*). The beads capture capacity was not improved when the bead concentration was increased to 20 μL (Figure 3B, *left*). Increasing the protein levels of the input exosomes linearly correlated with the protein level of captured $CD34^+$ exosomes (Figure 3B, *right and graph*). However, capture efficiency was only about 40% (Figure 3B, *graph*). To improve capture efficiency, additional CD34 microbeads were added after the removal of captured $CD34^+$ exosomes. As shown in Figure 4, this second step resulted in capture of additional Kasumi-1-derived $CD34^+$ exosomes, but the final *unbound* exosomal fraction still contained $CD34^+$ exosomes. However, AML plasma-derived $CD34^+$exosomes were completely captured by the first co-incubation with microbeads (Figure 4). The unbound fraction did not contain any $CD34^+$ exosomes, although it did contain other exosomal proteins such as CD81. Control exosomes derived from ND plasma did not contain $CD34^+$ exosomes. While two repetitions of immunocapture with 10 μL of CD34 microbeads

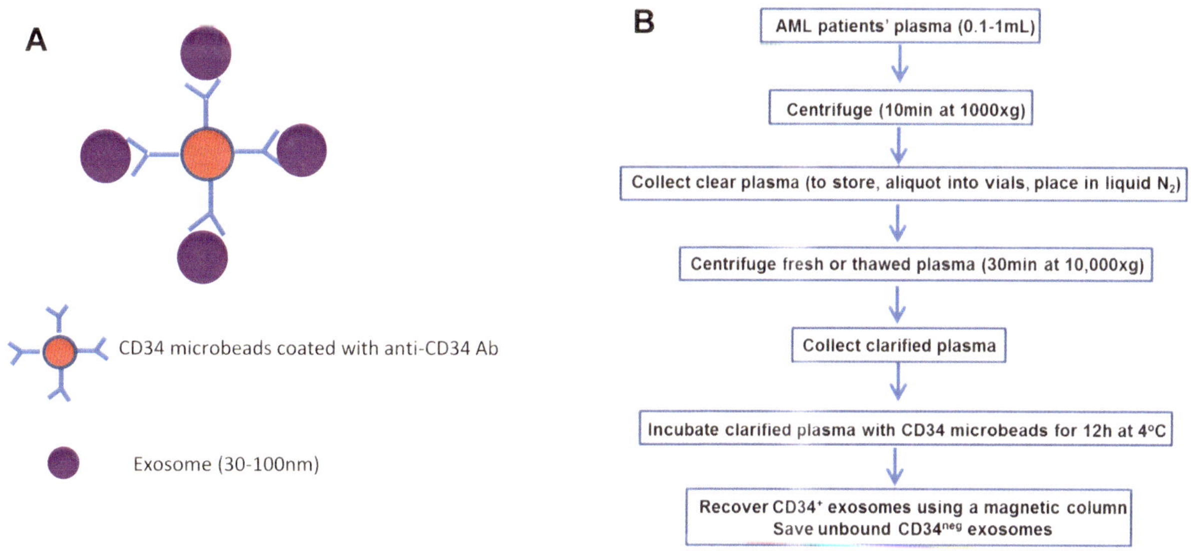

Figure 1. The strategy for capture of $CD34^+$ exosomes using anti-CD34 Ab-coated microbeads purchased from Miltenyi (A) and a schema for capture of $CD34^+$ exosomes directly from AML patients' plasma (B).

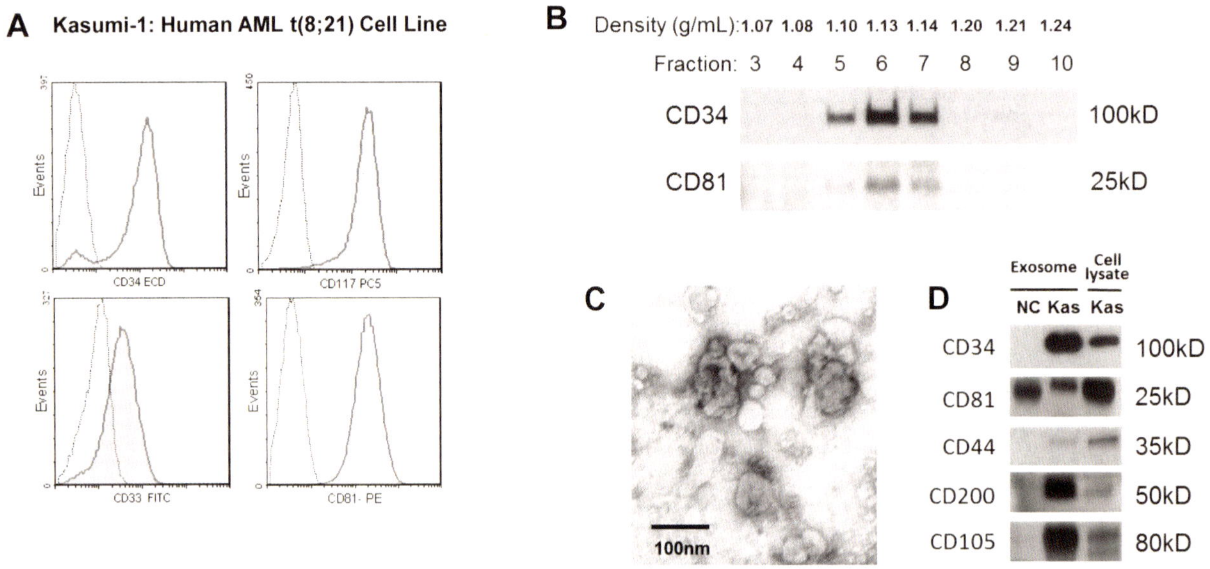

Figure 2. Studies with the Kasumi-1 cell line and with exosomes derived from Kasumi-1 culture supernatants. A) Flow cytometry of Kasumi-1 cells shows expression of blast markers, CD34, CD117 and CD33 and of CD81 (tetraspanin). Dotted lines indicate isotype controls. B) Kasumi-1 exosomes were separated on a continuous sucrose density gradient, and the collected gradient fractions were tested in Western blots for CD34 and CD81. $CD34^+$ and $CD81^+$ exosomes were recovered at the density of 1.10–1.14. C) An electron microscope image of isolated and negatively stained Kasumi-1 exosomes. D) Western blots of isolated Kasumi-1 exosomes (Kas) and of exosomes isolated from plasma of a normal donor (NC). Each lane was loaded with 10 μg exosomal protein.

each were necessary to capture about 75% $CD34^+$ exosomes present in 100 μg of supernatant-derived exosomes, one 10 μL aliquot of CD34 microbeads was sufficient for capture of all $CD34^+$ exosomes from 100 μg of exosomes obtained from AML plasma.

Capture of $CD34^+$ blast-derived exosomes directly from AML plasma

Anti-CD34 Ab-coated microbeads were next used to capture exosomes directly from AML patients' plasma. For direct exosome capture, an aliquot (0.1–1 mL) of freshly-harvested or frozen/thawed plasma was co-incubated with a 10 μL aliquot of microbeads coated with anti-CD34 Ab. CD34+ exosomes were captured using a magnetic column as described in Materials and

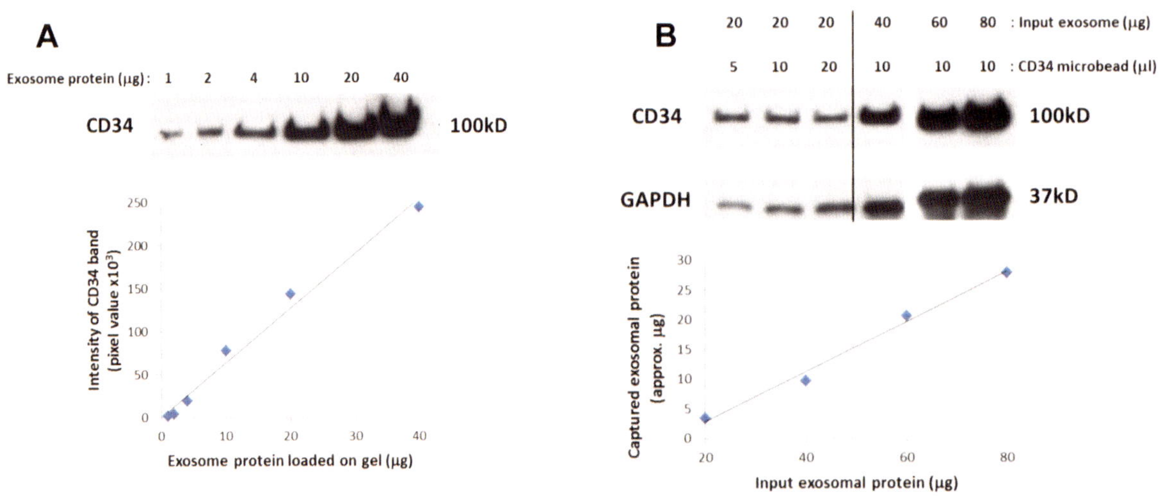

Figure 3. Calibration experiments with $CD34^+$ Kasumi-1 exosomes isolated by ultracentrifugation. A) Isolated exosomes were loaded at increasing protein concentrations onto gels and blotted using anti-CD34 Ab. Intensity of each band was measured in pixels. The graph illustrates a linear relationship between exosomal protein levels and pixel intensity in Western blots. B) Isolated exosomes (20 μg protein) were added to increasing volumes of CD34 microbeads (*left*). Five or 10 μL of microbeads were sufficient to capture 20 μg of exosomes. Next, a 10 μL aliquot of beads was used to capture increasing concentrations of Kasumi-1 exosomes (*right*). The graph shows that the capacity of CD34 microbeads to capture up to 80 μg of input exosomes increased linearly. However, at 80 μg only about 40% of exosomal proteins were captured, suggesting that additional microbeads are necessary for capture of all Kasumi-1 exosomes.

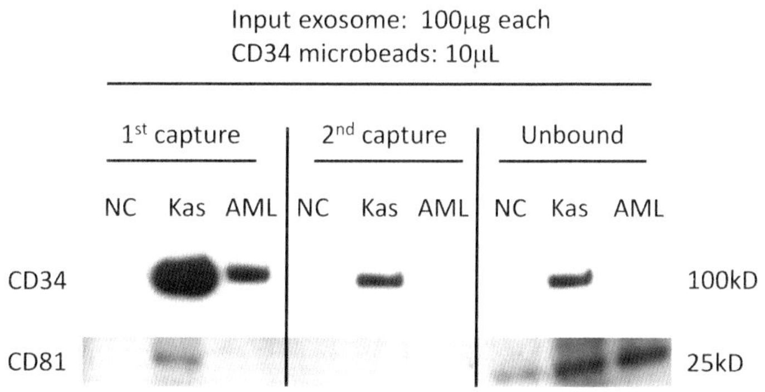

Figure 4. Capture of CD34+ exosomes from total exosomal fractions by CD34+ microbeads. Isolated Kasumi-1 exosomes (Kas) and total exosome fractions isolated by ultracentrifugation from normal donor plasma (NC) or from CD34$^+$ AML patient plasma (AML) were used for capture with CD34 microbeads. After the 1st capture and removal of beads, 2nd capture was performed with a fresh aliquot of CD34 microbeads. The final unbound fractions were ultracentrifuged to collect remaining exosomes. While the 2nd capture was necessary to recover all CD34$^+$ Kasumi-1 exosomes, a single capture was sufficient to recover all CD34$^+$ exosomes from the bulk of exosomes isolated from the AML plasma. There were no CD34$^+$ exosomes captured from the bulk exosomal fraction isolated from a normal donor's plasma. CD81 expression indicates that the unbound fractions still contain CD34^{neg} exosomes.

Methods (Figure 1). The TEM images of the recovered fraction showed cup-shaped exosomes attached to microbeads (Figure 5A). The capture capacity of CD34$^+$ exosomes from AML plasma correlated linearly with the input volume (in µL) of plasma (Figure 5B). Therefore, using 10 µL of CD34 microbeads, we were able to capture all CD34$^+$ exosomes from 100 µL to 1000 µL of AML patients' plasma. This capture procedure was reproduced with five different AML plasma- and five ND plasma- derived exosomes (data not shown). To determine whether protein levels of captured CD34$^+$ exosomes reflect the percentage of CD34$^+$ blasts in the peripheral circulation of AML patients, exosomes were captured from plasma of 5 patients with high or low blast counts as shown in Figure 5C. Patients with ~60% circulating CD34$^+$ blasts had the highest exosome recovery relative to the patients with fewer blasts in the periphery. Incidentally, CD34+ exosomes carry highly variable quantities of CD81, as shown, e.g., in Figure 5C. For this reason, we prefer to use GAPDH or CD63 as markers of AML exosomes (Figures 5B or D).

Potential interference of platelet derived exosomes

Since platelets are one of the major producers of exosomes found in plasma [15], an attempt was made to determine whether platelet-derived exosomes non-specifically bind to CD34 microbeads. We attempted to remove platelet-derived exosomes from plasma using anti-CD61 Ab-coated microbeads. These beads effectively captured exosomes positive for glycoprotein IIb/IIIa as seen in Figure 5D *(left)*. Following the removal of CD61$^+$ exosomes, CD34 microbeads were added to the remaining plasma to capture CD34+ exosomes. The recovered CD34$^+$ exosomes did not contain glycoprotein IIb/IIIa (Figure 5D, right). This experiment showed that unwanted exosomes, which potentially could interfere with capture of CD34+ exosomes or compromise their purity, may be removed by an additional immunocapture step with selected Ab-coated microbeads.

Characteristics of captured CD34$^+$ blast-derived exosomes

Western blots of CD34$^+$ exosomes captured from AML patients' plasma show that in addition to CD34, these exosomes carry proteins known as AML prognostic markers, including CD105 and CD200 (Figure 6A). The same markers were detected in exosomes captured from supernatants of the Kasumi-1 cell line (Figure 2D).

To determine whether the captured CD34$^+$ exosomes are biologically active, purified normal human NK cells were co-incubated with captured CD34$^+$ exosomes or CD34^{neg} exosomes and analyzed by flow cytometry for expression of NK cytotoxicity receptors. Captured CD34$^+$ exosomes inhibited NKG2D expression in the NK cells, while CD34^{neg} exosomes reduced the expression of NKp46 (Figure 6B). These results indicate that the CD34$^+$ and CD34^{neg} exosomes have differential effects on NK cells.

Discussion

The rationale for development of the method for immunocapture of AML blast-derived exosomes from plasma of patients with CD34$^+$ AML is based on existing evidence for selective ability of tumor-derived exosomes (TEX) to mediate immunosuppression [3–6]. Given that anti-tumor functions of immune cells are critical for the control of tumor progression in solid and hematological cancers [18,19]; TEX-mediated immunosuppression could promote tumor growth and increase the rate of recurrence. Exosomes present in cancer patients' plasma are derived from normal as well as malignant cell, and true biologic effects of such mixed populations may be difficult to discern. As only TEX are expected to carry tumor-derived signals responsible for altering functions of immune cells, capture of TEX and their separation from the bulk of plasma exosomes is a necessary and potentially important step.

Several studies have previously tried to immunocapture exosomes from plasma. For example, the widely-advertised Exotest kit uses a sandwich ELISA in which anti-Rab-5b Abs are immobilized in wells of 96-well plates and the captured exosomes are detected with anti-CD63 Abs [20]. For capture of exosomes in supernatants of colon cancer cell lines, anti-A33 Ab-coated Dynabeads or anti-EpCAM Ab-coated microbeads have been used prior to proteomics-based analyses [21,22]. These studies showed that the immunoaffinity-based capture was the most effective method for obtaining exosomes suitable for protein profiling, because these exosomes carried clinically-relevant tumor-specific proteins.

Based on this rationale and using somewhat different capturing strategy, we utilized AML patients' plasma, which was previously

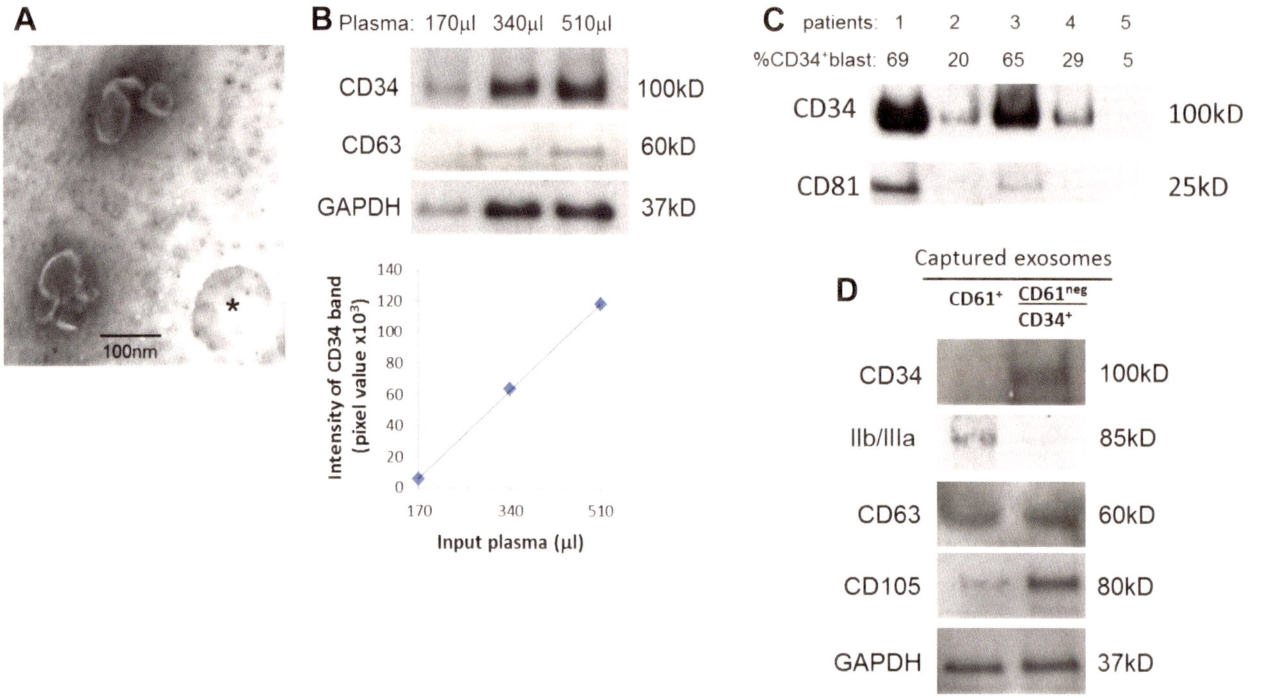

Figure 5. Capture of CD34^{+} blast-derived exosomes directly from AML patients' plasma. A) Negatively stained electron microscope images of exosomes captured on CD34 microbeads (* shows a vacant microbead). B) Increasing AML plasma volumes were used for capture of CD34^{+} exosomes by microbeads and recovered exosomes were studied by Western blots. The graph shows a linear relationship between the input plasma volumes and pixel densities of captured and blotted CD34^{+} exosomes. C) Exosomes were captured from plasma samples obtained from five CD34^{+} AML patients and were analyzed by Western blots. The percentage of leukemic blasts in the peripheral circulation of each of the patients is shown. CD81 serves as the exosome marker. D) Removal of platelet-derived exosomes from plasma using anti-CD61 Ab-coated microbeads prior to capture of CD34^{+} exosomes. Exosomes captured with CD61 microbeads (*left*: CD61^{+}) and CD34^{+} exosomes captured after removing CD61^{+} exosomes (*right*: CD61neg/CD34^{+}) are shown in a representative Western blot of three evaluated.

shown to be a rich source of exosomes [13,14], to separate CD34^{+} from CD34^{neg} exosomes. Titration experiments with different quantities of the anti-CD34 Ab-coated beads and input exosomes allowed for quantification of the capture method and estimations of exosome recovery. In fact, the method allows for recovery of immunocaptured as well as non-captured exosomes and their comparisons in Western blots or functional assays. The identity of captured exosomes was confirmed by TEM. In addition, Western blots of captured exosomes showed they carried not only CD34 but also other AML blast markers in addition to the usual exosome markers. In AML, several markers are available for identification of leukemic blasts by flow cytometry or immunohistochemistry, including CD34, CD33, CD117, CD133, CD90, CD99, CCL-1 and others [2]. Among them, CD34 has been most extensively studied and shown to be associated with unfavorable outcome [23]. CD34^{+} blasts, like primitive leukemic stem cells, are resistant to apoptosis induced by chemotherapy and can transfer the disease in xenograft transplant models [2,24,25]. Although CD34 is

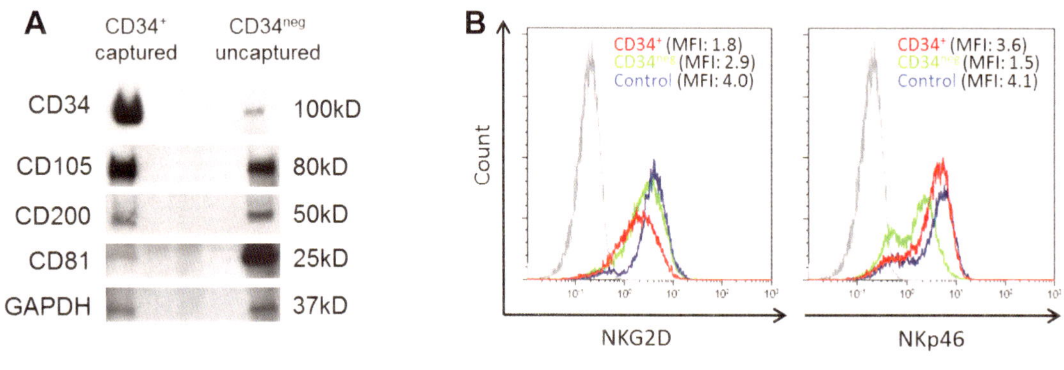

Figure 6. Characteristics of captured exosomes. A) A representative Western blot profile of the captured CD34^{+} exosomes and of non-captured CD34^{neg} exosomes which were isolated by ultracentrifugation from the same AML plasma sample. B) After co-incubation of NK cells with CD34^{+} exosomes captured directly from AML plasma or CD34^{neg} exosomes as described in materials and Methods, NKG2D expression (in MFI) was found to be down-regulated only with CD34+ exosomes (*red*) compared to CD34^{neg} exosomes (*green*) or control without exosomes (*blue*). The *gray* peak denotes isotype control. In contrast, NKp46 expression was down-regulated by co-incubation with CD34^{neg} exosomes.

expressed on normal hematopoietic precursor cells, AML blasts overexpress CD34, and only exosomes isolated from AML patients' plasma but not plasma of ND carried CD34. Therefore, selection of CD34 for immune capture of blast-derived exosomes is justified. However, only about 40% of AML patients have $CD34^+$ blasts [26,27]. For immunocapture of blast-derived exosomes in $CD34^{neg}$ AML, beads coated with Abs to other blast markers, e.g., CCL-1 or CD99, or beads coated with a mix of several Abs could be used, pending a further modification of the capturing method. This strategy should allow for a broader application of this method to exosome capture in all AML patients.

We developed and optimized this procedure for immunocapture of $CD34^+$ blast-derived exosomes from AML plasma in expectation that it will provide a specific tool for separation of tumor-derived immunologically-active exosomes from the bulk of those present in plasma and for discrimination of their potentially different biologic activities. Interestingly, preliminary experiments with NK cells used as targets for exosomes indicated that blast-derived captured exosomes had distinct biological activity from that mediated by non-captured exosomes. The former down-regulated NKG2D but not NKp46 expression levels, while the latter down-regulated NKp46 but not NKG2D expression levels. These data suggest that immunocaptured vs non-captured AML exosomes may have distinct biological effects. Having previously shown that TGF-β1carried by AML exosomes down-regulates NKG2D on NK cells [13], we are now attempting to show that these differential effects might reflect differences in TGF-β1 levels on CD34+ vs CD34negative exosomes. This is consistent with our hypothesis that isolation of blast-derived exosomes may be important for their use as future biomarkers. For AML patients with $CD34^+$ blasts, this immunocapture method will now be used to perform molecular profiling of AML blast-derived exosomes and of non-captured, non-blast derived exosomes. This should indicate whether blast-derived exosomes could more effectively serve as indicators of the presence of leukemic blasts in the bone marrow or as biomarkers of response to therapies. We have already shown that the protein levels of total plasma exosomes and their molecular profiles dramatically change in the course of chemotherapy [14]. These data emphasized the potential clinical significance of AML plasma-derived exosomes (isolated but not selectively captured) as a sensitive biological measure of leukemic blast persistence after chemotherapy and as a potential predictor of relapse in AML. The ability to immunocapture blast-derived exosomes is expected to improve the diagnostic and prognostic potential of exosomes in AML.

Author Contributions

Conceived and designed the experiments: MB TLW CSH LM. Performed the experiments: CSH LM. Analyzed the data: MB TLW CSH LM. Contributed reagents/materials/analysis tools: MB TLW CSH LM. Contributed to the writing of the manuscript: MB TLW CSH LM.

References

1. Burnett A, Wetzler M, Lowenberg B (2011) Therapeutic advances in acute myeloid leukemia. J Clin Onc 29(5): 487 94.
2. Horton SJ, Huntly BJ (2012) Recent advances in acute myeloid leukemia stem cell biology. Haematologica 97: 966 74.
3. EL Andaloussi S, Mäger I, Breakefield XO, Wood MJ (2013) Extracellular vesicles: biology and emerging therapeutic opportunities. Nat Rev Drug Discov 12: 347 57.
4. Peinado H, Aleckovic M, Lavotshkin S, Matei I, Costa-Silva B, et al. (2012) Melanoma exosomes educate bone marrow progenitor cells toward a pro-metastatic phenotype through MET. Nat Med 18: 883 91.
5. Filipazzi P, Burdek M, Villa A, Rivoltini L, Huber V (2012) Recent advances on the role of tumor exosomes in immunosuppression and disease progression. Semin Cancer Biol 22: 342 9.
6. Whiteside TL (2013) Immune modulation of T-cell and NK (natural killer) cell activities by TEXs (tumour-derived exosomes). Biochem Soc Transact 41: 245 51
7. Thery C, Zitvogel L, Amigorena S (2002) Exosomes: composition, biogenesis and function. Nat Rev Immunol 2: 569 79
8. Zhang HG, Zhuang X, Sun D, Liu Y, Xiang X, et al. (2012) Exosomes and immune surveillance of neoplastic lesions: a review. Biotech Histochem 87: 161 8.
9. Taylor DD, Gercel-Taylor C (2011) Exosomes/microvesicles: mediators of cancer-associated immunosuppressive microenvironments. Semin Immunopathol 33: 441 54.
10. Martínez-Lorenzo MJ, Anel A, Alava MA, Piñeiro A, Naval J, et al. (2004) The human melanoma cell line MelJuSo secretes bioactive FasL and APO2L/TRAIL on the surface of microvesicles. Possible contribution to tumor counterattack. Exp Cell Res 295: 315 29.
11. Andreola G, Rivoltini L, Castelli C, Huber V, Perego P, et al. (2002) Induction of lymphocyte apoptosis by tumor cell secretion of FasL-bearing microvesicles. J Exp Med 195: 1303 16.
12. Valenti R, Huber V, Filipazzi P, Pilla L, Sovena G, et al. (2006) Human tumor-released microvesicles promote the differentiation of myeloid cells with transforming growth factor-beta-mediated suppressive activity on T lymphocytes. Cancer Res 66: 9290 8.
13. Szczepanski MJ, Szajnik M, Welsh A, Whiteside TL, Boyiadzis M (2011) Blast-derived microvesicles in sera from patients with acute myeloid leukemia suppress natural killer cell function via membrane-associated transforming growth factor-beta1. Haematologica 96: 1302 9.
14. Hong CS, Muller L, Whiteside TL, Boyiadzis M (2014) Plasma Exosomes as Markers of Therapeutic Response in Patients with Acute Myeloid Leukemia. Front Immunol 5: 160
15. Muller L, Hong C-S, Stolz DR, Watkins S, Whiteside TL (2014) Isolation of biologically active exosomes from human plasma. Ms. submitted.
16. Aatonen M, Grönholm M, Siljander PR (2012) Platelet-derived microvesicles: multitalented participants in intercellular communication. Semin Thromb Hemost 38: 102 13.
17. Asou H, Tashiro S, Hamamoto K, Otsuji A, Kita K, et al. (1991) Establishment of a human acute myeloid leukemia cell line (Kasumi-1) with 8;21 chromosome translocation, Blood 77: 2031 2036.
18. Larizza L, Magnani I, Beghini A (2005) The Kasumi-1 cell line: a t(8;21)-kit mutant model for acute myeloid leukemia. Leuk Lymphoma 46: 247 55.
19. Teague RM, Kline J (2013) Immune evasion in acute myeloid leukemia: current concepts and future directions. J Immunother Cancer 1(13).
20. Whiteside TL (2014) Regulatory T cell subsets in human cancer: are they regulating for or against tumor progression? Cancer Immunol Immunother 63: 67 72.
21. Logozzi M1, De Milito A, Lugini L, Borghi M, Calabrò L, et al. (2009) High levels of exosomes expressing CD63 and caveolin-1 in plasma of melanoma patients. PLoS One 4(4):e5219.
22. Mathivanan S, Lim JW, Tauro BJ, Ji H, Moritz RL, et al. (2010) Proteomics analysis of A33 immunoaffinity-purified exosomes released from the human colon tumor cell line LIM1215 reveals a tissue-specific protein signature. Mol Cell Proteomics 9: 197 208.
23. Tauro BJ, Greening DW, Mathias RA, Mathivanan S, Ji H, et al. (2013) Two distinct populations of exosomes are released from LIM1863 colon carcinoma cell-derived organoids. Mol Cell Proteomics 12: 587 98.
24. van Stijn A, van der Pol MA, Kok A, Bontje PM, et al. (2003) Differences between the CD34+ and CD34- blast compartments in apoptosis resistance in acute myeloid leukemia. Haematologica 88: 497 508.
25. Ishikawa F1, Yoshida S, Saito Y, Hijikata A, Kitamura H, et al. (2007) Chemotherapy-resistant human AML stem cells home to and engraft within the bone-marrow endosteal region. Nat Biotechnol 25: 1315 21.
26. Oyan AM, Bo TH, Jonassen I, Ulvestad E, Gjertsen BT, et al. (2005) CD34 expression in native human acute myelogenous leukemia blasts: differences in CD34 membrane molecule expression are associated with different gene expression profiles. Cytometry B Clin Cytom 64: 18 27.
27. Blair A, Hogge DE, Sutherland HJ (1998) Most acute myeloid leukemia progenitor cells with long-term proliferative ability in vitro and in vivo have the phenotype CD34+/CD71-/HLA-DR+. Blood 92: 4325 4335.

8

MNK1-Induced eIF-4E Phosphorylation in Myeloma Cells: A Pathway Mediating IL-6-Induced Expansion and Expression of Genes Involved in Metabolic and Proteotoxic Responses

Yijiang Shi[1,2,3], Patrick Frost[1,2,3], Bao Hoang[1,2,3], Yonghui Yang[1,2,3], Carolyne Bardeleben[1,2,3], Joseph Gera[1,2,3], Alan Lichtenstein[1,2,3]*

1 Department of Medicine, Hematology-Oncology, Greater Los Angeles VA Healthcare Center, Los Angeles, California, United States of America, **2** Department of Medicine, UCLA School of Medicine, Los Angeles, California, United States of America, **3** Jonsson Comprehensive Cancer Center, Los Angeles, California, United States of America

Abstract

Because multiple myeloma (MM) cells are at risk for endoplasmic reticulum (ER) stress, they require a carefully regulated mechanism to promote protein translation of selected transcripts when proliferation is stimulated. MAPK-interacting kinases (MNKs) may provide this mechanism by enhancing cap-dependent translation of a small number of critical transcripts. We, thus, tested whether MNKs played a role in MM responses to the myeloma growth factor interleukin-6 (IL-6). IL-6 activated MNK1 phosphorylation and induced phosphorylation of its substrate, eIF-4E, in MM lines and primary specimens. MNK paralysis, achieved pharmacologically or by shRNA, prevented MM expansion stimulated by IL-6. A phosphodefective eIF-4E mutant also prevented the IL-6 response, supporting the notion that MNK's role was via phosphorylation of eIF-4E. Both pharmacological MNK inhibition and expression of the phosphodefective eIF-4E mutant inhibited MM growth in mice. Although critical for IL-6-induced expansion, eIF-4E phosphorylation had no significant effect on global translation or Ig expression. Deep sequencing of ribosome-protected mRNAs revealed a repertoire of genes involved in metabolic processes and ER stress modulation whose translation was regulated by eIF-4E phosphorylation. These data indicate MM cells exploit the MNK/eIF-4E pathway for selective mRNA translation without enhancing global translation and risking ER stress.

Editor: Venugopalan Cheriyath, Texas A&M University, United States of America

Funding: National Institutes of Health grants 2RO1CA111448, 1RO1CA132778 and 1R21CA168491; research funds of the Veteran's Administration; The Multiple Myeloma Research Foundation. The funders had no role in study design, data collection and analysis, decision to publish or preparation of the manuscript.

Competing Interests: The authors have declared that no competing interests exist.

* E-mail: alan.lichtenstein@med.va.gov

Introduction

Regulation of protein translation is important in MM because the significant rate of Ig production places the malignant plasma cell at risk for endoplasmic reticulum (ER) stress-induced death. Thus, the MM cell faces a dilemma: although unrestrained translation may be injurious due to enhanced ER stress, the cell requires a regulated mechanism to promote translation when proliferative signals arise. Such a mechanism would allow for the temporary upregulated translation of specific proliferation-dependent proteins but still retain control over global translation. The eIF-4E translation initiation factor could play such a role as it mediates tight regulation of expression of selected proteins [1].

The MAP kinase-interacting kinases 1 and 2 (MNK1 and MNK2) initially bind to eIF-4G and subsequently phosphorylate eIF-4E on S209, thus promoting eIF-4E's activity [2]. Although the physiologic function of such phosphorylation has been unclear because MNK1/2 double knock out mice exhibit a normal phenotype despite absence of eIF-4E phosphorylation [2], other data support the notion that the MNKs promote tumorigenesis [3–5]. They are highly expressed in several tumor types [6–8] and enhanced eIF-4E phosphorylation is also observed [3,9,10]. Genetic manipulation of MNKs and with phosphodefective eIF-4E constructs in pre-clinical models [3,11,12] also support a role for MNKs in tumor development. MNK-induced eIF-4E phosphorylation correlates with an increased translational efficiency of a subset of mRNAs encoding tumor-promoting proteins [4].

One particular scenario where the MNK kinases and eIF-4E may promote MM tumor growth is during Interleukin-6 (IL-6)-mediated expansion. IL-6-induced MM cell proliferation is mediated by signaling through the ERK MAPK pathway [13] and MNKs are activated downstream of this pathway [14]. Furthermore, since MNK activity and eIF-4E phosphorylation have minimal effects on overall translation in non-transformed cells [2], this pathway could be exploited by MM cells for translation of specific transcripts for a proliferative response while preventing marked increases in ER stress. We, thus, initiated the current study to test this hypothesis. Our results confirm the notion that MNK activity and eIF-4E phosphorylation are required for IL-6-induced MM cell expansion but do not stimulate significant increases in global translation. Deep sequencing of ribosome-protected transcripts identified a surprising number of genes involved in metabolism and ER stress whose translation was regulated by eIF-4E phosphorylation. These results identify MNK-induced eIF-4E phosphorylation as a promising therapeutic target in MM.

Materials and Methods

Cell lines, plasmids, transfections

The MM cell lines were obtained from ATCC. The lentiviral vectors targeting MNK1 were purchased from Sigma-Aldrich. The HA-tagged eIF-4E full length coding sequence was isolated from pHA-eIF4E (obtained from Addgene, plasmid 17343) by PCR. Insert from pLenti6/gfp-lc3 vector was removed by Spe1/Xho1digestion and replaced with Spe/Xho1-digested HA-eIF-4E to yield pLenti6HA-eIF4E. The serine to alanine (SA) and serine to aspartic acid eIF-4E mutants were constructed using the QuikChange site-directed mutagenesis kit (Stratgene). Lentiviral infection of MM cells was performed as previously described [15].

Primary myeloma specimens and ethics statement

Primary cells were purified from marrow of patients as described [16]. The purity by microscopy and CD138 flow analysis was >95% plasma cells. Marrow samples were obtained after informed consent in accordance with the Declaration of Helsinki, as approved by the West LA VA Institutional Review Board (IRB). The IRB of the VA West LA Medical Center approved this study. Written informed consent was obtained from all patients for use of their bone marrow sample in the research.

MNK In vitro kinase assay

The MNK kinase assay was carried out as described [17] with modifications. Cells were lysed with lysis buffer. Direct covalent attachment of MNK1 (Santa Cruz) and MNK2 (Sigma) antibodies to the agarose beads were performed with Pierce Direct IP Kit (Thermo Fisher Scientific). Labeled beads were washed with kinase buffer before 1 ug purified GST fusion eIF-4E protein (purchased from BPS Bioscience) was added. Reaction mixtures were incubated at 30°C for 30 minutes in the presence of 25 mM ATP. After SDS–PAGE, phosphorylated eIF-4E proteins were detected by Western blots.

Xenograft experiments

8226 cells (10^7/mouse) were injected subcutaneously (SQ) admixed with matrigel into NOD/SCID mice as described [18]. When tumor volume reached 200 mm^3, mice were randomized to control (0.5%DMSO), low dose 4-amino-3-(p-fluorophenylamino)pyrazolo (3,4-d)pyrimidine (CGP57380) (20 mg/kg) or high dose CGP57380 (50 mg/kg) groups and received daily intraperitoneal (IP) injections. Tumor volume was calculated as previously described [18]. Mice were also challenged SQ with 10^7 EV-transfected 8226 cells in the right flank versus 10^7 8226 cells transfected with a dominant negative eIF-4E construct. This study was carried out in strict accordance with the recommendations in the Guide for the Care and Use of Laboratory Animals in the NIH. The protocol was approved by the IACUC committee of the West LA VA Hospital. All efforts were made to minimize suffering to animals.

AHA incorporation assay

The AHA incorporation assay for estimating global translation was performed as previously described [19]. Briefly, cells were treated with IL-6 or pp242 in methionine-free media (Invitrogen), followed by a 30 minute exposure to 100 uM AHA (Azidohomoalanine, (Invitrogen)), a methionine analog to pulse label newly

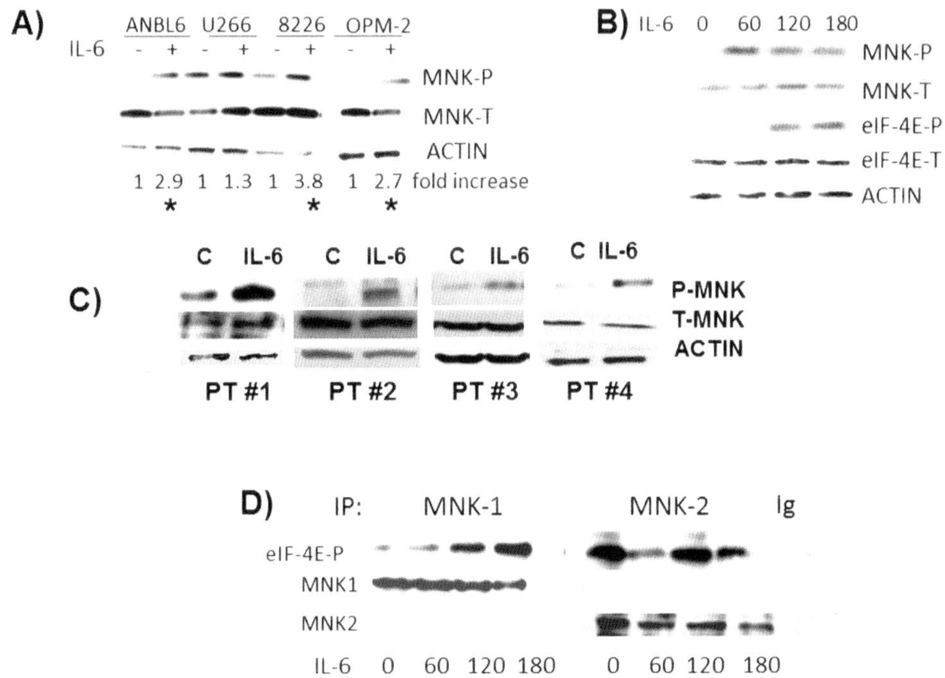

Figure 1. Activation of MNK kinases. A) MM lines exposed to IL-6 (100 U/ml) for 3 hrs followed by immunoblot assay for phospho-MNK and total MNK expression. Fold increase is determined by densitometric ratio of MNK-P/MNK-total and represents the mean of 3 independent experiments. * denotes IL-6-induced increase is statistically significant ($p<0.05$). **B**) ANBL-6 cells exposed to IL-6 for 0, 60, 120 or 180 mins, followed by immunoblot assay. **C**) Primary cells from 4 patients exposed to IL-6 or media (C) followed by immunoblot assay. **D**) ANBL-6 cells treated with IL-6 for increasing durations, followed by immunoprecipitation with anti-MNK1, MNK2 or control IgG. Immunoprecipitates tested for phosphorylation of eIF-4E in vitro.

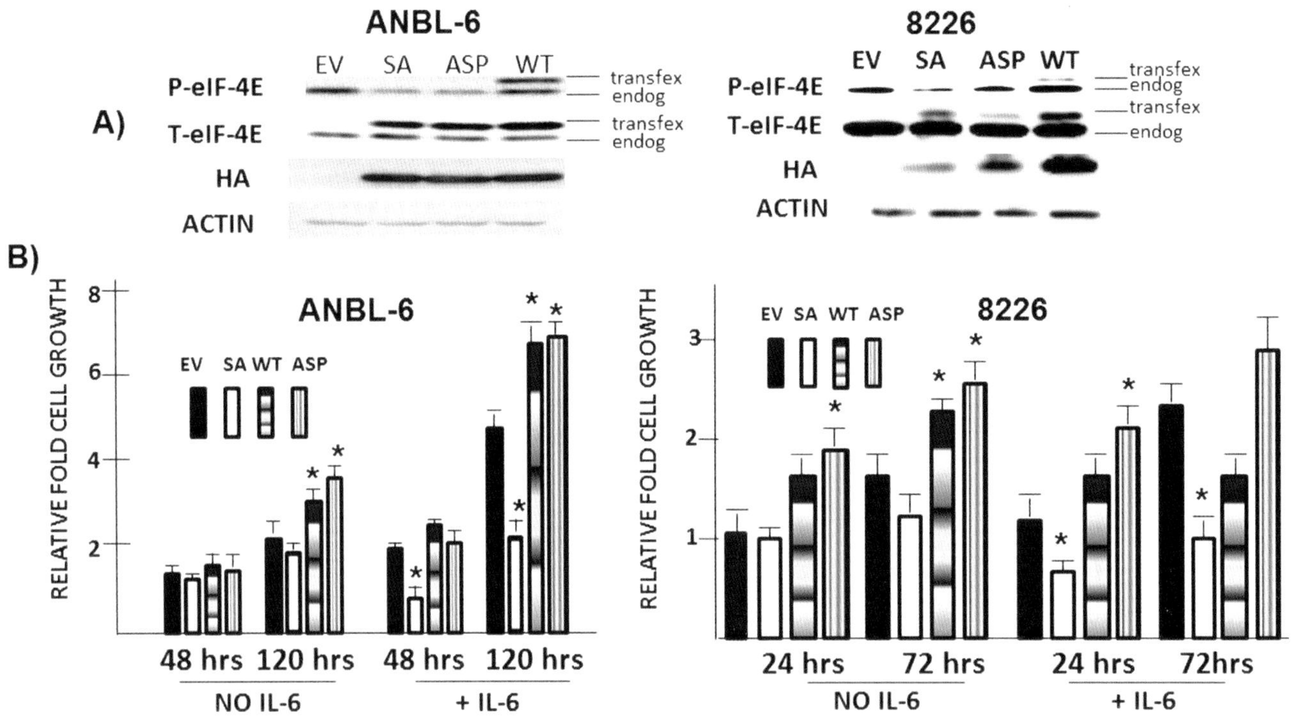

Figure 4. Effect of eIF-4E mutants. A) ANBL-6 or 8226 cells transfected with empty vector (EV), serine-to-alanine phosphodefective eIF-4E (SA), serine-to-aspartic acid phosphomimetic eIF-4E (ASP) or wild type (WT) eIF-4E, followed by immunoblot assay. Transfected (transfex) vs endogenous (endog) eIF-4E denoted. **B**) Above described ANBL-6 and 8226 transfected cell lines treated +/− IL-6 (100 U/ml) for varied durations and viable cell recovery enumerated. Results are relative cell growth compared to number of cells present at time 0 (mean+/−SD (n = 3)). * denotes statistically significant ($p<0.05$) alteration in cell recovery versus empty vector-transfected cells.

We also had the opportunity to test the effect of the CGP57380 inhibitor against two primary MM cell specimens (fig 2C), cultured for 96 Hrs. In contrast to the results described above in ANBL-6 and 8226 cells, CGP57380 at 25 or 50 uM significantly inhibited short term 1° MM cell survival in the absence of IL-6 in both specimens as well as when IL-6 was present.

Although frequently used experimentally as a MNK inhibitor, CGP57380 can inhibit additional kinases as potently as MNK [27]. We, thus, also tested cercosporamide, a MNK inhibitor with greater specificity. Cercosporamide has very limited activity against a panel of 76 other kinases [28]. Cercosporamide inhibited phosphorylation of eIF-4E in 8226 cells in the presence or absence of IL-6 as well as in IL-6-treated ANBL-6 MM cells (fig 2D). Very significant inhibition was present with the lowest concentration tested, 3.7 uM. This inhibitor also prevented IL-6-stimulated 8226 and ANBL-6 in vitro growth as shown in fig 2E while having little effect on MM cell growth in the absence of IL-6, similar to what was shown with the CGP57380 inhibitor. Thus, two independent inhibitors prevent MNK-induced phosphorylation of eIF-4E, which correlated nicely with their ability to prevent IL-6-stimulated MM cell growth.

We next used shRNA to knockdown MNK1, MNK2 or both. As shown in fig 3A, targeting 2 separate MNK1 sequences with shRNA (clone 1 & 2; (cl1 & cl2)) resulted in a significant decrease in MNK1 protein expression while having no effect on MNK2. Similarly, targeting MNK2 resulted in inhibited MNK2 expression while having no effect on MNK1. These cell lines were then treated with or without IL-6 and viable cell recovery enumerated 72 hrs later. As shown in fig 3B, in control (C) cells, IL-6 stimulated growth, allowing for an approximate doubling of cell numbers. In IL-6-stimulated MM cells, targeting MNK1 with both shRNAs significantly inhibited the IL-6 response although MNK1 knockdown in the absence of IL-6 had little effect. In contrast, targeting MNK2 with shRNAs had no effect on the IL-6 response.

Effects of eIF-4E mutants

To test if MNKs regulate expansion of MM cells via their phosphorylation of eIF-4E, we stably transfected wild type (WT), a serine-to-alanine (SA) mutant (at S209) or serine-to-aspartic acid (ASP) phosphomimetic eIF-4E mutant into ANBL-6 and 8226 MM cells. Figure 4A demonstrates successful expression of the transgenes by immunoblot assay for the HA tag and total eIF-4E compared to empty vector (EV)-transfected cells. As can be seen in fig 4A, ectopic expression of both SA and ASP mutants significantly inhibited phosphorylation of endogenous eIF-4E in both lines. Although the ectopic expression of the phosphomimetic ASP mutant should maintain normal-to-heightened eIF-4E function in transfected cells (as expected, it is not recognized by an antibody specific for eIF-4E phosphorylated on serine 209 (fig 4A)), the SA mutant should act as a dominant negative. The transfected MM clones were then cultured with or without IL-6 for 48–120 hrs. As shown in fig 4B, IL-6 was successful in stimulating expansion of MM clones in EV-, WT- and phosphomimetic ASP-transfected cells. In ANBL-6 cells, ectopic expression of WT and phosphomimetic eIF-4E significantly enhanced cell growth in the absence or presence of IL-6 at the 120 hr time point. Likewise, WT and phosphomimetic eIF-4E enhanced 8226 cell growth in the absence or presence of IL-6 (latter at 24 hrs). However, the SA dominant negative-transfected cells were significantly curtailed in their IL-6 response for ANBL-6 cells (left panel) and 8226 cells (right panel).

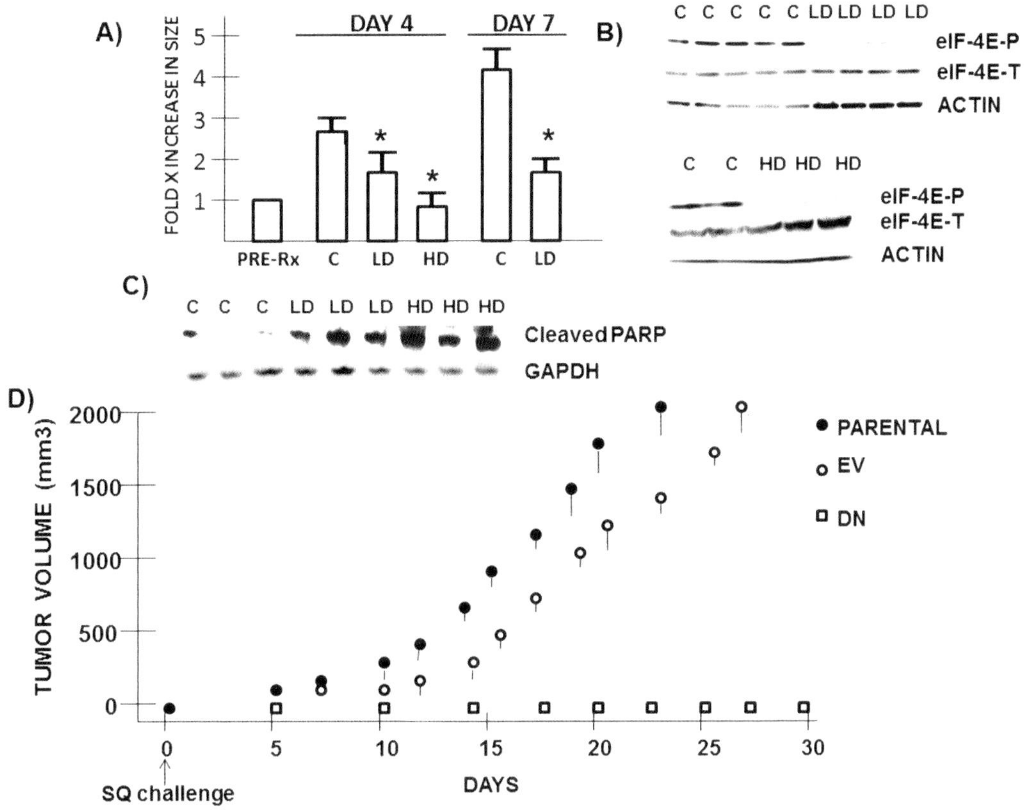

Figure 5. Effect of MNK/eIF-4E inhibition in vivo. A) 8226 cells injected SQ and mice randomized to control (C) group, low dose CGP57380 (LD, 20 mg/kg) or high dose (HD, 50 mg/kg). Treatment is daily IP injections. At day +4 and +7 of treatment, tumors were measured. Data is tumor volume, mean+/−SD (n = 8). * = significantly ($p<0.05$) smaller tumor vs control. **B and C**) Individual control (C), high dose (HD)-treated or low dose (LD)-treated tumors harvested after 3 days of treatment for Western blot, assaying phospho-eIF-4E, total eIF-4E, GAPDH and PARP that has been cleaved by caspase (AB #954 from Cell Signaling). **D**) Mice challenged SQ with 8226 cells transfected with EV (right flank) and 8226 cells transfected with dominant negative eIF-4E (left flank). A separate cohort of mice were challenged with non-transfected parental 8226 cells. Tumor growth is mean+/−SD tumor volume, n = 8.

Although the above described inhibitory effects of our dominant negative eIF-4E mutant strongly support the notion that IL-6-induced, MNK-dependent MM cell growth is, in part, due to a MNK-specific phosphorylation of eIF-4E, MNKs have other substrates that could be playing a role. In particular, MNK kinases can phosphorylate hn RNP A1 (A1) [26] and we have previously shown that A1 function in MM cells participates in IL-6-mediated growth [29]. It was also possible that our ectopically expressed SA mutant could out-compete A1 for binding to MNK1 and, thus, effectively prevent MNK phosphorylation of A1. Since antibodies for detecting A1 phosphorylation are not available, we investigated this issue indirectly. A1 binds to the 3′UTR of TNF-alpha at AU-rich elements (AREs) and, in so doing, restrains TNF expression. The one reported effect of MNK1-induced phosphorylation of A1 is to decrease its binding to TNF-alpha AREs resulting in upregulated TNF expression [26]. We, thus, reasoned that, if the SA eIF-4E phosphomutant prevented MNK1 phosphorylation of hn RNP A1, it would prevent or inhibit TNF expression. In MM cells infected with shRNA to silence hn RNP A1 (fig S3A), significantly enhanced TNF-alpha expression occurred (fig S3B), confirming a regulatory role of A1. Thus, A1 regulates TNF-alpha expression in our cells, presumably via its binding to the 3′UTR AREs. When we tested TNF-alpha expression in SA phospho-mutant-expressing cells, TNFα expression was not curtailed (fig S3B). As the LPS TNF-alpha response is dependent upon MNK1-induced A1 phosphorylation [26], these data support the hypothesis that the SA mutant is not preventing A1 phosphorylation as an off-target effect.

Effects of MNK/eIF-4E inhibition in vivo

In xenograft models, 8226 tumor cells were injected SQ and, when tumor volume reached 200 mm^3, mice were randomized to receive DMSO vehicle alone IP daily, or CGP57380 at 20 mg/kg (low dose (LD)) or 50 mg/kg (high dose (HD)). While MM growth progressed in control mice, both CGP57380 dose cohorts demonstrated an anti-tumor effect which was significant by 4 days of treatment (Fig 5A). Unfortunately, 50 mg/kg of CGP57380 was also toxic with weight (wt) loss and hunched over posture being evident. By 8 days of high dose CGP57380, 50% of treated mice succumbed although without significant tumor growth. At the lower dose of CGP57380, mice remained healthy without wt loss and with obvious anti-tumor effects at day+7 (fig 5A). When mice with equal-sized tumors were either treated with HD or LD CGP57380 (fig 5B) or DMSO (control) for 3 days followed by Western blot assay on extracted tumor protein, it is evident that the MNK inhibitor prevented eIF-4E phosphorylation in vivo (fig 5B). This was associated with a caspase-dependent cleavage of PARP (fig 5C), signifying activation of apoptosis. It is unclear to us why CGP57380 used in vivo resulted in MM cell apoptosis but not during in vitro exposure (fig S2). CGP57380

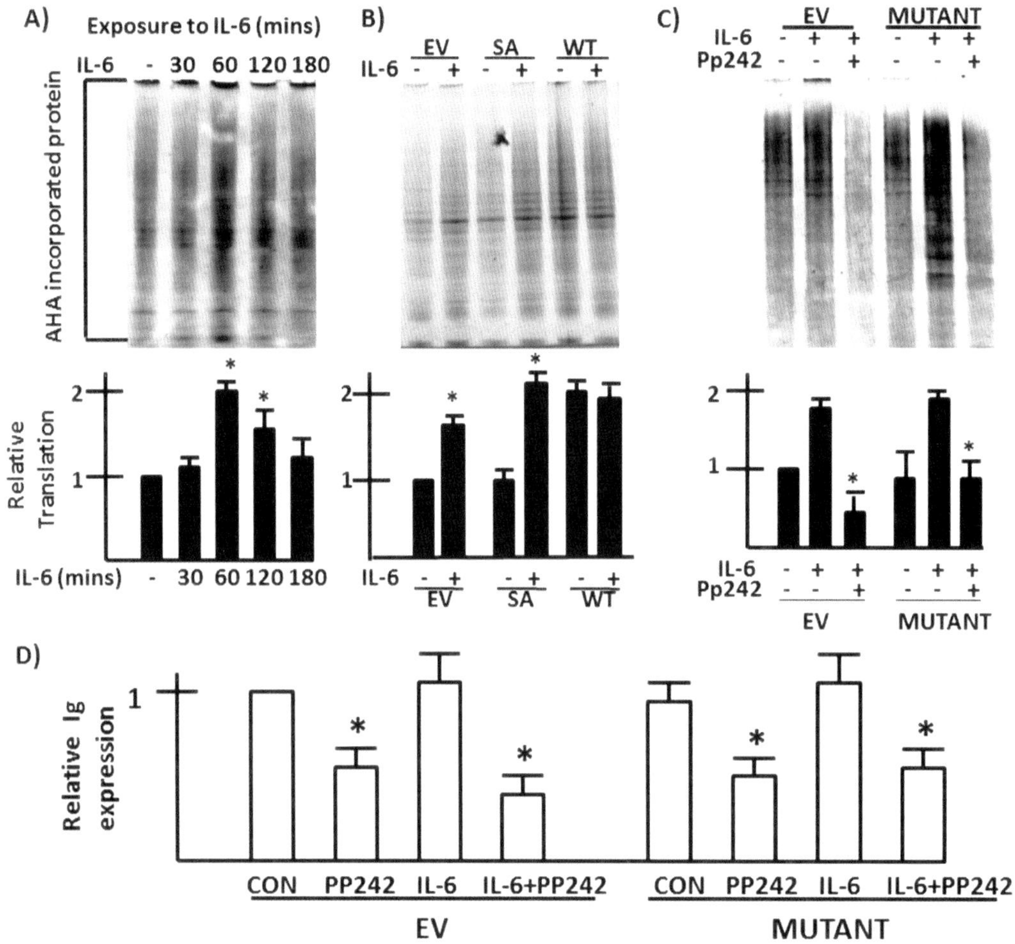

Figure 6. Effects on global translation and lambda light chain synthesis. A) AHA incorporation is tested in MM cells stimulated with IL-6 for 30, 60, 120 or 180 mins. In **B**), AHA incorporation is tested in IL-6-stimulated EV-, WT or mutant SA eIF-4E-transfected MM cells. In **C**), EV or SA mutant-expressing cells are pre-treated +/− pp242, followed by IL-6. Bar graphs under panels are means+/−SD of 4 separate experiments. * denotes statistically significant increase in AHA incorporation induced by IL-6 in A and B and decrease versus IL-6-stimulated control in C). **D**) Lambda light chain ELISA assay in MM cell lysates, comparing EV- vs mutant eIF-4E-transfected cells +/− IL-6 and +/− pp242. Data are means+/−SD, n = 4. * denotes statistically significant difference from corresponding controls.

injection of mice may disrupt some key viability pathways in vivo which involve interaction of MM cells with their milieu.

Mice were also challenged SQ with 10^7 8226 cells either transfected with an empty vector (EV) or the dominant negative eIF-4E mutant (DN). As shown in figure 5D, EV-transfected cells successfully grew out in mice, albeit at a slightly slower rate than parental inocula. In contrast, cells expressing the eIF-4E SA mutant were prevented from in vivo growth. Thus, either inhibiting MNK kinase activity (with CGP57380) or curtailing eIF-4E phosphorylation (with the phosphomutant) will prevent MM growth in mice.

Effects on protein translation

To assess effects on global translation, we utilized the methionine analog azidohomoalanine (AHA) to label newly translated proteins. By using click chemistry, the AHA-incorporating nascent proteins are labeled with a fluorescent dye as described in Materials & Methods. The fluorescent intensity is determined as an assessment of global translation. Protein loading in the gels is controlled by concurrent immunoblot for GAPDH (see Materials and Methods). ANBL-6 MM cells stimulated with or without IL-6 were incubated with AHA in a short 30 minute time window to assess newly made proteins. As shown in the representative experiment (Figure 6A) and the bar graph below depicting mean+/−SD increases in translation from 4 experiments, a modest increase in translation occurred which peaked after 60 mins of exposure to IL-6 (1.8 x fold) and returned to baseline by 180 mins. To assess any effect of eIF-4E phosphorylation on the IL-6-upregulated global protein synthesis, we stimulated ANBL-6 cells expressing the dominant negative eIF-4E phosphomutant (vs wild type (WT) eIF-4E-transfected and empty vector cells). As shown in a representative experiment and mean values from 3 independent experiments in the bar graph (Fig 6B), expression of the eIF-4E SA mutant did not decrease basal translation (no IL-6) as compared to empty vector-transfected cells. Furthermore, the ability of IL-6 to modestly enhance (approx 2 x fold) translation was also retained in mutant SA-expressing cells. Wild type (WT) eIF-4E-expressing cells demonstrated enhanced global translation in the absence of IL-6 without further increase when the cytokine was added. Although prevention of IL-6-induced eIF-4E phosphorylation in the SA mutant-expressing cells did not affect global translation, inhibition of mTOR by addition of pp242 ablated translation as shown in fig 6C.

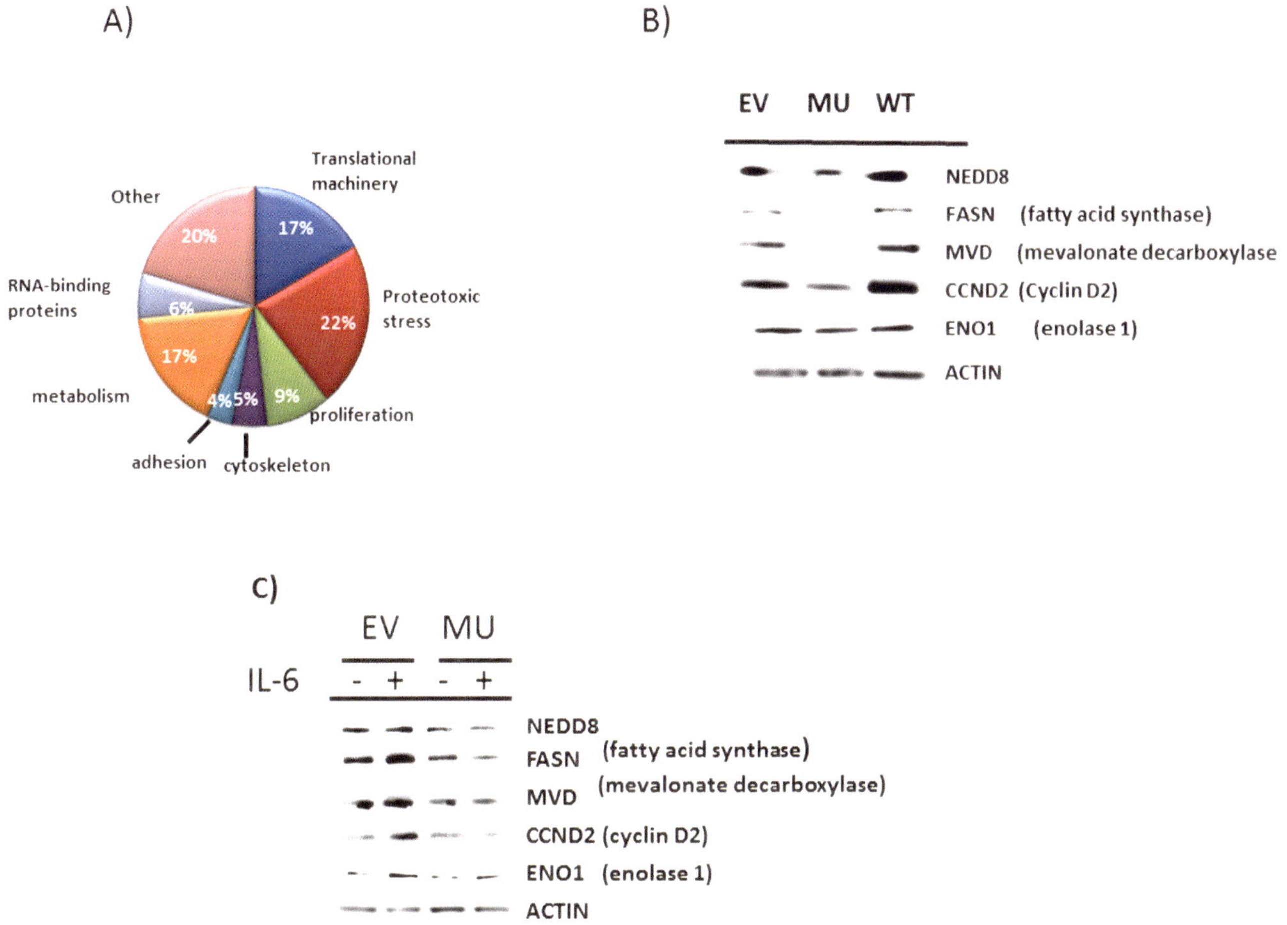

Figure 7. Ribosome profiling of EV vs mutant eIF-4E-transfected MM cells. A) Different categories of 166 genes demonstrating significantly inhibited translation in mutant-expressing cells. **B**) Immunoblot analysis of protein expression in EV-, WT and mutant (MU)-expressing MM cells. **C**) Immunoblot analysis of protein expression in EV vs mutant (MU) eIF-4E-expressing MM cells +/− IL-6 for 48 hrs.

Since immunoglobulin (Ig) synthesis is a significant portion of protein expression in MM cells, we also tested the effect of the eIF-4E mutant on Ig synthesis. We, thus, tested transfected 8226 cells which synthesize lambda light chains. As shown in figure 6D, IL-6 had a minimal effect on Ig synthesis in 8226 cells while pp242 significantly inhibited. Notably, when compared to EV-transfected 8226 cells, the eIF-4E mutant-transfected cells demonstrated no inhibition of Ig synthesis in the basal or IL-6-stimulated cultures. Collectively, these data indicate that eIF-4E phosphorylation does not affect global basal and IL-6-stimulated protein translation or Ig synthesis.

Ribosome-protection assay

To identify mRNAs susceptible to translation inhibition due to prevention of eIF-4E phosphorylation, we utilized transcriptome-scale ribosome profiling as previously described [20,21,30]. Ribosome profiling allows accurate quantification of mRNA fragments undergoing translation (ribosome footprints) as they are protected by ribosomes during digestion with RNase. To identify the mRNAs translationally regulated by eIF-4E phosphorylation, we calculated the induced changes in translational efficiency of each mRNA by normalizing footprint density of each gene to the abundance of the corresponding transcript. We studied control EV-transfected ANBL-6 cells and isogenic cells expressing the dominant negative eIF-4E both in the presence of IL-6. We detected 14-22 million reads per sample. In total, this corresponded to 1350 unique mRNAs that could be monitored for alterations in their translation. Ribosome profiling revealed 166 target mRNAs whose translation was significantly decreased ($\log_2 \leq -1.5$, false discovery rate <0.05) in mutant-containing MM cells compared to control ANBL-6 cells. A second ribosome profiling experiment gave similar results (correlation coefficient $R = 0.941$).

Figure 7A depicts the categories of genes whose expression is regulated by eIF-4E phosphorylation. A large fraction (17%) participate in the translational machinery such as ribosome proteins and elongation factors. This is not surprising since previous results in prostate cancer cells [30] also determined this category of genes was most sensitive to translational inhibition resulting from an active site mTOR inhibitor and we anticipated that eIF-4E phosphorylation-regulated genes would be included in the larger number of mTOR-regulated genes. However, we were surprised to find two additional categories highly represented consisted of metabolism genes (17%) and those involved in ER function and proteotoxic stress responses (22%). These latter genes are listed in figs 8 & 9. All these latter genes demonstrated inhibited translation ($\log_2 \leq -1.5$) but with little effect on mRNA abundance ('RNA' columns in figs 8 & 9) with few exceptions (#8, 17 and 23 in fig 8 (increased transcript level) and #25 and #29 in fig 9 (decreased level of mRNA abundance)). It was also notable

	Gene	Description	RNA
1	ASS1	Argininosuccinate synthase 1	-0.14
2	ATP5L	ATP synthase, H+ transporting, mitochondrial Fo complex, subunit G	1.42
3	ATP6V1G1	ATPase, H+ transporting, lysosomal 13kDa, V1 subunit G1	0.17
4	cytochrome b	Clone 35w unknown mRNA, mitochondrial.	-0.16
5	ENO1	Enolase 1, (alpha)	-0.17
6	FASN	Fatty acid synthase	-0.45
7	GUK1	Guanylate kinase 1	-0.14
8	KARS	Lysyl-tRNA synthetase	4.52
9	LSS	Lanosterol synthase (2,3-oxidosqualene-lanosterol cyclase)	0.26
10	MTND5	NADH dehydrogenase subunit 5	0.18
11	MVD	Mevalonate (diphospho) decarboxylase	0.34
12	NAA10	N(alpha)-acetyltransferase 10, NatA catalytic subunit	-0.39
13	NDUFA11	NADH dehydrogenase (ubiquinone) 1 alpha subcomplex, 11, 14.7kDa	0.35
14	NDUFA13	NADH dehydrogenase (ubiquinone) 1 alpha subcomplex, 13	-0.08
15	NDUFA3	NADH dehydrogenase (ubiquinone) 1 alpha subcomplex, 3, 9kDa	-0.23
16	NDUFB11	NADH dehydrogenase (ubiquinone) 1 ß subcomplex, 11, 17.3kDa	-0.24
17	NDUFB6	NADH dehydrogenase (ubiquinone) 1 beta subcomplex, 6, 17kDa	6.28
18	NDUFS3	NADH dehydrogenase (ubiquinone) Fe-S protein 3, 30kDa	0.15
19	NDUFV2	NADH dehydrogenase (ubiquinone) flavoprotein 2, 24kDa	0.21
20	OAZ1	Ornithine decarboxylase antizyme 1	0.48
21	OGT	O-linked N-acetylglucosamine (GlcNAc) transferase	0.30
22	P4HB	(P4HB), mRNA.	0.53
23	PNP	Purine nucleoside phosphorylase	2.57
24	PSAP	Prosaposin	0.31
25	PYGB	Phosphorylase, glycogen; brain	0.44
26	SCD	Stearoyl-CoA desaturase (delta-9-desaturase)	0.41
27	TPST2	Tyrosylprotein sulfotransferase 2	-0.08
28	UQCRH	Ubiquinol-cytochrome c reductase hinge protein	0.65

Figure 8. Metabolism genes whose translation is inhibited in mutant eIF-4E-containing MM cells. List of all genes related to metabolism with significant decreases in translational efficiency. 'RNA" value given is $\log_2$ change in RNA abundance in mutant-expressing cells vs EV-cells.

that the translationally inhibited metabolism genes (fig 8) included enzymes involved in lipid biosynthesis, such as fatty acid synthetase (FASN, #6), stearoyl-coA desaturase (SCD, #26), lanosterol synthetase (LSS #9) and mevalonate decarboxylase (MVD, #11). Proteotoxic stress response genes (fig 9) included genes responsible for proper folding of proteins (ie., PP1A, HSP90, HSP70, nucleophosmin (NPM1)), in proteasome function (NEDD8, PSMc3, PSMD7), in UPR responses (CALR) and in translocation of proteins across ER membranes (SSR4, Sec11c, Sec11a, BCAP31, SPCS2, SPCS3, LMAN1). Many of these genes are specifically upregulated at the RNA level in MM [31], supporting their important roles in myelomagenesis.

The remaining genes, transitionally inhibited by the mutant eIF-4E, are listed in figs S4 & S5. They include genes encoding RNA-binding proteins (6%), adhesion proteins (4%), cytoskeleton proteins (5%), miscellaneous proteins (17%) and those involved in proliferation/survival (11%). The latter include cyclin D2, SMAP42, defender against cell death (DAD1), PIM2 and POU2AF1. Cyclin D2 is the D cyclin used by these myeloma cells for cell cycle transit and its curtailed expression would certainly contribute to the inhibited growth response to IL-6 caused by the SA dominant negative mutant.

To confirm some of the ribosome profiling data, we utilized Western blot analysis which confirmed the dominant negative eIF-4E phosphomutant inhibited expression of several genes identified with ribosome profiling. Immunoblot assay performed on extracts of IL-6-stimulated EV-transfected and WT-transfecetd ANBL-6 cells vs stimulated mutant eIF-4E-containing cells (fig 7B) confirms the inhibitory effect of the SA mutant as seen in the ribosome profiling. In addition, ectopic expression of wild type (WT) eIF-4E appeared to increase expression of several of these proteins (ie., NEDD8, FASN, MVD and CCND2). An additional experiment (fig 7C) demonstrates the variable stimulation of expression of these genes in IL-6-treated EV cells (most marked for FASN, MVD, CCND2 and ENO1) which was prevented in mutant eIF-4E-containing MM cells.

Discussion

MM plasma cells have developed several strategies to deal with the risk of ER stress. They have efficient proteasome function, expanded ER membrane development and a heightened UPR mechanism [32,33]. MM cells also exploit mechanisms for repressing generalized TORC1 activity to limit unnecessary protein expression for prevention of further ER stress. For example, MM cells transcriptionally upregulate ARK5 and DEPTOR [34,35], two proteins that suppress TORC1 [35,36] function and global cap-dependent translation. However, when stimulated for proliferative responses, enhanced translation of key

	Gene	Description	RNA
1	TPT1	Tumor protein, translationally-controlled 1	0.07
2	MZB1	Marginal zone B and B1 cell-specific protein	0.15
3	TSPO	Translocator protein (18kDa) (TSPO), transcript variant PBR-S	0.30
4	NEDD8	Neural precursor cell expressed, developmentally down-regulated 8	0.15
5	SSR4	Signal sequence receptor, delta	0.10
6	SEC11C	SEC11 homolog C	-0.01
7	CALM2	Calmodulin 2 (phosphorylase kinase, delta)	-0.25
8	PRDX1	Peroxiredoxin 1	0.14
9	HSP90B1	Heat shock protein 90kDa beta (Grp94), member 1	0.55
10	SEC11A	SEC11 homolog A (S. cerevisiae) (SEC11A)	0.31
11	PSMC3	Proteasome (prosome, macropain) 26S subunit, ATPase, 3	0.44
12	SPCS3	Signal peptidase complex subunit 3 homolog	0.31
13	TRAM1	Translocation associated membrane protein 1	0.24
14	SPCS2	Signal peptidase complex subunit 2 homolog	0.01
15	BCAP31	B-cell receptor-associated protein 31 (BCAP31)	-0.21
16	CALR	Calreticulin (CALR)	0.25
17	PSMD7	Proteasome (Prosome, Macropain) 26S Subunit, Non-ATPase, 7	-0.15
18	UFM1	Ubiquitin-fold modifier 1	0.16
19	PPIA	Peptidylprolyl isomerase A (cyclophilin A)	-0.22
20	LMAN1	Lectin, mannose-binding, 1	-0.09
21	COPG	Coatomer protein complex, subunit gamma	0.00
22	NPM1	Nucleophosmin (nucleolar phosphoprotein B23, numatrin)	0.16
23	HSPA8	Heat shock 70kDa protein 8	-0.75
24	SQSTM1	Sequestosome 1	0.68
25	ERP29	Endoplasmic reticulum protein 29	-1.74
26	PSMA3	Proteasome (prosome, macropain) subunit, alpha type, 3	-0.69
27	PSME2	Proteasome (prosome, macropain) activator subunit 2 (PA28 beta)	0.03
28	ARF1	ADP-ribosylation factor 1 (ARF1), transcript variant 4	0.29
29	CYTH1	Cytohesin 1 (CYTH1), transcript variant 2	-1.59
30	FBXW5	F-box and WD repeat domain containing 5	1.04
31	GNB2L1	Guanine nucleotide binding protein (G protein), beta polypeptide 2-like 1	-0.31
32	NFE2L1	Nuclear factor (erythroid-derived 2)-like 1	0.69
33	ORMDL3	ORM1-like 3	0.10
34	SRPR	Signal recognition particle receptor (docking protein)	-0.14
35	TRIM28	Tripartite motif containing 28	1.25
36	YKT6	YKT6 v-SNARE homolog	0.31
37	HSP90AB1	Heat shock protein 90kDa alpha (cytosolic), class B member 1	-0.52

Figure 9. Proteotoxicity response genes whose translation is inhibited in mutant eIF-4E-containing MM cells. List of genes involved in proteotoxic responses with significant decreases in translational efficiency.

proteins must occur. Our results suggest that the MNK/eIF-4E pathway may provide one mechanism for this response while maintaining the repressed level of overall global translation. Furthermore, the high percentage of genes regulated transationally by eIF-4E phosphorylation involved in ER function and responses to proteotoxic stress underscore the fine line that the MM cell must walk between translation required for clonal expansion and translation that is toxic.

An important clinical issue is whether MNK activity is only important in IL-6 MM responses or is similarly involved in constitutive growth or MM cell growth stimulated by other factors like IGF-1 or triggers from the marrow microenvironment. Although CGP57380 and MNK knockdown did not significantly affect MM cell growth in the absence of IL-6 in cell lines,in two primary MM specimens there was significant cytoreduction induced by CGP57380 in the absence of IL-6. Additional primary specimens will have to be tested to address this issue.

MM cell growth requires lipids to replicate cellular membranes. Additional responses to continued ER stress require lipids for maintenance of an expanded ER membrane capacity. Thus, maintenance of lipid synthesis during IL-6 stimulation would be critical to allow for cell growth. It is not surprising, therefore, that several of the eIF-4E phopshorylation-dependent genes are involved with lipid metabolism, including fatty acid synthetase (FASN), stearoyl-coA desaturase (SCD) lanosterol synthase (LSS) and mevalonate decarboxylase (MVD). Indeed, interruption of

MM cell lipid metabolism is the hypothetical goal of several new therapeutic strategies in myeloma [37,38]. EIF-4E phosphorylation also regulated translation of the enolase gene (ENO1, (#5 in fig 7A)), a glycolytic enzyme, also known as c-myc promoter binding protein (MBP-1). In U266 and ANBL-6 MM cells, IL-6 is known to upregulate ENO1/MBP-1 mRNA levels [39] supporting the notion that it is important in IL-6 responses. Our data indicate that after IL-6-induced transcription, ENO1/MBP-1 translation depends upon the phosphorylation status of eIF-4E.

Although several genes specifically involved in proliferation and viability were regulated by eIF-4E phosphorylation, such as cyclin D2 and PIM-2, it was notable that expression of some well known myeloma-associated genes like c-myc and VEGF were not. Immunoblot assay of eIF-4E-mutation-containing MM cells (vs EV cells) confirmed expression of these genes was independent of eIF-4E function (data not shown). One possible explanation for these results is that these genes are translated during IL-6 stimulation through alternative pathways. They have well-defined internal ribosome entry site (IRES) sequences in their 5′UTRs which are highly active in the MM tumor model [40,41]. For example, in our prior work [29], we documented the importance of the c-myc IRES in upregulated myc translation secondary to IL-6 exposure. In addition, in similar ribosome protection profiling of cells treated with the mTOR inhibitor torin, genes containing known IRESes were resistant to inhibited translation [21]. It is, thus, not surprising that translation of these key genes is not regulated by eIF-4E phosphorylation.

In summary, our data underscores the importance of MNK kinase activation in the IL-6-induced growth response of MM cells. MNK-induced phosphorylation of eIF-4E upregulates translation of a select number of transcripts, which are important for the response, but does not significantly increase global translation. As the MNKs are dispensable for normal physiology [2], they may be good targets for therapy in myeloma. There are several MNK/eIF-4E inhibitors identified in pre-clinical studies [28,42] that are under development. Multiple myeloma is a promising tumor model for their study.

Supporting Information

Figure S1 ANBL-6 MM cells cultured +/− CGP (25 uM) for 72 hrs in the presence or absence of increasing concentrations of rIL-6. Data represent number of viable cells recovered, mean+/−SD, n = 3. CGP significantly ($p<0.05$) reduced the number of viable cells at all concentrations of IL-6 (but not in the absence of IL-6).

Figure S2 ANBL-6 or 8226 cells cultured +/− IL-6 (500 U/ml) and +/− CGP (25 uM) for 48 or 72 hrs after which apoptosis assayed by flow cytometric analysis of activated caspase 3. Data are means of 3 separate experiments. SDs were <10% of the means for all groups (not shown). As a positive control, staurosporine, at 1 uM, induced ANBL-6 and 8226 apoptosis (76% and 71% caspase 3+ cells, respectively).

Figure S3 A) shRNA-transfected 8226 MM cells to silence hn RNP A1 showing loss of A1 expression vs EV cells (transfected with shRNA expressing a scramble sequence (SCR)). **B**) MM cells expressing empty vectors (EVs) or shRNA for hn RNP A1 (sh1 or sh2) or wild type (WT) eIF-4E or SA dominant negative eIF-4E phospho-mutant. Cells stimulated +/− LPS and TNF-alpha expression assessed by ELISA. Data are means+/−SD of 3 experiments. *denotes statistically significant difference ($p<0.05$) from corresponding EV cells.

Figure S4 Proliferation, RNA-binding protein, and translational machinery genes showing inhibited translational efficiency due to eIF-4E mutation.

Figure S5 Cytoskeleton, adhesion proteins & other genes that demonstrate inhibited translational efficiency due to eIF-4E mutation.

Author Contributions

Conceived and designed the experiments: PF BH CB JG AL. Performed the experiments: YS YY. Analyzed the data: YS PF CB JG AL. Contributed reagents/materials/analysis tools: PF YY. Wrote the paper: AL.

References

1. Kentsis A, Topisirovic I, Culjkovic B, Shao L, Borden KLB (2004) Ribavirin suppresses eIF4E-mediated oncogenic transformation by physical mimicry of the 7-methyl guanosine mRNA cap. Proc Natl Acad Sci 101:18105–18110.
2. Ueda T, Watanabe-Fukunaga R, Fukuyama H, Nagata S, et al. (2004) MNK2 and MNK1 are essential for constitutive and inducible phosphorylation of eIF-4E but not for cell growth or development. Mol. Cell Biol. 24: 6539–6549.
3. Wendel HG, Silva RL, Malina A, Mills JR, Zhu H, et al. (2007) Dissecting eIF4E action in tumorigenesis. Genes & Dev 21:3232–3237.
4. Furic L, Rong L, Larsson O, Koumakpayi I, Yoshida K, et al. (2010) eIF4E phosphorylation promotes tumorigenesis and is associated with prostate cancer progression. Proc Natl Acad Sci 107:14134–14139.
5. Ueda T, Sasaki M, Elia AL, Chio I, Hamada K, et al. (2010) Combined deficiency for MAP kinase-interacting kinase 1 and 2 (MNK 1 and MNK 2) delays tumor development. Proc Natl Acad Sci 107:13984–13990.
6. Pellagatti A, Vetrie D, Langford CD, Gama S, Eagleton H, et al. (2003) Gene expression profiling in polycythemia vera using cDNA microarray technology. Cancer Res 63:3940–3944.
7. Worch J, Tickenbrock L, Schwable J, Steffen B, Cauvet T, et al. (2004) The serine-threonine kinase MNK1 is post-transationally stabilized by PML-RARalpha and regulates differentiation of hematopoietic cells. Oncogene 23:9162–9172.
8. Bredel M, Bredel C, Juric D (2005) High resolution genome-wide mapping of genetic alterations in human glial brain tumors. Cancer Res 65:4088–4096.
9. Fan S, Ramalingham SS, Kauh J, Xu Z, Khuri FR, et al. (2009) Phosphorylated eIF4E is elevated in human cancer tissues. Cancer Biol Ther 8:1463–1469.
10. Yoshizawa A, Fukuoka J, Shimizu S, Shilo K, Franks TJ, et al. (2010) Overexpression of phospho-eIF4E is associated with survival through AKT pathwy in non-small cell lung cancer. Clin Cancer Res 16:240–248.
11. Lazaris-Karatzas A, Montine KS, Sonenberg N (1990) Malignant transformation by a eukaryotic initiation factor subunit that binds to mRNA 5′cap. Nature 345:544–547.
12. Topisirovic I, Ruiz-Gutierrez M, Borden KL (2004) Phosphorylation of the eIF4E contributes to its transformation and mRNA transport activities. Cancer Res 64:8639–8642.
13. Ogata A, Chauhan D, Teoh G, Treon S, Urashima M, et al. (19997) IL-6 triggers cell growth via the RAS-dependent mitogen-activated protein kinase cascade. J Immunol 159:2212–2221.
14. Fukunaga R, Hunter T (1997) MNK1, a new MAP kinase-activated protein kinase, isolated by a novel expression screening method for identifying protein kinase substrates. EMBO J 16:1921–1997.
15. Hoang B, Frost P, Shi Y, Belanger E, Benavides A, et al. (2010) Targeting TORC2 in multiple myeloma with a new mTOR kinase inhibitor. Blood 116: 4560–4568.
16. Sharma S, Nemeth E, Chen Y, Goodnough J, Huston A, et al. (2008) Involvement of hepcidin in the anemia of multiple myeloma. Clin Cancer Res 14:3262–3267.
17. Waskiewicz AJ, Flynn A, Proud CG, Cooper JA (1997) Mitogen-activated protein kinases activate the serine/threonine kinses MNK1 and MNK2. EMBO J 16:1909–1920.

18. Frost P, Moatamed F, Hoang B, Shi Y, Gera J, et al. (2004) In vivo antitumor effects of the mTOR inhibitor CCI-779 against human multiple myeloma cells in a xenograft model. *Blood* 104(13):4181 87.
19. Lock R, Roy S, Kenific C (2011) Autophagy facilitates glycolysis during Ras-mediated oncogenic transformation. Mol Biol of the Cell 22:165 178.
20. Ingolia N, Ghaemmaghami S, Newman J, Weissman J (2009) Genome wide analysis in vivo of translation with nucleotide resolution using ribosome profiling. Science 324:218 223.
21. Thoreen C, Chantranupong L, Keys H, Wang T, Gray N, et al. (2012) A unifying model for mTORC1-mediated regulation of mRNA translation. Nature 485:109 113.
22. Jernberg-Wiklund H, Pettersson M, Carlsson M, Nilsson K (1992) Increase in IL-6 and IL-6 receptor expression in a human multiple myeloma cell line, U-266, during long term in vitro culture and the development of a possible autocrine IL-6 loop. Leukemia 6:310 318.
23. Parra JL, Buxade M, Proud CG (2005) Features of the catalytic domains and C termini of the MAPK signal-integrating kinases MNK1 and MNK2 determine their differing activities and regulatory properties. J. Biol. Chem. 280: 37623 37633.
24. Billadeau D, Jelinek DF, Shah N, LeBien TW, Van Ness B (1995) Introduction of an activated N-ras oncogene alters the growth characteristics of the IL-6-dependent myeloma cell line ANBL6. Cancer Res 55:3640 3646.
25. Knauf U, Tschopp C, Gram H (2001) Negative regulation of protein translation by mitogen-activated protein kinase-interacting kinases 1 and 2. Mol cell Biol 21:5500 5511.
26. Buxade M, Parra JL, Rousseau S, Shpiro N, Marquez R, et al. (2005) The MNKs are novel components in the control of TNF alpha biosynthesis and phosphorylate and regulate hnRNP A1. Immunity 23:177 189.
27. Bain J, Plater L, Elliot M, Shpiro N, Hastie CJ, et al. (2007) The selectivity of protein kinase inhibitors: a further update. Biochem J 408:297 315.
28. Konicek BW, Stephens JR, McNulty AM, Robichaud N, Peery RB, et al. (2011) Therapeutic inhibition of MAP kinase interacting kinase blocks eukaryotic initiation factor 4E phosphorylation and suppresses outgrowth of experimental lung metastases. Cancer Res 71: 1849 57.
29. Shi Y, Frost PJ, Hoang B, Gera J:Lichtenstein A (2008) IL-6-induced stimulation of c-myc translation in multiple myeloma cells is mediated by myc IRES function and the RNA-binding protein hnRNP A1. Cancer Res 68: 10215 10222.
30. Hsieh A, Liu Y, Edlind M, Ingoloa N, Janes M, et al. (2012) The translational landscape of mTOR signaling steers cancer initiation and metastasis. Nature 485:55 61.
31. Munshi N, Hideshima T, Carrasco D, Shammas M, Auclair D, et al. (2004) Identification of genes modulated in multiple myeloma using genetically identical twin samples. BLOOD 103:1799 1806.
32. Carrasco DR, Sukhdeo K, Protopopova M, Sinha R, EnoS M, et al. (2007) The differentiation and stress response factor XBP-1 drives multiple myeloma pathogenesis. Cancer Cell 11:349 360.
33. Obeng EA, Carlson LM, Gutman DM, Harrington WJ, Lee KP, et al. (2006) Proteasome inhibitors induce a terminal unfolded protein response in multiple myeloma cells. BLOOD 107:4907 4916.
34. Suzuki A, Iida S, Kato-Uranishi M, Tajima E, Zhan F, et al. (2005) ARK5 is transcriptionally regulated by the large MAF family and mediates IGF-1-induced cell invasion in multiple myeloma: ARK5 as a new molecular determinant of multiple myeloma. Oncogene 24:6936 6944.
35. Peterson TR, Laplante M, Thoreen CC, Sancak Y, Kang S, et al. (2009) DEPTOR is an mTOR inhibitor frequently overexpressed in multiple myeloma cells and required for their survival. Cell 137:873 886.
36. Liu L, Ulbrich J, Muller J, Wustfeld T, Aeberhard L, et al. (2012) Deregulated MYC expression induces dependence upon AMPK-related kinase 5. Nature 2012; 483:608 612.
37. Clendening J, pandyra A, Li Z, Boutros P, Martirosyan A, et al. (2010) Exploiting the mevalonate pathway to distinguish statin-sensitive multiple myeloma. BLOOD 115:4787 4797.
38. Tirado-Velez JM, Joumady I, Saez-Benito, Cozar-Castellano I, Perdomo G (2012) Inhibition of fatty acid metabolism reduces human myeloma cells proliferation. PLoS One 7:e46484.
39. Wen XY, Stewart A, Sooknanan RR (1999) Identification of c-myc promoter-binding protein and XBP-1 as interleukin-6 target genes in human myeloma cells. Int J Oncol 15:173 178.
40. Paulin FE, West MJ, Sullivan NF, Whitney RL, Lyne L, et al. (1996) Aberrant translational control of the c-myc gene in multiple myeloma. Oncogene 13:505 513.
41. Frost P, Shi Y, Hoang B, Lichtenstein A (2007) AKT activity regulates the ability of mTOR inhibitors to prevent angiogenesis and VEGF expression in multiple myeloma cells. Oncogene 26:2255 2262.
42. Assouline S, Culjkovic B, Cocolakis E, Rousseau C, Beslu N, et al. (2009) Molecular targeting of the oncogenic eIF-4E in AML: A proof of principle clinical trial with ribavirin. BLOOD 114:257 260.

9

Silencer of Death Domains Controls Cell Death through Tumour Necrosis Factor-Receptor 1 and Caspase-10 in Acute Lymphoblastic Leukemia

Adam Cisterne[1]‡, Rana Baraz[1]‡, Naveed I. Khan[1], Robert Welschinger[1], Jordan Basnett[1], Carina Fung[1], Helen Rizos[1], Kenneth F. Bradstock[2], Linda J. Bendall[1]*

1 Centre for Cancer Research, Westmead Millennium Institute, University of Sydney, Sydney, New South Wales, Australia, **2** Blood and Marrow Transplant Service, Department of Haematology, Westmead Hospital, Sydney, New South Wales, Australia

Abstract

Resistance to apoptosis remains a significant problem in drug resistance and treatment failure in malignant disease. NO-aspirin is a novel drug that has efficacy against a number of solid tumours, and can inhibit Wnt signaling, and although we have shown Wnt signaling to be important for acute lymphoblastic leukemia (ALL) cell proliferation and survival inhibition of Wnt signaling does not appear to be involved in the induction of ALL cell death. Treatment of B lineage ALL cell lines and patient ALL cells with NO-aspirin induced rapid apoptotic cell death mediated via the extrinsic death pathway. Apoptosis was dependent on caspase-10 in association with the formation of the death-inducing signaling complex (DISC) incorporating pro-caspase-10 and tumor necrosis factor receptor 1 (TNF-R1). There was no measurable increase in TNF-R1 or TNF-α in response to NO-aspirin, suggesting that the process was ligand-independent. Consistent with this, expression of silencer of death domain (SODD) was reduced following NO-aspirin exposure and lentiviral mediated shRNA knockdown of SODD suppressed expansion of transduced cells confirming the importance of SODD for ALL cell survival. Considering that SODD and caspase-10 are frequently over-expressed in ALL, interfering with these proteins may provide a new strategy for the treatment of this and potentially other cancers.

Editor: Halvard Boenig, German Red Cross Blood Service Frankfurt, Germany

Funding: This work was funded by a grant from NHMRC (Grant No. 352326) to LJB. LJB and HR are NHMRC Senior Research Fellows and recipients of Cancer Institute New South Wales Fellowships. The funders had no role in study design, data collection and analysis, decision to publish, or preparation of the manuscript.

* Email: linda.bendall@sydney.edu.au

‡ These authors contributed equally to this work.

Introduction

Acute lymphoblastic leukemia (ALL) is the most common malignancy in children and although remission is almost always attained, up to 20% of children will relapse, with subsequent poor prognosis [1]. Adult patients have a worse outlook, with more than half relapsing [2]. Current management of ALL in both children and adults is dependent on treatment with multiple chemotherapy drugs, such as corticosteroids and vincristine, which induce apoptosis in the leukemia cells. However, resistance to drug-induced apoptosis is a common problem, and there is an urgent requirement for new drugs with efficacy against leukemic cells in ALL.

Apoptosis can be mediated via the extrinsic death receptor-mediated pathway, or the intrinsic mitochondrial pathway. Cell death is ultimately mediated by activation of effector caspases including caspase-3 and -7. However, the initiator caspases differ between the two pathways, with caspases-8 and -10 being involved in the extrinsic, and caspase-9 in the intrinsic pathway [3]. Commitment to the intrinsic pathway occurs when cytochrome c is released from mitochondria as a result of mitochondrial outer membrane permeabilization (MOMP) [4]. This results in the formation of the apoptosome by recruitment of APAF-1 and pro-caspase-9 [5]. Here caspase-9 is activated by cleavage and in turn activates the effector caspases. The extrinsic death pathway is initiated by the binding of death ligands, such as tumour necrosis factor alpha (TNF-α), TNF-related apoptosis inducing ligand (TRAIL) or FasL to their respective cell surface death receptors, tumour necrosis factor receptor 1 (TNF-R1), death receptors (DR) 4 or 5, and Fas. Oligomerization of the death domains in the cytoplasmic regions of these receptors is the initial event in signalling through these receptors. This can be inhibited by silencer of death domain (SODD), alternatively known as BCL2-associated athanogene 4 (BAG4) in the case of TNF-R1, Fas and DR3 [6,7]. Once oligomerization has occurred, binding of the adaptor molecules, TNF-R1-associated death domain protein (TRADD) or Fas-associated protein with death domain (FADD), depending on the receptor involved, and pro-caspases-8 or -10 produces the death-inducing signaling complex (DISC) [8]. In some cells activation of caspases-8 or -10 within the DISC is sufficient to facilitate direct activation of effector caspases and cell death, while in others linkage to the intrinsic pathway is needed.

This occurs by caspase-8 or -10-mediated cleavage of Bid and induction of MOMP [9].

Despite expression of surface death receptors, including TNF-R1, Fas and TRAIL-R1 and R2, cells from a significant proportion of ALL patients are resistant to ligand-induced apoptosis when exposed to TNF-α, FasL or TRAIL [10–12]. The reasons for this are unclear but are thought to involve alterations to death receptor signalling pathways. The specific role of caspase-10 in the induction of cell death is not clear and in most settings it takes a subordinate role to caspase-8. Mice naturally lack caspase-10 [13] and in humans it can substitute for caspase-8 in certain cell types [14]. However, mutations in *CASP10* are associated with type II autoimmune lymphoproliferative syndrome suggesting it has a significant role in lymphoid cells [15]. Caspase-10 is highly expressed in lymphoid cells and can be mutated in lymphoid malignancies [16], including in ALL, although this appears to be rare [17]. Activity of caspase-10 has been implicated in the response to a number of chemotherapeutic agents including etoposide, doxorubicin, arsenic trioxide and paclitaxel [18–20]. This can be mediated by p53-dependent, or histone-H3 acetylation-dependent modulation of the *CASP10* locus [18].

We have previously reported that the nitric oxide donating non-steroidal anti-inflammatory drug (NO-NSAID) *para*-NO-aspirin (*para*-NO-ASA) has anti-leukemic activity against human ALL by induction of apoptosis in association with suppression of NF-κB signalling [21]. NO-NSAID drugs consist of traditional NSAID to which an NO-donating moiety is covalently attached via an aromatic or aliphatic spacer [22]. These compounds demonstrate substantial anti-cancer activity and are up to 20 fold more potent than the parental NSAID [23]. *para*-NO-ASA is the best characterized NO-NSAID and *para*-NO-ASA demonstrated a several hundred-fold increase in potency compared with aspirin [24].

In this study we examined the mechanisms involved in *para*-NO-ASA induced apoptosis. We found that *para*-NO-ASA resulted in caspase-10 dependent cell death. Although associated with caspase-10 binding to TNF-R1, there was no evidence to suggest that cell death was ligand dependent. Cell death was associated with suppression of SODD, suggesting that SODD provides protection from death receptor induced death. Agents that specifically suppress SODD may be of therapeutic benefit for the treatment of this disease. Furthermore SODD is overexpressed in a number of malignancies including ovarian and pancreatic cancers [25,26] and suppression of SODD has recently been associated with the induction of cell death in melanoma [27], suggesting that modulation of SODD may have broader application in cancer treatment.

Experimental Procedures

Chemicals and reagents

para-NO-ASA [2-(acetyloxy)benzoic acid 4-(nitrooxymethyl)-phenyl ester] was purchased from NicOx (Sophia Antipolis, France). The inhibitors of caspase-8 (Z-IETD-FMK) and caspase-9 (Z-LEHD-FMK), Fix/Perm and Perm/Wash solutions, mouse anti-human TNF-α PE, annexin V FITC and AlexaFluor 647, and 7AAD were obtained from Becton Dickinson (North Ryde, NSW, Australia). Tetramethylrhodamine methyl ester (TMRM) was purchased from Molecular Probes (Invitrogen, Grand Island, NY, USA), N-acetyl cysteine (NAC) from Sigma-Aldrich (St Louis, MO, USA), the InnoCyte Flow Cytometric Cytochrome C release Kit from Calbiochem (San Diego, CA, USA) and the Caspase-8 (BF4100) and caspase-9 (BF10100) activity assays were purchased from Bioscientific (Sydney, Australia). The following antibodies to human proteins were purchased: mouse anti-β-actin (Sigma-Aldrich); rabbit anti-SODD (Chemicon, Boronia, VIC, Australia); rabbit anti-PUMA, rabbit anti-Bcl-X_L Alexa Fluor-488, rabbit anti-BIM, rabbit anti-XIAP, rabbit anti-TNF-R1, rabbit anti-Bid, rabbit anti-cleaved caspase-9, rabbit anti-cleaved caspase-8, rabbit anti-full length caspase-10 (Cell Signaling Technologies, Boston, MA, USA); mouse anti-Noxa (Abcam, Cambridge, MA, USA). Goat anti-mouse Alexa Fluor-488 was purchased from Invitrogen. Human recombinant TNF-α was purchased from Millipore (Nth Ryde, NSW, Australia). Caspase-10 inhibitor AEVD-FMK was purchased from Biovision (Mountain View, CA, USA) and FAM Caspase-10 kit from AbD Serotec (Raleigh, NC, USA). Primers for PCR amplification were synthesized by Proligo (Lismore, NSW, Australia) or Sigma Aldrich.

Cells

Pre-B ALL cell lines NALM6 (DSMZ Braunschweig, Germany), Reh (ATCC, Manassas, VA, USA) and LK63 (gift of Prof A. Boyd, QMIR, Australia) [28], the Burkitt's lymphoma lines Raji and Daudi and T-ALL lines Jurkat and CEMT4 (ATCC) were cultured in RPMI medium with 10% fetal calf serum. The stromal-dependent cells were grown in RPMI with 10% fetal calf serum, on confluent layers of either a human bone marrow stromal cell line transformed with hTERT, here termed hTERT.BMS, (kind gift of Dr D. Campana, Memphis TN, USA) [29] or bone marrow stromal cells prepared as previously described [30].

Leukemic blasts were isolated from the bone marrow samples from five patients with B cell progenitor ALL and cryopreserved as previously described [31]. Samples were collected following informed written consent from the donor or guardian as appropriate and with ethics approval from the Sydney West Area Heath Service Human Research Ethics Committee. Details for 0407 cells have been previously published [32]. The details of the stromal-dependent lines, including the patient characteristics have been previously published [33,34]. A summary of the clinical information for all patient-derived samples and cell lines used in this study has been provided in Table S1 for convenience.

Proliferation and cell cycle analysis

Cell proliferation was determined by [^{3}H]-thymidine (Amersham Biosciences, NSW, Australia) incorporation as previously described [35]. The proliferation index = CPM of treated cells/ CPM of control cells. Cell cycle analysis was performed by assessment of DNA content after staining with propidium iodide as previously described [33].

Apoptosis and Caspase activation

Apoptosis was assessed by Annexin V/PI or 7AAD staining as previously described [35,36]. Cells negative for annexin V and PI (or 7AAD) were considered viable. Pan-caspase activation was measured by incubation of cells with 10 μM CaspACE^{TM} FITC-VAD-FMK (Promega) for 20 min in the dark at 37°C. Washed cells were analysis on FACSCalibur flow cytometer (Becton Dickinson) using Cell Quest software. Activation of specific caspases was assessed by flow cytometry using specific antibodies.

Assessment of TNF-α Production

For detection of TNF-α protein, cells were treated with 2 μM monensin and 1 μg/ml Brefeldin A for 4 h at 37°C prior to fixation with Fix/Perm solution for 20 min at 4°C. Cells were washed in Perm/Wash buffer and directly labelled for TNF-α using PE conjugated anti-TNF-α antibody.

Mitochondrial Depolarization and Cytochrome c Release

Mitochondrial depolarization was measured using 143 nM TMRM in PBS at 37°C for 20 mins, followed by labelling with annexin V Alexafluor 647 and 7AAD. A 5 min exposure to 12.5 mM CCCP (carbonyl cyanide 3-chlorophenylhydrazone) was used as a positive control. Cytochrome c release was performed using the InnoCyte Flow Cytometric Cytochrome C release Kit according to manufacturer's instructions except that goat anti-mouse Alexa Fluor 647 was used as the second layer.

RT-PCR and qRT-PCR

Total RNA was extracted using Trizol reagent and reverse transcribed. The relative expression ratio of the target genes was compared with the housekeeping gene glyceraldehyde-3-phosphate dehydrogenase (GAPDH) using the same cDNA. Values were then normalised to the untreated sample. All samples were run in quadruplicates. The primers for SODD were: Forward: acccaagtacatatcctgtaagacc; Reverse: aggagaagcccacgcatcttc. Those for GAPDH have been previously published (Khan, et al 2008).

For the qRT-PCR cDNA was prepared as above. SODD mRNA expression levels were quantitated from standard curves generated using cDNA prepared from NALM6 cells by real-time RT-PCR using SYBR Green JumpStart Taq Ready Mix (Sigma-Aldrich, Sydney, Australia) and a Corbett 6000 thermocycler (Corbett Life Science, NSW, Australia) and specific primers: SODD forward – acatgtgctggagagaaggtccagt; SODD reverse – acagagtcctggcccccagt. Values were normalised to the expression level of GAPDH using the same cDNA to generate the standard curve. The primers for GAPDH have been previously published (Bendall, et al 2004).

Immunoprecipitation and Western blotting

Cell lysates were prepared as previously described [35]. Immunoprecipitations were performed using Protein G Dynabeads (Invitrogen) according to the manufacturer's instructions. Beads were crosslinked to antibodies to TNF-R1 (Genesearch, Arundel, QLD, Australia) or Mouse IgG2b control (DakoCytomation), using bis(sulfosuccinimidyl)suberate reagent as described by the manufacturer. Immunoprecipitated material was eluted directly into SDS-PAGE reducing buffer. Western blotting was performed as previously described [35].

Lentiviral Knockdown of SODD

Lentiviral constructs were prepared as previously described [37] using the following shRNA sequences to SODD: SODD1 - acatatacttcatgtgtaatt or SODD2 - ccaacaatcaagatcaaagta. Lentiviral transduction was performed with Institutional Biosafety Committee approval. NALM6, LK63 or REH cells (1×10^6/mL) were transduced in RPMI containing 10% FCS, 8 µg/ml polybrene and 40×10^6 viral particles/ml containing shRNA for either SODD1 or SODD2 or empty vector (control) for 48 h. Viral particles were removed and the cells cultured in complete media for the indicated times. Successfully transduced cells were identified by GFP expression.

Statistical Analysis

Comparisons between 2 groups were performed using Student's t-tests and between multiple groups using ANOVA analysis. Pairwise comparisons between groups were adjusted for multiple comparisons using Bonferroni's method. Significance was defined as having a p value of less than 0.05.

Results

para-NO-ASA induces apoptotic cell death in pre-B ALL cell lines

We have recently shown that *para*-NO-ASA suppresses NF-κB signalling in ALL cells and that this is associated with apoptotic cell death [21]. Here we investigated the mechanism of this in more detail and extend the findings to primary patient cells. *para*-NO-ASA inhibited the proliferation of all three B cell progenitor ALL cell lines (NALM6, REH and LK63) tested in a dose dependent manner, with IC_{50} values in the low micromolar range (Fig 1A). Despite suppression of NF-κB signalling, changes in cell cycle distribution in response to *para*-NO-ASA were not consistently observed (Fig 1B and data not shown). However, a significant sub-$G_{0/1}$ peak was detected in all three cell lines, consistent with apoptotic cell death as previously reported in ALL cell lines [21]. *para*-NO-ASA also induced cell death in 5 freshly thawed patient samples ($p = 0.016$ for 5 µM and 0.006 for 10 µM *para*-NO-ASA) as well as 4 patient samples that had been expanded *in vitro* by co-culture with human stromal layers ($p = 0.029$ for 5 µM and $p = 0.0006$ for 10 µM *para*-NO-ASA) (Fig 1C), demonstrating that the effect is not confined to cell lines. Closer investigation of the cell death mechanism revealed activation of the executioner caspases -3 and -7 after 12 h (Fig 2A and data not shown) with cleavage of caspase-3 in response to 5 µM and 10 µM *para*-NO-ASA in NALM6 cells (Fig 2B) showing similar kinetics to those previously reported for pan-caspase detection by Z-VAD FITC [21]. Activation of caspase-3 correlated with a dose-dependent cleavage of PARP detected by Western blotting, 12 h after drug treatment in NALM6 cells (Fig 2C). These data are consistent with our previous demonstration that *para*-NO-ASA induced cell death is caspase dependent [21].

para-NO-ASA induces mitochondrial depolarisation ($\Delta\Psi_m$) and mitochondrial outer membrane permeabilization (MOMP)

Loss of the inner mitochondrial transmembrane potential ($\Delta\Psi_m$) and outer membrane permeablization (MOMP) are features of a number of cell death mechanisms including apoptotic cell death [38]. Treatment of cells with 5 µM *para*-NO-ASA resulted in a loss of $\Delta\Psi_m$ and release of cytochrome c. Loss of $\Delta\Psi_m$ occurred prior to the loss of plasma membrane integrity as determined by 7AAD staining (Fig 2D) and cytochrome c release (Fig 2E and F). Both occurred in close association with the induction of apoptosis as determined by annexin V staining. During cell death mediated by the intrinsic pathway, caspase activation occurs following loss of $\Delta\Psi_m$, MOMP and cytochrome c release and formation of the apoptosome [4]. In contrast, when death is mediated via the extrinsic pathway, loss of $\Delta\Psi_m$ and cytochrome c release is the result of caspase-8 and/or caspase-10 activation, and truncation of Bid [39]. Pan-caspase inhibition completely prevented mitochondrial depolarization implicating the extrinsic death mechanism (Fig 2G). We have previously reported that *para*-NO-ASA induced apoptosis is dependent on the generation of reactive oxygen species (ROS) [21] and here we found that inhibition of ROS by the anti-oxidant NAC also attenuated mitochondrial depolarization (Fig 2G).

para-NO-ASA activates the initiator caspases-8, -9 and -10 but only caspase-10 activation is required for cell death

para-NO-ASA treatment activated the initiator caspases of the extrinsic cell death mechanism, caspase-8, and -10, as well as the

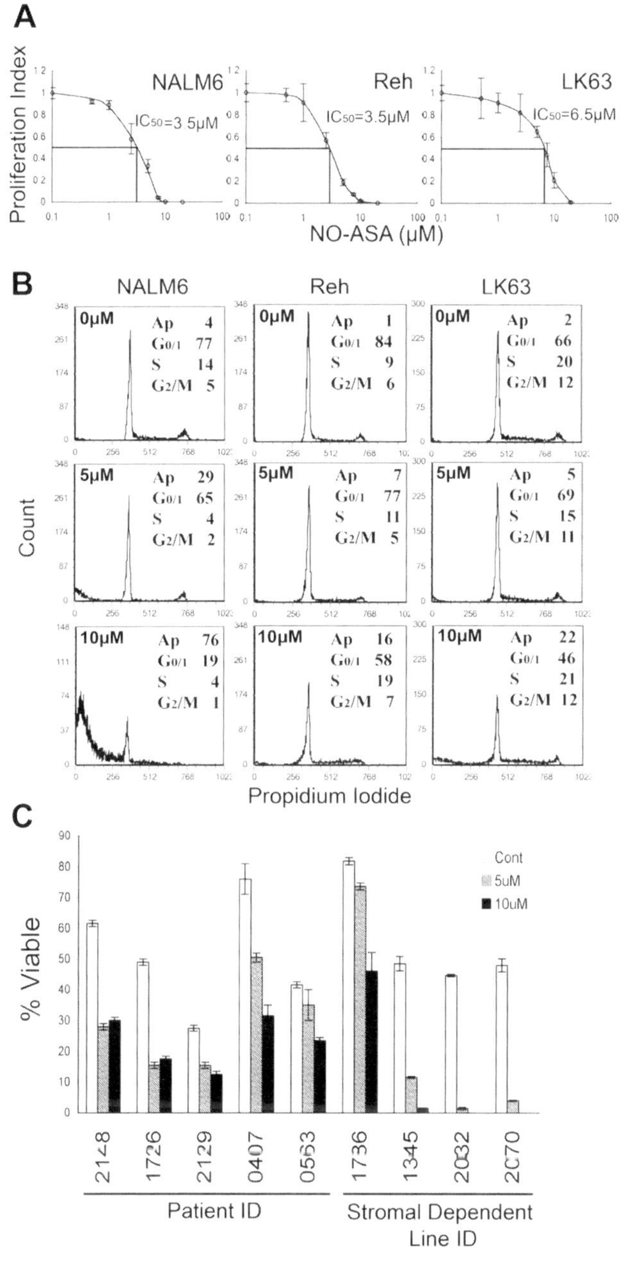

Figure 1. *para*-NO-ASA inhibit the proliferation and induces cell death in ALL cell lines and patient samples. (A) The proliferation of the indicated ALL cell lines as determined by ^{3}H-thymidine incorporation following 24 hours incubation with *para*-NO-ASA. Vertical bars represent standard deviation of quadruplicate determinations from one of 2 independent experiments. Curves were generated using the line of best fit in Excel software. IC_{50} values are indicated. (B) Cell cycle analysis of ALL cell lines treated with indicated concentrations of *para*-NO-ASA for 24 hours. Representative plots including the mean from duplicate assessments are shown. (C) The viability of pre-B ALL patient samples or patient derived stromal dependent cell lines was assessed after 24 hours of culture in the presence of DMSO (Cont), 5 or 10 μM *para*-NO-ASA by annexin V and 7AAD staining with dual negative cells being considered viable. Vertical bars represent standard deviation of quadruplicate determinations.

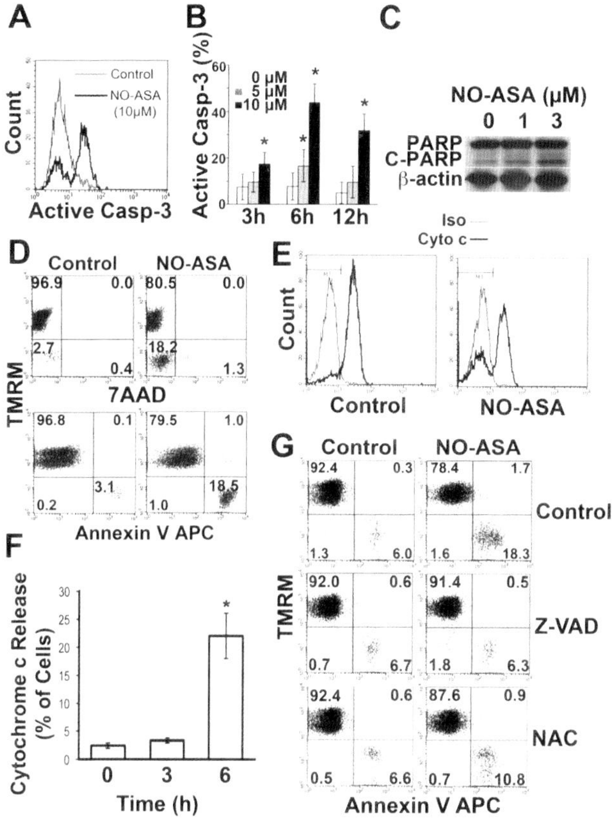

Figure 2. *para*-NO-ASA results in activation of executioner caspases and mitochondrial depolarization. (A) Cleavage of caspase-3 in NALM6 cells by intracellular flow cytometry following 6 hour exposure to 10 μM *para*-NO-ASA. (B) Caspase-3 activation as measured by flow cytometry, in NALM6 cells untreated or treated with 5 μM or 10 μM *para*-NO-ASA for the given time. Bars indicate the mean and s.d. of 3 independent experiments. (C) Western blot analysis of PARP activation in NALM6 cells stimulated with the indicated concentrations of *para*-NO-ASA for 12 hours. The cleaved (89 kD) and uncleaved (116 kD) forms of PARP are indicated. Data is representative of 2 independent experiments. (D) NALM6 cells were treated with 5 μM *para*-NO-ASA or vehicle for 6 hours and assessed for $\Delta\Psi_m$ using TMRM to label cells with polarized mitochondria, and apoptosis using annexin V and 7AAD. Representative plots are shown and the mean percentage of cells from 2 experiments in each quadrant indicated. (E) Representative histograms showing cytochrome c release following exposure of NALM6 cells to 5 μM para-NO-ASA for 6 hours. The thin line represents isotype control (Iso) staining and the heavy line cytochrome c (Cyto c) staining. (F) Quantitation of cytochrome c release at the indicated time points following addition of 5 μM *para*-NO-ASA. The mean and s.d. of replicates is shown. $^{*}p = 0.02$. (G) NALM6 cells were pre-treated with 100 μM Z-VAD or 2.5 mM NAC for 1 hour prior to exposure to 5 μM *para*-NO-ASA for 6 h the mean ± s.e. is shown (n≥5). $^{*}p < 0.05$ compared to NO-ASA alone.

initiator caspase for the intrinsic pathway, caspase-9. Cleavage of caspases-8 and -9, and loss of full-length caspase-10 following treatment with *para*-NO-ASA was demonstrated by Western blotting in NALM6 cells (Fig 3A). The activity of caspase-8 and -9 were confirmed using a colormetric activity assay (Fig 3B). The cleavage of caspase-10 could not be determined by western blotting as the antibody only recognised the full-length protein. However, activation of caspase-10 was demonstrated by flow cytometry (Fig 3C). Cleavage of all 3 caspases occurred between 1 and 3 h with no activation detectable at 1 h and some activation of all cases present at 3 h. Caspase cleavage preceded the disruption of mitochondrial function with greater than 60% of cells having activated caspase-10 by 6 h, but less than 30% of cells having disrupted mitochondria (Fig 3C&D). The percentage of cells with cleaved caspase-8 and -9 could not be determined, as Western blotting does not permit the identification of individual cells with activated caspases. Consistent with an extrinsic death mechanism Bid was processed to form tBid (Fig 3A). The presence of tBid, as well as the increase in Puma and Noxa (Fig 3A) provides a mechanism for inhibiting anti-apoptosis proteins including Bcl-2 and Bcl-X_L despite the lack of change in the level of these proteins (Fig S1). Furthermore, Mcl1 was down regulated in response to *para*-NO-ASA (Fig 3D). These results indicate that ultimately both intrinsic and extrinsic pathways are activated.

Surprisingly inhibition of caspase-8 and/or caspase-9 failed to completely inhibit apoptosis induced by *para*-NO-ASA, although caspase-9 inhibition did have a partial but statistically insignificant effect (Fig 4A left panel and data not shown). In contrast, inhibition of caspase-10 resulted in a complete block of *para*-NO-ASA-induced apoptosis (Fig 4A). Inhibition of caspase-10 also completely prevented $\Delta\Psi_m$ (Fig 4A right panel), suggesting that caspase-10 activation is an early and essential component of *para*-NO-ASA-mediated cell death. Indeed inhibition of caspase-10 also prevented activation of caspases-8 and -9 (Fig 4B). We have shown in Figure 1 that *para*-NO-ASA induces cell death in ALL cells from patients and as expected it also activated caspase-10 in these samples (Fig 4C).

Caspase-10 associates with TNF-R1 following treatment with para-NO-ASA

Caspase-10 forms part of the extrinsic death pathway, normally activated by factors such as TNF-α [40]. We were unable to detect any increase in TNF-R1 expression by quantitative RT-PCR (Fig 3D) or flow cytometry in response to *para*-NO-ASA (Fig 5A). Similarly there was no apparent induction of TNF-α expression in NALM6 cells following exposure to *para*-NO-ASA (Fig 5B) and there was no evidence of intracellular stores of the cytokine that could have been released following treatment. However, examination of complexes that co-precipitated with TNF-R1 demonstrated that addition of *para*-NO-ASA increases caspase-10 association with TNF-R1 (Fig 5C). We were unable to detect caspase-8 in the precipitated complexes (data not shown), however caspase-8 was also not detected in TNF-α induced complexes so it is possible this was a sensitivity issue and firm conclusions regarding the absence of caspase-8 should not be drawn from this data. Regardless, this suggests that TNF-R1 is involved in *para*-NO-ASA mediated apoptosis.

SODD is Over-expressed in ALL Cells and is Required for the Maintenance of Cell Viability. SODD is thought to prevent spontaneous, and suppress TNF-α-induced, trimerisation of TNF-R1 and signalling [6,7], and is also reportedly over-expressed in ALL cells [41], a finding which we have confirmed and extended here (Fig 6C). Interestingly the smaller isoform was predominant in leukemic cells, while the larger isoform was more abundant in normal peripheral blood mononuclear cells (PBMCs), although both forms were present in normal PBMC on longer exposure. *para*-NO-ASA resulted in down regulation of SODD mRNA and protein levels (Fig 6A&B). Consistent with SODD preventing activation of TNF-R1, ALL cells were found to be refractory to cell death induced by exogenous TNF-α (Fig S2). In contrast, a small but significant proliferative response to TNF-α was detected, probably via activation of TNF-R2 (Fig S2). Lentiviral based constructs to knockdown of SODD were prepared, and although both significantly reduced SODD expression, the first construct, SODD1, was superior, producing a log greater reduction in SODD mRNA expression in NALM6 cells on day 6 of the culture than SODD2 (Fig 6E): similar results were obtained for REH cells. In LK63 cells sufficient transduced

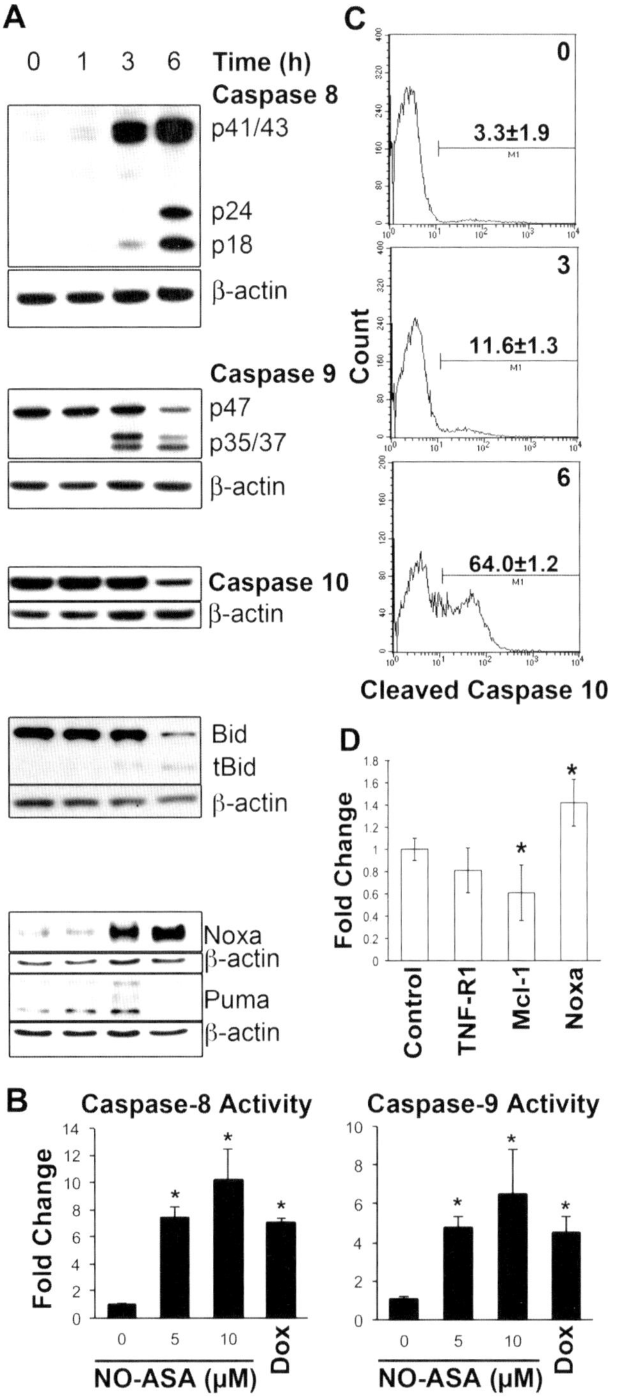

Figure 3. Multiple caspases are activated by *para*-NO-ASA. (A) Western blot of cell lysates from cells treated with *para*-NO-ASA for the indicated times. Western Blot of caspases-8 (cleaved forms only), -9 (full length, p47 and cleaved forms), caspase-10 (full length only), Bid (full length and cleaved forms) and full length Noxa and Puma are shown. Note that the caspase-8 antibody (#9496) only recognised the cleaved forms and not the intact protein, while the caspase-10 antibody only recognised the full-length form of the protein. (B) NALM6 cells were treated with 5 μM NO-ASA for 6 h and cell lysates analysed for caspase-8 or caspase-9 activity. The mean±SD of 3 experiments is shown. *$p<0.05$ compared to control. (C) Representative histograms showing *para*-NO-ASA mediated activation of caspase 10 as determined by flow cytometry. Time of exposure to *para*-NO-ASA is indicated on the histograms. The mean and s.d. from one of two independent experiments is shown. (D) Gene expression was assessed using quantitative RT-PCR in NALM6 cells treated with 10 μM *para*-NO-ASA for 12 hours. *$p<0.05$.

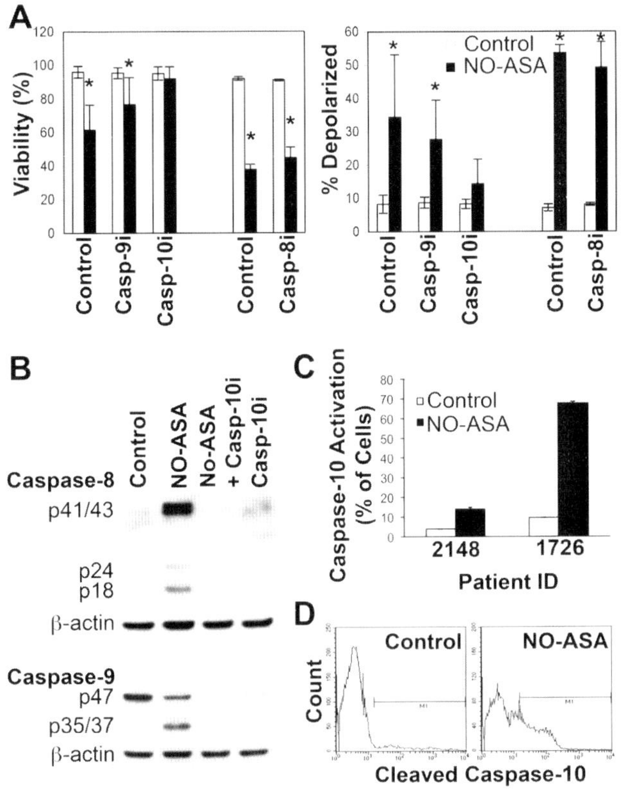

Figure 4. Caspase-10 activation is required for *para*-NO-ASA induced cell death. (A) The viability (top panel), as determined by 7AAD and annexin V staining, and mitochondrial depolarization (lower panel) of NALM6 cells treated with vehicle or 5 μM *para*-NO-ASA for the 30 min following pre-incubation with inhibitors of caspase-8, -9 or caspase-10. Mean and s.d. of 3 independent experiments is shown. *$p < 0.05$. (B) Western blot showing the cleavage of caspase-8 and -9 following treatment with 10 μM *para*-NO-ASA with or without a 30 min pre-incubation with the caspase-10 inhibitor. (C) Activation of caspase-10 in patient samples exposed to 5 μM *para*-NO-ASA for 6 h as assessed by flow cytometry. The mean and s.d. of duplicate samples is shown. (D) Activation of caspase-10 in control treated NALM6 cells (left) or NALM6 cells treated with 10 μM *para*-NO-ASA (right) for 6 h. The mean and s.d. of duplicate assessments of caspase-10 activation is shown in the lower right panel.

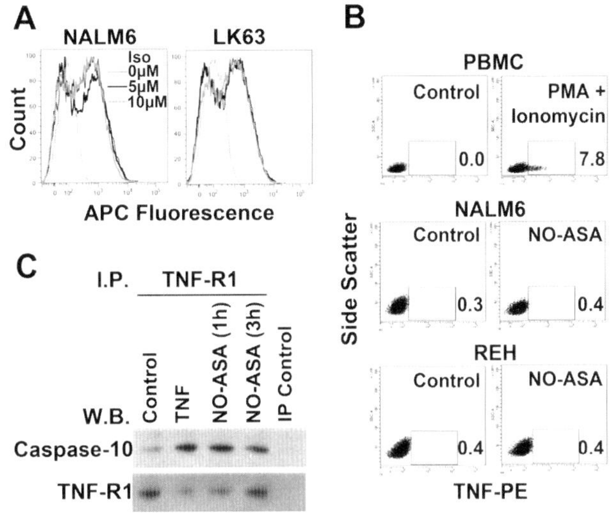

Figure 5. *para*-NO-ASA induces formation of the death initiating signalling complex containing caspase-10 and suppression of SODD. (A) NALM6 and LK63 cell lines were treated with 10 μM *para*-NO-ASA for 6 h and labelled for surface TNF-R1 (left panels). (B) NALM6 and REH cells were treated with *para*-NO-ASA for 6 h and assessed for TNF-α production by flow cytometry. PBMC treated with 50 ng/ml PMA and 1 μg/ml ionomycin are included as a positive control. The percentage of cells expressing TNF-α is shown on each plot. (C) NALM6 cells were treated with TNF-α (100 ng/ml), or *para*-NO-ASA (10 μM) as indicated and cell lysates prepared. TNF-R1 was immunoprecipitated and recovered complexes probed for caspase-10 or TNF-R1.

cells were obtained to examine the knockdown of the SODD protein. Here the SODD1 construct was also superior to SODD2 (Fig 6D), although neither reduced SODD to the level seen in normal peripheral blood cells (Fig 6D). Culture of NALM6, REH and LK63 cells following infection with the control and SODD2 lentiviral constructs resulted in the expected cell expansion, but those transduced with SODD1 showed significant growth retardation (Fig 6F, left panels). The transduction efficiency in cells transduced with control and SODD2 constructs was high and sustained over time, while that in cells transduced with the SODD1 construct was significantly lower, resulting in a major reduction in the number of GFP expressing cells in these cultures (Fig 6F, centre and left panels). In LK63 cells, where the culture time was further extended, the cells expressing the SODD2 construct also started to decline in the culture, albeit at a slower rate. This suggests that a threshold level of SODD is required for the survival of ALL cells and by inference that *para*-NO-ASA induced cell death is at least partially the result of the reduction of SODD expression.

Discussion

We report here that *para*-NO-ASA results in apoptotic cell death mediated through activation of caspase-10. The biochemical process appears to relate closely to death receptor mediated apoptosis, with activation of caspase-10 being the initiating event followed by cleavage of Bid, and loss of $\Delta\Psi_m$ and MOMP. Ultimately the intrinsic death mechanism is triggered with activation of caspase-9, and the executioner caspases-3 and -7. Cleavage of caspase-10 was subsequent to its association with TNF-R1. This demonstrates that *para*-NO-ASA is mediating cell death via activation of the extrinsic cell death mechanism.

Caspase-8 plays the predominant role in most scenarios involving extrinsic cell death, including those triggered by TNF-α. In contrast, *para*-NO-ASA resulted in caspase-10 dependent death in ALL cells with no measurable role for caspase-8. Caspase-10 is highly expressed in lymphoid cells and is frequently down regulated in lymphoid cell lines [40], and other cancers [42,43]. Mutations in caspase-10 are associated with autoimmune lymphoproliferative syndrome type II, suggesting that caspase-10 is important for the regulation of normal lymphoid cells [15]. Although mutations in caspase-10 have been demonstrated in Non-Hodgkin's lymphoma and are thought to contribute to disease pathogenesis [16], such mutations have not been detected in B lineage ALL [17], and are not associated with breast or ovarian cancer risk [44]. It is therefore likely that the majority of ALL samples will have functional caspase-10. Cell death that is exclusively or predominantly caspase-10 dependent has only rarely been reported, even within lymphoid populations. In most of these settings, caspase-10 activation occurred downstream of the mitochondria and independently of death receptors. Examples include cell death induced by Taxol in the human lymphoblastic

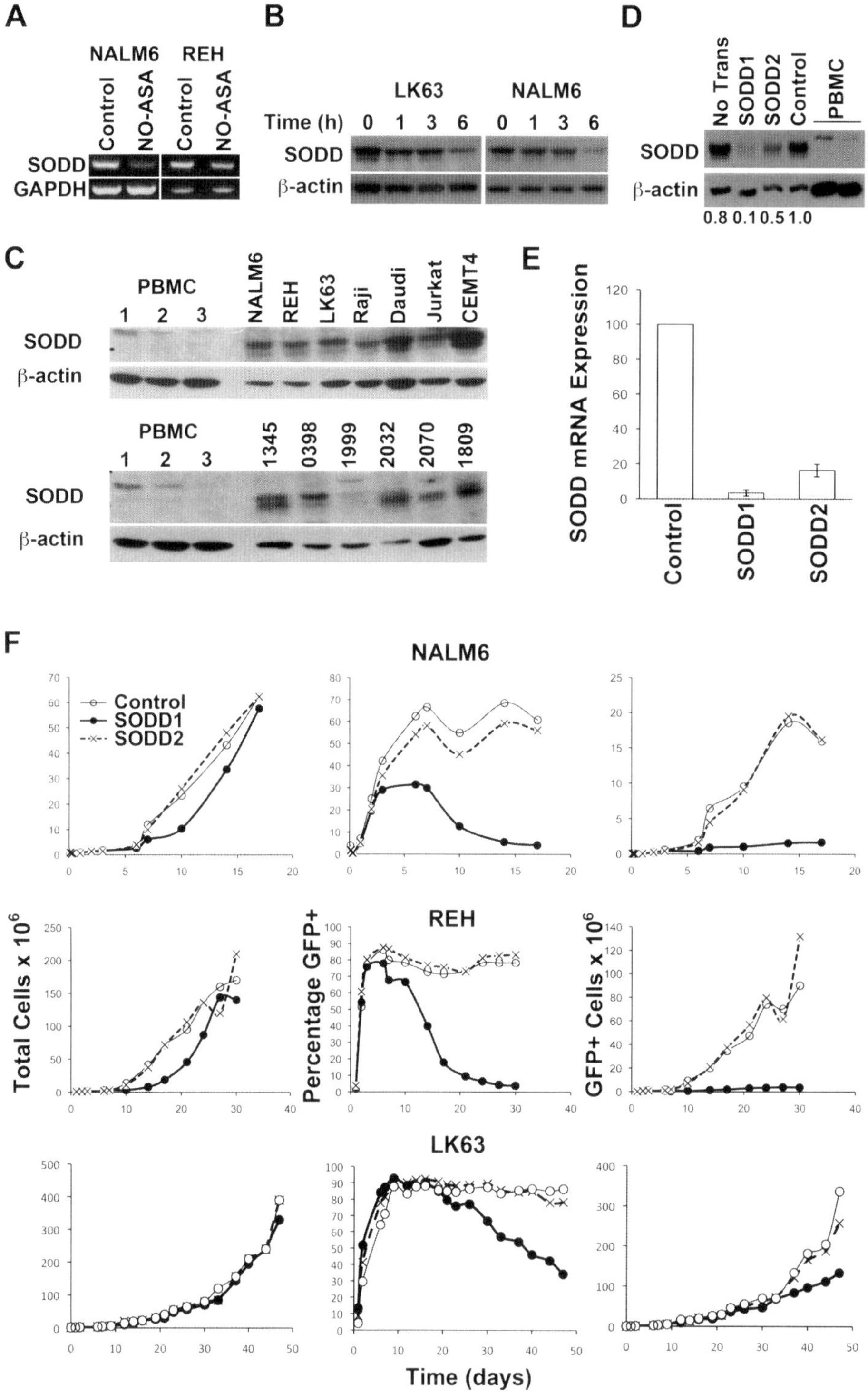

Figure 6. SODD is over-expressed in ALL cells and expression is required for ALL cell growth. (A) SODD expression was determined by semi-quantitative RT-PCR in NALM6 and REH cells treated with 10 μM *para*-NO-ASA for 12 h. (B) SODD expression was determined by western blotting following treatment with 10 μM *para*-NO-ASA for the indicated times. (C) Western blot analysis of SODD in normal peripheral blood mononuclear cells (PBMC), indicated cell lines (upper blots) or patient samples (lower blots). Patient samples had been expanded in NOD/SCID mice to obtain sufficient cells for Western blotting. (D) NALM6 transduced with lentiviral constructs expressing GFP alone (Control) or containing one of two shRNA specific for SODD (SODD1 and SODD2). The level of SODD protein (D) was determined in LK63 cells after 44 days in culture while mRNA levels were assessed in NALM6 cells on day 6 of culture by qRT-PCR and was normalised to the levels of GAPDH (E). The mean and s.e.m. of three independent experiments is shown. (F) The total cell number (left panels), and the percentage (centre panels) and total number of GFP+ transduced cells (right panels) was monitored over time. The mean and s.d. of duplicate cultures is shown.

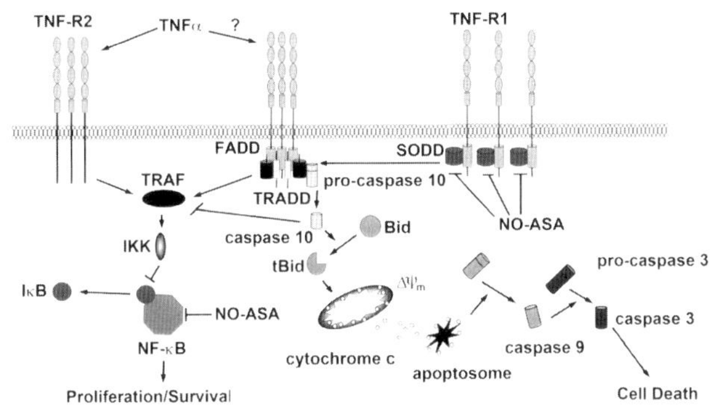

Figure 7. Schematic diagram illustrating the proposed mechanism of action of *para*-NO-ASA. *para*-NO-ASA down regulates SODD allowing self-aggregation, or enhancing TNF-α-induced, activation of signalling through TNF-R1. TNF-R1 signalling triggers the extrinsic apoptosis cascade including cleavage of pro-caspase-10 and Bid, mitochondrial depolarization, outer membrane permeabilization and release of cytochrome c. This is followed by cleavage of pro-caspase-9 and the executioner caspases-3 and -7. While signalling through TNF-R1 can activate NF-κB this may be suppressed by caspase-mediated cleavage of TRAF. In contrast, TNF-R2 signal induces cell survival and proliferation pathways, predominantly through NF-κB but also MAPK signalling. In ALL cells where SODD is over expressed, exogenous TNF-α is likely to predominantly signal through TNF-R2 resulting in increased survival and proliferation. Activating TNF-R1 by down regulation of SODD provides a mechanism for inducing cell death without increasing proliferation and survival signals. FADD, Fas-associated death domain; IKK, inhibitor of κB kinase; I-κB, inhibitor of κB; TRADD, TNF-R1-associated death domain; TRAF, TNF receptor-associated factor.

leukemia cell line, CCRF-HSB-2 [20], arsenic trioxide in acute promyelocytic leukemia cells [19], etoposide in U937 cells [45] and a number of other cell lines including Jurkat T cells [46], as well as in a colon cancer model [43]. In our study there was clear association between caspase-10 and TNF-R1, which preceded caspase activation, suggesting that TNF-R1 plays an active role in the process. However our inability to perform gene knockdown studies for caspase-10 and potential off target effects of the caspase-10 inhibitor used leaves room for the role of other caspases in *para*-NO-ASA induced cell death.

How the extrinsic death mechanism is triggered by *para*-NO-ASA is not entirely clear. B-lineage ALL cells only rarely express TNF-α [10,47], and we were unable to demonstrate any background, or *para*-NO-ASA-induced TNF-α production by NALM6 cells. This suggests that activation of TNF-R1 may be occurring in a ligand independent manner. Death receptors including TNF-R1 are known to self-aggregate, particularly when over-expressed and SODD is believed to play a role in keeping this in check [6]. Ligand-independent association has been previously reported in lung and breast carcinoma and although associated with DNA damage, DNA damage alone was not sufficient to activate TNF-R1 [48]. However the possibility remains that TNF-α, below the limit of detection, may be present and activates TNF-R1. We were unable to detect evidence of *para*-NO-ASA induced DNA damage using γ-H2AX staining prior to apoptosis driven DNA fragmentation (data not shown). This suggests that the DNA damage response is not involved. More recently ligand-independent activation of TNF-R1 has been associated with oxidative conditions and modification of cysteine residues within the extracellular cysteine rich domains of TNF-R1 in the model cell systems of renal and cervical cancer, most likely in the pre-ligand assembly domain (PLAD) [49]. This may be important in *para*-NO-ASA-induced cell death, as we have previously shown that reactive oxygen species are produced and are required for cell death in this setting [21].

Another possibility is that suppression of SODD by *para*-NO-ASA permits constitutive activation through TNF-R1 self-association. SODD is an anti-apoptotic protein that associates with the death domain of TNF-R1, Fas and death receptor-3 (DR3), and thereby negatively regulates cell death signalling [6,7]. The importance of SODD in maintaining TNF-R1 in an inactive conformation under physiological conditions has not been fully resolved, with one study finding no phenotype in SODD deficient mice, while another reported enhanced cytokine production [50,51]. Here we observed loss of SODD concomitantly with caspase-10 association with TNF-R1, which is consistent with SODD playing an active role in keeping TNF-R1 signalling in check. SODD is also reportedly over expressed in ALL [41], a finding that we confirmed in this study.

The death inducing ligands, TNF-α, Fas and TRAIL have not demonstrated the hoped for potency in killing malignant cells and methods to enhance the efficacy of these agents have been explored with varying degrees of success [52,53]. The role of TNF-α in ALL cell biology is unclear with the initial report showing suppression of ALL cell proliferation [47], while subsequent reports suggest that TNF-α enhances ALL cell growth [54]. The co-expression of TNF-R2, which lacks death domains in its cytoplasmic tail and hence only activates pro-survival NF-κB signalling [55], would also be expected to promote proliferation and survival in ALL cells. The pro-survival signals activated by NF-κB are known to limit the cytotoxic effects of TNF-α and other death ligands [56]. Over expression of SODD would be expected to further enhance ALL cell survival by preventing signalling through TNF-R1 and other death receptors such as Fas and DR3, but not TNF-R2 [6,41]. It is tempting to speculate that the potency of *para*-NO-ASA results from activation of signalling through TNF-R1, due to suppression of SODD, in the absence of any increase in NF-κB signalling through TNF-R2 (Fig 7). Furthermore, we have previously shown that *para*-NO-ASA suppresses NF-κB signalling [21]. Therefore, unlike TNF-α, *para*-NO-ASA activates death receptor signalling by inhibition of SODD while simultaneously suppressing pro-survival NF-κB signalling. We were surprised to discover that suppression of SODD expression alone was sufficient to significantly impair the growth of ALL cell lines. This finding is reminiscent of cells displaying oncogene addiction, which are killed following oncogene withdrawal, while normal cells are relatively unaffected. This suggests that targeting SODD may be a new therapeutic strategy for the treatment of ALL and other malignancies where SODD is overexpressed.

Acknowledgments

The authors would like to thank Dr Lisa Sedger for helpful discussions that assisted in the finalization of the study and the writing of the manuscript.

Author Contributions

Conceived and designed the experiments: NIK LJB KFB HR. Performed the experiments: AC RB NIK CF RW JB. Analyzed the data: AC RB LJB NIK. Contributed reagents/materials/analysis tools: HR CF. Wrote the paper: LJB KFB.

References

1. Pui CH (2010) Recent research advances in childhood acute lymphoblastic leukemia. J Formos Med Assoc 109: 777–787.
2. Gokbuget N, Hoelzer D (2009) Treatment of adult acute lymphoblastic leukemia. Semin Hematol 46: 64–75.
3. Movassagh M, Foo R (2008) Simplified apoptotic cascades. Heart Fail Rev 13: 111–119.
4. Goldstein J, Waterhouse N, Juin P, Evan G, Green D (2000) The coordinate release of cytochrome c during apoptosis is rapid, complete and kinetically invariant. Nat Cell Biol 2(3):156–62: 2(3):156–162.
5. Li P, Nijhawan D, Budihardjo I, Srinivasula SM, Ahmad M, et al. (1997) Cytochrome c and dATP-dependent formation of Apaf-1/caspase-9 complex initiates an apoptotic protease cascade. Cell 91: 479–489.
6. Jiang Y, Woronicz JD, Liu W, Goeddel DV (1999) Prevention of constitutive TNF receptor 1 signaling by silencer of death domains. Science 283: 543–546.
7. Eichholtz-Wirth H, Fritz E, Wolz L (2003) Overexpression of the 'silencer of death domain', SODD/BAG-4, modulates both TNFR1- and CD95-dependent cell death pathways. Cancer Lett 194: 81–89.
8. Kischkel FC, Hellbardt S, Behrmann I, Germer M, Pawlita M, et al. (1995) Cytotoxicity-dependent APO-1 (Fas/CD95)-associated proteins form a death-inducing signaling complex (DISC) with the receptor. EMBO J 14: 5579–5588.
9. Luo X, Budihardjo I, Zou H, Slaughter C, Wang X (1998) Bid, a Bcl2 interacting protein, mediates cytochrome c release from mitochondria in response to activation of cell surface death receptors. Cell 94: 481–490.
10. Pituch-Noworolska A, Gawlicka M, Wotoszyn M, Balwierz W, Strojny W, et al. (1998) Tumour necrosis factor alpha (TNF alpha) and leukaemic cells: secretion and response. Clin Lab Haematol 20: 231–238.
11. Karawajew L, Wuchter C, Ruppert V, Drexler H, Gruss H, et al. (1997) Differential CD95 expression and function in T and B lineage acute lymphoblastic leukemia cells. Leukemia 11: 1245–1252.
12. Ehrhardt H, Fulda S, Schmid I, Hiscott J, Debatin KM, et al. (2003) TRAIL induced survival and proliferation in cancer cells resistant towards TRAIL-induced apoptosis mediated by NF-kappaB. Oncogene 22: 3842–3852.
13. Reed JC, Doctor K, Rojas A, Zapata JM, Stehlik C, et al. (2003) Comparative analysis of apoptosis and inflammation genes of mice and humans. Genome Res 13: 1376–1388.
14. Kischkel FC, Lawrence DA, Tinel A, LeBlanc H, Virmani A, et al. (2001) Death receptor recruitment of endogenous caspase-10 and apoptosis initiation in the absence of caspase-8. J Biol Chem 276: 46639–46646.
15. Wang J, Zheng L, Lobito A, Chan FK, Dale J, et al. (1999) Inherited human Caspase 10 mutations underlie defective lymphocyte and dendritic cell apoptosis in autoimmune lymphoproliferative syndrome type II. Cell 98: 47–58.
16. Shin MS, Kim HS, Kang CS, Park WS, Kim SY, et al. (2002) Inactivating mutations of CASP10 gene in non-Hodgkin lymphomas. Blood 99: 4094–4099.
17. Rozenfeld-Granot G, Toren A, Amariglio N, Brok-Simoni F, Rechavi G (2001) Mutation analysis of the FAS and TNFR apoptotic cascade genes in hematological malignancies. Exp Hematol 29: 228–233.
18. Rikhof B, Corn PG, El-Deiry WS (2003) Caspase 10 levels are increased following DNA damage in a p53-dependent manner. Cancer Biol Ther 2: 707–712.
19. Li J, Chen P, Sinogeeva N, Gorospe M, Wersto RP, et al. (2002) Arsenic trioxide promotes histone H3 phosphoacetylation at the chromatin of CASPASE-10 in acute promyelocytic leukemia cells. J Biol Chem 277: 49504–49510.
20. Park SJ, Wu CH, Gordon JD, Zhong X, Emami A, et al. (2004) Taxol induces caspase-10-dependent apoptosis. J Biol Chem 279: 51057–51067.
21. Khan NI, Cisterne A, Baraz R, Bradstock KF, Bendall LJ (2012) Para-NO-Aspirin inhibits NF-κB and induces apoptosis in B-cell progenitor acute lymphoblastic leukemia. Exp Hematol 40: 207–215.
22. del Soldato P, Sorrentino R, Pinto A (1999) NO-aspirins: a class of new anti-inflammatory and antithrombotic agents. Trends Pharmacol Sci 20: 319–323.
23. Kashfi K, Ryan Y, Qiao L, Williams J, Chen J, et al. (2002) Nitric oxide-donating nonsteroidal anti-inflammatory drugs inhibit the growth of various cultured human cancer cells: evidence of a tissue type-independent effect. J Pharmacol Exp Ther 303: 1273–1282.
24. Williams J, Borgo S, Hasan I, Castillo E, Traganos F, et al. (2001) Nitric oxide-releasing nonsteroidal anti-inflammatory drugs (NSAIDs) alter the kinetics of human colon cancer cell lines more effectively than traditional NSAIDs: implications for colon cancer chemoprevention. Cancer Res 61: 3285–3289.
25. Annunziata CM, Kleinberg L, Davidson B, Berner A, Gius D, et al. (2007) BAG-4/SODD and associated antiapoptotic proteins are linked to aggressiveness of epithelial ovarian cancer. Clin Cancer Res 13: 6585–6592.
26. Ozawa F, Friess H, Zimmermann A, Kleeff J, Buchler MW (2000) Enhanced expression of Silencer of death domains (SODD/BAG-4) in pancreatic cancer. Biochem Biophys Res Commun 271: 409–413.
27. Reuland SN, Smith SM, Bemis LT, Goldstein NB, Almeida AR, et al. (2013) MicroRNA-26a is strongly downregulated in melanoma and induces cell death through repression of silencer of death domains (SODD). J Invest Dermatol 133: 1286–1293.
28. Boyd AW, Ward LD, Wicks IP, Simpson RJ, Salvaris E, et al. (1992) Isolation and characterization of a novel receptor-type protein tyrosine kinase (hek) from a human pre-B cell line. J Biol Chem 267: 3262–3267.
29. Mihara K, Imai C, Coustan-Smith E, Dome J, Dominici M, et al. (2003) Development and functional characterization of human bone marrow mesenchymal cells immortalized by enforced expression of telomerase. Br J Haematol 120: 846–849.
30. Kortlepel K, Bendall LJ, Gottlieb DJ (1993) Adhesion molecule expression on human myeloid leukemic cells:Regulation by growth factors. Leukemia 7: 1174–1179.
31. Bendall LJ, Kortlepel K, Gottlieb DJ (1993) Human acute myeloid leukemia cells bind to bone marrow stroma via a combination of beta 1 and beta 2 integrin mechanisms. Blood 82: 3125–3132.
32. Khan NI, Bradstock KF, Bendall LJ (2007) Activation of Wnt/beta-catenin pathway mediates growth and survival in B-cell progenitor acute lymphoblastic leukaemia. Br J Haematol 138: 338–348.
33. Juarez J, Baraz R, Gaundar S, Bradstock K, Bendall L (2007) Interaction of interleukin-7 and interleukin-3 with the CXCL12-induced proliferation of B-cell progenitor acute lymphoblastic leukemia. Haematologica 92: 450–459.
34. Crazzolara R, Cisterne A, Thien M, Hewson J, Baraz R, et al. (2009) Potentiating effects of RAD001 (Everolimus) on vincristine therapy in childhood acute lymphoblastic leukemia. Blood 113: 3297–3306.
35. Juarez J, Bradstock K, Gottlieb D, Bendall L (2003) Effects of inhibitors of the chemokine receptor CXCR4 on acute lymphoblastic leukemia cells in vitro. Leukemia 17: 1294–1300.
36. Saunders P, Cisterne A, Weiss J, Bradstock KF, Bendall LJ (2011) The mammalian target of rapamycin inhibitor RAD001 (everolimus) synergizes with chemotherapeutic agents, ionizing radiation and proteasome inhibitors in pre-B acute lymphocytic leukemia. Haematologica 96: 69–77.
37. Rizos H, Scurr L, Irvine M, Alling N, Kefford R (2007) p14ARF regulates E2F-1 ubiquitination and degradation via a p53-dependent mechanism. Cell Cycle 6: 1741–1747.
38. Green DR, Kroemer G (2004) The pathophysiology of mitochondrial cell death. Science 305: 626–629.
39. Li H, Zhu H, Xu C, Yuan J (1998) Cleavage of BID by caspase 8 mediates the mitochondrial damage in the Fas pathway of apoptosis. Cell 94: 491–501.
40. Wang J, Chun HJ, Wong W, Spencer DM, Lenardo MJ (2001) Caspase-10 is an initiator caspase in death receptor signaling. Proc Natl Acad Sci U S A 98: 13884–13888.
41. Tao H, Hu Q, Fang J, Liu A, Liu S, et al. (2007) Expression of SODD and P65 in ALL of children and its relationship with chemotherapeutic drugs. J Huazhong Univ Sci Technolog Med Sci 27: 326–329.
42. Shen XG, Wang C, Li Y, Zhou B, Xu B, et al. (2011) Downregulation of caspase-10 predicting poor survival after resection of stage II colorectal cancer. Int J Colorectal Dis 26: 1519–1524.
43. Meng L, Sefah K, O'Donoghue MB, Zhu G, Shangguan D, et al. (2010) Silencing of PTK7 in colon cancer cells: caspase-10-dependent apoptosis via mitochondrial pathway. PLoS One 5: e14018.
44. Engel C, Versmold B, Wappenschmidt B, Simard J, Easton DF, et al. (2010) Association of the variants CASP8 D302H and CASP10 V410I with breast and ovarian cancer risk in BRCA1 and BRCA2 mutation carriers. Cancer Epidemiol Biomarkers Prev 19: 2859–2868.
45. Filomenko R, Prevotat L, Rebe C, Cortier M, Jeannin JF, et al. (2006) Caspase-10 involvement in cytotoxic drug-induced apoptosis of tumor cells. Oncogene 25: 7635–7645.
46. Lee HJ, Pyo JO, Oh Y, Kim HJ, Hong SH, et al. (2007) AK2 activates a novel apoptotic pathway through formation of a complex with FADD and caspase-10. Nat Cell Biol 9: 1303–1310.
47. Zhou M, Findley H, Ma L, Zaki S, Hill T, et al. (1991) Effect of tumor necrosis factor-alpha on the proliferation of leukemic cells from children with B-cell precursor-acute lymphoblastic leukemia (BCP-ALL): studies of primary leukemic cells and BCP-ALL cell lines. Blood 77: 2002–2007.
48. Sheikh MS, Antinore MJ, Huang Y, Fornace AJ Jr (1998) Ultraviolet-irradiation-induced apoptosis is mediated via ligand independent activation of tumor necrosis factor receptor 1. Oncogene 17: 2555–2563.
49. Ozsoy HZ, Sivasubramanian N, Wieder ED, Pedersen S, Mann DL (2008) Oxidative stress promotes ligand-independent and enhanced ligand-dependent tumor necrosis factor receptor signaling. J Biol Chem 283: 23419–23428.
50. Takada H, Chen NJ, Mirtsos C, Suzuki S, Suzuki N, et al. (2003) Role of SODD in regulation of tumor necrosis factor responses. Mol Cell Biol 23: 4026–4033.
51. Endres R, Hacker G, Brosch I, Pfeffer K (2003) Apparently normal tumor necrosis factor receptor 1 signaling in the absence of the silencer of death domains. Mol Cell Biol 23: 6609–6617.

52. Bernhard D, Skvortsov S, Tinhofer I, Hubl H, Greil R, et al. (2001) Inhibition of histone deacetylase activity enhances Fas receptor-mediated apoptosis in leukemic lymphoblasts. Cell Death Differ 8: 1014–1021.
53. Balsas P, Lopez-Royuela N, Galan-Malo P, Anel A, Marzo I, et al. (2009) Cooperation between Apo2L/TRAIL and bortezomib in multiple myeloma apoptosis. Biochem Pharmacol 77: 804–812.
54. Makrynikola V, Kabral A, Bradstock KF (1991) Effects of recombinant human cytokines on precursor-B acute lymphoblastic leukemia cells. Exp Hematol 19: 674–679.
55. Faustman D, Davis M (2010) TNF receptor 2 pathway: drug target for autoimmune diseases. Nat Rev Drug Discov 9: 482–493.
56. Dutta J, Fan Y, Gupta N, Fan G, Gelinas C (2006) Current insights into the regulation of programmed cell death by NF-kappaB. Oncogene 25: 6800–6816.

Deregulation of COMMD1 Is Associated with Poor Prognosis in Diffuse Large B-cell Lymphoma

Minna Taskinen[1,2], Riku Louhimo[2], Satu Koivula[1,2], Ping Chen[2], Ville Rantanen[2], Harald Holte[3], Jan Delabie[4], Marja-Liisa Karjalainen-Lindsberg[5], Magnus Björkholm[6], Øystein Fluge[7], Lars Møller Pedersen[8¤], Karin Fjordén[9], Mats Jerkeman[9], Mikael Eriksson[9], Sampsa Hautaniemi[2], Sirpa Leppä[1,2]*

1 Department of Oncology, Helsinki University Central Hospital, Helsinki, Finland, 2 Genome Scale Biology Program, University of Helsinki, Helsinki, Finland, 3 Department of Oncology, Oslo University Hospital, Oslo, Norway, 4 Department of Pathology, Oslo University Hospital, Oslo, Norway, 5 Department of Pathology, Haartman Institute, University of Helsinki, Helsinki, Finland, 6 Department of Medicine, Karolinska University Hospital, Stockholm, Sweden, 7 Department of Oncology and Medical Physics, Haukeland University Hospital, Bergen, Norway, 8 Department of Hematology, Odense University Hospital, Odense, Denmark, 9 Department of Oncology, Lund University Hospital, Lund, Sweden

Abstract

Background: Despite improved survival for the patients with diffuse large B-cell lymphoma (DLBCL), the prognosis after relapse is poor. The aim was to identify molecular events that contribute to relapse and treatment resistance in DLBCL.

Methods: We analysed 51 prospectively collected pretreatment tumour samples from clinically high risk patients treated in a Nordic phase II study with dose-dense chemoimmunotherapy and central nervous system prophylaxis with high resolution array comparative genomic hybridization (aCGH) and gene expression microarrays. Major finding was validated at the protein level immunohistochemically in a trial specific tissue microarray series of 70, and in an independent validation series of 146 patients.

Results: We identified 31 genes whose expression changes were strongly associated with copy number aberrations. In addition, gains of chromosomes 2p15 and 18q12.2 were associated with unfavourable survival. The 2p15 aberration harboured *COMMD1* gene, whose expression had a significant adverse prognostic impact on survival. Immunohistochemical analysis of COMMD1 expression in two series confirmed the association of COMMD1 expression with poor prognosis.

Conclusion: COMMD1 is a potential novel prognostic factor in DLBCLs. The results highlight the value of integrated comprehensive analysis to identify prognostic markers and genetic driver events not previously implicated in DLBCL.

Editor: Joseph S. Pagano, The University of North Carolina at Chapel Hill, United States of America

Funding: This work was supported by the grants from the Finnish Academy of Sciences (SH, SL, MT), Finnish Cancer Societies (SH, SL, MT), Sigrid Jusélius Foundation (SH, SL), University of Helsinki (SL), Helsinki Biomedical Graduate Program (RL), Helsinki University Central Hospital (SL), Amgen (SL, HH) and Roche Norway (HH). The funders had no role in study design, data collection and analysis, decision to publish, or preparation of the manuscript.

Competing Interests: The authors have declared that no competing interests exist.

* E-mail: sirpa.leppa@helsinki.fi

¤ Current address: Department of Hematology, Roskilde University Hospital, Roskilde, Denmark

Introduction

Diffuse large B-cell lymphoma (DLBCL) is the most common lymphoid neoplasm. It is an aggressive lymphoma entity, and only 50% of patients can be cured with anthracycline-based CHOP (cyclophosphamide, doxorubicin, vincristine, and prednisone) or CHOP-like chemotherapy. However, following the addition of rituximab or etoposide to CHOP, or the administration of CHOP dose-densely at two-week intervals (CHOP-14), response rates and survival have significantly improved [1–5]. Despite these advances, 20–30% of patients experience disease relapses or have primary refractory disease. Such patients could benefit from alternative therapies if their clinical outcome could be more accurately predicted at the time of diagnosis. Therefore, the identification of biological prognostic factors that could identify high-risk DLBCL patients is a priority.

Genome-wide molecular profiling has revealed a high degree of complexity in DLBCL,and significantly accelerated the understanding of oncogenic mechanisms in lymphomagenesis [6,7]. On the basis of gene expression profiling (GEP), DLBCL is classified into distinct molecular subtypes [8–11]. Three major DLBCL entities, showing germinal center B-cell (GCB), activated B-cell (ABC)-like, and primary mediastinal B-cell lymphoma signatures have been recognized. Many oncogenic mechanisms distinguish GCB and ABC subtypes. For example, chromosomal translocations involving *BCL2* and the c-*REL* locus amplification on chromosome 2p occur predominantly in the GCB DLBCLs [10,12]. In contrast, ABC DLBCLs are characterized by transcriptional overexpression of *BCL2* and a constitutive activation of the NF-κB signaling pathway [10,13]. According to the gene expression based classification, the patients in the molecular subgroups also have different outcomes in response to chemo- and chemoimmunotherapy [9,10].

Over the past few years, progress in molecular genetics and sequencing technologies has also revealed several previously unrecognized genetic lesions and pathways that are involved in DLBCL [14–17]. For example, recurrent mutations inactivating histone and/or chromatin modifying genes, and genes involved in immune recognition have been identified. However, despite the rapidly growing number of genetic aberrations reported in DLBCL, association of these findings with treatment outcome remains to be shown.

We have integrated the information from high-resolution gene copy number and expression microarrays to identify the most likely "driver gene" candidates associated with DNA copy number aberrations (CNAs) and poor prognosis in DLBCL. Importantly, with our cohort of high-risk DLBCL patients treated homogenously in a phase II study with dose-dense chemoimmunotherapy and systemic CNS prophylaxis, we were able to identify a genomic region harbouring a gene that has a survival effect and thus is a candidate for a novel molecular marker for poor prognosis.

Materials and Methods

Ethics Statement

Written informed consent was obtained prior to treatment and sampling from all patients included in the NLG-LBC-04 study. Clinical protocol and sampling were approved in the participating countries at the national level by Regional Committee on Health Research Ethics in Glostrup, Denmark, the Hospital District of Helsinki and Uusimaa Regional Committee on Medical Research Ethics in Finland, Oslo Regional Committee for Medical and Health Research Ethics in Norway, and Lund Regional Ethics Committee in Sweden. The trial was registered at ClinicalTrials.-gov, number NCT01502982. For the retrospectively collected validation cohort, approval was obtained from the National Authority for Medicolegal Affairs, Finland and Helsinki University Central Hospital, Finland.

Patients

The prospectively collected screening (aCGH) and tissue microarray (TMA) cohorts consisted of DLBCL patients who were less than 65 years old and had primary high-risk (age-adjusted International Prognostic Index (aaIPI) score 2–3) disease. They were treated in the Nordic phase II NLG-LBC-04 protocol with six courses of R-CHOEP14 (rituximab, cyclophosphamide, doxorubicin, vincristine, etoposide, and prednisone supported with G-CSF) followed by systemic CNS prophylaxis with one course of high-dose methotrexate and one course of high-dose cytarabine [18]. The original clinical study included 156 eligible patients. Histological diagnosis was established from surgical or needle biopsy of the pretreatment tumour tissue by local pathologists according to current criteria of the World Health Organization classification [19], and subsequently reviewed by expert hematopathologists on a national basis. The patient selection for this molecular study was based on availability of fresh frozen tissue containing adequate material for DNA extraction and aGCH (screening cohort; n = 51), and for RNA extraction and gene expression profiling (n = 38). The infiltration of lymphoma cells in the tissue was assessed from frozen tissue section using hematoxylin eosin and toluidine blue stainings. Formalin-fixed paraffin-embedded (FFPE) tissue containing adequate material was used for the preparation of TMAs (TMA cohort; n = 70).

To validate the findings, an independent series of 146 primary DLBCL patients treated with chemoimmunotherapy at the Helsinki University Central Hospital between 2001 and 2010 was used. The patients were treated with R-CHOP (n = 126), R-CHOEP (*n* = 11) or other regimen (*n* = 9). The cases were selected based on the availability of FFPE tissue and clinical information.

Samples

RNA and DNA were extracted with Qiaqen AllPrep DNA/RNA/Protein Mini kit. CNAs were analysed from the DNA of 51 tumour samples hybridized onto Agilent Human (4×) 180 K CGH arrays. Tumour samples from 38 patients were eligible for mRNA analyses using Affymetrix Human Exon 1.0 ST arrays. All hybridizations were performed at the Biomedicum Genomics (University of Helsinki) according to manufacturer's instructions. Hybridization protocols and raw expression microarray data are available at ArrayExpress archive http://www.ebi.ac.uk/arrayexpress/experiments/E-MEXP-3488 and http://www.ebi.ac.uk/arrayexpress/experiments/E-MEXP-3463. All tissue samples were collected before treatment.

qRT-PCR

Expression of the *COMMD1* (Hs04190004_m1) and *XPO1* (Hs00418963_m1) genes were validated by quantitative real-time polymerase chain reaction (qRT-PCR) using TaqMan Gene Expression Assays (Assays-On-Demand, Applied Biosystems) and the ABI Prism 7500 Fast Sequence Detection System (Applied Biosystems) for 24 available tumour samples. Normalization for the quantity of DNA was done by performing simultaneous qRT-PCR for *GAPDH* (TaqMan Pre-Developed Assay Reagents, Applied Biosystems). Each assay was determined by a comparative cycle threshold method, using the arithmetic formula provided by the manufacturer. All assays were performed in triplicate.

Subgroup Classification by Gene Expression Profiling

Samples involved in exon array analysis were divided into germinal centre B-cell (GCB) and non-GCB subgroups by gene expression profiling (GEP). Briefly, we utilized the log ratios of 44 genes from the gene expression panel by Wright et al. [20] and agglomerative hierarchical clustering (complete linkage) to divide samples into two subgroups. The *IGHM* gene was not on our array and was subsequently dropped from the analysis. Following the Wright classification [20], samples in one main branch of the resulting cluster tree were categorized as GCB and samples in the other branch as non-GCB DLBCLs. In addition, all samples were classified into GCB and non-GCB phenotypes immunohistochemically (IHC) according to Hans algorithm [21].

Immunohistochemical Analyses of COMMD1

IHC stainings were performed on FFPE tissue sections on TMA slides containing 2–4 tissue cores/patient, with a core diameter of 1 mm (TMA cohort), or whole tissue sections (independent validation cohort). After deparaffinization, heat-induced epitope retrieval (121°C, 3 min), and blocking of endogenous peroxidase, the slides were incubated with anti-COMMD1 antibody (1:200, Sigma-Aldrich, Prestige Antibodies) at 4°C overnight. Staining was completed with Vectastain ABC kit reagents (Vector Laboratories) according to the manufacturer's instructions, and slides were counterstained with hematoxylin.

To score the stainings, COMMD1-positivity was evaluated from one to three high-power fields (hpf; x630 magnification) with the Leica DM LB bright-field microscope (Leica Microsystems GmbH) and a camera attached to it (Olympus DP50, InStudio 1.0.1 Software). The most representative areas with intense staining pattern were first selected with low magnification and further digitized with hpf, resulting in microscopic images with area size of 0.02 mm^2. Images were subsequently scored using computerized image analysis system [22]. All scorings were performed blindly.

Quantitative image analyses were performed using Anduril [22]. The colour space of each image was categorized to four expected representative colour classes: Brown, blue, white and background. The background class included faint brown and blue colours considered to be unspecific staining. The colour values were selected by pointing at 15 example colours for each class. All images were subjugated to use the same class specification. Each pixel was assigned to a class by finding the nearest example colour value, and a final staining coverage calculated from the area of each class present in each image.

Data Analysis

In copy number profiling the aCGH data were first normalized with locally weighted scatterplot smoothing (LOWESS) normalization (four iterations, 30% window) and the data were denoised with circular binary segmentation ($p<0.05$, split undo = none) [23]. The background noise level of copy number arrays was estimated by calculating the median probe signal of all arrays. An aberration was called significant if it was two standard deviations apart from the median. We identified minimal common CNA regions in which a CNA overlapped in 10% of the samples with both transcriptome and copy number data, and subsequent analysis were restricted to these regions. The Database of Genomic Variants (DGV, version 10, Nov 2010) [24] was used to determine locus specific copy number variants (CNVs). In short, for each gene in our CNA regions, the number of overlapping CNVs in the DGV according to genomic locus was counted. Genes with more than 10 CNVs were excluded from the subsequent analyses. Exon array expression data were normalized and transformed to gene expression level data by the Multiple Exon Array Preprocessing (MEAP) algorithm [25].

In order to find genes with a significant association of expression and CNA, all genes in the expression data, which were located in a minimal common CNA region, were first matched with their respective segmented copy number values. The samples were split into two groups based on their CNA status, separately for gains and losses, and a signal-to-noise statistic on the expression of each gene was calculated [26]. A p-value for each signal-to-noise score was calculated with a permutation test. Gain or deletion was associated with expression for genes that displayed up- or downregulation in CNA samples but stable expression in non-CNA samples ($p<0.05$). Moreover, only genes that exhibited CNA in at least three patients were analysed.

A Chi square test was performed to evaluate the differences in the frequency for the prognostic factors. Categorical data were compared using the Fisher's exact test (two-sided). Pearson correlation coefficient was calculated to evaluate the correlation between the expression values from microarray and qRT-PCR analyses. All genes with altered copy number levels in at least five samples were analysed for patient survival. Survival curves with corresponding p-values were calculated using Kaplan-Meier analysis with the log-rank test. Receiver operating characteristic (ROC) curve analysis was used to determine the ideal cutoff values for survival outcomes. Univariate analyses were performed according to the Cox proportional hazards regression model. The progression-free survival (PFS) was calculated as the period between the dates of registration and lymphoma progression or relapse. Otherwise, the patients were censored at the last date of follow-up. Patients in remission were censored at the last date they were known to be alive. Patients who died due to causes other than lymphoma were censored at the date of death. Overall survival (OS) was calculated as a period between registration date and date of death. Surviving patients were censored at the last date they were known to be alive. Lymphoma-specific OS was calculated as a period between registration date and the date of death due to lymphoma. P-values less than 0.05 were considered to indicate statistical significance. Data analyses were done with the computational framework Anduril [22], which is designed for systematic integration, analysis and result interpretation of large-scale molecular data, and with IBM SPSS Statistics 20.0.

Results

Clinical Characteristics of the Screening Cohort

The baseline characteristics of the screening (aCGH) cohort of 51 patients treated in the NLG-LBC-04 protocol [18] are shown in Table 1. Median age of the patients was 55 years (range, 20–65 years). The overall response rate (ORR; complete response (CR)+ partial response (PR)) in this study population was 98%. Median follow-up of the patient cohort was 55 months (range 31–101 months), 15 patients had relapsed, three experienced CNS relapse and 12 had died. Five of the deaths were not lymphoma-related. Predicted 5-year PFS was 69%, lymphoma-specific OS 85%, and OS 76%.

Gene Copy Number Aberrations

Genome-wide copy number analysis of 51 lymphoma samples with aCGH revealed several gains and losses. All patients had at least one abnormality with an average number of 17.5±9.8 CNAs per patient. The most frequently (≥10%) altered regions as well as their frequencies and possible target genes are shown in Table 2. Some samples exhibited narrower alterations than others, which caused the small variation in the CNA frequencies. Of the recurrent CNAs previously reported in DLBCL [27–30], gains in 3q, 7q22.1, and 19p13, and loss in 6q were observed in 9.8% of the patients.

The association of CNAs with molecular subgroups is summarized in Table S1 in File S1. Notably, GCB type DLBCL was characterized by more frequent gain of 2p15 and 2p16.1 including the well-known proto-oncogenes *REL* and *BCL11A* as compared to non-GCB DLBCL (15–19% vs. 5%, p = ns). Instead, the most frequently altered genomic regions in the non-GCB DLBCL subgroup in comparison to GCB DLBCL patients were gains of 18q12.2 (20% vs. 4%, p = ns) and 18q23 (20% vs. 4–7%, p = ns), and loss of 9p21.3 (30–35% vs. 7%, $p = 0.026$). Of the other genomic imbalances (<10% of all patients), only the gain of 18q21.2–33 in the non-GCB subgroup was significantly more frequent when compared to GCB subgroup (20% vs. 0%, $p = 0.027$).

Copy Number Associated Gene Expression Changes

To identify genes with altered expression due to large genomic aberrations, we combined the CNA and gene expression data obtained from 38 patients for whom both data sets were available. Our analysis showed that copy number gains and losses of 31 genes were associated with a simultaneous and significant increase or decrease in gene expression. The majority ($n = 29$) of the genes were over-expressed due to copy number gains in chromosomes 2

Table 1. Patient characteristics in the screening cohort.

	All n (%)	51 (100)
Gender	Female	19 (37)
	Male	32 (63)
Age	Median (range)	55 (20–65)
	<60	35 (69)
	60–65	16 (31)
	>65	0 (0)
Histology	GCB	27 (53)
	Non-GCB	20 (39)
	Other/Unclassified	4 (8)
Performance status	0–1	33 (65)
	2–3	18 (35)
B-symptoms		31 (61)
Elevated LDH		49 (96)
Stage	I–II	1 (3)
	III–IV	37 (97)
aaIPI	0	0 (0)
	1	0 (0)
	2	36 (71)
	3	15 (29)
mRNA analysis		38 (75)

(2p15 and 2p16.1) and 18 (18q21.2, 18q21.31–33, 18q23). In contrast, two genes were suppressed and located in regions of copy number losses at 9p21.3. The aforementioned CNA areas and target genes are presented in more detail in Table S2 in File S1 and at http://csbi.ltdk.helsinki.fi/pub/lymphoma. As an example, the patients with 2p15 amplification had elevated COMMD1 expression with a p-value and fdr <0.001.

Prognostic Significance of Chromosomal Alterations

In the whole series of 51 patients with the aGCH data, we found two chromosomal regions with genomic alterations associated with PFS and lymphoma-specific OS. Patients with amplification in chromosome 2p15 ($n = 6$; 12% of all patients) had inferior PFS in comparison to patients without this gain ($p = 0.010$; Figure 1A). In addition a non-significant difference towards poor lymphoma-specific OS was observed ($p = 0.131$; Figure 1B). Similarly, patients with amplification in 18q12.2 ($n = 6$) had worse PFS ($p = 0.044$) and lymphoma-specific OS ($p < 0.001$) than patients without this gain (Figures 1C and 1D). The survival associated gain in 2p15 contained the genes *B3GNT2* (UDP-GlcNAc:betaGal beta-1,3-N-acetylglucosaminyltransferase 2), *FAM161A* (family with sequence similarity 161, member A), *CCT4* (chaperonin containing TCP1 subunit 4), *COMMD1* (copper metabolism (Murr1) domain containing 1), and *XPO1* (exportin 1), and the amplification was associated with their over-expression (Figure 2). Association of *COMMD1* and *XPO1* over-expression with 2p15 amplification was further confirmed by qRT-PCR (Figure S1 in File S1). The amplification in 18q12.2 contained the *CELF4* gene but we found

Table 2. Genome-wide overview of recurrent gains and losses.

Band	Gain Freq %	Loss Freq %	Position (Mb)	Possible target genes
1q24.2	12	8	167.69–167.76	MPZL1
1q44	20	6	247.00–247.10	AHCTF1
2p16.1–p15	12	NA	60.68–63.27	BCL11A, PAPOLG, REL, PUS10, PEX13, KIAA1841, AHSA2, USP34, XPO1, FAM161A, CCT4, COMMD1, B3GNT2, TMEM17, EHBP1
9p21.3	NA	14–18	21.80–22.01	MTAP, CDKN2A, C9orf53, CDKN2B
14q11.2	2	12	22.938–22.939	TRDV3
18q12.2	12	NA	34.82–35.15	CELF4
18q21.1	12	4	44.06–44.34	LOXHD1, ST8SIA5
18q23	12–16	4	77.62–77.71	KCNG2, PQLC1
20q11.22	16	NA	33.13–33.15	MAP1LC3A

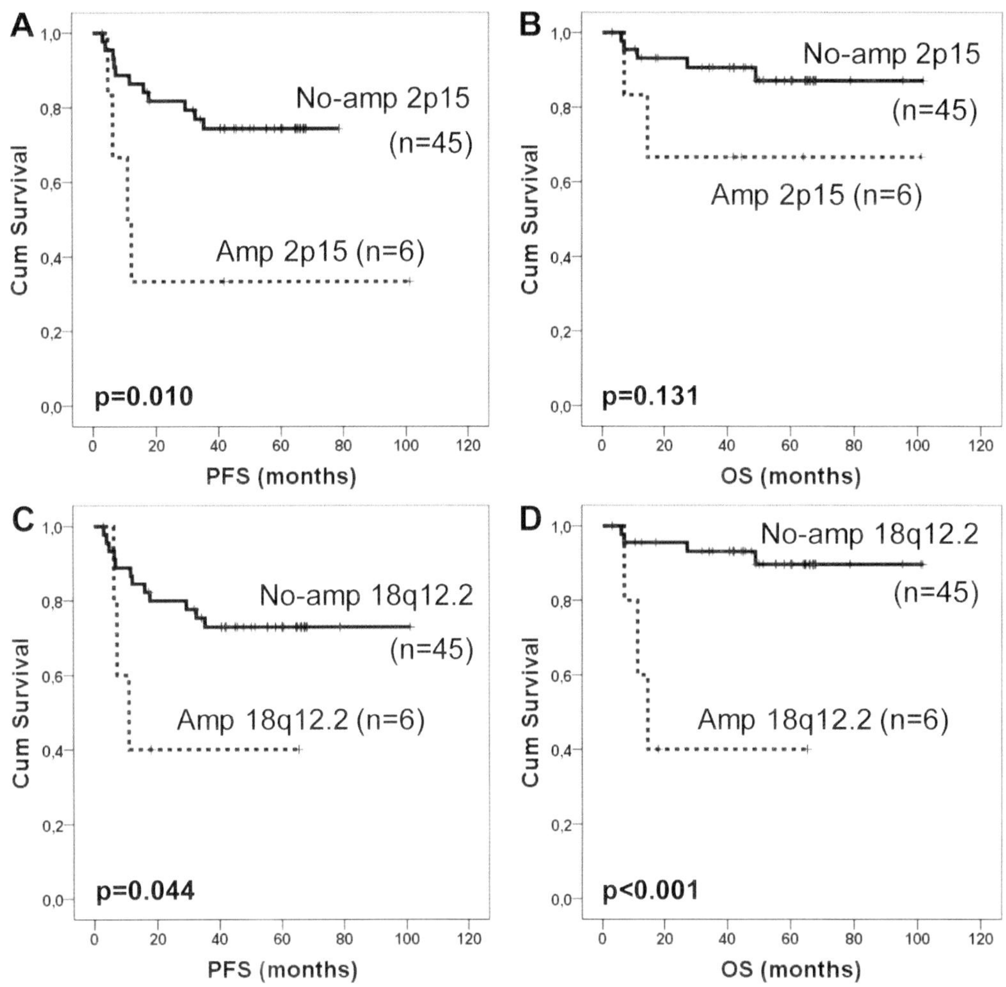

Figure 1. Survival of DLBCL patients according to genomic aberrations. PFS (A and C) and lymphoma-associated OS (B and D) rates according to indicated genomic aberration.

no correlation between the gain and *CELF4* gene expression (Figure 2).

Consistent with previous studies on lymphomas [27,28,31], we identified *REL* and *BCL11A* located at 2p16.1, and *BCL2* at 18q21.3 being among the genes, whose expression was linked with copy number gains (Table S2 in File S1). *CDKN2A* and *MTAP* genes, which have also been described in lymphomas, specifically in the chemoresistant and ABC type DLBCLs [27,28,30,32,33]}, were in turn located in the regions of copy number losses at 9p21.3. However, these genomic alterations were not associated with survival in our study population.

To further identify biomarker candidates located in the survival associated 2p15 amplification locus, we performed survival analysis for five genes whose expression values correlated with amplification. Using gene expression values as continuous variables in Cox univariate analyses, only *COMMD1* expression was identified to have prognostic impact on PFS ($p = 0.037$). When Kaplan-Meier analysis was performed, patients with high *COMMD1* expression had significantly inferior PFS as compared to patients with low expression (5-year PFS 65% vs. 100%, $p = 0.033$; Figure 3A). Association of *COMMD1* expression with the survival was further validated using qRT-PCR and Cox univariate analysis with continuous variables ($p = 0.009$) and Kaplan-Meier analysis with categorical data ($p = 0.031$, Figure 3B). In comparison, the expression of *XPO1*, another selected gene for qRT-PCR validation, was not significantly associated with survival ($p = 0.345$). Correlation coefficients between the expression arrays and qRT-PCR were 0.641 ($p < 0.001$) for *COMMD1* and 0.494 ($p = 0.037$) for *XPO1*.

COMMD1 Protein Expression is Associated with Outcome

Considering that our multi-level analysis revealed *COMMD1* to be amplified, over-expressed and survival associated gene in DLBCL, we extended COMMD1 analyses to the protein level. IHC stainings were performed on a TMA consisting of 70 lymphoma samples from the patients treated in the NLG-LBC-04 protocol (Table 3). Overall, intensity of COMMD1 positivity was highly variable (Figure 4A–B). COMMD1 immunoreactivity was primarily localized as perinuclear, granular, cytoplasmic pattern in lymphoma cells (Figure 4B), but also in endothelial cells and macrophages with more uniform cytoplasmic staining pattern.

The prognostic significance of COMMD1 expression and correlation with mRNA data were assessed by computerized image analysis of COMMD1 positivity in the tumour tissue. In the univariate analysis the increasing COMMD1 positivity was an adverse prognostic factor for PFS ($p = 0.003$). The cutoff point for survival outcomes was selected by ROC curve analysis, resulting in

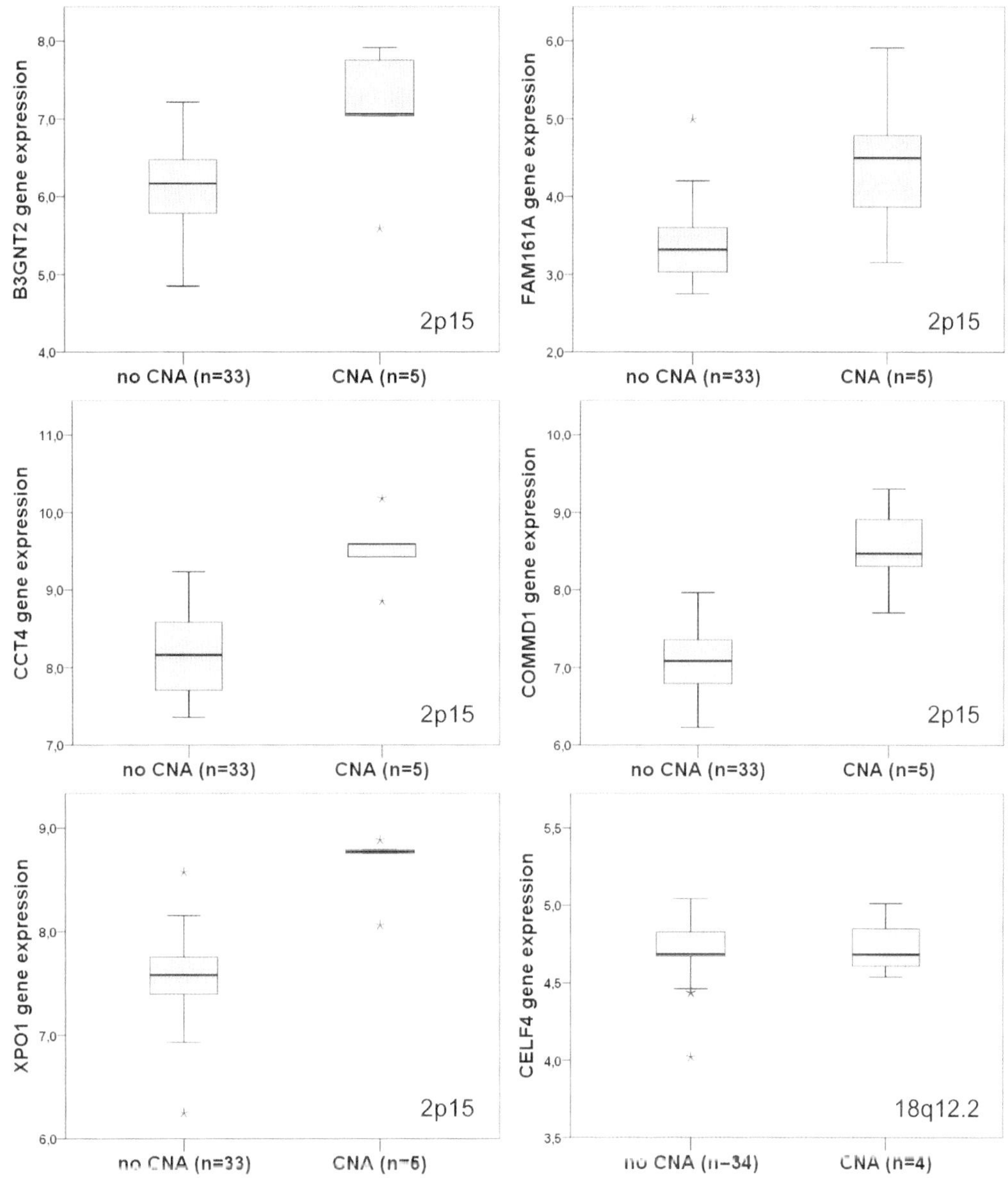

Figure 2. Expression of genes associated with amplifications in 2p15 and 18q12.2 locuses. Boxes contain expression values between the 25th and 75th percentile in the tumour subgroup. The extremes denoted by asterisks represent maximum and minimum expression values.

a staining coverage of 8.9% being the most discriminative value (median 7.3%, range 0–24%), with an area under the curve (AUC) value of 0.663 (95% CI 0.516–0.810, $p = 0.027$). In Kaplan-Meier analyses, the patients with high COMMD1 expression had a significantly worse PFS and a trend towards adverse lymphoma associated OS in comparison to the remaining patients with lower COMMD1 expression (5-year PFS 47% vs. 79%, $p = 0.005$ (Figure 4C) and 5-year OS 75% vs. 90%, $p = 0.081$). According to COMMD1 expression, the relative risk of relapse was 3.2 (95% CI 1.361–7.584, p = 0.008) and death 2.825 (95% CI 0.837–9.536, p = 0.094). In multivariate analysis with aaIPI, COMMD1 expression retained its prognostic value on PFS (RR 2,996; CI 1.210–7.418, p = 0.018). When clinical characteristics of the patients were compared according to COMMD1 expression, no differences in gender, subtype, age, LDH level or stage were observed between the subgroups (Table 3). However, low COMMD1 expression was associated with low performance status.

We also examined prognostic impact on COMMD1 expression according to molecular subtype, and found that a significant adverse prognostic impact of COMMD1 expression was restricted to the GCB subgroup (Fig. 4D; p = 0.029). The relative risk of relapse according to COMMD1 expression within the GCB subgroup was 3.434 (95% CI 1.056–11.164, p = 0.040). Overall, immunohistochemically defined molecular subgroup was not associated with survival.

In contrast to the results from genomic and transcriptomic levels, no correlation was found between COMMD1 protein levels and CNA or gene expression data (r = 0.236). The observation suggests that post-transcriptional mechanisms may be involved in the regulation of COMMD1 protein levels in DLBCL.

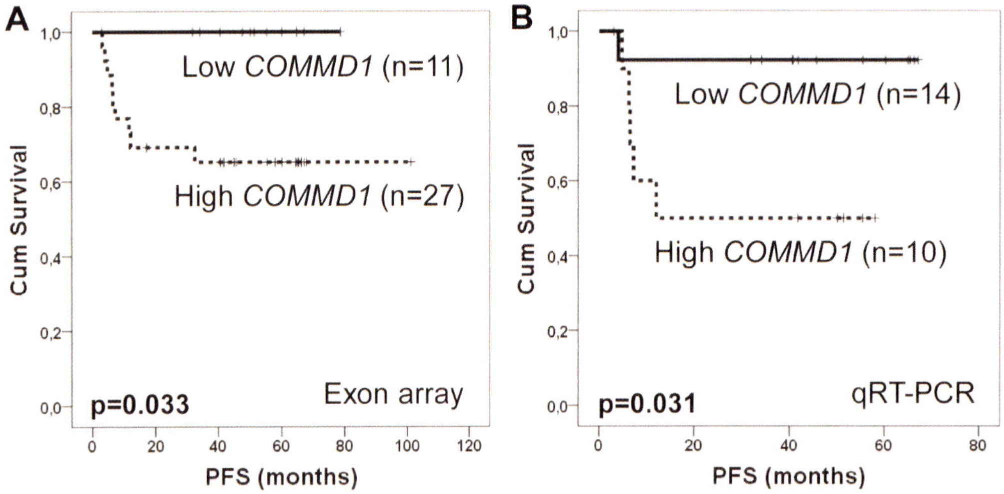

Figure 3. PFS according to *COMMD1* expression. A. PFS according to exon array based *COMMD1* expression values. B. PFS according to quantitative PCR analysis based *COMMD1* expression values. In both A and B, the ideal cutoff values have been calculated using ROC curve analyses. In A the estimated area under the curve (AUC) was 0.717 ($p = 0.063$, 95% CI 0.531–0.903). In B the AUC was 0.759 ($p = 0.062$, 95% CI 0.468–1.000).

COMMD1 Expression in an Independent DLBCL Series

In order to further validate the importance of COMMD1 in DLBCL, we analysed the prognostic significance of COMMD1 expression in a larger independent cohort of 146 DLBCL patients treated with chemoimmunotherapy (Table 3). Median age of the whole cohort was 63 years (range, 16–84 years), median follow-up 64 months (range 20–133 months), predicted 5-year PFS 74%, lymphoma-specific OS 79%, and OS 71%. While high IPI score was a strong predictor for survival ($p<0.001$), immunohistochemically defined molecular subgroup was not associated with outcome.

The clinical features of the patients according to COMMD1 expression (low versus high, cut-off defined according to TMA cohort) are summarized in Table 3. Accordingly, no differences were observed between COMMD1 low and high subgroups. In Kaplan-Meier analyses, PFS at five years for the patients with high

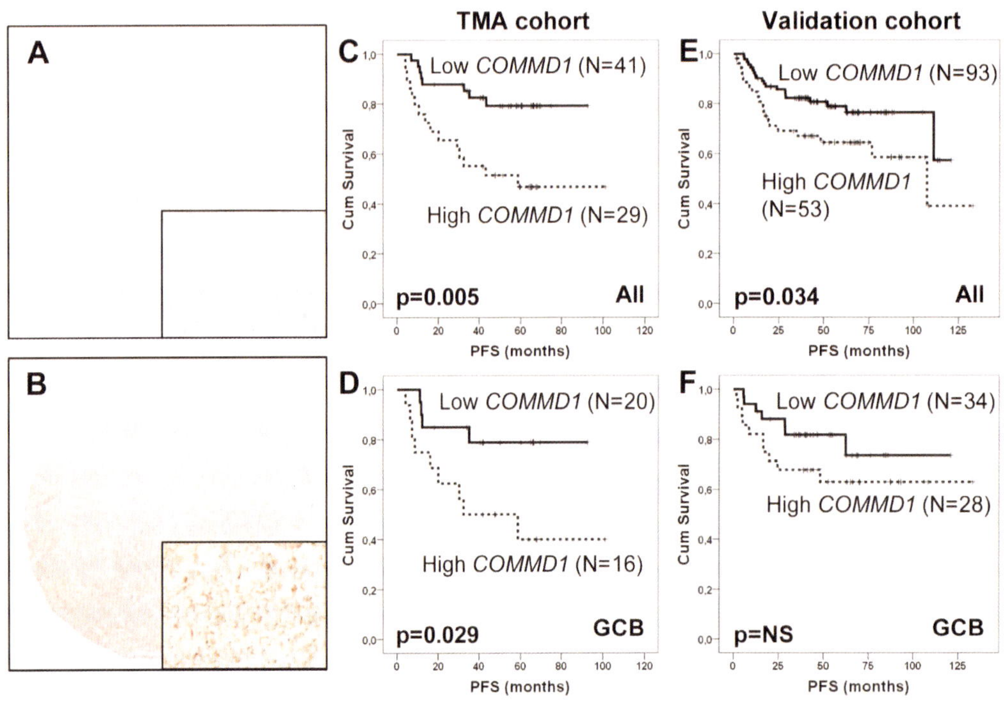

Figure 4. COMMD1 protein expression and outcome. Representative examples of low (A) and high (B) expression levels of COMMD1 in FFPE DLBCL tissue (original magnifications 100×, and 400×). C–D. Outcome according to COMMD1 expression in the trial specific TMA cohort. PFS in in the whole TMA cohort (C) and in the GCB subgroup (D). E–F. Outcome according COMMD1 expression in the validation cohort. PFS in in the whole validation cohort (E) and in the GCB subgroup (F). The cutoff point (staining coverage of 8.9%) for survival outcomes (COMMD1 low vs high) was selected by the ROC curve analysis in the training set, and then applied also to validation cohort.

Table 3. Baseline characteristics according to COMMD1 expression in TMA and validation cohorts.

		TMA cohort(n = 70)			Validation cohort (n = 146)		
	Number of patients	**COMMD1 low**	**COMMD1 high**	**p**	**COMMD1 low**	**COMMD1 high**	**p**
	All n (%)	41 (100)	29 (100)		93 (100)	53 (100)	
Gender	Female	13 (32)	11 (38)	0.618	34 (37)	26 (49)	0.163
	Male	28 (68)	18 (62)		59 (63)	27 (51)	
Subtype	GCB	20 (49)	16 (55)	1.000	34 (37)	28 (53)	0.115
	Non-GCB	10 (24)	9 (31)		52 (56)	24 (45)	
	FL grade 3B	4 (10)	1 (3)		2 (2)	1 (2)	
	Other/unknown	7 (17)	3 (10)		5 (5)	0 (0)	
Age	<60	27 (66)	22 (76)	0.434	40 (43)	22 (42)	1.000
	60–65	14 (34)	7 (24)		10 (11)	8 (15)	
	>65	0 (0)	0 (0)		43 (46)	23 (43)	
B-symptoms		24 (59)	13 (45)	0.333	23 (27)	13 (27)	1.000
Elevated LDH		38 (93)	29 (100)	0.261	57 (62)	41 (77)	0.067
Performance status	0–1	32 (78)	13 (45)	0.006	73 (79)	41 (77)	1.000
	2–4	9 (22)	16 (55)		20 (21)	12(23)	
Stage	I-II	0 (0)	1 (3)	0.414	46 (50)	21 (40)	0.301
	III-IV	41 (100)	28 (97)		47 (50)	32 (60)	
IPI	0–2	17 (41)	9 (31)	0.455	57 (65)	30 (59)	0.586
	3–5	24(59)	20 (69)		31 (35)	21 (41)	

COMMD1 expression was 64% compared with 79% for those with lower expression levels ($p = 0.034$; Figure 4E). When adjusted for IPI, COMMD1 expression maintained its prognostic effect on PFS ($p = 0.023$). In addition, when adjusted for age (<60 vs. ≥60), COMMD1 expression remained predictor for PFS ($p = 0.035$). According to COMMD1 expression, the relative risk or relapse was 1.9 (95% CI 1.040–3.606, $p = 0.037$). In multivariate analysis with IPI, COMMD1 retained its prognostic value on PFS (RR 2.0; 95% CI 1.037–3.730, $p = 0.038$).

Finally, when adjusted for molecular subgroups, COMMD1 expression was marginally predictive for PFS ($p = 0.066$). When COMMD1-related PFS was analysed separately for the patients in different molecular subtypes, there was a non-significant difference in PFS between COMMD1 high and low subgroups in the GCB DLBCLs (Fig. 4F; p = NS). Collectively, the results in our two independent cohorts provide evidence that COMMD1 is a novel survival-associated marker in DLBCLs.

Discussion

Although the addition of rituximab to chemotherapy has considerably improved the survival rates of DLBCL, the patients with high IPI scores still have a poor prognosis. Here we have studied genomic alterations and gene expression in freshly frozen lymphoma tissue collected prospectively from patients included in a Nordic phase II study for young high-risk DLBCL patients. With this comprehensive approach we have identified copy number gain at 2p15 driving *COMMD1* mRNA upregulation with impact on survival. The gain was more frequently seen in the GCB than ABC DLBCLs. Furthermore, we have validated the results at the protein level by IHC in the same patient cohort as well as in an independent larger series. These data show that COMMD1 is a novel biomarker candidate that may be useful in improving risk stratification for DLBCL patients.

In a previous prospective study of poor prognosis DLBCL patients treated uniformly with dose-escalated CHOP followed by high-dose chemotherapy with autologous stem cell transplantation, the amplification of 2p16.1 was suggested to be associated with poor treatment response [34]. Candidate genes mapped within this amplification include proto-oncogenes *REL* and *BCL11A*, with increased expression levels [31,35]. However, the functional correlation of this amplification event has not been illustrated [36]. Although *REL* and *BCL11A* expression levels were integrated with chromosomal amplification in our cohort, they were not associated with survival. Instead, we observed that the increased copy number in region 2p15 was associated with adverse PFS and lymphoma-specific OS. The region covers five genes, *CCT4*, *XPO1*, *COMMD1*, *FAM161A* and *B3GNT2*, which are all potentially important regulators of cellular growth. None of the genes, however, have previously been associated with DLBCL biology. While further investigation of the roles of these genes in DLBCL pathogenesis is needed, our results demonstrate that *COMMD1* is a candidate genetic prognostic biomarker in DLBCL.

COMMD1 is a pleiotropic factor that participates in multiple processes, including copper metabolism, sodium excretion, inflammatory responses, and adaptation to hypoxia [37]. Recent mechanistic studies have revealed that COMMD1 suppresses NF-kB- and HIF-mediated gene expression [38,39]. *COMMD1* is underexpressed in some carcinomas, and low *COMMD1* expression has been associated with inferior clinical outcome in patients with endometrial cancer [39]. In lymphomas, the prognostic role of COMMD1 has not previously been established. In the Oncomine database [40] the expression of *COMMD1* is increased in lymphomas in comparison to other cancers [41]. Furthermore, two independent studies showed that *COMMD1* expression is higher in DLBCLs than follicular lymphomas [41,42], whereas no differences in the *COMMD1* expression were observed between molecular subtypes of DLBCL [9]. At the present time, it remains unclear how COMMD1 is involved in a variety of seemingly unrelated and even opposite cellular activities. However, in most instances including lymphomas, the mechanism is likely via protein-protein interactions and ubiquitination [39,43,44].

To confirm whether COMMD1 expression could be useful to recognize DLBCLs with a more aggressive clinical course, we studied COMMD1 protein expression by IHC, which is a method that can be easily incorporated into a routine diagnostic approach. The predictive value of COMMD1 positivity was first defined in a training cohort of clinically high-risk DLBCL patients, and subsequently confirmed in an independent, larger and more heterogeneous DLBCL cohort. Thus, COMMD1 expression seems to represent a potential novel prognostic marker preferentially in the GCB type molecular subgroup.

Recently Monti and colleagues investigated gene expression and copy number data in 168 DLBCL patients, with the focus on the role of p53/cell cycle pathway in patient survival [28]. Interestingly, even though they reported that the region harboring *COMMD1* is the second highest region in their cohort, and *COMMD1* among the top genes in the region (Table1S in their publication [28]), they did not study its survival association. Additionally, our findings are supported by reports showing amplification of 2p15-p16 with the concordant elevated gene expression in DLBCL [28,31,34,35]. These indicate that while integration of copy number and expression data is known to be a powerful approach to find driver genes, carefully selected, homogenous patient cohort together with integrative analysis can produce clear and important findings that may not be evident in more heterogeneous cohorts.

Since CNA status was integrated with gene expression data, only the genes, whose expression correlated with the CNAs were identified. The results from the qRT-PCR also correlated with the exon array data. However, we found no correlation between COMMD1 protein and gene expression levels. The reason for this difference is currently unknown but based on the literature indicating a strong regulatory role for the processes downstream of transcription [45,46], it is plausible to speculate that post-transcriptional mechanisms may have a role in the regulation of COMMD1 protein levels in DLBCL. The work demonstrating that COMMD1 cellular levels are tightly controlled by ubiquitination [47] provides additional evidence that the regulatory level may be posttranslational. Together with the CNA data the results indicate that COMMD1 expression is regulated at multiple levels.

Amplification in 18q12.2 was found to be another significant CNA associated with inferior outcome. The gain has not been previously associated with survival in DLBCL, but its deletion has been reported to correlate with poor outcome in colorectal carcinoma. The CNA was found to harbour a single gene, *CELF4/CUGBP*, coding for a member of a family of RNA binding proteins playing an essential role in post-transcriptional gene regulation. However, despite the gain in 18q12.2 locus we were not able to demonstrate the over-expression of the *CELF4* gene. While more work is needed to establish the exact role of the 18q12.2 gain in DLBCL, our data supports the prognostic importance of this region in DLBCL.

Consistent with previous studies [27,30,32,33], expression of CDKN2A was associated with deletion of 9p21.3 in our patient cohort, and especially in the non-GCB subtype. However, overall incidence of the deletion was lower and no correlation with survival was found. Considering that aCGH and exon arrays were not performed on purified tumour samples it is possible that the presence of background material (tumour infiltrating non-malignant cells) could to some extent dilute tumour specific genetic alterations and explain a lower incidence of 9p21 deletions in our material. However, a more likely explanation for the differences in the results between different studies is that clinical and histopathological features of the study populations are not identical. The differences in the treatments may also contribute.

In conclusion, we have integrated copy number alteration and transcriptomic data in a carefully chosen high-risk DLBCL patient cohort to identify biological markers that could be used in risk stratification. We found two profiles with increased copy number of genes in chromosomes 2p15 and 18q12.2 that predicted a poor outcome for a subgroup of DLBCL patients. Furthermore, we identified a novel potential genetic driver event with prognostic significance. Notably, the prognostic impact of COMMD1 on survival was also observed at the protein level. The strengths of our study are a prospectively collected and homogenously treated study population, the availability of copy number, gene expression and IHC data from the same patients, the possibility to correlate the findings with clinical outcome, and validate the findings in an independent cohort of DLBCL patients. Our results demonstrate that it is possible to use relatively small but carefully designed prospective cohorts as a hypothesis generating material to identify a list of putative targets, and then validate and extend the major results to the protein level. Taken together, the results presented herein are promising and novel, and emphasize the importance of integrated genetic information and multilevel analyses for both the optimal use of existing combination therapies and the development of novel treatments for DLBCL.

Supporting Information

File S1 Table S1, The most recurrent CNAs distributed between molecular subgroups. Table S2, Gene expression changes associated with CNAs. Figure S1, Association of *COMMD1* (A) and *XPO1* (B) overexpression with 2p15 amplification according to qRT-PCR analysis based expression values.

Acknowledgments

We are grateful to NLG-LBC-04 study investigators, who provided samples and clinical data, members of the Leppä laboratory and Outi Monni for helpful discussions, and Maria Tikkala and Anne Aarnio for technical assistance. We also thank Biomedicum Imaging Unit (BIU) at the University of Helsinki for providing instruments and support with microscopy.

Author Contributions

Conceived and designed the experiments: MT RL SK PC SH SL. Performed the experiments: MT RL SK PC VR. Analyzed the data: MT RL SK PC VR SH SL. Contributed reagents/materials/analysis tools: HH JD MLKL ØF LMP MJ KF ME SL. Wrote the paper: MT SL. Coordinated research: HH ØF LMP MB MJ ME SL.

References

1. Coiffier B, Lepage E, Briere J, Herbrecht R, Tilly H, et al. (2002) CHOP chemotherapy plus rituximab compared with CHOP alone in elderly patients with diffuse large-B-cell lymphoma. N Engl J Med 346: 235–242.
2. Habermann TM, Weller EA, Morrison VA, Gascoyne RD, Cassileth PA, et al. (2006) Rituximab-CHOP versus CHOP alone or with maintenance rituximab in older patients with diffuse large B-cell lymphoma. J Clin Oncol 24: 3121–3127.
3. Pfreundschuh M, Schubert J, Ziepert M, Schmits R, Mohren M, et al. (2008) Six versus eight cycles of bi-weekly CHOP-14 with or without rituximab in elderly patients with aggressive CD20+ B-cell lymphomas: a randomised controlled trial (RICOVER-60). Lancet Oncol 9: 105–116.
4. Pfreundschuh M, Trumper L, Kloess M, Schmits R, Feller AC, et al. (2004) Two-weekly or 3-weekly CHOP chemotherapy with or without etoposide for the treatment of young patients with good-prognosis (normal LDH) aggressive lymphomas: results of the NHL-B1 trial of the DSHNHL. Blood 104: 626–633.
5. Pfreundschuh M, Trumper L, Osterborg A, Pettengell R, Trneny M, et al. (2006) CHOP-like chemotherapy plus rituximab versus CHOP-like chemotherapy alone in young patients with good-prognosis diffuse large-B-cell lymphoma: a randomised controlled trial by the MabThera International Trial (MInT) Group. Lancet Oncol 7: 379–391.
6. Lenz G, Staudt LM (2010) Aggressive lymphomas. N Engl J Med 362: 1417–1429.
7. Shaffer AL 3rd, Young RM, Staudt LM (2012) Pathogenesis of human B cell lymphomas. Annu Rev Immunol 30: 565–610.
8. Alizadeh AA, Eisen MB, Davis RE, Ma C, Lossos IS, et al. (2000) Distinct types of diffuse large B-cell lymphoma identified by gene expression profiling. Nature 403: 503–511.
9. Lenz G, Wright G, Dave SS, Xiao W, Powell J, et al. (2008) Stromal gene signatures in large-B-cell lymphomas. N Engl J Med 359: 2313–2323.
10. Rosenwald A, Wright G, Chan WC, Connors JM, Campo E, et al. (2002) The use of molecular profiling to predict survival after chemotherapy for diffuse large-B-cell lymphoma. N Engl J Med 346: 1937–1947.
11. Rosenwald A, Wright G, Leroy K, Yu X, Gaulard P, et al. (2003) Molecular diagnosis of primary mediastinal B cell lymphoma identifies a clinically favorable subgroup of diffuse large B cell lymphoma related to Hodgkin lymphoma. J Exp Med 198: 851–862.
12. Huang JZ, Sanger WG, Greiner TC, Staudt LM, Weisenburger DD, et al. (2002) The t(14;18) defines a unique subset of diffuse large B-cell lymphoma with a germinal center B-cell gene expression profile. Blood 99: 2285–2290.
13. Davis RE, Brown KD, Siebenlist U, Staudt LM (2001) Constitutive nuclear factor kappaB activity is required for survival of activated B cell-like diffuse large B cell lymphoma cells. J Exp Med 194: 1861–1874.
14. Lohr JG, Stojanov P, Lawrence MS, Auclair D, Chapuy B, et al. (2012) Discovery and prioritization of somatic mutations in diffuse large B-cell lymphoma (DLBCL) by whole-exome sequencing. Proc Natl Acad Sci U S A 109: 3879–3884.
15. Morin RD, Mendez-Lago M, Mungall AJ, Goya R, Mungall KL, et al. (2011) Frequent mutation of histone-modifying genes in non-Hodgkin lymphoma. Nature 476: 298–303.
16. Morin RD, Mungall K, Pleasance E, Mungall AJ, Goya R, et al. (2013) Mutational and structural analysis of diffuse large B-cell lymphoma using whole-genome sequencing. Blood 122: 1256–1265.
17. Pasqualucci L, Trifonov V, Fabbri G, Ma J, Rossi D, et al. (2011) Analysis of the coding genome of diffuse large B-cell lymphoma. Nat Genet 43: 830–837.
18. Holte H, Leppa S, Bjorkholm M, Fluge O, Jyrkkio S, et al. (2013) Dose-densified chemoimmunotherapy followed by systemic central nervous system prophylaxis for younger high-risk diffuse large B-cell/follicular grade 3 lymphoma patients: results of a phase II Nordic Lymphoma Group study. Ann Oncol 24: 1385–1392.
19. Swerdlow SH, Campo E, Harris NL, Jaffe E, Pileri A, et al. (2008) WHO Classification of tumours of hematopoietic and lymphoid tissues. Lyon: IARCH Press.
20. Wright G, Tan B, Rosenwald A, Hurt EH, Wiestner A, et al. (2003) A gene expression-based method to diagnose clinically distinct subgroups of diffuse large B cell lymphoma. Proc Natl Acad Sci U S A 100: 9991–9996.
21. Hans CP, Weisenburger DD, Greiner TC, Gascoyne RD, Delabie J, et al. (2004) Confirmation of the molecular classification of diffuse large B-cell lymphoma by immunohistochemistry using a tissue microarray. Blood 103: 275–282.
22. Ovaska K, Laakso M, Haapa-Paananen S, Louhimo R, Chen P, et al. (2010) Large-scale data integration framework provides a comprehensive view on glioblastoma multiforme. Genome Med 2: 65.
23. Olshen AB, Venkatraman ES, Lucito R, Wigler M (2004) Circular binary segmentation for the analysis of array-based DNA copy number data. Biostatistics 5: 557–572.
24. Iafrate AJ, Feuk L, Rivera MN, Listewnik ML, Donahoe PK, et al. (2004) Detection of large-scale variation in the human genome. Nat Genet 36: 949–951.
25. Chen P, Lepikhova T, Hu Y, Monni O, Hautaniemi S (2011) Comprehensive exon array data processing method for quantitative analysis of alternative spliced variants. Nucleic Acids Res 39: e123.
26. Hyman E, Kauraniemi P, Hautaniemi S, Wolf M, Mousses S, et al. (2002) Impact of DNA amplification on gene expression patterns in breast cancer. Cancer Res 62: 6240–6245.
27. Lenz G, Wright GW, Emre NC, Kohlhammer H, Dave SS, et al. (2008) Molecular subtypes of diffuse large B-cell lymphoma arise by distinct genetic pathways. Proc Natl Acad Sci U S A 105: 13520–13525.
28. Monti S, Chapuy B, Takeyama K, Rodig SJ, Hao Y, et al. (2012) Integrative analysis reveals an outcome-associated and targetable pattern of p53 and cell cycle deregulation in diffuse large B cell lymphoma. Cancer Cell 22: 359–372.

29. Tagawa H, Suguro M, Tsuzuki S, Matsuo K, Karnan S, et al. (2005) Comparison of genome profiles for identification of distinct subgroups of diffuse large B-cell lymphoma. Blood 106: 1770–1777.
30. Takeuchi I, Tagawa H, Tsujikawa A, Nakagawa M, Katayama-Suguro M, et al. (2009) The potential of copy number gains and losses, detected by array-based comparative genomic hybridization, for computational differential diagnosis of B-cell lymphomas and genetic regions involved in lymphomagenesis. Haematologica 94: 61–69.
31. Bea S, Zettl A, Wright G, Salaverria I, Jehn P, et al. (2005) Diffuse large B-cell lymphoma subgroups have distinct genetic profiles that influence tumor biology and improve gene-expression-based survival prediction. Blood 106: 3183–3190.
32. Kreisel F, Kulkarni S, Kerns RT, Hassan A, Deshmukh H, et al. (2011) High resolution array comparative genomic hybridization identifies copy number alterations in diffuse large B-cell lymphoma that predict response to immuno-chemotherapy. Cancer Genet 204: 129–137.
33. Jardin F, Jais JP, Molina TJ, Parmentier F, Picquenot JM, et al. (2010) Diffuse large B-cell lymphomas with CDKN2A deletion have a distinct gene expression signature and a poor prognosis under R-CHOP treatment: a GELA study. Blood 116: 1092–1104.
34. Robledo C, Garcia JL, Caballero D, Conde E, Arranz R, et al. (2009) Array comparative genomic hybridization identifies genetic regions associated with outcome in aggressive diffuse large B-cell lymphomas. Cancer 115: 3728–3737.
35. Fukuhara N, Tagawa H, Kameoka Y, Kasugai Y, Karnan S, et al. (2006) Characterization of target genes at the 2p15–16 amplicon in diffuse large B-cell lymphoma. Cancer Sci 97: 499–504.
36. Houldsworth J, Olshen AB, Cattoretti G, Donnelly GB, Teruya-Feldstein J, et al. (2004) Relationship between REL amplification, REL function, and clinical and biologic features in diffuse large B-cell lymphomas. Blood 103: 1862–1868.
37. Maine GN, Burstein E (2007) COMMD proteins: COMMing to the scene. Cell Mol Life Sci 64: 1997–2005.
38. Maine GN, Burstein E (2007) COMMD proteins and the control of the NF kappa B pathway. Cell Cycle 6: 672–676.
39. van de Sluis B, Mao X, Zhai Y, Groot AJ, Vermeulen JF, et al. (2010) COMMD1 disrupts HIF-1alpha/beta dimerization and inhibits human tumor cell invasion. J Clin Invest 120: 2119–2130.
40. Rhodes DR, Yu J, Shanker K, Deshpande N, Varambally R, et al. (2004) Large-scale meta-analysis of cancer microarray data identifies common transcriptional profiles of neoplastic transformation and progression. Proc Natl Acad Sci U S A 101: 9309–9314.
41. Ramaswamy S, Tamayo P, Rifkin R, Mukherjee S, Yeang CH, et al. (2001) Multiclass cancer diagnosis using tumor gene expression signatures. Proc Natl Acad Sci U S A 98: 15149–15154.
42. Shipp MA, Ross KN, Tamayo P, Weng AP, Kutok JL, et al. (2002) Diffuse large B-cell lymphoma outcome prediction by gene-expression profiling and supervised machine learning. Nat Med 8: 68–74.
43. Drevillon L, Tanguy G, Hinzpeter A, Arous N, de Becdelievre A, et al. (2011) COMMD1-mediated ubiquitination regulates CFTR trafficking. PLoS One 6: e18334.
44. Thoms HC, Loveridge CJ, Simpson J, Clipson A, Reinhardt K, et al. (2010) Nucleolar targeting of RelA(p65) is regulated by COMMD1-dependent ubiquitination. Cancer Res 70: 139–149.
45. Schwanhausser B, Busse D, Li N, Dittmar G, Schuchhardt J, et al. (2011) Global quantification of mammalian gene expression control. Nature 473: 337–342.
46. Vogel C, Marcotte EM (2012) Insights into the regulation of protein abundance from proteomic and transcriptomic analyses. Nat Rev Genet 13: 227–232.
47. Maine GN, Mao X, Muller PA, Komarck CM, Klomp LW, et al. (2009) COMMD1 expression is controlled by critical residues that determine XIAP binding. Biochem J 417: 601–609.

11

Circulating Mediators of Inflammation and Immune Activation in AIDS-Related Non-Hodgkin Lymphoma

Brian M. Nolen[1], Elizabeth Crabb Breen[2,3], Jay H. Bream[4], Frank J. Jenkins[1,5], Lawrence A. Kingsley[6], Charles R. Rinaldo[5], Anna E. Lokshin[1,5,7,8]*

1 University of Pittsburgh Cancer Institute, University of Pittsburgh, Pittsburgh, Pennsylvania, United States of America, **2** Department of Psychiatry & Biobehavioral Sciences, David Geffen School of Medicine at UCLA, University of California Los Angeles, Los Angeles, California, United States of America, **3** UCLA AIDS Institute, University of California Los Angeles, Los Angeles, California, United States of America, **4** Department of Molecular Microbiology and Immunology, Johns Hopkins Bloomberg School of Public Health, Johns Hopkins University, Baltimore, Maryland, United States of America, **5** Department of Pathology, School of Medicine, University of Pittsburgh, Pittsburgh, Pennsylvania, United States of America, **6** Department of Infectious Diseases and Microbiology, Graduate School of Public Health, University of Pittsburgh, Pittsburgh, Pennsylvania, United States of America, **7** Department of Medicine, School of Medicine, University of Pittsburgh, Pittsburgh, Pennsylvania, United States of America, **8** Department of Ob/Gyn, School of Medicine, University of Pittsburgh, Pittsburgh, Pennsylvania, United States of America

Abstract

Background: Non-Hodgkin lymphoma (NHL) is the most common AIDS-related malignancy in developed countries. An elevated risk of developing NHL persists among HIV-infected individuals in comparison to the general population despite the advent of effective antiretroviral therapy. The mechanisms underlying the development of AIDS-related NHL (A-NHL) are not fully understood, but likely involve persistent B-cell activation and inflammation.

Methods: This was a nested case-control study within the ongoing prospective Multicenter AIDS Cohort Study (MACS). Cases included 47 HIV-positive male subjects diagnosed with high-grade B-cell NHL. Controls were matched to each case from among participating HIV-positive males who did not develop any malignancy. Matching criteria included time HIV+ or since AIDS diagnosis, age, race and CD4+ cell count. Sera were tested for 161 serum biomarkers using multiplexed bead-based immunoassays.

Results: A subset of 17 biomarkers, including cytokines, chemokines, acute phase proteins, tissue remodeling agents and bone metabolic mediators was identified to be significantly altered in A-NHL cases in comparison to controls. Many of the biomarkers included in this subset were positively correlated with HIV viral load. A pathway analysis of our results revealed an extensive network of interactions between current and previously identified biomarkers.

Conclusions: These findings support the current hypothesis that A-NHL develops in the context of persistent immune stimulation and inflammation. Further analysis of the biomarkers identified in this report should enhance our ability to diagnose, monitor and treat this disease.

Editor: Derya Unutmaz, New York University, United States of America

Funding: Data in this manuscript were collected by the Multicenter AIDS Cohort Study (MACS) with centers (Principal Investigators) at: Johns Hopkins University Bloomberg School of Public Health (Joseph Margolick), U01-AI35042; Northwestern University (Steven Wolinsky), U01-AI35039; University of California, Los Angeles (Roger Detels), U01-AI35040; University of Pittsburgh (Charles Rinaldo), U01-AI35041; the Center for Analysis and Management of MACS, Johns Hopkins University Bloomberg School of Public Health (Lisa Jacobson), UM1-AI35043. The MACS is funded primarily by the National Institute of Allergy and Infectious Diseases (NIAID), with additional co-funding from the National Cancer Institute (NCI). Targeted supplemental funding for specific projects was also provided by the National Heart, Lung, and Blood Institute (NHLBI), and the National Institute on Deafness and Communication Disorders (NIDCD). MACS data collection is also supported by UL1-TR000424 (JHU CTSA). The funders had no role in study design, data collection and analysis, decision to publish, or preparation of the manuscript.

Competing Interests: The authors have declared that no competing interests exist.

* E-mail: lokshina@pitt.edu

Introduction

Non-Hodgkin lymphoma (NHL) is the most common AIDS-related malignancy in developed countries [1], where it accounts for 23–30% of AIDS-related death [2–4]. Although NHL also affects HIV-uninfected individuals, the risk of developing AIDS-associated NHL (A-NHL) is estimated to be 60 times greater in HIV-infected (HIV+) persons [5,6]. A recent study regarding the incidence of AIDS-related cancer in the years prior to and during widespread administration of highly active antiretroviral therapy (HAART) indicated that while HAART implementation is associated with a reduction in NHL rates among HIV+ persons, rates of A-NHL development remain significantly higher than those observed in uninfected populations [7]. Immunosuppression of any type appears to be a major risk factor for NHL development, with duration of HIV infection and nadir CD4-positive (CD4+) T cell counts positively and inversely associated with the risk of A-NHL, respectively [8,9]. The incidence of primary central nervous system lymphoma (PCNSL), a less prevalent subtype of NHL associated with immune deficiency, has been reported to be over 1000 times higher in persons with AIDS compared to the general population [10,11], although recent evidence suggests that this incidence is declining dramatically with the advent of HAART [12].

The precise pathogenic mechanism underlying A-NHL development is a current focus of intense scrutiny, and several basic themes have emerged. Immune deficiency appears to contribute to the development of A-NHL through the loss of T-cell mediated control over B-cell proliferation. This mechanism appears to be particularly important in the development of Epstein-Barr virus (EBV)-positive A-NHL (reviewed in [13]). The persistently elevated incidence of A-NHL despite the advent of HAART argues for additional pathogenic mechanisms including hyperactivation of B-cells. Chronic B-cell hyperactivation associated with genetic abnormalities due to EBV or human herpesvirus-8 (HHV-8) infection, c-MYC and BCL-6 rearrangements, RAS or p53 mutations, and 6 q deletions is believed to play a role in A-NHL [6,14,15]. Direct integration of HIV into the genome of malignant B-cells has not been observed experimentally, however persistent antigenic stimulation of B-cells during HIV infection may promote hyperactivation and transformation [16–19]. Another proposed mechanism suggests that HIV-infected macrophages contribute stimulatory signals in order to create a microenvironment permissive to malignant B-cell growth [20].

The proposed pathogenic pathways underlying the development of A-NHL suggest a complex network of interactions between various components of the immune system. Cytokines and other inflammatory mediators represent the chief means by which these components mediate those interactions. A number of groups have evaluated serum biomarkers in an effort to more fully characterize the dysregulated cytokine signalling underlying the immunological mechanisms at work in the development of A-NHL. A number of proteins involved in B-cell activation, stimulation and other inflammatory functions have been implicated by the findings of those groups including: IL-6 [21,22], IL-10 [21–23], IP-10 [22], neopterin [22], immunoglobulin free light chains [22], sCD30 [21,24], sCD23 [21,25], sCD44 [26], CRP [21], CXCL13 [27,28] and TNFα [22]. Many of these proteins were observed at elevated serum levels in subjects prior to the diagnosis of A-NHL with a lead time ranging from several months to several years [21,23,24,26]. These findings suggest that the analysis of serum biomarker levels in HIV+ individuals may help in risk assessment strategies for NHL or in the development of prophylactic or preventive measures through an improved understanding of the early events of malignancy.

In the current study, we sought a broad evaluation of serum biomarkers that could possibly be associated with the development of NHL in HIV+ individuals. To that end, multiplexed bead-based immunoassays were utilized in the evaluation of serum levels of 161 proteins in subjects diagnosed with A-NHL and controls.

Materials and Methods

Ethics Statement

All subjects involved in this study were over the age of 18 and provided written informed consent. Specimen collection procedures were approved by the respective Institutional Review Board (IRB) at each collection site: Johns Hopkins Medicine IRB, Northwestern University IRB, University of California, Los Angeles IRB, University of Pittsburgh IRB. The current study was approved by the University of Pittsburgh IRB.

Study Population

The Multicenter AIDS Cohort Study (MACS) is an ongoing prospective study of the natural and treated histories of HIV-1 infection in homosexual and bisexual men conducted at sites located in Baltimore, Chicago, Pittsburgh and Los Angeles [29]. A total of 6,972 men have been enrolled. For the current analysis we obtained archived sera from HIV+ subjects diagnosed with high grade B-cell NHL (according to the MACS data repository) for which serum was available either immediately prior to (≤12 months, n = 37) or shortly after (≤3 months, n = 10) NHL diagnosis. For each case, a single matched control was identified from among HIV+ participants who did not develop any malignancy. Cases for which NHL was AIDS-defining (n = 25) were matched to controls who had not yet received an AIDS diagnoses at the time of blood collection, based on duration of HIV+ status (+/−1 year). Cases for which NHL developed subsequent to an AIDS diagnosis (n = 22) were matched to controls who had developed an AIDS-defining opportunistic infection (OI), based on time since AIDS diagnosis (+/−1 year). Matching criteria also included age (+/−5 yrs) and absolute CD4+ T cell count (+/−100 cells/mm^3) at the time of blood collection in the case or matched visit in the control, and race (white or black). Following matching, a total of 49 cases and 49 controls were selected. Sera obtained for three subjects (2 cases, 1 control) were not evaluable due to insufficient volume or hemolysis. In the resulting groups of 47 cases and 48 controls (Table 1), age, race distribution, CD4+ T cell counts, and duration of HIV positivity did not differ significantly ($p>0.05$), reflecting the original matching criteria. The final experimental cohort included 46 matched pairs. 46 of the cases included in the current study overlap with those used in recent studies utilizing the MACS cohort [21,27,30]. In the majority of overlapping cases, the date of serum collection for the current study was closer to or after the A-NHL diagnosis date, compared to previous studies, as determined by the specific selection criteria. Information on NHL subtypes was obtained from the MACS data repository. HIV viral load values obtained at time of blood draw for biomarker analysis were available from the MACS data repository for 36 case and 22 control subjects. Viral load values were not utilized for matching but were utilized in subsequent biomarker analyses. Information on antiretroviral therapy was obtained from the MACS data repository for each case and control. HAART regimens were defined according to the DHHS/Kaiser guidelines [31]. Subjects were classified as current recipients if they received HAART at the same visit as their blood draw or during the interim time in between this visit and the previous MACS visit. Subjects were classified as former recipients if they received HAART prior to but not during this time period. Subjects classified as never receiving HAART may have received other antiretroviral therapy not classified as HAART. The characteristics of the study population are presented in Table 1.

Sources of bead-based immunoassays

A combination of 161 bead-based immunoassays for a diverse set of serum biomarkers available on the Luminex platform was utilized in this study (Table 2). This list of biomarkers was assembled based on a literature review of proteins and families of proteins of interest in all areas of HIV and NHL research. Biomarkers were selected from this list on the basis of suitable immunoassay availability. A total of 29 multiplexed and individual assays were utilized (Table S1). Bead-based immunoassays

Table 1. Characteristics of Study Population.

	A-NHL Cases (n = 47)	Controls (n = 48)
Age (years), range (median)	25–56 (42)	26–56 (40)
Race, n (%)		
White	46 (98)	47 (98)
Black	1 (2)	1 (2)
CD4+ T Cell Count (cells/mm^3), range (mean)	7–788 (146)	6–794 (193)
Receiving HAART [31], n (%)		
Current	6 (13)	5 (10)
Former	1 (2)	1 (2)
Never	38 (81)	42 (87.5)
Unknown	2 (4)	0 (0)
HBV Serology, n (%)		
Positive	41 (87)	42 (87.5)
Negative	3 (6)	6 (12.5)
Unknown	3 (6)	0 (0)
HHV-8 Serology, n (%)		
Positive	28 (57)	35 (73)
Negative	9 (19)	9 (19)
Unknown/Indiscriminate	10 (21)	4 (8)
NHL Subtype, n (%)		
B-cell Diffuse	20 (43)	
CNS	11 (23)	
BL, BL-like	7 (15)	
NHL, NOS	6 (13)	
Other	3 (6)	

HAART – highly active antiretroviral therapy; HBV/HHV-8 status obtained at time of blood draw; CNS – central nervous system; BL – Burkitt's lymphoma; NOS – not otherwise specified.

targeting ErbB2, EGFR, Cytokeratin 19(Cyfra 21-1), mesothelin (MSLN), AFP, CA 72-4, MICA, SCC, HSP 70, EPCAM, PSA, transthyretin (TTR), angiostatin (AS), thrombospondin (TSP), endostatin (ES), TgII, HE4, CA 15-3, CA 125, CEA, and Kallikrein 10 (Klk10) were developed by the UPCI Luminex Core Facility according to strict quality control standards[32]. Assays for MMP 1, 2, 3, and 7 and TIMP 1–4 were obtained from R&D Systems (Minneapolis, MN). Assays for PDGF-BB, RANTES, SCGF-B, and NGF were obtained from Bio-Rad (Hercules, CA). Assays for HSP27, IL-1α, IL-1β, IL-3, IL-5, IL-7, IL-8, IL-12p40, IL-15, IL-17, TNF-α, IFNα, GM-CSF, MCP-1, MCP-3, MIP-1α, MIP-1β, IP-10, Eotaxin (CCL11), RANTES, DR5, EGF, FGFb, G-CSF, HGF, VEGF, and GROα were obtained from Life Technologies/Biosource (Grand Island, NY). All other assays were obtained from Merck/Millipore (Durmstadt, Germany). All commercial immunoassays were performed according to manufacturer's protocols while UPCI Luminex Core Facility assays were performed as previously described [32,33].

Collection and statistical analysis of biomarker data

Each serum sample was analyzed for each multiplex immunoassay using the Bio-Plex suspension array system and the Bio Plex Manager software (version 4.1) (Bio-Rad Laboratories, Hercules, CA). For each analyte, 100 beads were analyzed and the median fluorescence intensity was determined. Analysis of serum sample biomarker data was performed using five-parameter logistic curve fitting to standard analyte values. A number of samples fell below lower limit of extrapolation of the Bio-Plex Manager software for certain analytes and were therefore reported as out of range low (OOR <). The percentages of cases and controls classified in this manner for each analyte are listed in Table S2. Observed concentration values were assigned to each of the OOR < samples by manual extrapolation using the curve fitting parameters determined by the Bio-Plex software. Hence, no samples were excluded from the analysis on the basis of undetectability. The entire biomarker dataset has been deposited with the Center for Analysis and Management of Multicenter AIDS Cohort Study (CAMACS).

Biomarker distributions among the A-NHL and control groups were analyzed using both parametric and non-parametric statistical tests. In each analysis the minimum level of significance was $p<0.05$. For the parametric analysis, exact conditional logistic regression was performed on the biomarker data obtained for the A-NHL and control groups (n = 46 matched case-control pairs). The results were further analyzed using the Bonferroni Step-Down (Holm) correction for multiple comparisons. For the non-parametric analysis, the Mann-Whitney U test was utilized on data from 47 cases and 48 controls without regards to matching. Here, the False Discovery Rate (FDR) was controlled at 5% according to the method described by Benjamini and Hochberg[34]. Biomarker variations among several subtypes of NHL were evaluated using a one-way ANOVA with Tukey's multiple

Table 2. Complete List of Evaluated Biomarkers.

Tumor Markers	AFP, CA 15-3, CA 19-9, CA125, CA72-4, CEA, EPCAM, HE4, Kallikrein-10 (Klk10), Mesothelin (MSLN), PSA, squamous cell carcinoma antigen (SCC), tissue transglutaminase (TgII)
Growth/Angiogenesis Factors	Angiostatin (AS), EGF, EGFR, Endostatin (ES), ErbB2, FGFb, HGF, IGFBP 1-7, NGF, PDGF-BB, SCGF-B, sVEGF-1, sVEGFR2-3, TGFα, Thrombospondin (TSP)
Hormones	ACTH, Cortisol, FSH, GH, Insulin, LH, Prolactin, PTH, TSH
Apoptosis Factors	Cyfra 21-1, Fas, FasL
Cytokines/Chemokines/ Receptors	6CKine/CCL21, CTACK/CCL27, DR5, ENA-78/CXCL5, EOTAXIN-1 (CCL11), EOTAXIN-2/CCl24/MPIF-2, EOTAXIN-3/CCL26, FLT3, Fractalkine, GCP-2/CXCL6/LIX, G-CSF, GM-CSF, GROα, HCC-1/CCL14a, I-309/CCL1, IFNα, IL-1α, IL-1β, IL-3,5,7,8,11, IL-12p70, IL-12p40, IL-15-17,20, IL-28α, IL-29, IL-33/NF-HEV(mat), IP-10, I-TAC/CXCL11, LIF, Lymphotactin, MCP-1-4, M-CSF, MDC, MIF, MIP-1α, MIP-1β, MIP-1δ/MIP-5/CCL15, MIP-3α/CCL20, MIP-3β/CCL19, MIP-4, MPO, NAP-2/CXCL7, RANTES, sCD40L, SCF, SDF-1a+b/CXCL12, sIL-1RI,II, sIL-4R, sIL-6R, sRAGE, sTNF –RI, sTNF-RII, TARC/CCL17, TNFα, TNFβ, TPO, TRAIL/TNFSF10, TSLP
Adhesion Molecules	E-Selectin, Fibronectin (FN), sICAM, sVCAM
MMPs/TIMPs	MMP-1-3, 7-9, 12,13, TIMP-1-4
Bone Factors	Osteoprotegerin (OPG), Osteocalcin (OC), Osteopontin (OPN), RANKL
Apolipoproteins	Apo A1, Apo CIII, Apo E
Acute Phase Proteins	α1-Antitrypsin (A1A), α2-Macroglobulin, Complement C3 (C3), Complement C4, Complement Factor H (CFH), Fibrinogen (FBN), Haptoglobin (HPN), human serum albumin (HSA), transthyretin (TTR), serum amyloid A (SAA), serum amyloid P (SAP)
Adipokines	Adiponectin, aPAI-1, Leptin, Resistin, tPAI-1
Other	HSP 70, Involucrin, pan-Keratin (1,10,11), Keratin-6, LPS, MICA, PEDF

comparison test. Correlations between biomarker levels and HIV viral load were evaluated using the Spearman test for correlation.

Pathway Analysis

The Ingenuity Pathway Analysis (IPA) software package (Ingenuity Systems, Inc., Redwood City, CA) was used to examine pathways and interactions associated with the most promising biomarkers identified in our analysis described above. Additional serum biomarkers demonstrating associations with A-NHL in previous reports, which were not measured in the current investigation, were also included in this analysis. The list of additional biomarkers included IL-6 [21], IL-10 [21,23,30], sCD30 [21,24], sCD23 [21], sCD44 [26], sCD27 [21], CRP [21], and CXCL13 [27,28]. Some of these reports utilized a number of overlapping MACS NHL cases as described above. The IPA analysis identifies interactions based solely on the identity of the biomarkers inputted into the software and did not utilize biomarker concentrations.

Results

Biomarker alterations among A-NHL cases and controls

The non-parametric analysis of biomarker distributions among all cases and controls revealed that 19 out of the 161 biomarkers tested were significantly altered in the comparison of A-NHL cases and controls (Table 3). Among these 19 significant biomarkers, two (MMP-9, OC) were observed to be decreased in the A-NHL group in comparison to the controls, while the remaining 17 were increased. The parametric statistical analysis on 46 case-control pairs yielded a larger list of 37 significant biomarkers (Table 4) which included all but two biomarkers (FBN, A1A) identified in the non-parametric analysis. Among the 37 significant biomarkers in this analysis, four (OC, ApoA1, MMP-9, IGFBP-6) were observed to be decreased in the A-NHL subjects relative to the control groups, while the remaining 33 biomarkers were all increased. All trends in biomarker alterations between the cases and controls were consistent among the non-parametric and parametric analyses despite the differential use of median and mean values, respectively, and slightly different numbers of subjects. The application of the Bonferroni Step-down (Holm) correction to our parametric analyses yielded a restricted list of three biomarkers (IL-11, CXCL11, IL-29) which were observed to be highly significant (Table 4). A comparison of the non-parametric and parametric analyses prior to Bonferroni correction (overlap between tables 3 and 4) yielded a consensus list of 17 serum biomarkers significantly altered in the comparison of the A-NHL and control groups. The consensus list included cytokines/chemokines (CCL19, CXCL11, MCP-2, MIP-1δ, IFNα, IL-11, IL-29, IP-10, M-CSF, sIL-1R1), acute phase proteins (C3, HPN, SAA, SAP), tissue remodeling factors (MMP-9, TIMP-1), and the bone metabolic factor OC.

Correlation with HIV viral load

Biomarker measurements from the A-NHL and control groups were combined in order to identify correlations between specific biomarkers and HIV viral load. Among the complete panel of 161 biomarkers, a total of 17 biomarkers exhibited significant correlations with HIV viral load (data not shown). Most notably, 11 of the significantly correlated biomarkers were among the consensus biomarkers described above, and are presented in Table 5. With the notable exception of MMP-9, each of the significant correlations among the consensus biomarkers was consistent with HIV progression, i.e., higher biomarker concentrations were correlated with higher HIV viral load.

A-NHL subtype specific biomarker alterations

Each of the 17 consensus biomarkers were evaluated in case subsets including subjects diagnosed with B-cell diffuse, CNS, or Burkitt's Lymphoma (BL)/BL-like NHL using pair-wise one-way ANOVA. As this analysis included cases only, biomarker levels were normalized to CD4 counts prior to ANOVA to account for variations in disease severity. In a comparison of BL/BL-like and CNS NHL cases, OC and Timp-1 were significantly different with $p<0.05$. In the comparison of CNS and B-cell diffuse NHL cases, three significant alterations were observed including OC, SAP and Timp-1 (data not shown). In each comparison, significantly

Table 3. Serum biomarker levels in AIDS-NHL subjects and controls evaluated by Non-parametric Statistics.

	A-NHL (n = 47)		Control (n = 48)		A-NHL vs. Control	
Biomarker	**Median**	**IQR**	**Median**	**IQR**	**MWU p value (trend)**	
CCL19/MIP-3β	238	133	197	112	6.89E-03	(I)
C3†	111	53.7	80.9	33.0	1.52E-03	(I)
CXCL11/I-TAC	266	393	132	128	9.31E-05	(I)
FBN†	161	151	84.6	95.1	8.20E-04	(I)
HPN†	4054	3284	3041	2546	8.23E-03	(I)
IFN-α	34.1	43.6	20.5	13.9	1.89E-03	(I)
IL-11	278	163	146	145	9.97E-06	(I)
IL-29/IFNλ1	284	193	200	100	6.97E-04	(I)
IP-10	98.2	96.0	60.2	53.4	1.48E-03	(I)
MCP-2	71.3	56.1	53.5	35.8	8.32E-03	(I)
M-CSF	317	554	86.8	250	2.45E-03	(I)
MIP-1δ	3720	2267	2816	1941	8.05E-03	(I)
MMP-9†	81.0	76.5	128	133	5.88E-03	(D)
OC	3811	2644	4536	2808	7.79E-03	(D)
SAA†	591	3361	295	462	9.69E-03	(I)
SAP†	4934	1962	3647	1207	2.69E-04	(I)
sIL-1R1	26.8	15.7	21.1	8.10	7.37E-03	(I)
TIMP-1†	160	50.6	137	33.8	4.57E-03	(I)
A1A†	1769	2124	1062	810	3.28E-03	(I)

IQR – interquartile range; MWU - Mann Whitney U test with 5% False Discovery Rate; Biomarkers in bold represent consensus markers also selected by parametric statistics;
†values expressed in ng/ml, all others expressed in pg/ml; Trends: I – increased in A-NHL group, D – decreased in A-NHL group.

elevated levels of each biomarker were observed in CNS NHL relative to the other subtypes.

Pathway Analysis

The IPA software package was first used to analyze the consensus list of 17 serum biomarkers identified in this study. The top biological functions associated with the consensus list included Cellular Movement (14/17 molecules, $p = 1.6\times10^{-14}$–1.9×10^{-3}), Cell-to-Cell Signaling and Interaction (13/17 molecules, $p = 1.4\times10^{-10}$–1.9×10^{-3}), Hematological System Development and Function (14/17 molecules, $p = 1.6\times10^{-14}$–1.9×10^{-3}), and Immune Cell Trafficking (14/17 molecules, $p = 1.6\times10^{-14}$–1.9×10^{-3}). Interactions between molecules were then examined for each biomarker included in the consensus list and several biomarkers examined in association with A-NHL in previous studies including IL-6, sCD30, IL-10, sCD23, sCD44, sCD27, CRP, CXCL13, and IgE. An extensive array of interactions within and among the two lists of biomarkers was identified (Figure 1). With the exceptions of MIP-1δ, IFNα, and OC, each of the newly identified biomarkers was found to interact with at least one previously identified biomarker. MMP-9 demonstrated the most extensive network of interactions including six interactions with other newly identified biomarkers and four interactions with previously identified biomarkers. Other newly identified biomarkers demonstrating more than five interactions included IP-10 (7 new/2 previous), M-CSF (3 new/4 previous), sIL-1R1 (4 new/2 previous), TIMP-1 (3 new/3 previous), C3 (3 new/3 previous), and SAP (2 new/4 previous). Many of the previously identified biomarkers also displayed numerous interactions within and among the groups.

Discussion

A diverse analysis of serum proteins in samples collected just before or after the time of A-NHL diagnosis identified a consensus list of potential A-NHL biomarkers, assembled through rigorous statistical analysis, which included various inflammatory mediators, acute phase proteins and tissue remodeling agents. Although our panel of candidate biomarkers was considerably large and composed primarily of inflammatory and immune-modulating factors, a relatively small subset was observed to be altered, suggestive of some level of specificity for A-NHL with respect to HIV+ status or other AIDS defining illness. Increased levels of a number of circulating proteins have previously been reported up to 3–5 years prior to the diagnosis of A-NHL including IL-6, IL-10, sCD23, sCD27, sCD30, sCD44, IgE, CRP, and BCA-1/CXCL13[21–24,26–28,30,35,36]. While the current study did not include a direct examination of these biomarkers, an analysis of biomarker interactions revealed a number of mechanistic links between and among those biomarkers identified both previously and currently (Figure 1). The most recent longitudinal study of A-NHL risk in HIV+ persons identified IP-10 and TNFα, in addition to several others, as potential biomarkers [22]. The current cross-sectional analysis evaluated both of these biomarkers but found only IP-10 to be significantly altered.

The conservative use of the Bonferroni correction as part of our parametric statistical analysis suggested that serum levels of IL-11, CXCL11 and IL-29 demonstrated the strongest associations with A-NHL in our study. These findings further agree with the hypothesized immune activating origins of this disease. IL-11, an important mediator of hematopoiesis, has been investigated as an

Table 4. Conditional Logistic Regression Analyses with Bonferroni Step-down Adjustment of Serum Biomarker Levels of AIDS-NHL and control subjects.

Biomarker	A-NHL (n = 46)		Controls (n = 46)		Exact p-value	Bonferroni Adjusted p-value
	Mean	SD	Mean	SD		
ApoA1	1267	252	1374	213	0.0111	NS
CA 19-9	4.97	26.9	0.490	0.197	0.0013	NS
CCL19/MIP-3β	648	2777	196	77.5	0.0025	NS
CCL20/MIP-3α	47.2	188	11.5	7.51	0.0056	NS
C3	111	47.3	81.9	30.3	0.0003	NS
CFH	559	169	473	94.8	0.0016	NS
CXCL11/I-TAC	436	535	175	151	0.0001	0.017
CXCL6/GCP-2	342	1362	114	51.7	0.0138	NS
CCL11	212	145	190	70.7	0.0061	NS
G-CSF	176	325	73.8	71.9	0.0023	NS
HPN†	5110	4037	3148	2284	0.0093	NS
I-309	11.3	29.9	3.39	3.52	0.0126	NS
IFNα	13365	87796	65.5	189	0.0407	NS
IGFBP-3†	1524	248	1420	328	0.0085	NS
IGFBP-5†	120	72.6	90.8	58.3	0.0124	NS
IGFBP-6†	149	42.0	169	64.0	0.0274	NS
IL-11	5663	36435	176	97.9	<0.0001	<0.017
IL-20	115	253	56.8	34.3	0.0177	NS
IL-28A	555	3128	16.0	20.4	0.0249	NS
IL-29	11685	76491	232	127	0.0001	0.017
IL-7	49.7	146	18.4	7.37	0.0066	NS
IP-10	130	93.0	86.8	91.4	0.0173	NS
MCP-2	88.0	66.9	61.5	36.1	0.025	NS
M-CSF	15887	105262	277	405	0.0065	NS
MIF	964	2916	246	181	0.0402	NS
MIP-1δ	5617	7942	3295	2265	0.0056	NS
MIP-4†	22.2	19.4	16.0	7.88	0.0205	NS
MMP-3†	57.5	163	18.1	7.30	0.0453	NS
MMP-9†	108	94.1	154	103	0.0171	NS
OC	3996	2421	5375	3116	0.006	NS
PEDF†	1777	424	1604	339	0.0379	NS
SAA†	18574	67358	582	1020	0.0008	NS
SAP†	4759	1623	3867	1307	0.004	NS
SCGF-B†	60.3	49.4	45.9	15.7	0.0464	NS
sIL-1RI	45.2	106	24.3	8.43	0.0041	NS
sTNF-RII†	10.5	4.56	8.43	3.56	0.0172	NS
TIMP-1†	199	174	148	40.4	0.0096	NS

SD – standard deviation, NS - non-significant;
†concentration expressed as ng/ml, all others expressed in pg/ml; Biomarkers in bold represent consensus markers also selected by non-parametric statistics.

experimental treatment for hematological malignancies [37]. CXCL11 is a chemokine known to mediate the migration of activated T-cells, and has been described as an immunomodulatory target of miRNA in primary lymphoma and has also demonstrated potent antitumor activity in an animal model [38,39]. The type III interferon IL-29 is the focus of considerable interest in the setting of hepatitis C viral infection and was recently shown to impede HIV-1 infection in T-cells [40,41]. A role in the development of A-NHL for IL-29 has not yet been described.

A number of additional proteins with varying biological functions but unifying roles in inflammation and immune activation were also associated with A-NHL in univariate analyses in the current study, but were not statistically significant after Bonferroni correction. In such a broad survey, this is not unexpected, but the data does confirm previous reports of some of these proteins being associated with inflammatory processes around the time of A-NHL or NHL diagnosis. Several of the chemoattractant proteins (CCL19/MIP-3β, MCP-2, CXCL9/

Table 5. Spearman Correlations of Consensus Biomarkers and HIV Load among all subjects.*

Biomarker	Spearman *r*	*p*
CCL19/Mip-3β	0.67	0.0001
CXCL11/I-TAC	0.52	0.0001
IL-11	0.50	0.0001
IP-10	0.46	0.0003
MCP-2	0.42	0.001
IFN-α	0.42	0.0011
M-CSF	0.41	0.0013
SAP	0.40	0.0019
MMP-9	−0.38	0.0029

*Analysis included all subjects with available HIV load measurement (n = 58).

MIG) have been reported to have an association with various forms of leukemia and lymphoma [42,43], [11]. Of particular interest for A-NHL is IP-10, a leukocyte chemoattractant implicated in the development and progression of B-cell lymphoma. In two recent studies, elevated levels of IP-10 in the sera of HIV-positive individuals were associated with the development of B-cell lymphoma within 0–5 years [22], [44]. Elevated pretreatment serum levels of IP-10 were also associated with increased likelihood of disease relapse and diminished survival in HIV-uninfected patients with diffuse large B-cell lymphoma [45]. The gelatinase MMP-9 and its inhibitor TIMP-1 mediate breakdown of the extracellular matrix during inflammatory and other responses, and one or both have been linked to lymphoma at the time of diagnosis [46] [47,48]. The acute phase protein, SAA has been shown to be overexpressed in B-cell NHL associated with SIV infection in monkeys [49], and complement components (C3 and CR2) may be involved in lymphomagenesis and/or complement activation [50], [51]. IFNα is currently under investigation as a potential therapeutic agent in lymphoma, including A-NHL, stemming from its ability to mediate apoptosis in malignant cells[52–54].

Biological roles related to the development of lymphoma have not been conclusively described for MIP-1δ, M-CSF, sIL-1R1, HPN, SAP, and OC and, to the best of our knowledge, we are the first to report on these associations. Each of these proteins does possess functions relating them to inflammation and were linked mechanistically to other potential biomarkers in our pathway analysis. Further investigation into the precise activity of each of these proteins in lymphoma would be of great interest.

Many of the biomarkers found to be significantly altered in A-NHL subjects appear to be positively associated with HIV disease progression, as indicated by their observed correlation with HIV viral load (Table 5). Each of the biomarkers found to be positively correlated with viral load were also observed to be elevated in the sera of A-NHL cases in comparison to the controls. As CD4 count was included in our matching criteria and was not significantly different between the two experimental groups, we propose that varying degrees of control of HIV (or lack thereof) within each experimental group, as opposed to among the groups, led to our observations. These observations are in line with the hypothesis that increases in HIV viral burden result in elevated levels of immune stimulation and inflammation which then promotes NHL pathogenesis. Based on these findings, we may also hypothesize that HIV-driven alterations in immune response are augmented in A-NHL, a phenomenon that warrants additional investigation. In contrast to other biomarkers, higher MMP-9 levels correlated with lower viral load and control (non-malignancy) status. A direct relationship between increased MMP-9 activity and immune competence and/or protection from lymphoma has not been described, leading us to speculate that the relationship between MMP-9 and A-NHL may be a protective one which warrants further exploration.

When A-NHL subjects of differing disease subtypes were evaluated separately, relatively few significant alterations were found. Several biomarkers including OC, SAP, and Timp-1 were found to be significantly elevated in CNS NHL in comparison to other subtypes. To the best of our knowledge, we are the first to report on such associations. For the vast majority of the biomarkers examined, we were not able to detect any significant differences between NHL subtypes, although this may be due to the relatively small sample size of each subset and the amount of variability within both case and control groups. Our results are similar to the recent findings of Breen et al. in which no significant differences were observed when comparing biomarker levels of diffuse large B cell cases to BL cases; however, in that study all significantly increased biomarker levels in cases compared to controls were associated with the systemic form of NHL but not CNS NHL [21]. While utilizing many of the same MACS A-NHL cases, the current investigation in general examined different time points (closer to or after NHL diagnosis), and each study evaluated a distinct set of biomarkers.

The results of the pathway analysis indicate the existence of a complex network of interactions among the collective list of biomarkers identified in the current and previous investigations. An examination of this network suggests central roles for two previously identified biomarkers, IL-6 and IL-10 (Figure 1). Several newly identified biomarkers including MMP-9, IP-10, and M-CSF also appear to play central roles. Each of the three biomarkers demonstrating the strongest associations with A-NHL in the current study (IL-11, CXCL11, and IL-29) were found to interact with biomarkers from both the current and previous reports. In the course of further development of potential A-NHL biomarkers, many candidate proteins are likely to be eliminated based on technical and/or biological limitations. A more complete understanding of the network of interactions displayed in this analysis should enable us to more effectively identify potential alternatives to those biomarkers which work in close proximity within disease processes.

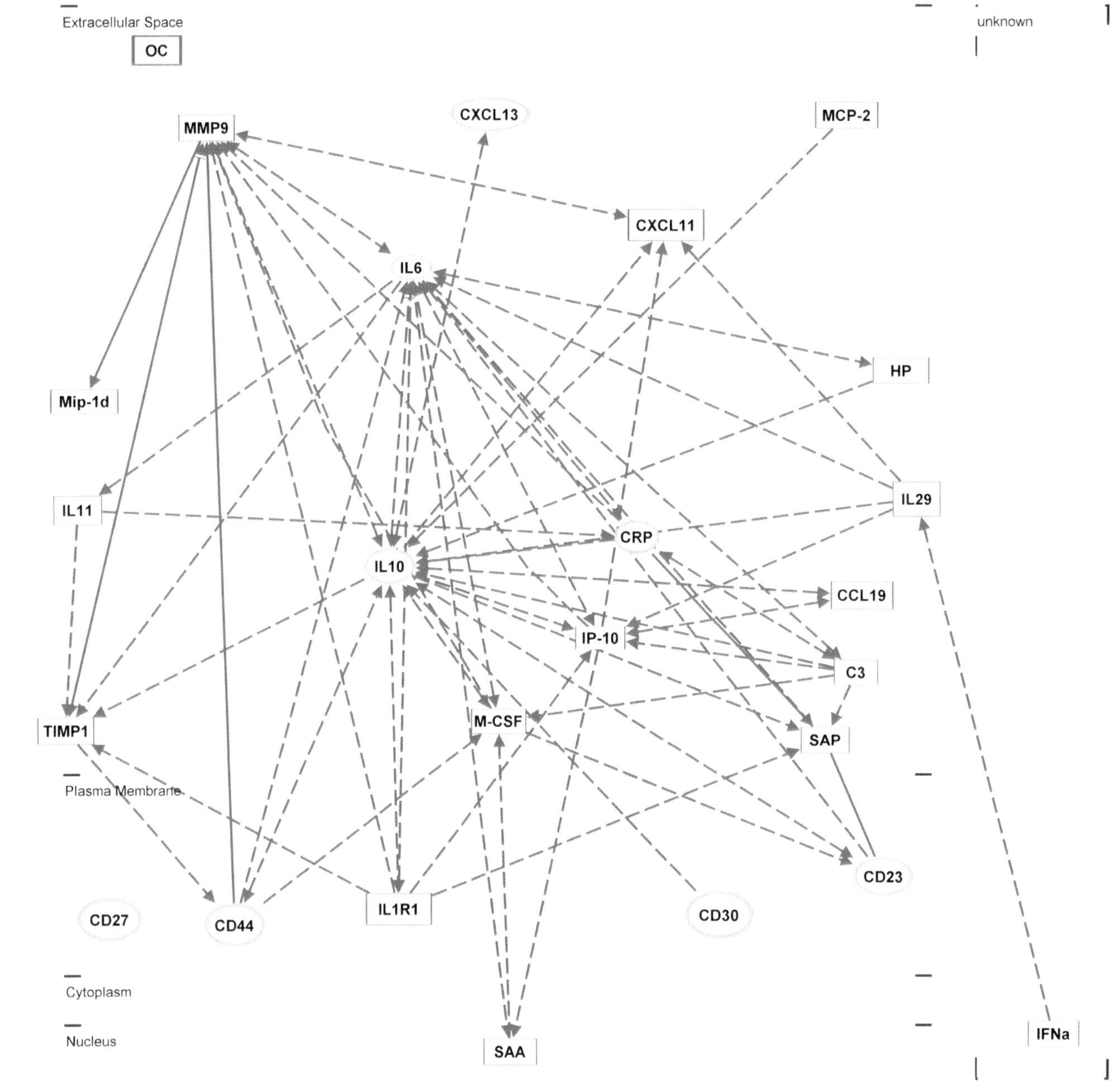

Figure 1. A-NHL biomarker pathway analysis. The Ingenuity Pathway Analysis (IPA) software package was utilized to identify pathways and specific interactions associated with the serum biomarkers identified in the current and previous reports. Biomarkers evaluated from the current study (rectangles) included CCL19, CXCL11, MCP-2, MIP-1δ, IFN-α, IL-11, IL-29, IP-10, M-CSF, sIL-1R1, C3, HPN, SAA, SAP, MMP-9, TIMP-1 and OC. Biomarkers evaluated based on previous findings (ovals) included IL-6, sCD30, IL-10, sCD23, sCD44, sCD27, CRP, BCA-1/CXCL13 and IgE. Solid lines indicate direct interactions, dashed lines indicate indirect interactions.

In the current study, an analysis of a broad array of circulating proteins yielded a relatively small but robust collection of inflammatory mediators associated with the development of A-NHL in comparison to controls. Many of the identified biomarkers were positively correlated to HIV viral load and indicate heightened immune responses in A-NHL with respect to HIV infection and/or AIDS in the absence of lymphoma. A minority of the subjects included in the current study were former or current recipients of HAART. Although the distribution of HAART recipients was similar among cases and controls, we cannot rule out some effect of treatment on our biomarker findings. Our findings further support the hypothesis that A-NHL develops in response to persistent immune activation and inflammation and adds new points of focus for further investigation. Ongoing analysis into the precise role of each of the biomarkers identified in our report should enhance our ability to diagnose, monitor and treat this disease.

Supporting Information

Table S1 Description of Biomarker assays utilized in the current study.

Table S2 Percentage of samples classified as out of range low according to the Bioplex Manager software.

Author Contributions

Conceived and designed the experiments: BMN ECB LAK CRR AEL. Performed the experiments: BMN AEL. Analyzed the data: BMN ECB FJJ LAK CRR AEL. Contributed reagents/materials/analysis tools: ECB JHB CRR AEL. Contributed to the writing of the manuscript: BMN ECB JHB FJJ LAK CRR AEL.

References

1. Grulich AE, Li Y, McDonald AM, Correll PK, Law MG, et al. (2001) Decreasing rates of Kaposi's sarcoma and non-Hodgkin's lymphoma in the era of potent combination anti-retroviral therapy. AIDS 15: 629–633.
2. Bonnet F, Balestre E, Thiebaut R, Morlat P, Pellegrin JL, et al. (2006) Factors associated with the occurrence of AIDS-related non-Hodgkin lymphoma in the era of highly active antiretroviral therapy: Aquitaine Cohort, France. Clin Infect Dis 42: 411–417.
3. Bonnet F, Lewden C, May T, Heripret L, Jougla E, et al. (2004) Malignancy-related causes of death in human immunodeficiency virus-infected patients in the era of highly active antiretroviral therapy. Cancer 101: 317–324.
4. Matthews GV, Bower M, Mandalia S, Powles T, Nelson MR, et al. (2000) Changes in acquired immunodeficiency syndrome-related lymphoma since the introduction of highly active antiretroviral therapy. Blood 96: 2730–2734.
5. Beral V, Peterman T, Berkelman R, Jaffe H (1991) AIDS-associated non-Hodgkin lymphoma. Lancet 337: 805–809.
6. Rabkin CS (2001) AIDS and cancer in the era of highly active antiretroviral therapy (HAART). European Journal of Cancer 37: 1316–1319.
7. Seaberg EC, Wiley D, Martinez-Maza O, Chmiel JS, Kingsley L, et al. (2010) Cancer incidence in the multicenter AIDS Cohort Study before and during the HAART era: 1984 to 2007. Cancer 116: 5507–5516.
8. Beral V, Jaffe HW, Weiss RA (1991) Cancer, HIV and AIDS. Cancer Surveys: 1–5.
9. Bower M, Fife K (2001) Current issues in the biology of AIDS-related lymphoma. HIV Medicine 2: 141–145.
10. Cote TR, Manns A, Hardy CR, Yellin FJ, Hartge P (1996) Epidemiology of brain lymphoma among people with or without acquired immunodeficiency syndrome. AIDS/Cancer Study Group. J Natl Cancer Inst 88: 675–679.
11. Knowles DM (2003) Etiology and pathogenesis of AIDS-related non-Hodgkin's lymphoma. Hematology/Oncology Clinics of North America 17: 785–820.
12. Polesel J, Clifford GM, Rickenbach M, Dal Maso L, Battegay M, et al. (2008) Non-Hodgkin lymphoma incidence in the Swiss HIV Cohort Study before and after highly active antiretroviral therapy. AIDS 22: 301–306.
13. Epeldegui M, Widney DP, Martinez-Maza O (2006) Pathogenesis of AIDS lymphoma: role of oncogenic viruses and B cell activation-associated molecular lesions. Curr Opin Oncol 18: 444–448.
14. Carbone A (2002) AIDS-related non-Hodgkin's lymphomas: From pathology and molecular pathogenesis to treatment. Human Pathology 33: 392–404.
15. Gaidano G, Carbone A, Dalla-Favera R (1998) Pathogenesis of AIDS-related lymphomas: Molecular and histogenetic heterogeneity. American Journal of Pathology 152: 623–630
16. Cunto-Amesty G, Przybylski G, Honczarenko M, Monroe JG, Silberstein LE (2000) Blood 95: 1393–1399.
17. Grulich AE (2000) Update: Cancer risk in persons with HIV/AIDS in the era of combination antiretroviral therapy. AIDS Reader 10: 341–346.
18. Grulich AE, Wan X, Law MG, Milliken ST, Lewis CR, et al. (2000) B-cell stimulation and prolonged immune deficiency are risk factors for non-Hodgkin's lymphoma in people with AIDS. AIDS 14: 133–140.
19. Kirk O, Pedersen C, Cozzi-Lepri A, Antunes F, Miller V, et al. (2001) Non-Hodgkin lymphoma in HIV-infected patients in the era of highly active antiretroviral therapy. Blood 98: 3406–3412.
20. Killebrew D, Shiramizu B (2004) Pathogenesis of HIV-associated non-Hodgkin lymphoma. Curr HIV Res 2: 215–221.
21. Breen EC, Hussain SK, Magpantay L, Jacobson LP, Detels R, et al. (2011) B-cell stimulatory cytokines and markers of immune activation are elevated several years prior to the diagnosis of systemic AIDS-associated non-Hodgkin B-cell lymphoma. Cancer Epidemiol Biomarkers Prev 20: 1303–1314.
22. Vendrame E, Hussain SK, Breen EC, Magpantay LI, Widney DP, et al. (2014) Serum Levels of Cytokines and Biomarkers for Inflammation and Immune Activation, and HIV-Associated Non-Hodgkin B-Cell Lymphoma Risk. Cancer Epidemiol Biomarkers Prev 23: 343–349.
23. Breen EC, Boscardin WJ, Detels R, Jacobson LP, Smith MW, et al. (2003) Non-Hodgkin's B cell lymphoma in persons with acquired immunodeficiency syndrome is associated with increased serum levels of IL10, or the IL10 promoter -592 C/C genotype. Clin Immunol 109: 119–129.
24. Breen EC, Fatahi S, Epeldegui M, Boscardin WJ, Detels R, et al. (2006) Elevated serum soluble CD30 precedes the development of AIDS-associated non-Hodgkin's B cell lymphoma. Tumor Biology 27: 187–194.
25. Schroeder JR, Saah AJ, Hoover DR, Margolick JB, Ambinder RF, et al. (1999) Serum soluble CD23 level correlates with subsequent development of AIDS-related non-Hodgkin's lymphoma. Cancer Epidemiol Biomarkers Prev 8: 979–984.
26. Breen EC, Epeldegui M, Boscardin WJ, Widney DP, Detels R, et al. (2005) Elevated levels of soluble CD44 precede the development of AIDS-associated non-Hodgkin's B-cell lymphoma [4]. AIDS 19: 1711–1712.
27. Hussain S, Zhu W, Chang SC, Crabb Breen E, Vendrame E, et al. (2013) Serum levels of the chemokine CXCL13, genetic variation in CXCL13 and its receptor CXCR5, and HIV-associated non-Hodgkin B cell lymphoma risk. Cancer Epidemiol Biomarkers Prev 22: 295–307.
28. Widney DP, Gui D, Popoviciu LM, Said JW, Breen EC, et al. (2010) Expression and Function of the Chemokine, CXCL13, and Its Receptor, CXCR5, in Aids-Associated Non-Hodgkin's Lymphoma. AIDS Res Treat 2010: 164586.
29. Kaslow RA, Ostrow DG, Detels R, Phair JP, Polk BF, et al. (1987) The Multicenter AIDS Cohort Study: rationale, organization, and selected characteristics of the participants. Am J Epidemiol 126: 310–318.
30. Wong HL, Breen EC, Pfeiffer RM, Aissani B, Martinson JJ, et al. (2010) Cytokine signaling pathway polymorphisms and AIDS-related non-Hodgkin lymphoma risk in the multicenter AIDS cohort study. AIDS 24: 1025–1033.
31. (2008) Panel on Antiretroviral Guidelines for Adults and Adolescents. Guidelines for the use of antiretroviral agents in HIV-1-infected adults and adolescents. Department of Health and Human Services.
32. UPCI Luminex Core Facility. http://www.upci.upmc.edu/cbf/luminex.cfm
33. Yurkovetsky Z, Skates S, Lomakin A, Nolen B, Pulsipher T, et al. (2010) Development of a multimarker assay for early detection of ovarian cancer. J Clin Oncol 28: 2159–2166.
34. Benjamini Y, Hochberg Y (1995) Controlling the false discovery rate: a practical and powerful approach to multiple testing. Journal of the Royal Statistical Society, Series B (Methodological) 57: 289–300.
35. Pagès F, Galon J, Karaschuk G, Dudziak D, Camus M, et al. (2005) Epstein-Barr virus nuclear antigen 2 induces interleukin-18 receptor expression in B cells. Blood 105: 1632–1639.
36. Purdue MP, Lan Q, Martinez-Maza O, Oken MM, Hocking W, et al. (2009) A prospective study of serum soluble CD30 concentration and risk of non-Hodgkin lymphoma. Blood 114: 2730–2732.
37. Ellis M, Hedstrom U, Frampton C, Alizadeh H, Kristensen J, et al. (2006) Modulation of the systemic inflammatory response by recombinant human interleukin-11: a prospective randomized placebo controlled clinical study in patients with hematological malignancy. Clin Immunol 120: 129–137.
38. Hensbergen PJ, Wijnands PG, Schreurs MW, Scheper RJ, Willemze R, et al. (2005) The CXCR3 targeting chemokine CXCL11 has potent antitumor activity in vivo involving attraction of CD8+ T lymphocytes but not inhibition of angiogenesis. J Immunother 28: 343–351.
39. Xia T, O'Hara A, Araujo I, Barreto J, Carvalho E, et al. (2008) EBV microRNAs in primary lymphomas and targeting of CXCL-11 by ebv-mir-BHRF1-3. Cancer Res 68: 1436–1442.
40. Dolganiuc A, Kodys K, Marshall C, Saha B, Zhang S, et al. (2012) Type III Interferons, IL-28 and IL-29, Are Increased in Chronic HCV Infection and Induce Myeloid Dendritic Cell-Mediated FoxP3+ Regulatory T Cells. PLoS One 7: e44915.
41. Tian RR, Guo HX, Wei JF, Yang CK, He SH, et al. (2012) IFN-lambda inhibits HIV-1 integration and post-transcriptional events in vitro, but there is only limited in vivo repression of viral production. Antiviral Res 95: 57–65.
42. Corcione A, Arduino N, Ferretti E, Raffaghello L, Roncella S, et al. (2004) CCL19 and CXCL12 trigger in vitro chemotaxis of human mantle cell lymphoma B cells. Clin Cancer Res 10: 964–971.
43. Wang X, Yuling H, Yanping J, Xinti T, Yaofang Y, et al. (2007) CCL19 and CXCL13 synergistically regulate interaction between B cell acute lymphocytic leukemia CD23+CD5+ B Cells and CD8+ T cells. J Immunol 179: 2880–2888.
44. Ouedraogo DE, Makinson A, Kuster N, Nagot N, Rubbo PA, et al. (2013) Increased T-Cell Activation and Th1 Cytokine Concentrations Prior to the Diagnosis of B-Cell Lymphoma in HIV Infected Patients. J Clin Immunol 33: 22–29.
45. Ansell SM, Maurer MJ, Ziesmer SC, Slager SL, Habermann TM, et al. (2012) Elevated pretreatment serum levels of interferon-inducible protein-10 (CXCL10) predict disease relapse and prognosis in diffuse large B-cell lymphoma patients. Am J Hematol 87: 865–869.
46. Bozkurt C, Ertem U, Oksal A, Sahin G, Yuksek N, et al. (2008) Expression of matrix metalloproteinase-9 (MMP-9) and tissue inhibitor of matrix metalloproteinase (TIMP-1) in tissues with a diagnosis of childhood lymphoma. Pediatr Hematol Oncol 25: 621–629.

47. Citak EC, Oguz A, Karadeniz C, Akyurek N (2008) Role of gelatinases (MMP-2 and MMP-9), TIMP-1, vascular endothelial growth factor (VEGF), and microvessel density on the clinicopathological behavior of childhood non-Hodgkin lymphoma. Pediatr Hematol Oncol 25: 55-66.
48. Hottinger AF, Iwamoto FM, Karimi S, Riedel E, Dantis J, et al. (2011) YKL-40 and MMP-9 as serum markers for patients with primary central nervous system lymphoma. Ann Neurol 70: 163-169.
49. Tarantul VZ, Nikolaev AI, Martynenko A, Hannig H, Hunsmann G, et al. (2000) Differential gene expression in B-cell non-Hodgkin's lymphoma of SIV-infected monkey. AIDS Res Hum Retroviruses 16: 173-179.
50. Bassig BA, Zheng T, Zhang Y, Berndt SI, Holford TR, et al. (2012) Polymorphisms in complement system genes and risk of non-Hodgkin lymphoma. Environ Mol Mutagen 53: 145-151.
51. Marquart HV, Olesen EH, Johnson AA, Damgaard G, Leslie RG (1997) A comparative study of normal B cells and the EBV-positive Burkitt's lymphoma cell line, Raji, as activators of the complement system. Scand J Immunol 46: 246-253.
52. Harrington WJ Jr, Cabral L, Cai JP, Chan ASS, Wood C (1996) Azothymidine and interferon-alpha are active in AIDS-associated small non-cleaved cell lymphoma but not large-cell lymphoma. Lancet 348: 833.
53. Lee RK, Cai JP, Deyev V, Gill PS, Cabral L, et al. (1999) Azidothymidine and interferon-alpha induce apoptosis in herpesvirus-associated lymphomas. Cancer Res 59: 5514-5520.
54. Toomey NL, Deyev VV, Wood C, Boise LH, Scott D, et al. (2001) Induction of a TRAIL-mediated suicide program by interferon alpha in primary effusion lymphoma. Oncogene 20: 7029-7040.

12

Evolution of Treatment Regimens in Multiple Myeloma: A Social Network Analysis

Helen Mahony[1], Athanasios Tsalatsanis[1], Ambuj Kumar[1], Benjamin Djulbegovic[1,2]*

1 Department of Internal Medicine, Division of Evidence-Based Medicine & Health Outcomes Research, University of South Florida, Tampa, Florida, United States of America, **2** H. Lee Moffitt Cancer Center & Research Institute, Department of Hematology and Health Outcomes and Behavior, Tampa, Florida, United States of America

Abstract

Background: Randomized controlled trials (RCTs) are considered the gold standard for assessing the efficacy of new treatments compared to standard treatments. However, the reasoning behind treatment selection in RCTs is often unclear. Here, we focus on a cohort of RCTs in multiple myeloma (MM) to understand the patterns of competing treatment selections.

Methods: We used social network analysis (SNA) to study relationships between treatment regimens in MM RCTs and to examine the topology of RCT treatment networks. All trials considering induction or autologous stem cell transplant among patients with MM were eligible for our analysis. Medline and abstracts from the annual proceedings of the American Society of Hematology and American Society for Clinical Oncology, as well as all references from relevant publications were searched. We extracted data on treatment regimens, year of publication, funding type, and number of patients enrolled. The SNA metrics used are related to node and network level centrality and to node positioning characterization.

Results: 135 RCTs enrolling a total of 36,869 patients were included. The density of the RCT network was low indicating little cohesion among treatments. Network Betweenness was also low signifying that the network does not facilitate exchange of information. The maximum geodesic distance was equal to 4, indicating that all connected treatments could reach each other in four "steps" within the same pathway of development. The distance between many important treatment regimens was greater than 1, indicating that no RCTs have compared these regimens.

Conclusion: Our findings show that research programs in myeloma, which is a relatively small field, are surprisingly decentralized with a lack of connectivity among various research pathways. As a result there is much crucial research left unexplored. Using SNA to visually and analytically examine treatment networks prior to designing a clinical trial can lead to better designed studies.

Editor: Yu-Kang Tu, National Taiwan University, Taiwan

Funding: The authors have no support or funding to report.

Competing Interests: The authors have declared that no competing interests exist.

* Email: bdjulbeg@health.usf.edu

Introduction

Multiple myeloma (MM) is a hematological malignancy, which accounts for 1% of cancer deaths and 10% of all hematological malignancies in the US. [1] Several advances in the treatment of MM have been possible due to testing of newer agents in randomized controlled trials (RCTs). As a result of these advancements, MM has transformed into a chronic disease.

The first randomized controlled trial (RCT) in MM was published in 1966. [2] Since then over 300 RCTs have been published and nearly half have been conducted in an induction and transplant setting. [3] While there is a vast body of research involving RCTs in MM as well as systematic reviews and meta-analyses [4–7], there has been no formal assessment of patterns of treatment discoveries in the context of RCTs. That is, it is not known how a new treatment regimen makes its way through the translational cycle to be tested in an RCT. Understanding the process of this translational cycle, specifically in relation to the choice of new regimens for the treatment of MM in RCTs, is important and has several benefits. At the highest level, it can provide investigators interested in assessing the efficacy of similar treatment regimens with collaborative opportunities, thereby avoiding duplication of research efforts. Avoiding duplication can result in not only consolidation of research efforts and allocation of limited resources, but can also lead to averting patients from participating in trials where the answers to the treatment efficacy may already be known.

Using methodologies that provide analytical as well as visual representations of existing research in MM, prior to conducting new RCTs, could lead to better designed studies and enable researchers to address more relevant clinical and research questions. In this paper, we propose using social network analysis (SNA) to study the patterns of interactions between treatment regimens in RCTs, to identify potential limitations, and draw future research directions. SNA provides a "bird's-eye view" of the overall RCT universe, which enables us to examine relationships, directions, and importance of different treatment regimens in the network. Such an approach could allow industry and government to save valuable healthcare dollars by focusing resources on relevant research.

We have previously reported on a preliminary SNA on RCTs of autologous stem cell transplant (ASCT) and novel agents for MM [8]. Our analyses showed that research programs in myeloma, which is a relatively small field, were surprisingly decentralized and various research pathways suffered by lack of connectivity. We hypothesize that this finding is attributed to lack of interaction among researchers performing RCTs and the absence of policies that enforce consolidation of the totality of existing evidence prior to designing new RCTs. In this paper, we expand our initial analyses to include all RCTs of induction or ASCT among patients with MM and we illustrate a novel application of SNA to study the topology of RCT treatment networks.

Methods

Dataset

We searched MEDLINE for any relevant RCTs published until April 2012 using the searching strategies described by Haynes et al. [9] No limits of any kind were imposed. Abstracts from the American Society of Hematology and the American Society of Clinical Oncology were also searched. All references from relevant publications were scanned manually to identify additional candidate studies. Any MM RCT studying the treatment regimens of induction or ASCT was eligible for our analysis. We extracted data on treatments used for experimental arm and control arm, year of publication, funding type, and number of patients enrolled. For funding type, we categorized the funding source into the broad categories of public, private for profit, or private not for profit. If the funding source were a mix of these categories, funding type was recorded as mixed. For publications that did not report a funding source, we labeled their funding type as unclear.

Social networks

A social network is represented as a set of nodes denoting different entities such as individuals or organizations and their interactions denoted as ties [10,11]. SNA is the theoretical framework developed to understand social networks and to reveal hidden and potentially useful information regarding entities and their interactions. SNA has been used extensively to explain phenomena such as (among others) scientific interaction [12], information exchange [13], and treatment success [14]. In this paper, we use SNA to study the RCTs of MM universe focusing on the treatment regimen interactions as they appear in each RCT. Such modeling can provide an in-depth understanding of how treatments and comparisons are distributed and identify the factors associated with development of research questions. [10] We define a treatment network as the set of nodes denoting each treatment tested in an RCT connected with ties denoting a direct comparison between treatments in RCTs (Figure S1 in File S1). The direction of a tie in the treatment network is used to distinguish treatments as experimental and as control. That is, the ties are directed away from the experimental node and toward the control node. Using SNA we can measure the properties of the entire treatment network as well as the properties of each node individually. [15] These measures help us understand how nodes interact and identify opportunities and constraints for future research.

Node-level properties

Not all nodes in a network are of the same importance. Nodes with a certain position in the network can interact easier/harder with particular nodes and faster/slower with others. To measure the ability of the node to interact with other nodes in the network or to facilitate interactions between nodes we use the *centrality* measures of *degree*, *closeness*, and *betweenness*. In general, centrality measures describe key attributes of the position of a node representing a treatment regimen in the treatment network. [10] Degree measures the number of different comparisons a treatment regimen has participated in; closeness measures the ease at which a treatment regimen can reach other treatment regimens in a network [16], and it is directly associated with the ability to extract information about regimen superiority outside an RCT environment (i.e. indirect meta-analyses); betweenness [17] represents the ability of a treatment regimen to link other treatment regimens, a property that is particularly desirable in indirect meta-analyses. Degree and closeness are further classified into *in-* and *out-degree* and *in-* and *out-closeness* respectively. In the RCT network, in- and out-degree show the number of times a particular regimen has been participating in an RCT as control or experimental respectively. In-closeness shows the easiness at which a node can be reached and out-closeness the easiness at which a node can reach others in the network. When measuring degree and closeness we need to differentiate between control and experimental treatments. Therefore, degree and closeness calculations are performed on the directed treatment networks. On the other hand, when measuring betweenness, we are interested only in the position of the node. Therefore, betweenness calculations were performed on the undirected networks. Note that directed and undirected networks have the same structure (i.e. same number of nodes and number of ties); however, directed networks are represented with directional ties, while undirected networks are represented with bidirectional ties.

Network level properties

Network level properties are associated with the topology of the entire treatment network. We compute measures such as the network's *density*, *maximum geodesic distance*, *clustering coefficient*, *centrality measures*, *KeyPlayer function*, and the *Girvan-Newman Algorithm* as indicators of the network structure. [10] Density reports the actual treatment interactions in the network as a fraction of all possible interactions (e.g. each regimen is compared to all other regimens). A density value of 15% to 25% indicates that a very small portion of all available comparisons have been achieved and that any changes to the interactions between treatments would have a profound effect on the cohesion of the network. [10] Conversely, values greater than 50% demonstrate that a significant number of comparisons have been made and that changes to interactions will have no or little effect on the cohesion of the network. The maximum geodesic distance corresponds to the network's diameter and it measures the maximum distance between any two treatments in the network. The clustering coefficient is the degree at which treatments in the network form clusters. [10] The clustering coefficient takes values between 0 and 1 where 1 indicates a fully connected network (e.g. each treatment is connected to all the rest). Smaller values of clustering coefficient reveal a rather random pattern of connectivity. [10] The network level centralization measures such as closeness, betweenness, and degree provide an overall impression of network centrality. Interpretation of the network level centralization values is similar to their node level centrality counterparts. For example, a network with low betweenness does not facilitate sharing of information. The Girvan-Newman

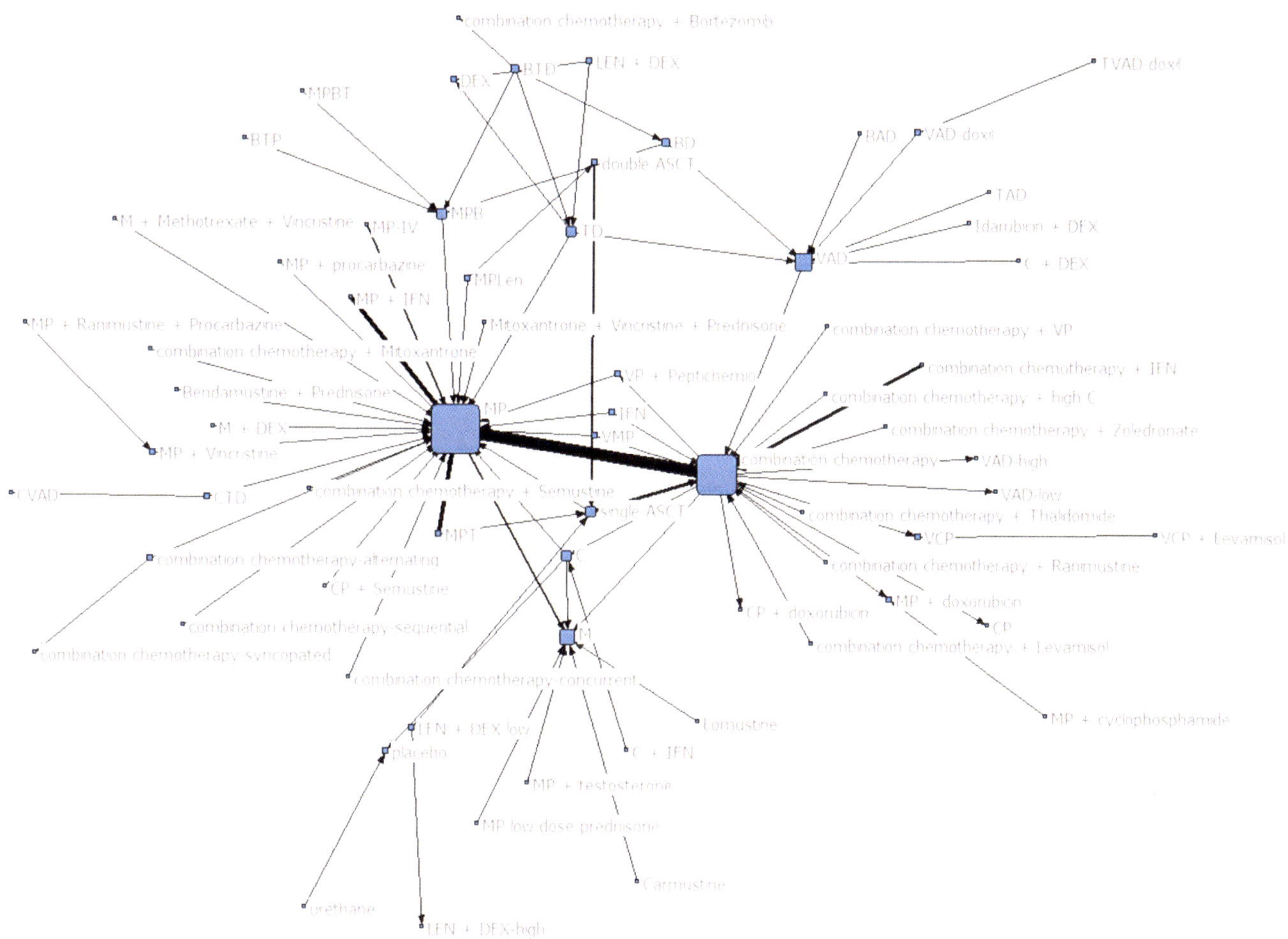

Figure 1. Connected component of RCT treatment network. Each node is associated with a treatment tested in an RCT and each tie denotes a comparison between two treatments. The width of the ties among treatments denotes the number of times two treatments have been tested in RCTs. The network represents the connected component of the network depicted in Figure S1 in File S1 and it is comprised of 155 treatment comparisons. The most frequently tested comparison is between *combination therapy* and *MP*.

Algorithm identifies *communities* of treatment regimens. Communities are loosely connected groups of tightly interconnected nodes. [18] The existence of multiple communities may be an indicator of research in isolation. The KeyPlayer function determines the optimal set of treatments in the sense that if an optimal set of nodes were to be removed from the network, this would have a crippling effect. Additionally, the KeyPlayer function determines the most well-connected treatment regimens. Changes to these regimens can influence other treatment regimens. [19]

2-mode networks

In addition to the treatment network described in the previous subsections we formed and studied a different category of networks. 2-Mode networks are used to report and analyze the relationships between two different classes of entities. While the treatment network presented previously is used to analyze the relationships between all treatment regimens, the 2-mode network is built to analyze the relationships between treatment regimens and an additional entity such as the funding source or the publication year. We have generated two 2-mode networks. The first 2-mode network (treatment – year) provides a visual association of treatment regimens and the decade they have been used. Similarly, the second 2-mode network (treatment – funding) provides a representation of the funding mechanisms used for each regimen. In the 2-mode networks, the direction of the ties is formed from the experimental and control nodes towards either year of publication or funding type.

Data analysis

The main analysis included calculation of the following measures: *betweenness*, *density*, *clustering coefficient*, *closeness*, *degree*, *Girvan-Newman Algorithm*, *KeyPlayer*, *maximum geodesic distance* and *distance* among treatments. For the analysis of the node-level and network level properties, we included only treatment regimens from the connected component of the treatment network (e.g. disregarded isolated sets of nodes). The first well-designed RCT of ASCT versus chemotherapy was published in 1996. [20] In order to examine the effect of the first important breakthrough (ASCT) on the evolution of treatment regimens, we also conducted a subgroup analysis of trials published in 1996 or later. Additionally, a time series analysis of the networks with trials from 1996 to 2012 was conducted to compare network properties through time. All networks ware analyzed with UCINET 6 [21] and KeyPlayer 1.44 [19]. Visual representations of the networks were created with NetDraw 2.119. [21]

Table 1. Abbreviations of Treatment Regimens.

Abbreviation	Name of Treatment Regimens
M	melphalan
P	prednisone
C	cyclophosphamide
V	vincristine
MP	melphalan, prednisone
ASCT	autologous stem cell transplant
LEN	lenalidomide
DEX	dexamethasone
TD	thalidomide, dexamethasone
MPT	melphalan, prednisone, thalidomide
MPB	melphalan, prednisone, bortezomib
MPLen	melphalan, prednisone, lenalidomide
BTP	bortezomib, thalidomide, prednisone
BD	bortezomib, dexamethasone
VAD	vincristine, doxorubicin, dexamethasone
MPBT	melphalan, prednisone, bortezomib, thalidomide
TAD	thalidomide, doxorubicin, dexamethasone
TVAD	thalidomide, vincristine, doxorubicin, dexamethasone
BTD	bortezomib, thalidomide, dexamethasone
CTD	cyclophosphamide, thalidomide, dexamethasone
VP	vincristine, prednisone
Q	quinine
IFN	interferon
Combination chemotherapy	vincristine, doxorubicin, melphalan, cyclophosphamide, prednisone
	vincristine, BCNU, doxorubicin, melphalan, prednisone
	vincristine, BCNU, melphalan, cyclophosphamide, prednisone
	vincristine, BCNU, doxorubicin, dexamethasone
	BCNU, doxorubicin, melphalan, cyclophosphamide
	BCNU, melphalan, cyclophosphamide, prednisone
	vincristine, BCNU, doxorubicin, prednisone
	vincristine, doxorubicin, cyclophosphamide, prednisone

Table 2. Node-level properties of RCT treatment network (connected component).

Treatment	Betweenness	In-Closeness	Out-Closeness	In-Degree	Out-Degree
MP	1399.8	4.572	1.471	72	4
Combination chemotherapy	1129.5	2.209	1.753	23	39
VAD	451.3	1.694	1.779	7	1
TD	264.3	1.493	1.838	3	4
MPB	207.167	1.538	1.492	4	1
C	197	2.293	1.515	2	4
Single ASCT	188.5	1.538	1.779	7	9
M	262.0	5.732	1.449	11	0
VAD-doxil	67	1.471	1.805	1	1

Table 3. Distances between selected treatment regimens.

Measure	Value
Distance from:	
MPT to combination chemotherapy	2
MPB to combination chemotherapy	2
MPLen to combination chemotherapy	2
MPT to MPB	2
MPT to MPLen	2
MPB to MPLen	2
MPT to single ASCT	1
MPB to single ASCT	2
MPLen to single ASCT	2

Results

Study selection

We found 135 trials which examined induction or ASCT therapies among patients with MM. Because of multi-arm RCTs, these 135 trials represented 165 comparisons and enrolled 36,869 patients. The entire treatment network is shown in Figure S1 in File S1. Figure 1 depicts the connected portion (connected component) of the entire treatment network that includes 155 comparisons and disregards the unconnected regimens. The treatment regimen abbreviations are listed in Table 1.

Node-level properties

Table 2 shows selected node-level properties for treatment regimens in the network depicted in Figure 1. The tie thickness, in Figure 1, denotes the frequency that two trials have been compared in an RCT. For example, the treatment regimen of *combination chemotherapy* was frequently compared to the treatment regimen of *MP*. The size of a node represents the number of different comparisons a regimen has been included in (node degree). The larger the size of the node, the greater the number of trials the associated treatment was compared to. The treatment participated in most trials was *MP* followed by *combination chemotherapy*. Also, based on the measures for in- and out-degree we see that MP (in-degree of 72) and combination chemotherapy (in-degree of 23) are the regimens used most often as controls in RCTs. Combination chemotherapy has also been frequently used as experimental therapy in RCTs (out-degree of 39).

Regarding closeness (measured using directed network), all nodes had small, relatively similar closeness measures demonstrating a large distance between each node in the network and all other nodes in the network (Table 2). The node-level betweenness (measured using undirected network) was largest for the treatment regimens of *combination chemotherapy*, *MP*, and *VAD*, indicating that these regimens and those directly connected to them are excellent candidates for indirect meta-analysis.

Distances between selected treatment regimens (undirected network) are reported in Table 3. The majority of the distance between many important treatment regimens (e.g. *MP* to *combination chemotherapy*; *MPT* to *MPB*; *MPT* to *MPLen*; *MPB* to *MPLen*; and *MPB* to *single ASCT)* is equal to 2. This demonstrates that these treatment regimens can reach each other in two "steps", a property of significance in indirect meta-analyses. This also indicates that these treatment regimens have never been tested in a head-to-head comparison in an RCT.

Network level properties

The network level properties of *density*, *geodesic distance*, *clustering coefficient*, and the *centrality* measures are reported in Table 4. The density of the network was low, indicating there is

Table 4. Results of network level analysis for myeloma treatment network.

Measure	RCT network	Erdos-Renyi (random network) value
Density (%)	2.5	2.5
Average Geodesic Distance	3	4.33
Maximum Geodesic Distance	6	10
Clustering Coefficient	3.4	0.025
Network Centralization Metrics		
Betweenness	55.3	78
in-Closeness	1.69	24.1
out-Closeness	1.59	24.1
in-Degree	2.36	4.2
out-Degree	2.13	4.2

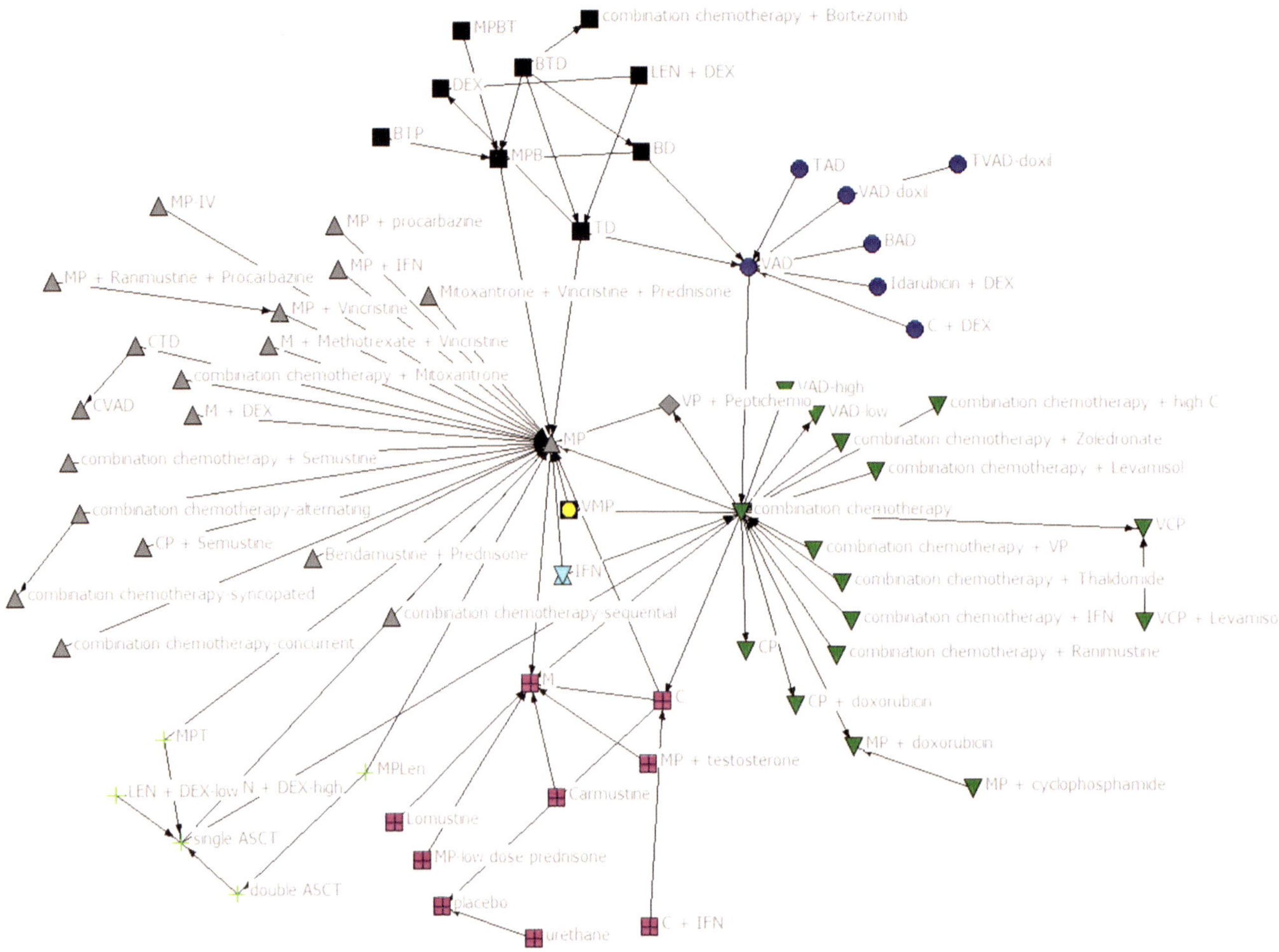

Figure 2. Girvan-Newman Algorithm. The algorithm identified 9 research communities that are loosely connected with each other.

little cohesion among the treatments studied. The maximum geodesic distance was equal to 6, indicating that all connected treatments could reach each other in six "steps" within the same pathway of development. All centrality measures are much lower than a similar random network (e.g. Erdos-Renyi with same number of nodes and same density). This shows that the RCT network is decentralized.

The KeyPlayer function identified that the treatment regimens of *MP*, *combination chemotherapy*, and *VAD* are vital to the network. The Girvan-Newman Algorithm (Figure 2) identified 9 research communities that are loosely connected with each other. These communities would be completely disconnected if the nodes: *MP*, *combination chemotherapy*, and *VAD* were to be removed.

For our subgroup analysis, we focused on trials published in 1996 or later to determine the effect of the publication by Attal et al., [20] on evolution of treatment regimens. The associated network is shown in Figure S2 in File S1. The KeyPlayer function identified again the *combination chemotherapy*, *MP*, and *VAD* as vital to the network. As in the complete treatment network, the Girvan-Newman Algorithm (Figure 3) shows that there are six research communities that are loosely connected to each other. A visual inspection of Figure 3 shows that these communities would be completely disconnected if the MP, combinational chemotherapy, TD and VAD therapies were to be removed.

2-mode network

Figure 4 demonstrates trends in treatment regimens over time and Figure S4 in File S1 displays the treatment comparisons by funding source. In these figures, degree is represented by the size of the node i.e. the larger the node the more comparisons are directed toward that node. All treatment comparisons were used in these networks, which included 165 comparisons.

In Figure 4, the largest number of treatment regimens was studied in the decades of the 1990s and 2000s, which corresponds to these nodes being the largest out of the six decades in which RCTs of MM patients have existed. As shown in Figure S4 in File S1, the highest number of comparisons came from trials which were publicly funded while the fewest trials were funded by private for profit funding organizations. Out of the 47 trials which did not report funding source, the majority (77%) were trials reported in either abstracts only (full publication not available) at the time this search was conducted or in trials published prior to 1996 when the CONSORT statement [22] was published.

The funding trends have changed for RCTs conducted after 1996. Figure 5 demonstrates the results of our subgroup analysis, where it is clear that the majority of RCTs are funded by both public and private entities (mixed). However, there are many trials that did not clearly report their funding mechanisms. The number of these trials is larger than the trials with mixed funding

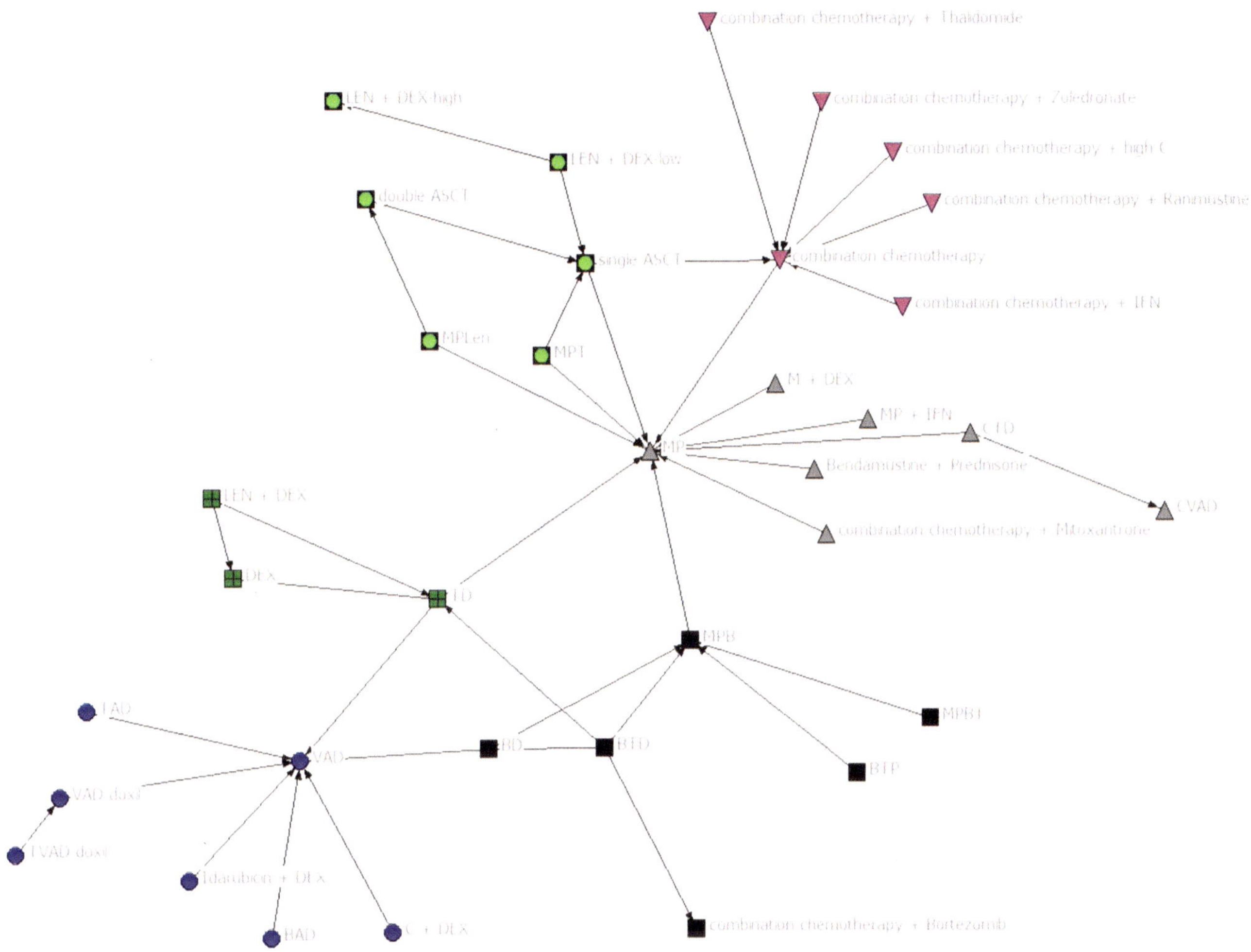

Figure 3. Girvan-Newman Algorithm of RCTs published 1996–2012. The algorithm 6 research communities that are loosely connected with each other.

(Figure 6). Even though the evidence is missing, we believe that these trials have been funded by private entities.

Finally, Figure 6 presents the evolution of different centrality measures as the treatment network is constructed over time (Figure S3 in File S1). It is interesting to note that even with the addition of multiple treatment regimens over time, there is very little change in the network's centrality, which stresses the fact that there is no coordinated research effort in MM.

Discussion

We have analyzed a diverse network of induction and transplant treatment regimens compared in RCTs. Our main finding is that new therapies are compared against established treatments over and over again and not proceeding within a logical framework of testing the most relevant hypotheses. This is demonstrated by the low closeness at both the node and network level and the high betweenness for *MP*, *combination chemotherapy*, *VAD*, and *single ASCT* that do not fully extend to novel agents such as bortezomib, lenalidomide, and thalidomide. This is further exemplified by the fact that there are no direct comparisons between many new regimens, which draws future research directions for RCTs in indirect meta-analysis.

One surprising finding was that through the KeyPlayer function and Girvan-Newman Algorithm we identified two newer treatment regimens, *TD* and *MPB*, which in addition to *combination chemotherapy* and *VAD*, are crucial in maintaining the network structure. However, lenalidomide was not identified as being important in the network even though it is widely used in contemporary practice as first line treatment. These findings point to the discrepancy in regimens being tested in RCTs versus regimens used in practice by the treating Oncologists. The results also demonstrate that researchers tend to compare experimental treatments to inferior regimens. That is, researchers do not compare the most active experimental treatments in head to head trials.

The results of our subgroup analyses show that since 1996 the MM treatment network has evolved in such a way that the novel agents of thalidomide and bortezomib have become very important in maintaining network cohesion. In 1996, Attal et al. [20] demonstrated that ASCT was superior to chemotherapy. This is considered to be the first important breakthrough in the treatment of MM. This subgroup analysis also indicates that chemotherapy and MP are of mostly historical importance.

We also found that the largest number of treatment regimens was studied in the decades of the 1990s and 2000s. The three

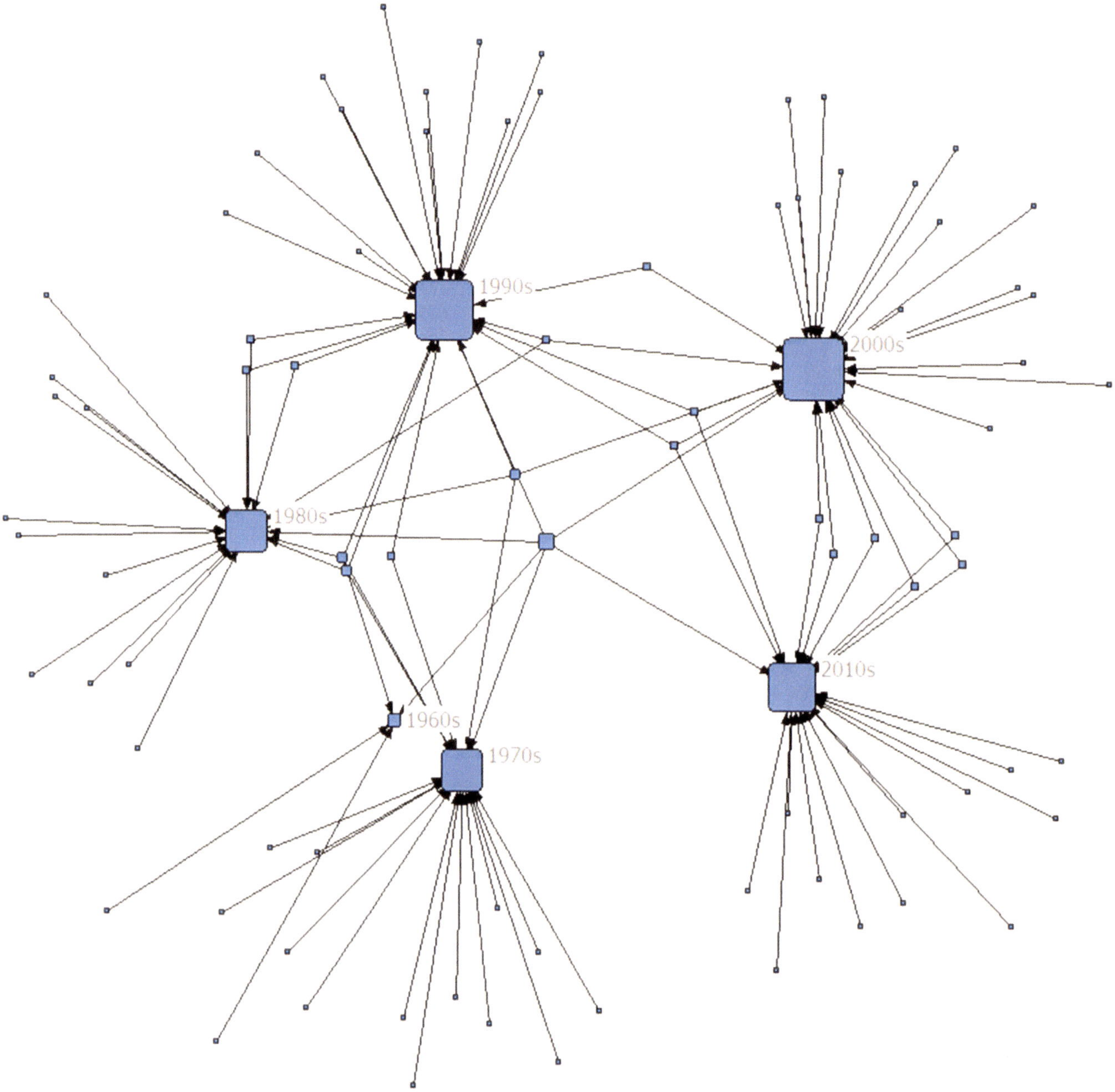

Figure 4. Decades in which treatments have been tested. Most treatment comparisons have been implemented in the decades of the 1990s and 2000s.

novel agents of *thalidomide*, *bortezomib*, and *lenalidomide* were developed in the late 1990s and early 2000s which may explain this increase in comparisons of treatment regimens during this time. Additionally, funding source has changed in recent years (since 1996) from being predominately publically funded to a mix of both private and public funding sources.

In this treatment network, designing trials which compare these treatment regimens to each other directly has been avoided by researchers and funders. As a result, better treatment regimens may not be discovered. The fastest rate of discovery occurs when a few hypotheses are tested sequentially. The lack of attention to the entire network is likely the reason that there is current confusion in the field and as a result guideline panels [23] are not able to provide conclusive recommendations on the best first-line treatment from a list of 83 regimens.

Our analysis has some limitations. The main limitation is that we are inferring reasons from published trials on why researchers and funders choose which treatment to study. Since we only included trials examining treatment regimens used in induction or transplant setting, we cannot decipher how this treatment network fits into the larger network of all MM trials. Future research should focus on conducting a SNA on other areas of MM treatment such as supportive, maintenance, and salvage therapies. Nevertheless, our network analysis focuses on giving insight into first-line treatment, which is the practitioner's best attempt to slow down the progression of disease.

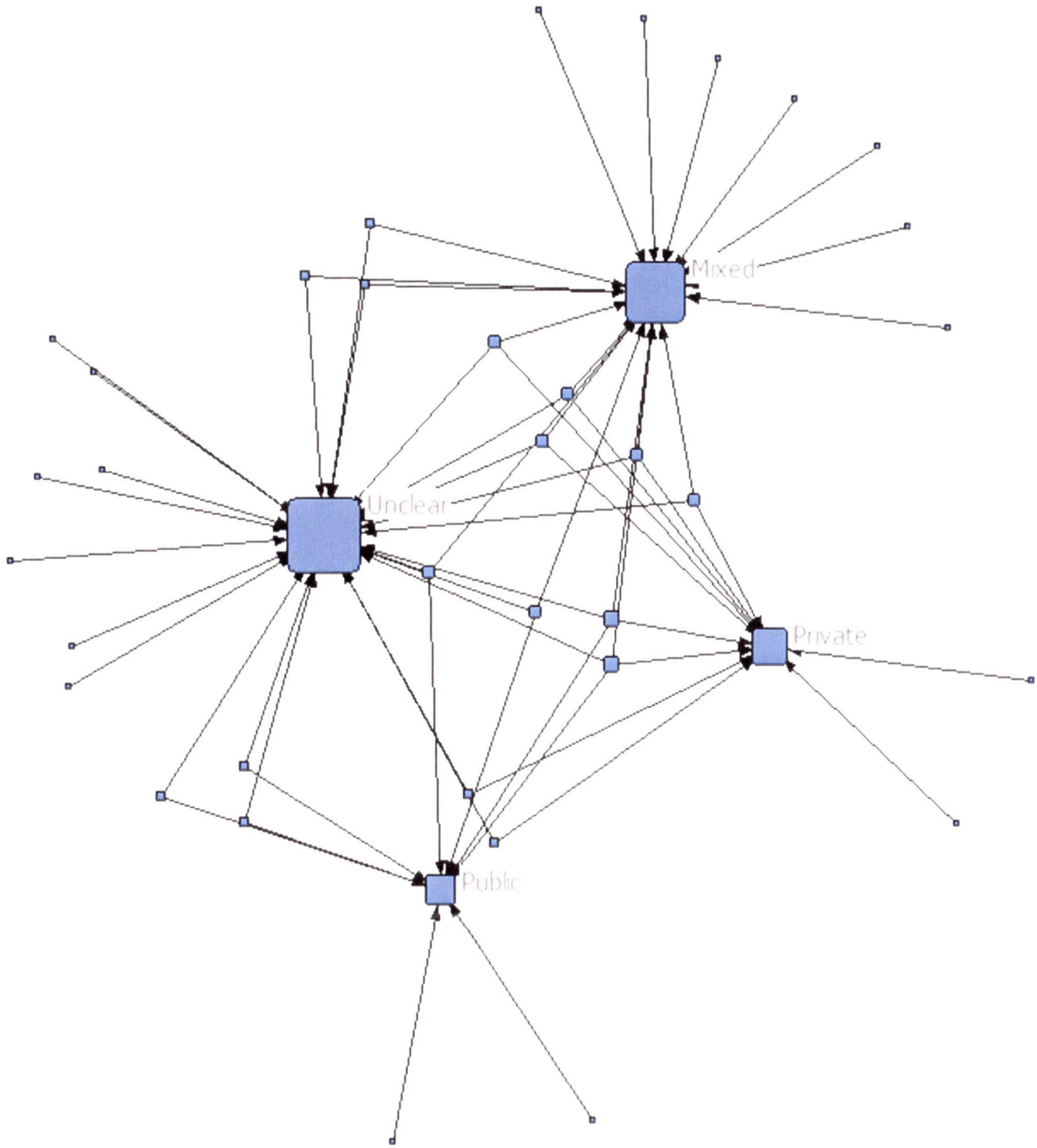

Figure 5. Funding type of trials published in the period 1996–2012. Most treatment comparisons have been funded by a mix of public and private entities. Even though the evidence is missing, we believe that the trials within the unclear funding node have been funded by private entities.

Furthermore, the current design does not allow for analysis of single arm RCTs, which may provide valuable information regarding a regimen's efficacy in MM, and does not include phase I or phase II trials. Finally, since this is the first SNA study on RCT treatments, it is impossible to compare our findings with similar networks in different diseases, which forced us to use random networks for comparison.

Performing SNA in RCTs may provide both funders and researchers with the overall assessment of existing evidence in a given field within the totality of research efforts that may help avoid isolation and duplication. Once performed, researchers may visualize the overall research network and determine the relevance of their hypotheses and if necessary derive future research directions such as those suggested in this study (e.g. MP to

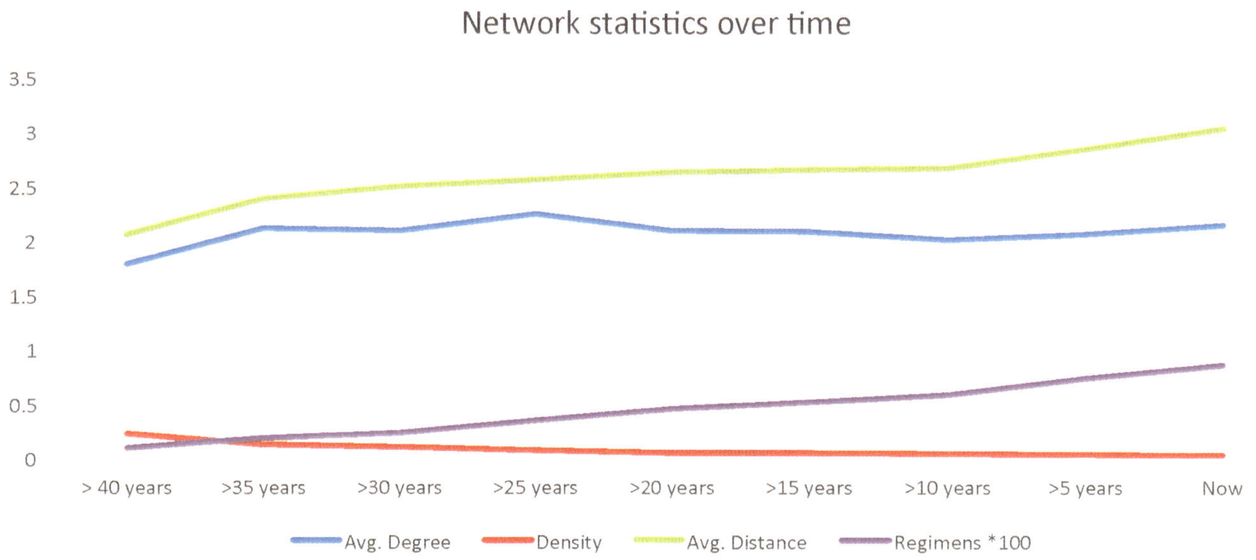

Figure 6. Evolution of centrality measures over time. There is little change in the network's centrality which stresses the fact that there is no coordinated research effort in MM.

combination chemotherapy; MPT to MPB; MPT to MPLen; MPB to MPLen; and MPB to single ASCT).

We conclude that research programs in myeloma are decentralized with a lack of connectivity among various research pathways. This results in lack of head-to-head RCTs of novel agents compared to each other or single ASCT. We have demonstrated that by using SNA to visually and analytically examine treatment networks prior to designing a clinical trial, researchers can better design studies to address more relevant clinical and research questions.

Supporting Information

File S1 Contains the following files: **Figure S1.** Entire treatment network. Each node is associated with a treatment participating in an RCT and each tie denotes a comparison between two treatments. The width of the ties among treatments denotes the number of times two treatments have been tested in RCTs. The network is comprised of 165 treatment comparisons. **Figure S2.** Connected component of network of RCTs published between1996–2012. The width of the ties among treatments denotes the number of times two treatments have been tested in RCTs. **Figure S3.** Evolution of the treatment network over time. The figure presents the network's topology 40, 30, 20 and 1 year ago. **3a.** RCT network that includes trials performed more than 40 years ago; **3b.** RCT network that includes trials performed more than 30 years ago; **3c.** RCT network that includes trials performed more than 20 years ago; **3d.** RCT network that includes trials performed more than 1 year ago. **Figure S4** Funding type of all trials. Most treatment comparisons have been funded by the public sector.
(DOCX)

Author Contributions

Conceived and designed the experiments: BD HM AT. Performed the experiments: HM AT. Analyzed the data: HM AT BD. Contributed reagents/materials/analysis tools: HM AT BD AK. Contributed to the writing of the manuscript: HM AT BD AK.

References

1. Breitkreutz I, Lokhorst HM, Raab MS, Holt B, Cremer FW, et al. (2007) Thalidomide in newly diagnosed multiple myeloma: influence of thalidomide treatment on peripheral blood stem cell collection yield. Leukemia 21: 1294–1299.
2. Holland JF, Hosley H, Scharlau C (1966) A Controlled Trial of Urethane Treatment in Multiple Myeloma. Blood 27: 328–342.
3. Mahony H, Kumar A, Berndt D, Chemudu S, Djulbegovic B (2012) Database of Randomized Trials in Myeloma (DRAM). University of South Florida and Millennium Pharmaceuticals, Inc., The Takeda Oncology Company.
4. Djulbegovic B, Kumar A (2008) Multiple myeloma: detecting the effects of new treatments. The Lancet 371: 1642–1644.
5. Kumar A, Hozo I, Wheatley K, Djulbegovic B (2011) Thalidomide versus bortezomib based regimens as first-line therapy for patients with multiple myeloma: A systematic review. American journal of hematology 86: 18–24.
6. Kumar A, Kharfan-Dabaja MA, Glasmacher A, Djulbegovic B (2009) Tandem versus single autologous hematopoietic cell transplantation for the treatment of multiple myeloma: a systematic review and meta-analysis. Journal of the National Cancer Institute 101: 100–106.
7. Kumar A, Loughran T, Alsina M, Durie BGM, Djulbegovic B (2003) Management of multiple myeloma: a systematic review and critical appraisal of published studies. The lancet oncology 4: 293–304.
8. Georgiev H, Tsalatsanis A, Kumar A, Djulbegovic B (2011) Social Network Analysis (SNA) of Research Programs in Multiple Myeloma (MM) American Society of Hematology Annual Meeting and Exposition. San Diego.
9. Haynes RB, McKibbon KA, Wilczynski NL, Walter SD, Werre SR (2005) Optimal search strategies for retrieving scientifically strong studies of treatment from Medline: analytical survey. Bmj 330: 1179.
10. Valente T (2010) Social networks and health: models, methods, and applications. New York Oxford University Press.
11. Wasserman S, Faust K (1994) Social Network Analysis. Cambridge: Cambridge University Press.
12. Newman MEJ (2001) The structure of scientific collaboration networks. Proceedings of the National Academy of Sciences 98: 404.
13. Friedkin NE (1982) Information flow through strong and weak ties in intraorganizational social networks. Social networks 3: 273–285.
14. Tsalatsanis A, Hozo I, Djulbegovic B (2010) Small world networks and treatment discovery process in cancer. pp. 6086.
15. Skvoretz J (2011) Workshop on Basic Network Methods. pp. 1–84.
16. Jackson M (2008) Social and Economic Networks. Princeton, New Jersey: Princeton University Press.
17. Freeman LC (1979) Centrality in social networks conceptual clarification. Social networks 1: 215–239.

18. Girvan M, Newman ME (2002) Community structure in social and biological networks. Proceedings of the National Academy of Sciences 99: 7821-7826.
19. Borgatti S (2003) KeyPlayer 1.44 ed. Boston, MA: Analytic Technologies.
20. Attal M, Harousseau JL, Stoppa AM, Sotto JJ, Fuzibet JG, et al. (1996) A prospective, randomized trial of autologous bone marrow transplantation and chemotherapy in multiple myeloma. Intergroupe Francais du Myelome. N Engl J Med 335: 91-97.
21. Borgatti SP (2002) Netdraw Network Visualization. 2.119 ed. Harvard, MA: Analytic Technologies.
22. Begg C, Cho M, Eastwood S, Horton R, Moher D, et al. (1996) Improving the quality of reporting of randomized controlled trials. The CONSORT statement. Jama 276: 637-639.
23. National Comprehensive Cancer Network (2013) Multiple Myeloma. version 1.2013 version 1.2013.

No Survival Improvement for Patients with Angioimmunoblastic T-Cell Lymphoma over the Past Two Decades: A Population-Based Study of 1207 Cases

Bei Xu[1], **Peng Liu**[2]*

1 Department of Medical Oncology, the First Affiliated Hospital of Nanjing Medical University, Nanjing, PR China, **2** Department of Hematology, the First Affiliated Hospital of Nanjing Medical University, Nanjing, PR China

Abstract

Angioimmunoblastic T-cell lymphoma (AITL) is a rare lymphoid malignancy with dismal prognosis. We conducted a large population-based study using the Surveillance, Epidemiology, and End Results (SEER) database (1973–2010) to determine the temporal survival trends and prognostic factors of AITL patients. A total of 1207 patients with AITL were included in this study, with a median age at diagnosis of 69 years. At presentation, most patients (79.5%) had an advanced-stage disease. Overall survival (OS) probabilities at 2, 5 and 10 years were 46.8%, 32.9%, and 21.9% respectively. Two-year, 5-year, and 10-year disease-specific survival (DSS) rates were 56.1%, 44.0%, and 35.9% respectively.On multivariate analysis, age older than 70 years, advanced-stage disease and male sex were identified adverse predictors for OS and DSS. We failed to find any survival differences among subgroups diagnosed in the 5 periods studied (1992 to 1998, 1999 to 2001, 2002 to 2004, 2005 to 2007, and 2008 to 2010). The current study represents the largest specific series of patients with AITL and the first investigation on temporal changes in survival of AITL patients. There has been no survival improvement for AITL patients over the past two decades. Further investigations are warranted to develop more effective treatment for AITL.

Editor: Masaru Katoh, National Cancer Center, Japan

Funding: This work was supported by National Natural Science Foundation of China (81170486, 81101498), Natural Science Fund for Distinguished Young Scholars of Jiangsu Province (BK20130049), Scientific Research Foundation from the Ministry of Education of China (43-NJYKDX-3), Jiangsu Province's Medical Elite Program (RC2011168), Key Project of Jiangsu Province Health Agency (K201107), "Liu Da Ren Cai Gao Feng" Project (2012-WS-017), A Project Funded by the Priority Academic Program Development of Jiangsu Higher Education Institute (JX10231801). Web site: http://www.nsfc.gov.cn/Portal0/default152.htm. The funders had no role in study design, data collection and analysis, decision to publish, or preparation of the manuscript.

Competing Interests: The authors have declared that no competing interests exist.

* E-mail: liupeng9098@163.com

Introduction

Angioimmunoblastic T-cell lymphoma (AITL) is a rare lymphoid malignancy, accounting for approximately 2% of all non-Hodgkin lymphomas [1]. AITL represents the second most common form (18.5%) of peripheral T-cell lymphoma (PTCL) worldwide [2,3]. It displays an aggressive course and is clinically characterized by sudden onset of constitutional symptoms, generalized lymphadenopathy, hepatosplenomegaly, anemia and polyclonal hypergammaglobulinemia. Also, this disease is frequently associated with autoimmune phenomena, such as hemolytic anemia and thrombocytopenia [1].

The standard approach for treating patients with AITL has not yet been clearly established. Treatment options consist of steroids, immunomodulators, single-agent cytotoxic drugs as well as combination chemotherapy [1,2]. Of these, Anthracycline-based chemotherapy has been recommended as first line therapy. Additional treatment modalities have been employed to obtain better outcomes, including novel agents (Alemtuzumab [4], Bortezomib [5], rituximab [6], histone deacetylase inhibitors [7], antifolic drugs [8], etc.), more intensive chemotherapeutic regimens, consolidation with autologous stem-cell transplantation (ASCT) [9,10], and even allogeneic stem-cell transplantation (alloSCT) [11–13]. However, there is little evidence from randomized controlled trials that these therapies have improved survival of patients with AITL. Several retrospective studies were conducted, with reported 5-year overall survival (OS) rates ranging from 25% to 41% (Table 1). Because of the rarity of AITL, all these series based their conclusions on limited numbers of patients (range, 45 to 243).

Administrative data sources, which provide access to large numbers of patients, are particularly well suited for the study of rare diseases such as AITL. Using data from the Surveillance, Epidemiology, and End Results (SEER) program, we evaluated the temporal survival trends in a large population-based cohort of AITL patients in the United States and determined the prognostic factors of this disease.

Subjects and Methods

Study Population

This retrospective study was conducted using the SEER public-use database 1973 to 2010 (November 2012 Submission) [19]. The SEER Program, sponsored by the National Cancer Institute, currently collects and publishes cancer incidence and survival data from 18 population-based cancer registries covering approximately 27.8% of the United States population. For more information about SEER, one is referred to its Web site (http://seer.cancer.

Table 1. Large series of patients with AITL reported in the literature.

Study	No. of Patients	Median age, years	Stages III to IV, %	Overall survival, %
Siegert 1995 [14]	62	64	90	36 at 4 years
Park 2007 [15]	65	60	95	25 at 5 years
Mourad 2008 [16]	157	62	81	51 at 2 years; 33 at 5 years; 29 at 7 years
Kyriakou* 2008 [10]	146	53#	73※	67 at 2 years; 59 at 4 years
Kyriakou§ 2009 [13]	45	48	69	66 at 1 years; 64 at 3 years
Tokunaga 2012 [17]	207	67	90	54 at 3 years; 41 at 5 years; 35 at 7 years
Federico 2013 [18]	243	65	89	33 at 5 years

Abbreviations: AITL, angioimmunoblastic T-cell lymphoma.
*Patients were treated with high-dose therapy followed by autologous stem-cell transplantation.
#Age at stem-cell transplantation.
※Stages IV, %.
§Patients were treated with allogeneic stem-cell transplantation.

gov/). Patients with AITL were identified using the third edition of the International Classification of Diseases for Oncology (ICD-O-3) histology code 9705. We obtained the following patient-specific data: age at diagnosis, sex, race, stage, year of diagnosis, diagnostic confirmation, vital status recode, length of survival, and cause of death. We excluded cases without microscopically confirmed diagnosis, those identified only through autopsy or death certificate, and those without follow-up records. For analyses requiring stratification by stage of disease, patients for whom no stage information was provided were excluded. Figure 1 outlines the inclusion process that was used to select cases with AITL for analysis.

The study was performed in accordance with the Declaration of Helsinki. Approval was obtained from the Institutional Review Board of the First Affiliated Hospital of Nanjing Medical University.

Outcome assessment

In current study, the follow-up cutoff was December 31, 2010. OS was calculated from the date of diagnosis to the date of death from any cause or the follow-up cutoff. Disease-specific survival (DSS) was calculated from the date of diagnosis to the date of death from non-Hodgkin's lymphoma or the follow-up cutoff. Patients who died from causes other than non-Hodgkin's lymphoma were considered censored at their date of death in DSS analysis.

Statistical Analysis

For survival analysis, the whole period of evaluation was segmented into five consecutive time periods based on date of diagnosis (1992 to 1998, 1999 to 2001, 2002 to 2004, 2005 to 2007, and 2008 to 2010). For the November 2012 submission, the survival time was calculated in months using complete dates (month, day, and year components) and the results were always rounded down. One hundred and twenty cases had a SEER-assigned survival time of 0 months after the exclusion process described above. To minimize any bias that could result from excluding these cases from the analysis, we assigned each case with zero survival time a survival time of 0.5 month. Survival outcomes were estimated using the Kaplan-Meier method. Log-rank test was used to compare survival distributions. We also studied the prognostic effect of the various clinical variables using univariate and multivariate Cox proportional hazards models. All statistical analysis was performed using STATA/SE 12.0 (Stata Corp,

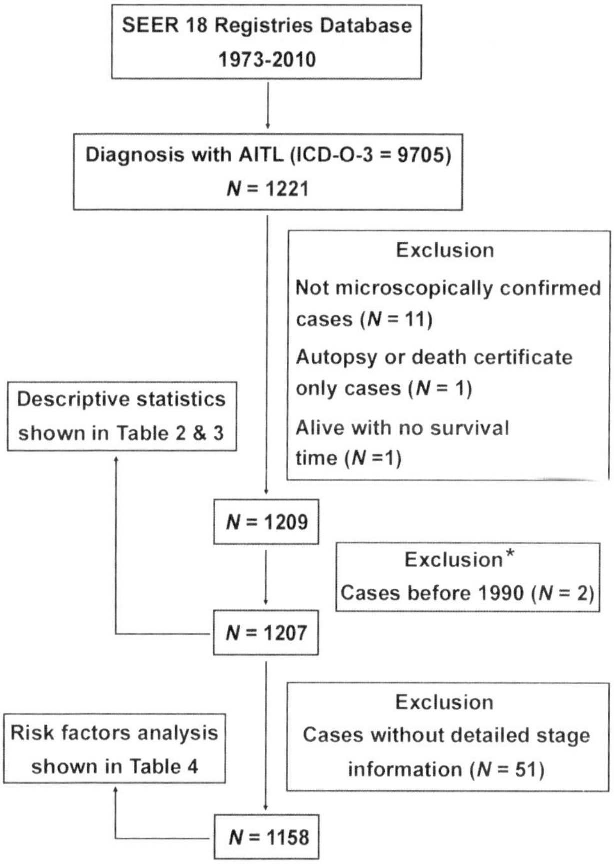

Figure 1. Patient selection flowchart. ICD-O-3, International Classification of Diseases for Oncology, 3rd edition; AITL, angioimmunoblastic T-cell lymphoma; SEER, Surveillance, Epidemiology, and End Results. *The histology code 9705 first appeared as a code for AITL in ICD-O-2, which was published in 1990 [20]. We excluded 2 cases diagnosed before 1990, which might be found late and abstracted after the introduction of the ICD-O-2 codes.

College Station, TX). Results were considered significant if a two-sided $P<0.05$ was obtained.

Results

Patient characteristics

From 1973 through 2010, 1221 AITL cases were ascertained by the SEER program. A total of 1207 patients with AITL matching the specified criteria described in Figure 1 were included in the final sample for this investigation. Demographic and clinical data for the entire study population are presented in Table 2.

AITL is generally a disease of the elderly, with a median age at diagnosis of 69 years (range, 10 to 96 years). Of the cohort of patients, 51.5% were male, and 48.5% female. The racial/ethnic distribution of this study was 81.2% white, 10.9% Asian/Pacific Islander, 7.5% black, and 0.5% other or unknown. At presentation, the overwhelming majority of patients (79.5%) had an advanced-stage (III to IV) disease by Ann Arbor classification. The proportion of patients diagnosed in 1992 to 1998, 1999 to 2001, 2002 to 2004, 2005 to 2007, and 2008 to 2010 was 8.4%, 10.5%, 20.0%, 27.1%, and 34.1% respectively.

Table 2. Patient Characteristics (N = 1207).

Characteristic	No. of Patients	%
Age, years		
Median (range)	69 (10 to 96)	
10 or less	1	0.1
11–20	1	0.1
21–30	12	1.0
31–40	36	3.0
41–50	110	9.1
51–60	238	19.7
61–70	262	21.7
71–80	357	29.6
81–90	179	14.8
91 or more	11	0.9
Sex		
Male	622	51.5
Female	585	48.5
Race		
White	980	81.2
Black	90	7.5
Asian/Pacific Islander	131	10.9
Other or unknown	6	0.5
Stage		
I	101	8.4
II	98	8.1
III	507	42.0
IV	452	37.5
Unstaged	49	4.1
Year of diagnosis		
1992–1998	101	8.4
1999–2001	127	10.5
2002–2004	241	20.0
2005–2007	327	27.1
2008–2010	411	34.1

Survival Outcomes

The median follow-up of the study was 13 months (range, 0 to 220 months). Among 1207 AITL cases, 742 deaths were observed as of December 31, 2010. Of these, 552 (74.4%) were because of non-Hodgkin's lymphoma and were considered disease-specific deaths. The second major cause of death (5.1%) was heart disease.

Overall survival probabilities at 2, 5 and 10 years were 46.8% (95% CI, 43.8% to 49.8%), 32.9% (95% CI, 29.8% to 36.0%), and 21.9% (95% CI, 18.2% to 25.9%), respectively. Two-year, 5-year, and 10-year DSS rates were 56.1% (95% CI, 52.9% to 59.1%), 44.0% (95% CI, 40.5% to 47.5%), and 35.9% (95% CI, 31.3% to 40.5%), respectively (Figure 2). Table 3 reflects the OS and DSS according to the demographic and clinical characteristics of AITL patients.

Prognostic factors

Analyses of prognostic factors are listed in Table 4. On univariate analysis, older age and advanced-stage (III to IV) disease were associated with an increased risk of all-cause mortality and disease-specific death.

On multivariate analysis, no statistically significant differences in OS ($P=0.460$) and DSS ($P=0.304$) were identified between patients diagnosed at 51 to 60 years and those at 61 to 70 years. Cases age 50 years or younger had a significantly lower incidence of all-cause (hazard ratio [HR], 0.7; 95% CI, 0.5 to 0.9; $P=0.011$) and disease-specific mortality (HR, 0.7; 95% CI, 0.5 to 0.9; $P=0.017$) than did those diagnosed between the ages of 51 and 60 years. Patients diagnosed at 71 to 80 years had a markedly higher risk of all-cause (HR, 1.7; 95% CI, 1.4 to 2.1; $P<0.001$) and disease-specific death (HR, 1.6; 95% CI, 1.2 to 2.0; $P=0.001$) than did those in the 51- to 60-year age category.

Although having no influence on survival in univariate analysis, male sex conferred a significantly worse OS (HR, 1.3; 95% CI, 1.1 to 1.5; $P=0.003$) and DSS (HR, 1.2; 95% CI, 1.0 to 1.4; $P=0.041$) in multivariate analysis. Patients with advanced-stage disease had a markedly higher risk of all-cause (HR, 1.5; 95% CI, 1.2 to 1.8; $P<0.001$) and disease-specific death (HR, 1.9; 95% CI, 1.5 to 2.5; $P<0.001$) in comparison to those with early stage disease.

Of note, no significant differences in OS were observed with more modern treatment eras in our multivariable model (all $P>0.05$). It seems that patients diagnosed during the 1992–1998 period experienced a reduced DSS (HR, 1.5; 95% CI, 1.0 to 2.1; $P=0.033$) compared with the baseline group (1999–2001 period). However, when performing joint test to determine the overall effect of the 5 categorical variables of treatment eras, we cannot reject the null hypothesis that all of the coefficients are zero (joint significance test, $P=0.138$), indicating the absence of changes in AITL patient survival over time.

Discussion

Although recognized as one of the most common forms of PTCL, AITL is a rare clinicopathologic entity according to the 2008 WHO classifications, with an estimated incidence of 0.05 cases per 100 000 person-years in the United States [21]. So far, limited data are available on clinical features, survival patterns, and prognostic factors in AITL. To the best of our knowledge, the current study represents the largest specific series of patients with AITL and the first investigation on temporal changes in survival of AITL patients.

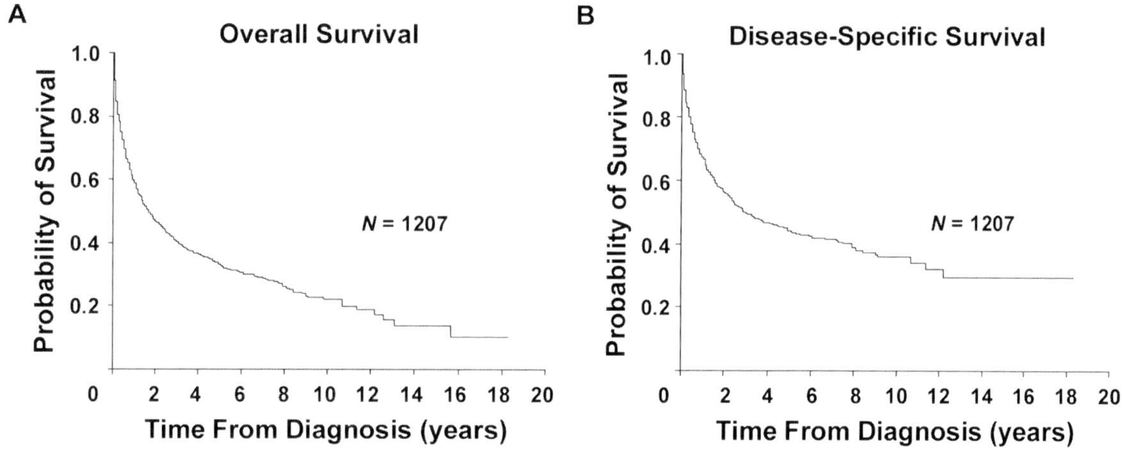

Figure 2. Survival of patients with angioimmunoblastic T-cell lymphoma. OS (A) and DSS (B).

Numerous clinical and pathologic classification schemes have been introduced over the past 3 decades, particularly for non-Hodgkin lymphomas. The histology code 9705 first appeared as a code for AITL in the second edition of the International Classification of Diseases for Oncology (ICD-O-2), which was published in 1990 [20]. In the current study, we excluded 2 cases diagnosed before 1990, which might be found late and abstracted after the introduction of the ICD-O-2 codes.

Table 3. Overall and Disease-Specific Survival (N = 1207).

Characteristic	Overall Survival			Disease-Specific Survival		
	2 Year, % (95% CI)	5 Year, % (95% CI)	10 Year, % (95% CI)	2 Year, % (95% CI)	5 Year, % (95% CI)	10 Year, % (95% CI)
All	46.8 (43.8 to 49.8)	32.9 (29.8 to 36.0)	21.9 (18.2 to 25.9)	56.1 (52.9 to 59.1)	44.0 (40.5 to 47.5)	35.9 (31.3 to 40.5)
Age, years						
50 or less	67.0 (58.9 to 73.9)	57.5 (48.7 to 65.3)	47.6 (36.7 to 57.7)	74.4 (66.3 to 80.9)	64.6 (55.4 to 72.4)	58.6 (47.8 to 68.0)
51–60	54.5 (47.5 to 60.9)	38.8 (31.3 to 46.2)	31.0 (22.2 to 40.3)	62.7 (55.5 to 69.0)	48.4 (40.1 to 56.2)	40.7 (30.0 to 51.2)
61–70	52.7 (45.9 to 59.1)	39.6 (32.5 to 46.6)	19.5 (11.2 to 29.5)	57.4 (50.5 to 63.8)	46.7 (39.2 to 53.9)	31.5 (21.3 to 42.3)
71–80	39.7 (34.4 to 45.0)	22.9 (18.0 to 28.2)	12.5 (7.6 to 18.7)	49.8 (43.9 to 55.3)	35.9 (29.6 to 42.3)	30.3 (22.4 to 38.6)
81 or more	25.1 (18.8 to 31.7)	14.4 (9.0 to 21.0)	12.3 (6.9 to 19.5)	40.6 (32.2 to 48.8)	29.9 (21.3 to 39.0)	25.6 (15.6 to 36.9)
Sex						
Male	44.1 (40.0 to 48.2)	28.1 (24.0 to 32.3)	19.3 (14.8 to 24.3)	54.2 (49.8 to 58.5)	40.7 (35.8 to 45.5)	32.0 (25.8 to 38.3)
Female	49.7 (45.4 to 53.9)	38.3 (33.7 to 42.9)	24.9 (18.9 to 31.4)	58.0 (53.5 to 62.3)	47.6 (42.5 to 52.5)	40.6 (34.0 to 47.1)
Race						
White	47.6 (44.2 to 50.8)	33.2 (29.7 to 36.7)	22.4 (18.2 to 26.9)	56.9 (53.4 to 60.2)	44.0 (40.1 to 47.9)	35.8 (30.6 to 41.0)
Other	43.7 (36.9 to 50.3)	31.4 (24.6 to 38.4)	19.8 (12.4 to 28.6)	52.7 (45.4 to 59.6)	43.9 (35.9 to 51.6)	36.0 (25.8 to 46.3)
Stage						
I	50.5 (40.1 to 60.0)	43.7 (33.3 to 53.6)	34.7 (22.6 to 47.0)	66.0 (54.8 to 75.0)	62.4 (50.7 to 72.0)	56.1 (39.8 to 69.6)
II	63.3 (52.3 to 72.4)	39.5 (27.6 to 51.2)	24.7 (10.7 to 41.7)	76.5 (65.5 to 84.4)	56.8 (43.1 to 68.4)	47.3 (26.8 to 65.4)
III	45.5 (40.9 to 50.0)	32.5 (27.8 to 37.4)	23.0 (17.6 to 28.8)	54.4 (49.5 to 59.1)	44.1 (38.7 to 49.4)	35.1 (28.0 to 42.2)
IV	42.2 (37.3 to 47.1)	28.3 (23.5 to 33.3)	18.7 (13.2 to 25.0)	49.1 (43.8 to 54.1)	36.3 (30.7 to 41.8)	30.2 (23.3 to 37.4)
Unstaged	60.1 (44.8 to 72.5)	40.1 (25.0 to 54.8)	16.7 (4.1 to 36.7)	74.8 (58.9 to 85.3)	52.5 (33.9 to 68.2)	39.4 (19.6 to 58.7)
Year of diagnosis						
1992–1998	44.6 (34.7 to 53.9)	28.7 (20.3 to 37.7)	15.8 (9.5 to 23.6)	53.1 (42.5 to 62.7)	41.7 (31.2 to 51.8)	25.4 (16.2 to 35.6)
1999–2001	51.2 (42.2 to 59.5)	35.4 (27.2 to 43.7)	26.0 (18.7 to 33.8)	60.4 (50.8 to 68.7)	46.7 (37.2 to 55.8)	43.3 (33.7 to 52.5)
2002–2004	42.7 (36.4 to 48.9)	27.8 (22.3 to 33.6)	NR	55.2 (48.3 to 61.5)	41.6 (34.7 to 48.4)	NR
2005–2007	48.9 (43.4 to 54.2)	37.7 (31.9 to 43.6)	NR	59.1 (53.2 to 64.5)	48.5 (41.9 to 54.8)	NR
2008–2010	45.1 (38.8 to 51.2)	NR	NR	51.2 (44.6 to 57.4)	NR	NR

Abbreviations: NR, not reached.

Table 4. Cox Proportional Hazards Regression Analysis for Overall and Disease-Specific Survival (N = 1158).

Variable	Univariate Analysis						Multivariate Analysis					
	Overall Survival			Disease-Specific Survival			Overall Survival			Disease-Specific Survival		
	HR	95% CI	*P*	HR	95% CI	*P*	HR	95% CI	*P*	HR	95% CI	*P*
Age, years												
50 or less	0.7	0.5 to 0.9	0.012	0.7	0.5 to 0.9	0.018	0.7	0.5 to 0.9	0.011	0.7	0.5 to 0.9	0.017
51–60	Reference			Reference			Reference			Reference		
61–70	1.1	0.9 to 1.4	0.442	1.2	0.9 to 1.5	0.267	1.1	0.9 to 1.4	0.460	1.2	0.9 to 1.5	0.304
71–80	1.7	1.4 to 2.1	<0.001	1.6	1.2 to 2.0	<0.001	1.7	1.4 to 2.1	<0.001	1.6	1.2 to 2.0	0.001
81 or more	2.5	2.0 to 3.2	<0.001	2.2	1.6 to 2.9	<0.001	2.7	2.1 to 3.4	<0.001	2.3	1.7 to 3.0	<0.001
Sex												
Male	1.1	1.0 to 1.3	0.107	1.1	0.9 to 1.3	0.348	1.3	1.1 to 1.5	0.003	1.2	1.0 to 1.4	0.041
Female	Reference			Reference			Reference			Reference		
Race												
White	0.9	0.8 to 1.1	0.328	0.9	0.7 to 1.1	0.421	0.8	0.7 to 1.0	0.064	0.8	0.7 to 1.0	0.113
Other	Reference			Reference			Reference			Reference		
Stage												
I to II	Reference			Reference			Reference			Reference		
III to IV	1.4	1.1 to 1.7	0.001	1.8	1.4 to 2.4	<0.001	1.5	1.2 to 1.8	<0.001	1.9	1.5 to 2.5	<0.001
Year of diagnosis												
1979–1998	1.3	1.0 to 1.7	0.097	1.4	1.0 to 2.0	0.064	1.3	1.0 to 1.8	0.058	1.5	1.0 to 2.1	0.033
1999–2001	Reference			Reference			Reference			Reference		
2002–2004	1.2	0.9 to 1.6	0.135	1.2	0.9 to 1.6	0.276	1.3	1.0 to 1.6	0.073	1.2	0.9 to 1.7	0.188
2005–2007	1.0	0.8 to 1.3	0.832	1.0	0.7 to 1.4	0.997	1.0	0.8 to 1.3	0.952	1.0	0.8 to 1.4	0.808
2008–2010	1.1	0.8 to 1.4	0.695	1.2	0.9 to 1.6	0.284	1.1	0.8 to 1.4	0.647	1.2	0.9 to 1.6	0.291

Abbreviations: HR, hazard ratio.

The clinicobiologic features of AITL observed in our study were similar to those described by other researchers [16–18]. AITL chiefly affected elderly adults in their seventh (21.7%) or eighth (29.6%) decades, at a median age of 69 years. The incidence in males (51.5%) was slightly higher than that in females (48.5%). Eighty percent of patients presented with advanced-stage (III to IV) disease. Of 1207 patients, most cases were diagnosed during or after the year 2002 (81%).

AITL is an aggressive neoplasm with a poor survival outcome. In 157 AITL patients retrieved from the Groupe d'Etude des Lymphomes de l'Adulte (GELA) trials [16], the 2-, 5-, and 7-year OS rates were 51%, 33%, and 29% respectively. Tokunaga et al described a multicenter retrospective study of 207 AITL patients in Japan [17]. In their analysis, the 3-, 5-, and 7-year OS rates were 54%, 41%, and 35% respectively. More recently, Federico et al presented the data of 243 AITL cases from the International Peripheral T-Cell Lymphoma Project, reporting an OS of 33% at 5 years [18].

In the current study, we showed that the OS rates at 2, 5 and 10 years were 46.8%, 32.9%, and 21.9% respectively, which were similar to those reported by previous researches mentioned above. Interestingly, our 5-year OS probability was almost the same as those in GELA study and International Peripheral T-Cell Lymphoma Project, with a narrower 95% CI (25.6% to 41.0% in GELA trials vs 29.8% to 36.0% in the present study). Our results, together with those from other researchers, confirmed the dismal prognosis of AITL with current treatment strategies.

A number of clinicobiologic and pathological characteristics, including age, stage, systemic symptoms, skin rush/pruritus, edema, ascites, lactate dehydrogenase, hemoglobin [14], lymphocyte value [22], presence of clear and convoluted cells [23], achievement of complete remission [24,25], drug exposure history [25] and cytogenetic findings [26], have been reported to be associated with survival of AITL patients, with controversial results. The International Prognostic Index (IPI), the widely used predictive model for many types of non-Hodgkin lymphoma, was shown to be significantly related to treatment outcomes of AITL patients [17]. A recently proposed prognostication score system for PTCL, not otherwise specified (PIT) also seemed to impact survival of patients with AITL [17]. However, the prognosis significance of both models for AITL have not been be supported by other investigations [3,16,18,27,28]. In report from GELA trials, only male sex, mediastinal lymphadenopathy, and anemia were suggestive of decreased survival [16]. Tokunaga et al showed that age older than 60 years, elevated white blood cell and IgA levels, the presence of anemia and thrombocytopenia, and extranodal involvement at more than 1 site adversely affected OS [17]. Federico et al recently suggested a new predictive model for AITL (PIAI), using five significant prognostic factors: age>60 years, PS>2, extranodal sites more than one, B symptoms, and platelet count<150×10^9/L. They showed that the novel prognostic index system did better compared with IPI and PIT in identifying AITL patient subsets with different outcomes [18].

In the present study, older age, advanced-stage disease and male sex were identified adverse predictors for OS and DSS of AITL patients. Patients diagnosed at 71 to 80 years had a 70% higher risk of death than did those at 51 to 60 years, while cases age 50 years or younger had a 30% lower risk of mortality compared with the reference group. However, we failed to find any difference in survival outcome between patients diagnosed at 51 to 60 years and those at 61 to 70 years. Advanced-stage (III to IV) disease was associated with a 50% higher risk of death compared with early stage lymphoma. In addition, we demonstrated in the largest cohorts of cases to date that male sex is an independent poor prognostic marker for patients with AITL ($P = 0.003$ and $P = 0.041$ for OS and DSS, respectively), which is consistent with the results from GELA study.

In the present study, older age, advanced-stage disease and male sex were identified adverse predictors for OS and DSS of AITL patients. Patients diagnosed at 71 to 80 years had a 70% higher risk of death than did those at 51 to 60 years, while cases age 50 years or younger had a 30% lower risk of mortality compared with the reference group. However, we failed to find any difference in survival outcome between patients diagnosed at 51 to 60 years and those at 61 to 70 years. Advanced-stage (III to IV) disease was associated with a 50% higher risk of death compared with early stage lymphoma. In addition, we demonstrated in the largest cohorts of cases to date that male sex is an independent poor prognostic marker for patients with AITL ($P = 0.003$ and $P = 0.041$ for OS and DSS, respectively), which is consistent with the results from GELA study.

An important finding in our study is the trend toward better OS for white patients in comparison to other ethnic groups ($P = 0.064$). To our knowledge, our report represents the first study addressing the prognostic role of race/ethnicity in AITL patients, while comprehensively controlling for other variables. Actually, there has been a large body of data describing racial and economic disparities in cancer treatment and outcomes over the last decade. Poor prognosis for black compared with white patients was reported across many types of malignancy. Underuse of effective treatment has been indicated to play a key role for this difference in survival among ethnic groups [29].

Various strategies have been proposed for the management of AITL, ranging from the watch-and-wait attitude to intensive chemotherapy followed by ASCT. However to date, no convincing results from large series of randomized trials have demonstrated that one treatment is superior to others. Our large sample size allowed us to examine the temporal trends in survival of patients with AITL, with acceptable statistical power. In the present study, we failed to find any survival rate differences among subgroups diagnosed in the 5 periods spanning 19 years, indicating the lack of survival improvement after the sequential attempts made for AITL treatment. Thus, novel management approaches are warranted.

Several groups have reported the benefit of high dose chemotherapy with ASCT (HDT-ASCT) for AITL patients. Data from the Lymphoma Working Party of the European Group for Blood and Marrow Transplantation (EBMT), which included 146 AITL patients treated with HDT-ASCT, reported a 59% OS and 42% progression-free survival at 4 years after transplantation. Best survival outcomes were observed in those patients who underwent ASCT during first complete remission [10]. Limited data so far are available regarding the use of alloSCT in AITL patients. A recently published retrospective study from the Lymphoma Working Party of EBMT showed encouraging results. Forty-five patients with AITL underwent an alloSCT, with a median age of 48 years. Of those, 25 patients underwent a myeloablative alloSCT, while 20 underwent a reduced-intensity alloSCT. OS and PFS rates at 3 years were 64% and 53%, respectively. Relapse rate was estimated as 16% and 20% at 2 and 3 years, respectively [13]. Prospective multicenter clinical trials are much needed to determine the role of ASCT and alloSCT in AITL.

Clinical outcomes among AITL patients remain dismal in part because of the lack of understanding of genetics of this disease. Odejide et al recently showed that AITL is characterized by high frequencies of overlapping mutations in epigenetic modifiers, including TET2, IDH2 and DNMT3A. This study defines the first genetic landscape of AITL across over 200 genes known to be recurrently mutated in hematologic neoplasms. The complement of genes frequently mutated in AITL resembles myeloid diseases more than other lymphomas, which could help explain the poor outcomes after treatment with regimens developed against B cell lymphomas [30].

A major concern for the epidemiological cancer study based on information from population-based cancer registries is diagnosis reliability. SEER collects information on incidence, prevalence, and survival from specific geographic areas representing 27.8% of the US population. Thus, cancers may have been diagnosed and classified by numerous independent pathologists, perhaps using diverse methodologies. Excellent agreement in diagnosis between the expert review and the SEER registry record has been reported for small-cell carcinoma of the lung. Agreement of registry and expert diagnoses was nearly 80% for the most common non-Hodgkin's lymphoma (NHL) subtype, diffuse large B cell lymphoma. Another subtype of NHL, chronic lymphocytic leukemia, might be underreported in certain cancer registries [31,32].

The SEER program registries routinely collect data on patient demographics, primary tumor site, tumor morphology and stage at diagnosis, first course of treatment, and follow-up for vital status. Unfortunately, detailed treatment data are not collected by the SEER. Since there is a known heterogeneity in the management of AITL, this limitation made it impossible to evaluate interactions between clinical outcome and specific treatment modalities used for AITL directly. Moreover, the SEER database does not provide enough clinicopathologic information needed for calculating IPI and PIT scores. Therefore, we failed to analyze survival outcomes according to these prognostic models, although several previous studies showed that both index systems were not predictive of survival for AITL patients [3,16,18,27,28]. Nevertheless, the present study provides novel information on AITL and the grounds for further research.

In conclusion, AITL is a rare lymphoid neoplasm with dismal prognosis, even when treated intensively. There has been no survival improvement for patients with AITL over the past two decades. Further investigations are warranted to develop more effective treatment for this disease.

Acknowledgments

We wish to acknowledge Prof. Qinhe Fan and Dr. Zhihong Zhang for their help in lymphoma diagnosis.

Author Contributions

Conceived and designed the experiments: BX PL. Performed the experiments: BX PL. Analyzed the data: BX PL. Contributed reagents/materials/analysis tools: BX. Wrote the paper: BX PL.

References

1. Iannitto E, Ferreri AJ, Minardi V, Tripodo C, Kreipe HH (2008) Angioimmunoblastic T-cell lymphoma. Crit Rev Oncol Hematol 68:264–271.
2. de Leval L, Gisselbrecht C, Gaulard P (2010) Advances in the understanding and management of angioimmunoblastic T-cell lymphoma. Br J Haematol 148:673–689.
3. Rüdiger T, Weisenburger DD, Anderson JR, Armitage JO, Diebold J, et al. (2002) Peripheral T-cell lymphoma (excluding anaplastic large-cell lymphoma): results from the Non-Hodgkin's Lymphoma Classification Project. Ann Oncol 13:140–149.
4. Gallamini A, Zaja F, Patti C, Billio A, Specchia MR, et al. (2007) Alemtuzumab (Campath-1H) and CHOP chemotherapy as first-line treatment of peripheral T-cell lymphoma: results of a GITIL (Gruppo Italiano Terapie Innovative nei Linfomi) prospective multicenter trial. Blood 110:2316–2323.
5. Delmer A, Fitoussi O, Gaulard P, Laurent G, Bordessoule D, et al. (2009) A phase II study of bortezomib in combination with intensified CHOP-like regimen (ACVBP) in patients with previously untreated T-cell lymphoma: results of the GELA LNH05–1T trial. Journal of Clinical Oncolology (ASCO Meeting Abstracts), 27 (Suppl. 15):8554.
6. Delfau-Larue MH, de Leval L, Joly B, Plonquet A, Challine D, et al. (2012) Targeting intratumoral B cells with rituximab in addition to CHOP in angioimmunoblastic T-cell lymphoma. A clinicobiological study of the GELA. Haematologica 97:1594–1602.
7. Piekarz RL, Frye R, Turner M, Wright JJ, Allen SL, et al. (2009) Phase II multi-institutional trial of the histone deacetylase inhibitor romidepsin as monotherapy for patients with cutaneous T-cell lymphoma. J Clin Oncol 27:5410–5417.
8. O'Connor OA, Hamlin PA, Portlock C, Moskowitz CH, Noy A, et al. (2007) Pralatrexate, a novel class of antifol with high affinity for the reduced folate carrier-type 1, produces marked complete and durable remissions in a diversity of chemotherapy refractory cases of T-cell lymphoma. Br J Haematol 139:425–428.
9. Schetelig J, Fetscher S, Reichle A, Berdel WE, Beguin Y, et al. (2003) Long-term disease-free survival in patients with angioimmunoblastic T-cell lymphoma after high-dose chemotherapy and autologous stem cell transplantation. Haematologica 88:1272–1278.
10. Kyriakou C, Canals C, Goldstone A, Caballero D, Metzner B, et al. (2008) High-dose therapy and autologous stem-cell transplantation in angioimmunoblastic lymphoma: complete remission at transplantation is the major determinant of Outcome-Lymphoma Working Party of the European Group for Blood and Marrow Transplantation. J Clin Oncol 26:218–224.
11. Corradini P, Dodero A, Zallio F, Caracciolo D, Casini M, et al. (2004) Graft-versus-lymphoma effect in relapsed peripheral T-cell non-Hodgkin's lymphomas after reduced-intensity conditioning followed by allogeneic transplantation of hematopoietic cells. J Clin Oncol 22:2172–2176.
12. Le Gouill S, Milpied N, Buzyn A, De Latour RP, Vernant JP, et al. (2008) Graft-versus-lymphoma effect for aggressive T-cell lymphomas in adults: a study by the Société Francaise de Greffe de Moëlle et de Thérapie Cellulaire. J Clin Oncol 26:2264–2271.
13. Kyriakou C, Canals C, Finke J, Kobbe G, Harousseau JL, et al. (2009) Allogeneic stem cell transplantation is able to induce long-term remissions in angioimmunoblastic T-cell lymphoma: a retrospective study from the lymphoma working party of the European group for blood and marrow transplantation. J Clin Oncol 27:3951–3958.
14. Siegert W, Nerl C, Agthe A, Engelhard M, Brittinger G, et al. (1995) Angioimmunoblastic lymphadenopathy (AILD)-type T-cell lymphoma: prognostic impact of clinical observations and laboratory findings at presentation. The Kiel Lymphoma Study Group. Ann Oncol 6:659–664.
15. Park BB, Ryoo BY, Lee JH, Kwon HC, Yang SH, et al. (2007) Clinical features and treatment outcomes of angioimmunoblastic T-cell lymphoma. Leuk Lymphoma 48:716–722.
16. Mourad N, Mounier N, Brière J, Raffoux E, Delmer A, et al. (2008) Clinical, biologic, and pathologic features in 157 patients with angioimmunoblastic T-cell lymphoma treated within the Groupe d'Etude des Lymphomes de l'Adulte (GELA) trials. Blood 111:4463–4470.
17. Tokunaga T, Shimada K, Yamamoto K, Chihara D, Ichihashi T, et al. (2012) Retrospective analysis of prognostic factors for angioimmunoblastic T-cell lymphoma: a multicenter cooperative study in Japan. Blood 119:2837–2843.
18. Federico M, Rudiger T, Bellei M, Nathwani BN, Luminari S, et al. (2013) Clinicopathologic characteristics of angioimmunoblastic T-cell lymphoma: analysis of the international peripheral T-cell lymphoma project. J Clin Oncol 31:240–246.
19. Surveillance, Epidemiology, and End Results (SEER) Program (www.seer.cancer.gov) SEER*Stat Database: Incidence - SEER 18 Regs Research Data + Hurricane Katrina Impacted Louisiana Cases, Nov 2012 Sub (1973-2010 varying) - Linked To County Attributes - Total U.S., 1969-2011 Counties, National Cancer Institute, DCCPS, Surveillance Research Program, Surveillance Systems Branch, released April 2013, based on the November 2012 submission.
20. Percy C, Van Holten V, Muir C (1990) International Classification of Diseases for Oncology. 2nd ed. Geneva:World Health Organization.
21. Morton LM, Wang SS, Devesa SS, Hartge P, Weisenburger DD, et al. (2006) Lymphoma incidence patterns by WHO subtype in the United States, 1992–2001. Blood 107:265–276.
22. Pangalis GA, Moran EM, Nathwani BN, Zelman RJ, Kim H, et al. (1983) Angioimmunoblastic lymphadenopathy. Long-term follow-up study. Cancer 52:318–321.
23. Aozasa K, Ohsawa M, Fujita MQ, Kanayama Y, Tominaga N, et al. (1989) Angioimmunoblastic lymphadenopathy. Review of 44 patients with emphasis on prognostic behavior. Cancer 63:1625–1629.
24. Ch'ang HJ, Su IJ, Chen CL, Chiang IP, Chen YC, et al. (1997) Angioimmunoblastic lymphadenopathy with dysproteinemia—lack of a prognostic value of clear cell morphology. Oncology 54:193–198.
25. Archimbaud E, Coiffier B, Bryon PA, Vasselon C, Brizard CP, et al. (1987) Prognostic factors in angioimmunoblastic lymphadenopathy. Cancer 59:208–212.
26. Schlegelberger B, Zwingers T, Hohenadel K, Henne-Bruns D, Schmitz N, et al. (1996) Significance of cytogenetic findings for the clinical outcome in patients with T-cell lymphoma of angioimmunoblastic lymphadenopathy type. J Clin Oncol 14:593–599.
27. Lin HN, Liu CY, Hong YC, Pai JT, Yang CF, et al. (2010) Clinical features and prognostic factors of angioimmunoblastic T-cell lymphoma in Taiwan: a single-institution experience. Leuk Lymphoma 51:2208–2214.
28. Lee SS, Rüdiger T, Odenwald T, Roth S, Starostik P, et al. (2003) Angioimmunoblastic T cell lymphoma is derived from mature T-helper cells with varying expression and loss of detectable CD4. Int J Cancer 103:12–20.
29. Hershman DL, Wright JD (2012) Comparative effectiveness research in oncology methodology: observational data. J Clin Oncol 30:4215–4222.
30. Odejide O, Weigert O, Lane AA, Toscano D, Lunning MA, et al. (2013) A targeted mutational landscape of angioimmunoblastic T cell lymphoma. Blood. Dec 17. [Epub ahead of print] PMID: 24345752
31. Clarke CA, Glaser SL, Dorfman RF, Bracci PM, Eberle E, et al. (2004) Expert review of non-Hodgkin's lymphomas in a population-based cancer registry: reliability of diagnosis and subtype classifications. Cancer Epidemiol Biomarkers Prev 13:138–143.
32. Yu JB, Gross CP, Wilson LD, Smith BD. (2009) NCI SEER public-use data: applications and limitations in oncology research. Oncology (Williston Park) 23:288–295.

14

Matrix Metalloproteinase-9 Is Involved in Chronic Lymphocytic Leukemia Cell Response to Fludarabine and Arsenic Trioxide

Irene Amigo-Jiménez[1], Elvira Bailón[1], Estefanía Ugarte-Berzal[1], Noemí Aguilera-Montilla[1], José A. García-Marco[2], Angeles García-Pardo[1]*

1 Cellular and Molecular Medicine Department, Centro de Investigaciones Biológicas, Consejo Superior de Investigaciones Científicas (CSIC), Madrid, Spain, **2** Hematology Unit, Hospital Universitario Puerta de Hierro, Madrid, Spain

Abstract

Background: Matrix metalloproteinase-9 (MMP-9) contributes to chronic lymphocytic leukemia (CLL) pathology by regulating cell migration and preventing spontaneous apoptosis. It is not known if MMP-9 is involved in CLL cell response to chemotherapy and we address this in the present study, using arsenic trioxide (ATO) and fludarabine as examples of cytotoxic drugs.

Methods: We used primary cells from the peripheral blood of CLL patients and MEC-1 cells stably transfected with an empty vector or a vector containing MMP-9. The effect of ATO and fludarabine was determined by flow cytometry and by the MTT assay. Expression of mRNA was measured by RT-PCR and qPCR. Secreted and cell-bound MMP-9 was analyzed by gelatin zymography and flow cytometry, respectively. Protein expression was analyzed by Western blotting and immunoprecipitation. Statistical analyses were performed using the two-tailed Student's t-test.

Results: In response to ATO or fludarabine, CLL cells transcriptionally upregulated MMP-9, preceding the onset of apoptosis. Upregulated MMP-9 primarily localized to the membrane of early apoptotic cells and blocking apoptosis with Z-VAD prevented MMP-9 upregulation, thus linking MMP-9 to the apoptotic process. Culturing CLL cells on MMP-9 or stromal cells induced drug resistance, which was overcome by anti-MMP-9 antibodies. Accordingly, MMP-9-MEC-1 transfectants showed higher viability upon drug treatment than Mock-MEC-1 cells, and this effect was blocked by silencing MMP-9 with specific siRNAs. Following drug exposure, expression of anti-apoptotic proteins (Mcl-1, Bcl-xL, Bcl-2) and the Mcl-1/Bim, Mcl-1/Noxa, Bcl-2/Bax ratios were higher in MMP-9-cells than in Mock-cells. Similar results were obtained upon culturing primary CLL cells on MMP-9.

Conclusions: Our study describes for the first time that MMP-9 induces drug resistance by modulating proteins of the Bcl-2 family and upregulating the corresponding anti-apoptotic/pro-apoptotic ratios. This is a novel role for MMP-9 contributing to CLL progression. Targeting MMP-9 in combined therapies may thus improve CLL response to treatment.

Editor: Andreas Villunger, Innsbruck Medical University, Austria

Funding: This work was supported by grants SAF2012-31613 (AGP) and RTICC (Red Temática de Investigación Cooperativa en Cáncer) RD12/0036/0061 (AGP), from the Ministry of Economy and Competitiveness (MINECO), Spain; S2010/BMD-2314-Neoplasbim (AGP) from the Comunidad de Madrid/European Union; and by a grant from the Fundacioen Puerta de Hierro, Madrid (JAGM). IAJ and EB were were supported by the Junta de Ampliación de Estudios program, CSIC/EU, Spain. The funders had no role in study design, data collection and analysis, decision to publish, or preparation of the manuscript.

Competing Interests: The authors have declared that no competing interests exist.

* Email: agarciapardo@cib.csic.es

Introduction

Chronic lymphocytic leukemia (CLL) is characterized by the accumulation of malignant $CD5^+$ B lymphocytes in the peripheral blood and their progressive infiltration of lymphoid tissues [1,2]. Frontline therapies for CLL consist in the administration of the purine analogue fludarabine, alone or in combination with other drugs such as anti-CD20 monoclonal antibodies or kinase inhibitors [3–5]. Because CLL is a heterogeneous disease, patients carrying specific molecular markers such as del17p13, unmutated IgV_H and/or high expression of ZAP-70 or CD38, do not respond well to these treatments [4], making it crucial to continue searching for new compounds useful in these cases. In this regard, arsenic trioxide (ATO), an efficient therapy in acute promyelocytic leukemia [6,7], has been shown to induce apoptosis in all CLL cases including those with unfavorable prognosis [8]. We previously reported that the mechanism by which ATO induces CLL cell death is via c-jun N-terminal kinase activation and PI3K/Akt downregulation and this was observed in all samples tested, regardless of their prognostic markers [9]. ATO may thus constitute an efficient alternative/complementary treatment for CLL.

As with most tumors, CLL cell response to therapy is influenced by the microenvironment, whose cellular and molecular components provide survival signals that favor drug resistance [10,11]. A consistent component of CLL niches is matrix metalloproteinase-9 (MMP-9) [12], which is also produced by CLL cells and upregulated by several stimuli [13–15]. Endogenous or/and exogenous MMP-9 binds to CLL cells via specific docking receptors and regulates cell migration [16]. Surface-bound MMP-9 also prevents CLL cell spontaneous apoptosis by a non-catalytic mechanism, consisting in Lyn/STAT3 activation and Mcl-1 upregulation [17], thus contributing to CLL progression.

It is not known if MMP-9 affects CLL cell response to chemotherapy. This is important to elucidate since MMP-9, as other MMPs, may play dual roles in apoptosis, either facilitating or antagonizing drug action [18,19]. To approach this issue, we have studied whether MMP-9 is modulated by fludarabine or ATO treatment and whether it is involved in the CLL cell response to these compounds. Using primary CLL cells and a CLL-derived cell line stably expressing MMP-9 [20], we show that MMP-9 contributes to chemoresistance by preventing downregulation of anti-apoptotic proteins.

Materials and Methods

Patients, cells and cell culture

Approval was obtained from the CSIC Bioethics Review Board for these studies. All patients signed an informed consent before blood was drawn. B-lymphocytes were purified from the 20 CLL samples listed in Table 1 as reported [9,17], using Ficoll-Paque PLUS (GE Healthcare, Uppsala, Sweden) centrifugation and, if necessary, negative selection with anti-CD3-conjugated Dynabeads (Invitrogen Dynal AS, Oslo, Norway). The resulting B cell population was mostly >90% $CD19^+$, determined on a Coulter Epics XL flow cytometer (Beckman Coulter, Fullerton, CA). Primary stromal cells were obtained from a bone marrow sample of one CLL patient after 3 week culture in IMDM (Lonza, Amboise, France)/15% FBS, and used for up to 4 weeks. The HS-5 stromal cell line was obtained from Dr. Atanasio Pandiella (Cancer Research Center, Salamanca, Spain) and cultured in RPMI/10% FBS. The MEC-1 cell line, established from a CLL patient [21], was obtained from Dr. Enrique Ocio (Cancer Research Center, Salamanca), authenticated by short tandem repeat DNA typing (Secugen S.L., Madrid, Spain) and cultured in IMDM/10% FBS. MMP-9- and Mock-MEC-1 cells were generated by lentiviral transfection exactly as described [20]. Briefly, full-length human proMMP-9 DNA cloned in the pEGFP-N1 vector was amplified by PCR using cloned Pfu DNA polymerase (Agilent Technologies, Waldbronn, Germany) and inserted into the pCR-Blunt vector (Blunt Zero PCR cloning kit, Invitrogen). After restriction enzyme digestion, DNA sequences were inserted into the pRRL sin18.CMV.IRES.eGFP lentiviral vector (Dr. Juan Carlos Ramírez, Viral Vector Unit, Centro de Investigaciones Cardiovasculares, Madrid). Control constructs (Mock) contained only GFP DNA. Viral stocks were obtained after vector transfection of HEK293T cells and used to infect MEC-1 cells. GFP-expressing cells were selected by several cell sorting steps until more than 95% of the cells were clearly positive for expression. Cells were maintained in IMDM medium (Lonza, Basel, Switzerland), 10% fetal bovine serum (FBS).

Antibodies and reagents

Rabbit polyclonal antibodies (RpAb) to MMP-9 (sc-6841R), Mcl-1 (sc-819), Bax (sc-526), Noxa (sc-52), Bcl-xL (sc-634), RhoGDI (sc-360), and mouse monoclonal Ab (mAb) to Bcl-2 (sc-509) were from Santa Cruz Biotechnology (Santa Cruz, CA). RpAb to Bim (559685) was from BD Pharmingen (Franklin Lakes, NJ). Rp IgG (isotype control for flow cytometry) was from Immunostep (Salamanca, Spain). mAb to vinculin (#V9131) was from Sigma-Aldrich (St. Louis, MO, USA). mAbs to CD19 and CD5 were from Diaclone (Besançon, France). mAbs against CD38 (16BDH), CD44 (HP2/9), α4 integrin subunit (HP2/1, function blocking), α4 integrin subunit (HP1/7, inactive control, isotype matched for HP2/1 and HP2/9), CD45, and β1 integrin subunit (Alex1/4) were from Dr. F. Sánchez-Madrid (Hospital de la Princesa, Madrid, Spain). HRP-labeled Abs to rabbit or mouse Ig (used for Western blotting) were from Dako (Glostrup, Denmark). Alexa 488- and Alexa 647-labeled Abs (used for flow cytometry) were from Molecular Probes (Eugene, OR). Rabbit TrueBlot (18-8816-31) was from Rockland Immunochemicals (Gilbertsville, PA). Bovine serum albumin (BSA) was from Roche Diagnostics GmbH (Mannheim, Germany). Propidium iodide (PI), MTT (3-(4,5-dimethylthiazolyl-2)-2,5-diphenyltetrazoliumbromide), actinomycin D, arsenic trioxide (ATO), fludarabine (2-fluoroadenine-9-β-D-arabinofuranoside) and the pan-caspase inhibitor Z-VAD-FMK were from Sigma-Aldrich. FITC-Annexin V was from Immunostep. MMP-9 was isolated from the conditioned medium of MMP-9-MEC-1 transfectants by gelatin-Sepharose affinity chromatography, as previously reported [17,22]. Purity and identity of the protein was assessed by gelatin zymograhy and Western blotting analyses (see below).

RT-PCR and RNA stabilization assays

Total RNA isolation and cDNA amplification were performed as described [17] using the following primers: MMP-9: 5′-TGGGCTACGTGACCTATGAC-3′ and 5′-CAAAGGTGAGAAGAGAGGGC-3′; *c-fos*: 5′-TACTACCACTCACCCGCAGA-3′ and 5′-CAGGTTGGCAATCTCGGTCT-3′; *c-jun*: 5′-CGACAAGTAAGAGTGCGGGA-3′ and 5′-CCCGTTGCTGGACTGGATTA-3′; glyceraldehyde-3-phosphate dehydrogenase (GAPDH): 5′- GGCTGAGAACGGGAAGCTTGTCA-3′ and 5′-CGGCCATCACGCCACAGTTTC-3′. PCR analyses were performed for 25 cycles consisting of 1 min denaturation-95°C, 1 min annealing-59°C, 1 min polymerization-72°C (MMP-9/GAPDH) or 30 s denaturation-95°C, 30 s anneling-60°C, 45 s polymerization-72°C (*c-fos/c-jun*). To assess mRNA stability, CLL cells were cultured with or without 3 μM ATO and after 20 h, 5 μM actinomycin D was added. At various time points samples were collected and mRNA levels of MMP-9 and GAPDH were measured by RT-PCR. Bands were visualized by ethidium bromide staining and quantified using the MultiGauge V3.0 program (Fujifilm Global Lifescience, Düsseldorf, Germany).

Quantitative PCR (qPCR)

Quantitative PCR (qPCR) was performed using iQ SYBR Green Supermix (Bio-Rad Laboratories, Hercules, CA), and the primers described above for MMP-9. The primers for TATA binding protein (TBP) were: 5′-CGGCTGTTTAACTTCGCTTC-3′ and 5′-CACACGCCAAGAAACAGTGA-3′. Triplicate assays were performed, and results were normalized according to the expression levels of TBP RNA and expressed by using the ΔΔCT method for quantization.

RNA interference experiments

The siRNA sequence targeting human proMMP-9 was: sense 5′-CAUCACCUAUUGGAUCCAAdTdT-3′ (targets bases 377–403); the siRNA sequence for negative control was: sense 5′-AUUGUAUGCGAUCGCAGACdTdT-3′. siRNA duplexes were verified to be specific for their targets by Blast search against the

Table 1. Clinical characteristics of CLL patients.

Patient	Sex/Age	Stage[a]	CD19[b]	CD5[b]	CD38/ZAP70[c]	Membrane MMP-9[b]	Ig Status	p53 status
P1	M/69	C/IV	88.0	11.2	−/+	15.8	ND	ND
P2	F/72	C/IV	95.0	97.6	−/+	18.4	Mutated	-
P3	M/70	B/II	91.5	99.5	+/+	2.5	Unmutated	-
P4	M/65	A/I	86.7	98.8	−/−	11.7	Mutated	-
P5	M/79	A/I	96.4	98.1	−/+	14.5	Unmutated	-
P6	M/79	B/II	96.2	83.2	+/−	6.6	Unmutated	-
P7	M/77	A/0	90.0	ND	+/ND	4.9	Unmutated	del+/mut+
P8	M/59	C/IV	95.9	86.6	+/+	1.0	ND	del+/mut+
P9	M/85	C/IV	91.5	5.0	+/ND	18.4	Unmutated	-
P10	F/73	A/II	97.3	26.2	−/−	1.9	Mutated	del-/mut+
P11	M/48	B/I	97.0	15.8	+/+	8.4	Unmutated	ND
P12	M/68	ND	95.6	26.6	+/ND	2.7	ND	-
P13	F/54	A/0	96.4	73.6	+/ND	15.8	Unmutated	-
P14	F/82	ND	95.3	52.9	+/ND	6.8	Unmutated	del-/mut+
P15	F/70	C/IV	93.0	91.0	+/ND	7.3	ND	ND
P16	F/ND	ND	93.1	95.1	+/ND	ND	ND	ND
P17	M/71	B/II	91.3	98.8	+/−	9.1	ND	-
P18	M/80	ND	90.1	44.1	+/ND	15.5	ND	ND
P19	M/62	ND	90.8	84.8	+/ND	11.5	ND	ND
P20	M/68	C/IV	90.7	83.7	−/ND	20.4	Mutated	-

[a]Clinical stage according to references [1,2].
[b]Percentage of cells expressing this marker.
[c]The coexpression of CD38 and ZAP-70 has clinical prognostic value [1,2].
ND, not determined.

human genome and were custom-made by Sigma-Aldrich. 15×10^6 Mock- or MMP-9-MEC-1 cells were nucleofected with 30 nM siRNAs using solution V and programme T-01 (Amaxa, Cologne, Germany), and assayed 24 h after transfection. Efficiency of transfection was confirmed by gelatin zymography and Western blot analyses.

Cell viability assays

1.5×10^5 CLL cells in RPMI/0.1% FBS were incubated with ATO, fludarabine or vehicle and cell viability was determined after 24 (ATO) or 48 (fludarabine) h on a Coulter Epics XL flow cytometer (Beckman Coulter, Fullerton, CA), using FITC-Annexin V and PI. In some experiments, live (Annexin V^-/PI^-) and early apoptotic (Annexin V^+/PI^-) cells were separated on a FACS Vantage cell sorter (Becton Dickinson, Franklin Lakes, NJ). For MTT assays, 0.75×10^5 MEC-1 cells in IMDM/0.1% FBS were incubated with 50 µg MTT for 4 h in the dark. The blue MTT formazan precipitate was dissolved in isopropanol-HCl (24:1) and the absorbance at 540 nm was determined on a Multiskan Bichromatic microplate reader (Labsystems, Helsinki, Finland).

Cell fractionation

30×10^6 cells CLL cells were serum-starved for 1 h and incubated with 3 µM ATO or vehicle for 24 h. Cells were collected, washed 1× with cold PBS, and incubated (15 min, 4°C) in 250 µl of ice-cold hypotonic digitonin buffer (5 mM Tris pH 7.5, 10 mM NaCl, 0.5 mM $MgCl_2$, 1 mM EGTA, 20 µg/ml digitonin), containing a protease/phosphatase inhibitor cocktail (Roche Diagnostics). Cytosolic (soluble) and membrane (pellet) fractions were separated by centrifugation. The pellet was washed 1× with ice-cold PBS and extracted with 125 µl of NP-40 lysis buffer (10 mM Tris pH 7.5, 40 mM NaCl, 1 mM $MgCl_2$, 1% NP-40, protease inhibitors). After 20 min at 4°C lysates were clarified by centrifugation. For MEC-1 transfectants, 5×10^6 Mock- or MMP-9-cells were serum-starved for 3 h, washed with cold PBS, and incubated in 500 µl of ice-cold hypotonic digitonin buffer (containing 40 µg/ml digitonin). After separation of the cell fractions the pellet was extracted in 100 µl of NP-40 lysis buffer (containing 0.2% NP-40) and analysis continued as above. Soluble proteins in membrane and cytosolic fractions were quantitated using the Pierce BCA protein assay kit (Thermo Scientific, Rockford, IL) and analyzed by gelatin zymography. RhoGDI (typical cytosolic protein) and CD45 (typical membrane protein) were visualized by Western blotting and used as internal controls for the procedure.

Gelatin zymography

The conditioned medium of ATO untreated or treated CLL cells was collected and concentrated 20× using ultrafiltration spin columns fitted with 30 kDa MWCO membranes (Sartorius Stedim Biotech GmbH, Goettingen, Germany). This medium, as well as membrane and cytosolic cellular fractions were analysed on 7.5% polyacrylamide gels containing 0.1% gelatin (Sigma-Aldrich). After electrophoresis gels were rinsed 3×30 min in 2.5% Triton X-100 and 1×30 min in distilled water, followed by overnight incubation in 50 mM Tris pH 7.5, 200 mM NaCl, 10 mM $CaCl_2$ at 37°C. Gels were stained with 0.2% Coomassie blue and areas of gelatinolytic activity were visualized as transparent bands. Bands were quantitated using the MultiGauge V3.0 program.

Analysis of MMP-9 protein expression

5×10^6 CLL cells were cultured with or without 3 µM ATO (24 h) or 3 and/or 5 µM fludarabine (48 h). Secreted MMP-9 in the conditioned medium was analyzed by gelatin zymography. Surface-bound MMP-9 was determined by flow cytometry on the same cells, upon incubation with the anti-MMP-9 Ab or control rabbit IgG (1 h, 4°C), followed by Alexa 488- or 647- labeled Abs (20 min, 4°C). In some experiments, live (Annexin V^-PI^-) and early apoptotic (Annexin V^+PI^-) cells were separately analyzed for MMP-9 expression on a FACS Vantage cell sorter (Becton Dickinson, Franklin Lakes, NJ). Cells were also pre-incubated with anti-α4 integrin or anti-CD44 Abs for 1 h prior to ATO exposure, and subsequently analyzed for surface-bound MMP-9 by flow cytometry. Specific fluorescence (SF), also called "Generalized Integrated Mean Fluorescence Intensity (GiMFI) [23] and defined as mean fluorescence intensity (MFI)×% of positive cells, was chosen to represent MMP-9 expression. SF/GiMFI measurements have been previously used [24], as they may be more accurate than the individual MFI or % of positive cells values.

Immunoprecipitation and Western blotting

For immunoprecipitation, 3×10^7 Mock- or MMP-9-cells were serum-starved for 3 h and incubated with or without 5 µM ATO for 24 h. Cells were lysed in ice-cold 20 mM Tris-HCl pH 7.5, 150 mM NaCl, 1 mM EDTA, 0.5% NP-40, 1 mM PMSF, and protease inhibitors (IP buffer). After protein quantitation lysates were pre-cleared by incubating (1.5 h, 4°C) with 25 µl protein A-Sepharose (GE Healthcare Bio-Science, Uppsala, Sweden). Pre-cleared lysates were incubated (16 h, 4°C) with 3 µg primary or control Abs and mixed with 25 µl protein A-Sepharose for 2 h at 4°C. Pellets containing the immune complexes were washed with IP buffer and proteins extracted by boiling for 5 min in Laemmli buffer.

For Western blotting, samples were resolved by SDS-PAGE and transferred to nitrocellulose or PVDF membranes (Bio-Rad Laboratories, Hercules, CA). After electrophoresis, membranes were blocked with 5% BSA/TBS-Tween 20 for 1 h and incubated (4°C, 16 h) with primary Abs, followed by incubation for 1 h at room temperature with Rabbit TrueBlot HRP-labeled Abs (immune complexes) or HRP-labeled secondary Abs (whole lysates). To detect multiple proteins on the same membrane, after identification of the first protein, membranes were washed with TBS/0.1% Tween 20 for 10 min, followed by 3×30 min incubation in 1% glycine pH 2.2, 1% SDS, 0.0005% NP-40, at room temperature. Membranes were washed 1×10 min with TBS/Tween, blocked with 5% BSA for 1 h, and re-probed with subsequent primary and secondary Abs. Protein bands were developed using the enhanced chemiluminiscent detection method (Amersham) and quantitated as above.

Statistical analyses

Normal distribution of the data was confirmed by the Shapiro-Wilk's normality test, using the univariate procedure of SAS 9.3 software (SAS Institute, Cary, NC). Statistical significance of the data was determined using the two-tailed Student's t-test. A p value of ≤ 0.05 was considered significant. Analyses were performed using the GraphPad InStat v3.06 software (GraphPad Software, San Diego, CA, USA). All values are expressed as means ± standard deviation, except for the qPCR assays in which means ± standard error are shown.

Results

ATO transcriptionally upregulates MMP-9 in CLL cells via c-fos/c-jun activation

To first establish the best conditions to study ATO action, CLL cells (1.5×10^6/ml) were cultured for 24 h with or without various concentrations of ATO and apoptosis measured by flow cytometry, using FITC-Annexin V and PI. Figure 1A shows that the percentage of apoptotic cells (Annexin V^+PI^-) increased in a dose-dependent manner, reaching average values of 46.2% at 3 μM ATO (Figure 1A). 16.6% of the remaining cells were viable (Annexin V^-PI^-) and 37% were necrotic cells (Annexin V^+PI^+). As the 46.2% level of apoptosis seemed appropriate for biochemical studies, we chose 3 μM ATO concentration for subsequent experiments, except when indicated.

We next studied whether MMP-9, a protein previously shown to contribute to CLL survival [17], was modulated by ATO and involved in the cellular response to this agent. In initial experiments, 10–15×10^6/ml CLL cells from three different patients were treated or not with 3 μM ATO and MMP-9 mRNA analyzed by RT-PCR. Figure 1B shows that MMP-9 mRNA expression increased after 8 or 24 h of ATO treatment, compared to control cells. Due to the endogenous MMP-9 production in CLL cell cultures, MMP-9 mRNA was also slightly elevated in untreated cells compared to constitutive values, with similar levels at 8 and 24 h (Figure 1B). The same samples were then analyzed by qPCR, which also showed a significant increase in MMP-9 mRNA expression of 2.4-fold and 9.3-fold, respectively, after 8 or 24 h treatment (Figure 1C). The average percentage of Annexin V^+PI^- in ATO-treated cells at these times was 23.6% (8 h) and 37.6% (24 h), compared to 15% (8 and 24 h) in untreated cells (not shown).

To next study whether ATO affected the stability of MMP-9 mRNA, actinomycin D was added to CLL cells previously treated with 3 μM ATO for 20 h. RT-PCR analysis of these samples at various time points revealed that the increase in MMP-9 was not due to stabilization of MMP-9 mRNA (Figure 1D), indicating that ATO regulated MMP-9 at the transcriptional level.

Several transcription factors can activate the MMP-9 promoter including NF-κB and AP-1 [25]. Because we previously showed that ATO downregulates NF-κB and activates c-Jun N-terminal kinase (JNK) in CLL cells [9], we studied whether ATO regulated the JNK downstream effectors *c-fos* and *c-jun*, two components of the AP-1 heterodimer. RT-PCR analyses indicated that both, *c-fos* and *c-jun* mRNAs, were significantly upregulated upon cell exposure to 3 μM ATO, with maximun levels after 2 h (Figure 2A). At longer times expression declined but remained higher than control cells even at 24 h in the case of *c-jun* (Figure 2A). To determine whether this transcriptional modulation correlated with increased c-Fos and c-Jun protein expression, CLL cells from the same patients were treated with 3 μM ATO for various times, lysed and analyzed by Western blotting. Figure 2B shows the Western blot results for a representative sample and the average quantitation of the 3 patients studied. As observed, c-Fos increase was visible after 2 h, was maximal after 8 h and remained higher than the control after 24 h. Likewise, c-Jun phosphorylation was clearly observed after 8 h and remained elevated after 24 h of ATO treatment, compared to controls. As these times for c-Fos and phospho-c-Jun protein induction correlated with the upregulation of MMP-9 gene expression, these results strongly suggested that ATO regulated MMP-9 via AP-1 activation.

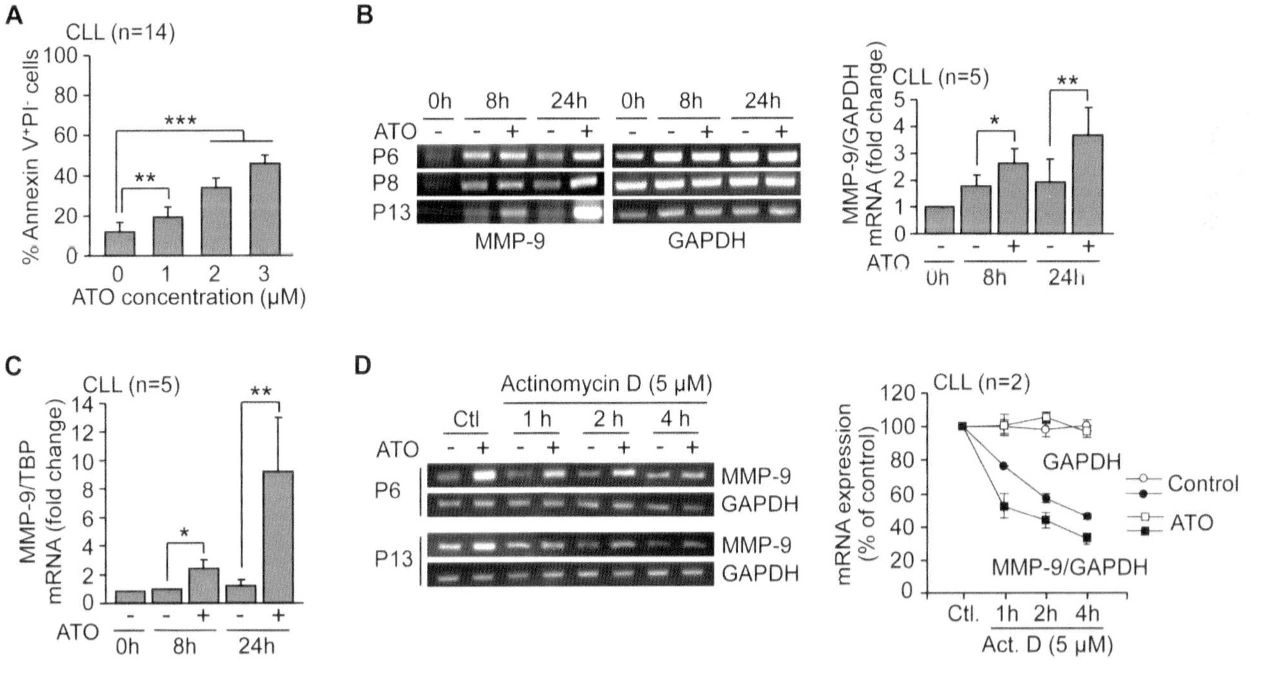

Figure 1. ATO transcriptionally upregulates MMP-9 in CLL cells. (A) 1.5×10^5 CLL cells in RPMI/0.1%FBS were incubated with or without the indicated concentrations of ATO. After 24 h, cells were analyzed by flow cytometry using FITC-Annexin V and PI. (B) 10–15×10^6 CLL cells were treated with 3 μM ATO for the indicated times and MMP-9 mRNA expression was analyzed by RT-PCR, using GAPDH mRNA as internal control. Normalized average values (fold change) are shown. (C) The same mRNA samples were also analyzed by qPCR using TBP as internal control and normalized average values (fold change) are shown. (D) 10–15×10^6 CLL cells were cultured with or without 3 μM ATO for 20 h. Cells were then treated or not (Control, Ctl) with 5 μM actinomycin D and mRNA expression was analyzed at the indicated times. Values represent the average MMP-9/GAPDH ratio from the two samples after normalizing control values to 100. Values for GAPDH mRNA are also shown. $^*P\leq0.05$; $^{**}P\leq0.01$; $^{***}P\leq0.001$.

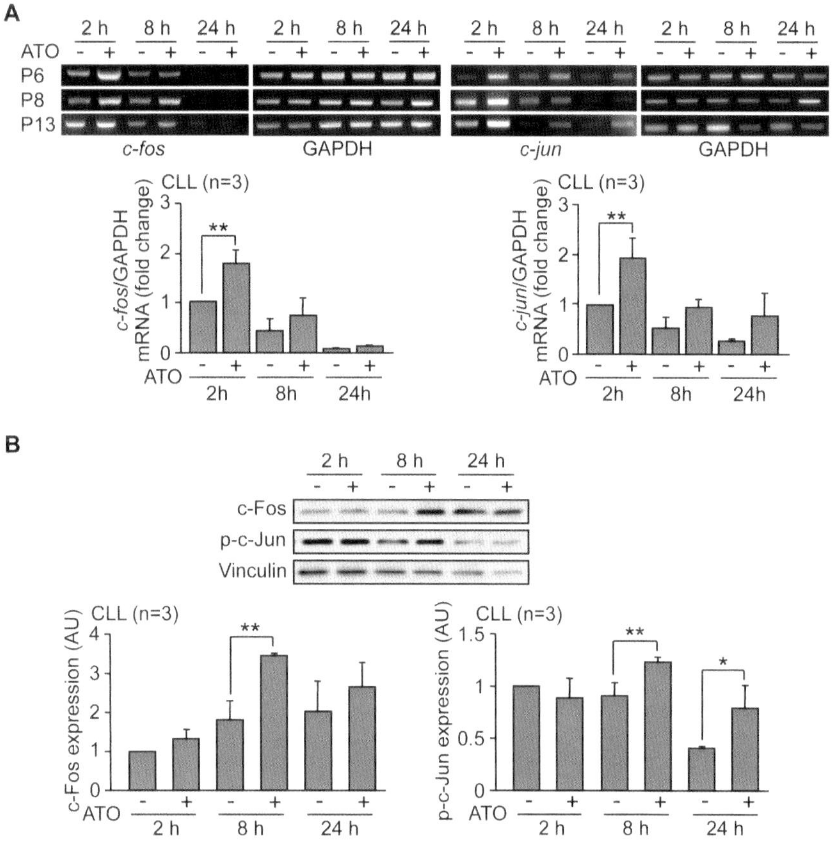

Figure 2. ATO treatment of CLL cells induces activation of the c-fos/c-jun transcription factors. (A) 10–15×10[6] CLL cells in RPMI/0.1%FBS from three different patients were treated with 3 μM ATO or vehicle. At the indicated times, *c-fos* and *c-jun* mRNA was analyzed by RT-PCR, using GAPDH as an internal control. Average values (fold change) were normalized with respect to the control at 2 h. (B) 10–15×10[6] CLL cells were treated as above, lysed at the indicated times and analyzed by Western blotting, using vinculin as internal control. The results for one representative sample and the normalized average values for the 3 samples studied, compared to the control at 2 h are shown. *P≤0.05; **P≤0.01.

ATO-induced MMP-9 mainly localizes at the cell membrane via interaction with α4β1 integrin and CD44

To determine if ATO also regulated MMP-9 at the protein level and because MMP-9 is mostly a secreted protein, we analyzed by gelatin zymography the conditioned media of equal number of CLL cells incubated with or without 3 μM ATO for 24 h. Figure 3A shows that, in contrast to what was expected, the levels of secreted MMP-9 in cells treated with ATO were significantly lower (2.6-fold average) than those in untreated cells. Since CLL cells also express MMP-9 on their surface [16] we studied whether cell-associated MMP-9 increased upon ATO treatment. CLL cells treated or not with ATO for 24 h were incubated with isotype control or anti-MMP-9 antibodies and analyzed by flow cytometry. The PI$^+$ (necrotic) cell population was excluded from these analyses to avoid false results due to non-specific antibody capture. As shown in Figure 3B for 6 representative patients and quantitated for all 10 cases studied, surface-bound MMP-9 was significantly increased in cells treated with ATO (24% average positive cells) compared to control cells (10%). Moreover, cell fractionation analyses on two representative CLL samples confirmed that, upon ATO treatment, expression of MMP-9 was much higher in the membrane fraction than in the cytosolic fraction (Figure 3C). Parallel zymographic analyses of the conditioned media of the same samples confirmed that secreted MMP-9 was reduced on ATO-treated cells compared to controls (Figure 3C).

To then study whether the observed MMP-9 membrane association was via interaction with its reported receptors α4β1 integrin and CD44v [16], we blocked these receptors with specific antibodies prior to cell incubation with 3 μM ATO. As shown in Figure 3D for 2 representative patients and quantitated for the 3 cases studied, these antibodies significantly reduced the levels of MMP-9 found at the cell surface from 30.4% to 11.5% and 8.1%, respectively, for anti-α4 and anti-CD44 Abs upon ATO treatment. Moreover, these Abs also decreased cell viability by 19% (anti-α4) and 20% (anti-CD44) with respect to the effect of the control Ab (results not shown), suggesting a correlation between cell-bound MMP-9 and increased cell viability. In parallel gelatin zymography analyses of the conditioned media of these cells we did not observe an increase in soluble MMP-9, compared to control cells (not shown). This is likely due to the small variation of secreted MMP-9 under these conditions, with the consequent difficulty in quantitating differences.

Next, we determined if increased transcription and surface expression of MMP-9 was associated to apoptosis, the main effect of ATO in CLL cells. To this end, live (Annexin V$^-$PI$^-$) and apoptotic (Annexin V$^+$PI$^-$) cells were analyzed on a cell sorter for MMP-9 surface expression after ATO exposure. The concentration of ATO in these experiments was adjusted to 2 μM to allow a more similar distribution between live and apoptotic cells and facilitate comparisons. Figure 4A shows for two representative cases that increased MMP-9 expression in response to ATO

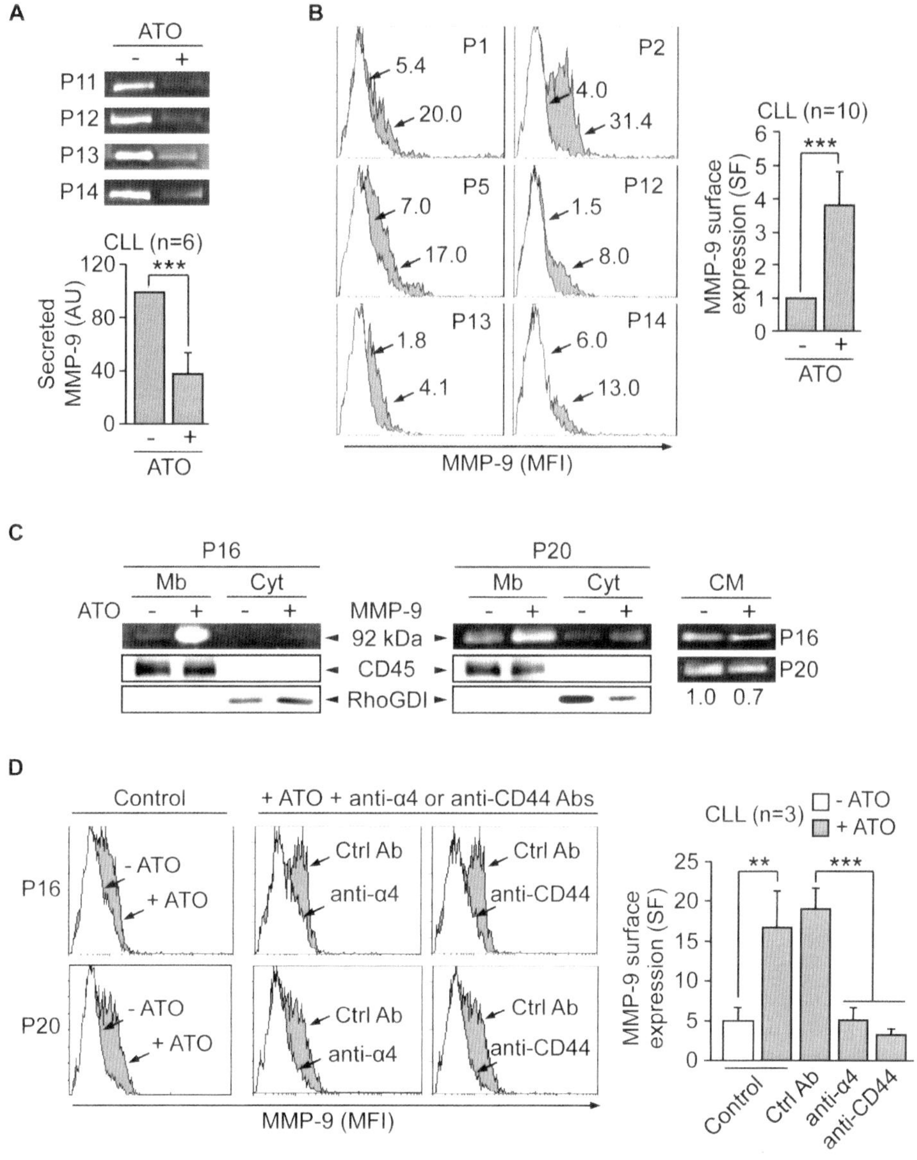

Figure 3. MMP-9 localizes to the CLL cell surface in response to ATO and in correlation with induction of apoptosis. (A) 5×10^6 CLL cells in RPMI/0.1% FBS were treated or not with 3 μM ATO for 24 h. The conditioned media was collected, concentrated 20× and analyzed by gelatin zymography. The results from four representative samples and the average normalized values (arbitrary units, AU) from all six samples studied are shown. (B) 1.5×10^5 CLL cells were incubated with or without 3 μM ATO for 24 h. MMP-9 surface expression was analyzed by flow cytometry using an anti-MMP-9 pAb or a control pAb. Histograms from six representative cases are shown, where white areas correspond to control/untreated cells and grey areas to ATO treated cells. Arrows indicate specific fluorescence (SF). Average normalized values from all ten samples analyzed are also shown. (C) 30×10^6 CLL cells in RPMI/0.1%FBS were incubated with or without 3 μM ATO for 24 h. Membrane (Mb) and cytosolic (Cyt) fractions were separated and analyzed by gelatin zymography. RhoGDI and CD45 detected by Western blotting in the same lysates were used as controls for the procedure. The conditioned media (CM) of these cells was also analyzed by gelatin zymography and the normalized average values of the quantitated bands are shown (D) 1.5×10^5 CLL cells in RPMI/0.1%FBS were incubated for 1 h with or without the indicated antibodies. 3 μM ATO was added and after 24 h, surface-bound MMP-9 was determined by flow cytometry using an anti-MMP-9 pAb or a control pAb. Histograms for two representative cases are shown. White areas correspond to untreated cells (−ATO) and grey areas (both light and dark) to ATO-treated cells (+ATO). Average normalized SF values are also shown. **$P\leq0.01$; ***$P\leq0.001$.

(35.3% and 37.5% positive cells, respectively, compared to 7.5% and 10.1%, respectively, in controls) was clearly coincident with the apoptotic cell population. To confirm these results CLL cells were incubated with the caspase-inhibitor Z-VAD-FMK prior to exposure to 2 μM ATO. This treatment prevented apoptosis and MMP-9 localization to the cell surface (Figure 4B). Moreover, the absence of membrane-bound MMP-9 correlated with the lack of MMP-9 mRNA upregulation by ATO, determined by qPCR analyses on these Z-VAD-FMK treated samples (Figure 4C).

To then determine if the observed MMP-9 gene induction and membrane localization preceded or was a consequence of the ongoing apoptosis, we lowered the ATO concentration to 1 μM, which had been previously shown to result in minimal apoptosis (see Figure 1A). Initial analysis by RT-PCR on 2 different samples clearly showed an increase in MMP-9 mRNA upon ATO

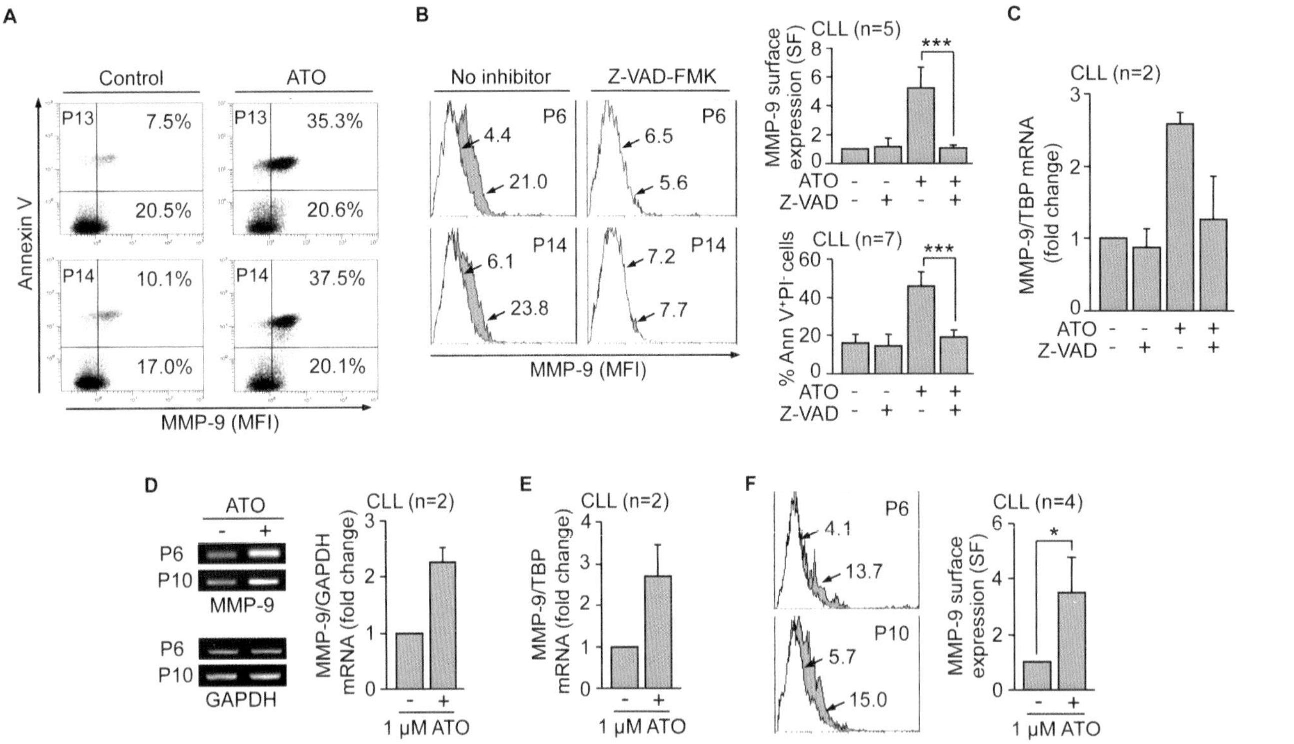

Figure 4. Upregulation and membrane localization of MMP-9 is an initial CLL cell response to the cytotoxic action of ATO. (A) Cell sorter biparametric diagrams of PI$^-$ CLL cells (1.5×10^5) treated or not with ATO for 24 h and analyzed for MMP-9 expression. Numbers indicate the percentage of cells expressing MMP-9 in the early apoptotic (Annexin V$^+$, top) and live (Annexin V$^-$, bottom) cell compartments. (B) Flow cytometric analysis of MMP-9 expression in control or ATO-treated CLL cells with or without previous incubation with 50 μM Z-VAD-FMK. Histograms from two representative cases are shown. White areas: control cells; grey areas: ATO-treated cells. Arrows indicate specific fluorescence (SF). Normalized average values for all five samples analyzed are shown. The average % of early apoptotic (Ann V$^+$/PI$^-$) cells in these samples is also shown. (C) 10–15×10^6 CLL cells treated as in (B) were analyzed for MMP-9 mRNA expression by qPCR, using TBP as an internal control. Average normalized values (fold change) are shown. (D,E) 10–15×10^6 CLL cells were treated with 1 μM ATO for 24 h and MMP-9 mRNA expression analyzed by RT-PCR (D) and qPCR (E). Normalized average values (fold change) are shown. (F) CLL cells treated as in (D, E) were analyzed for MMP-9 surface expression by flow cytometry with an anti-MMP-9 pAb or a control pAb. Histograms for the same samples used in (D, E) are shown. Arrows, white and grey areas are as in (B). Normalized average SF values of all four samples studied are shown. *P≤0.05; ***P≤0.001.

treatment (Figure 4D). These results were further confirmed by qPCR, which showed a 2.4-fold average increase in MMP-9 mRNA for the 2 patients studied (Figure 4E). Moreover, flow cytometric analyses of these and 2 additional samples demonstrated the enhanced presence (from 8.8% to 20.4% positive cells) of MMP-9 at the cell surface (Figure 4F). Parallel viability analyses showed that, at the time studied, 1 μM ATO did not decrease cell viability with respect to control cells (P6: 75% vs 79%; P10: 54% vs 55%, not shown). Altogether these results suggested that CLL cells responded to an apoptotic stimulus like ATO, by first upregulating MMP-9 and its membrane localization. Upon the onset of apoptosis, MMP-9 remained specifically associated to apoptotic cells.

MMP-9 upregulation and cell membrane localization in response to fludarabine treatment of CLL cells

To determine whether MMP-9 modulation was a particular feature of ATO exposure or a more general response to drug-induced apoptosis, we studied the effect of fludarabine, a front-line treatment for CLL, on MMP-9. CLL cells were incubated with or without 3 or 5 μM fludarabine for 48 h and MMP-9 mRNA analyzed by RT-PCR. Figure 5A shows that fludarabine increased MMP-9 transcription in a dose-dependent manner, compared to control cells. These results were confirmed by qPCR, which showed an increase on MMP-9 mRNA of 4.9-fold and 17.5-fold, respectively, for 3 and 5 μM fludarabine (Figure 5B). Parallel flow cytometric analyses indicated that the average percentage of apoptotic cells at this time was 45.2% and 48%, respectively, for 3 and 5 μM fludarabine (not shown). As observed in the case of ATO, MMP-9 expression at the cell surface was enhanced (15.5% to 26.6% positive cells) upon fludarabine treatment (Figure 5C). These results indicated that MMP-9 upregulation in correlation with CLL cell apoptosis was not restricted to ATO action.

MMP-9, isolated or present in stroma, induces resistance of CLL cells to ATO and fludarabine

Having established that MMP-9 was modulated by ATO and fludarabine and localized to the CLL cell surface, we aimed to determine whether MMP-9 had a role in the cellular response to these drugs. This was particularly relevant, given the dual role played by MMPs in apoptosis [18,19]. CLL cells were cultured on BSA (a control substrate that does not mediate cell adhesion or induce intracellular signaling) or MMP-9-coated wells for 1 h prior to exposure to ATO or fludarabine. Drug concentrations were lowered in these experiments to avoid excessive reduction in cell viability and allow comparisons. In control experiments in the absence of drug, MMP-9-cultures had significantly more live cells (Annexin V$^-$PI$^-$) than BSA-cultures (Figure 6A), in agreement

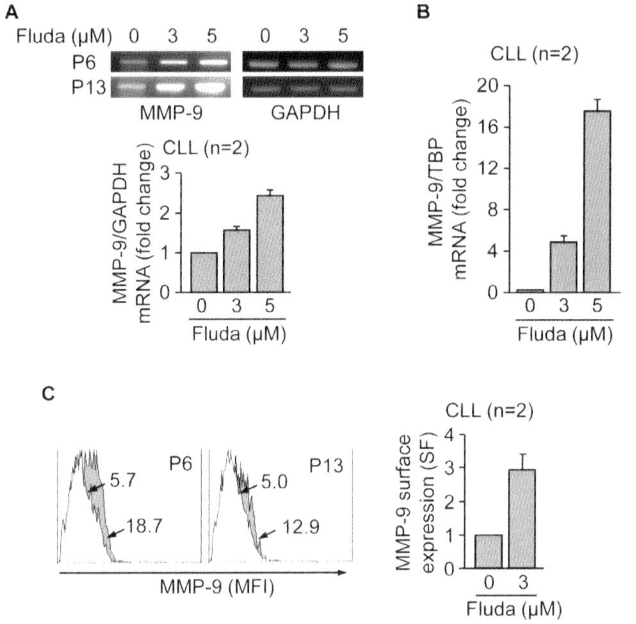

Figure 5. Fludarabine transcriptionally upregulates MMP-9 and induces its localization to the CLL cell membrane. (A,B) 10–15×10^6 CLL in RPMI/0.1% FBS cells from two different patients were treated with 3 or 5 μM fludarabine (Fluda) for 48 h and MMP-9 mRNA expression was analyzed by RT-PCR (A) and qPCR (B). Normalized average values (fold change) are shown. (C) 1.5×10^5 CLL cells from two different patients were incubated with or without 3 μM fludarabine for 48 h and MMP-9 surface expression was analyzed by flow cytometry. White areas, control/untreated cells; grey areas, fludarabine treated cells. Arrows indicate specific fluorescence (SF) values for each cell population. Normalized average values are also shown.

with our previous results in which MMP-9 prevented CLL cell spontaneous apoptosis [17]. Importantly, cells cultured on MMP-9 and treated with ATO or, for comparison, with fludarabine, also showed significantly higher viability compared to cells cultured on BSA (Figure 6A).

The above results indicated that adhesion to MMP-9 induced CLL cell resistance to ATO and to the commonly used drug fludarabine. MMP-9 is an abundant component of the stroma found in the CLL microenvironment and stromal cells contribute to CLL cell resistance to certain drugs [10,26]. We therefore studied whether stromal cells influenced the response of CLL cells to ATO and whether this involved MMP-9. CLL cells from 4 different patients were incubated on BSA (control) or HS-5 stromal cells and treated with or without ATO. Cell viability was determined after 48 h by flow cytometry and values for cells cultured on stromal cells in the absence of ATO (69.2% average) were normalized to 100. Figure 6B shows that in the absence of ATO, the anti-MMP-9 Ab significantly reduced the viability of CLL cells cultured on HS-5 cells compared to cells in the absence of Ab, while a control Ab had no effect. As in the case of isolated MMP-9 (Figure 6A), this confirmed our previous report showing that MMP-9 protects CLL cells from spontaneous apoptosis in culture [17]. Treatment with ATO reduced the viability of CLL cells cultured on BSA by 74.4% but had a limited effect (32.8% reduction) on HS-5 cultured-CLL cells (Figure 6B), indicating a protective effect by stromal cells. This was completely overcome by the anti-MMP-9 Ab, which reduced CLL viability to 15.5%, while a control Ab had no effect (Figure 6B).

To confirm and validate these results, the same experiments were carried out on CLL cells cultured on primary stromal cells derived from a CLL patient. Primary stromal cells protected CLL cells from spontaneous apoptosis (undergone in suspended cells) and this was significantly reverted by an anti-MMP-9 Ab, but not by a control Ab. Primary stromal cells also significantly induced CLL cell resistance to ATO (67.1% cell viability compared to 14.5% on suspended cells) and the anti-MMP-9 Ab clearly overcame this protective effect, reducing the stroma-induced survival to 18.8% (Figure 6C). Altogether these results established that stromal cells protected CLL cells from the cytotoxic effect of ATO and that MMP-9 had a role in this protection.

MEC-1 cells also upregulate MMP-9 in response to ATO and fludarabine

To further establish that MMP-9 conferred drug resistance in CLL cells we used the MEC-1 cell line, derived from a CLL patient and expressing very low constitutive levels of MMP-9. To first determine if these cells behave like primary CLL cells, we studied the response of MEC-1 cells to ATO and, for comparison, to fludarabine. The viability of untreated cells after 24 h and 48 h was 146% and 154%, respectively, compared to initial viability normalized to 100 (due to cell proliferation), and these values were normalized to 100. Figure 7A,B shows that after 24 h (ATO) or 48 h (fludarabine) treatment, the viability of MEC-1 cells, measured by the MTT assay, decreased in a dose-dependent manner. Because this assay primarily determines cell proliferation and, indirectly, cell viability, we also measured MEC-1 cell viability after ATO or fludarabine treatment by flow cytometry, using FITC-Annexin V and PI. In results not shown, ATO decreased cell viability by 39%, 58% and 79%, at 3, 5, and 8 μM, respectively. Likewise, fludarabine treatment reduced viability by 13%, 29%, and 32%, at 3, 5 and 8 μM, respectively. These results were very similar to those shown in Figure 7A,B, thus confirming the validity of the MTT assay to assess cell viability.

We next studied whether ATO also modulated MMP-9 in MEC-1 cells. Indeed, and as observed in primary CLL cells, ATO upregulated MMP-9 mRNA on MEC-1 cells after 8 and 24 h, compared to control cells (Figure 7C). These results were confirmed by qPCR, which showed a 4.2-fold and 4.4-fold MMP-9 mRNA increase, respectively, after 8 or 24 h treatment (Figure 7D). Moreover, MMP-9 surface expression on these cells also significantly increased (from 15.6% to 34.1% positive cells) upon ATO treatment (Figure 7E). These results confirmed the similar response of MEC-1 and primary CLL cells to ATO and validated the MEC-1 cell system for subsequent studies.

MMP-9 expression in MEC-1 cells confers resistance to ATO and fludarabine

Using the MEC-1 cell line, we recently established [20] stable transfectants expressing a GFP-lentiviral vector (Mock-cells) or a vector containing GFP-MMP-9 (MMP-9-cells), thus representing an unambiguous system to study MMP-9 functions. As recently reported [20], MMP-9-cells expressed cell-associated MMP-9, determined by flow cytometry (Figure 8A), thus resembling primary CLL cells [16]. This expression was further confirmed by cell fractionation, which clearly showed the presence of MMP-9 on the membrane (92 kDa and 86 kDa forms) and cytosol (92 kDa form) fractions of MMP-9-cells and its absence on Mock-cells (Figure 8B). Additionally, MMP-9-cells secreted high levels of MMP-9 into the medium, while secretion was very low in untransfected or MEC-1 Mock-cells (Figure 8B).

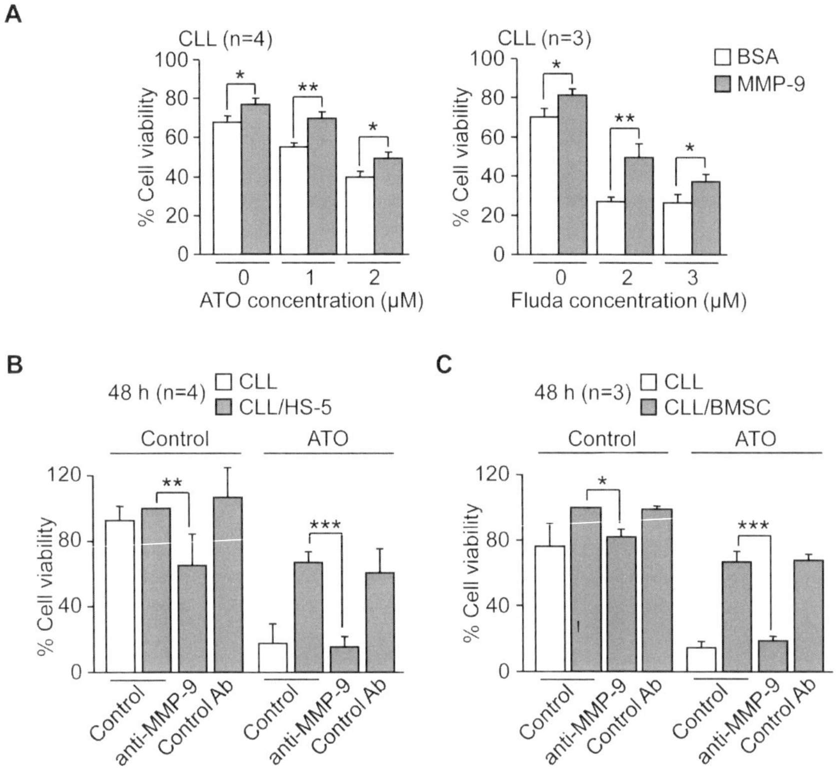

Figure 6. MMP-9, isolated or present in stroma, induces resistance of CLL cells to ATO and fludarabine. (A) 1.5×10^5 CLL cells RPMI/0.1% FBS were cultured on 0.5% BSA or 150 nM MMP-9 for 1 h prior to adding the indicated concentrations of ATO or fludarabine (Fluda). After 24 h (ATO) or 48 h (Fluda) cell viability was determined by flow cytometry using FITC-Annexin V and PI. (B) 1.5×10^5 CLL cells were treated or not with anti-MMP-9 pAbs or control pAbs for 1 h and added to wells coated with 0.5% BSA, HS-5 cells or primary stromal cells (BMSC). After 2 h at 37°C, 2 μM ATO was added and cells further incubated for 48 h. Cell viability was determined by flow cytometry using FITC-Annexin V and PI. The viability of CLL cells cultured over stroma in the absence of ATO was normalized to 100 and average values are shown. *P≤0.05; **P≤0.01; ***P≤0.001.

Mock- and MMP-9-cells where then incubated with various concentrations of ATO (24 h) or fludarabine (48 h) or vehicle and viability measured by the MTT assay. In the absence of drug, the viability of Mock-cells and MMP-9-cells was similar (155% vs 149% at 24 h and 154% vs 152% at 48 h, compared to initial viability) and these values were normalized to 100, for better assessment of the effect of the drugs. Treatment with ATO (Figure 8C) or fludarabine (Figure 8D) decreased cell viability in a dose-dependent manner in both cell types, but at all doses tested MMP-9-cells showed significantly higher viability than Mock-cells. To further confirm that this was due to the presence of MMP-9 (cell-associated and in soluble form), we performed gene silencing experiments using a specific siRNA for MMP-9 or a control siRNA. Gelatin zymographic analyses indicated that MMP-9 silencing inhibited the already low MMP-9 expression in Mock-cells, and produced an average 75% reduction in MMP-9-cells, also confirmed by Western blotting (Figure 8E). This procedure equally affected the viability of either transfectant cell type (35% reduction). siRNA-transfected Mock- and MMP-9-cells were then treated with several concentrations of ATO and the viability measured after 24 h by MTT. Although the effect of ATO was milder in these experiments, there were clear differences between Mock- and MMP-9-cells. As shown in Figure 8F, the viability of Mock-cells upon ATO exposure decreased in a dose-dependent manner with no differences between MMP-9 siRNA-transfected or control siRNA-transfected cells for all doses tested. The lack of functional effect of MMP-9 silencing in Mock-cells could be explained by the very low constitutive levels of MMP-9 in these cells (see Figure 8E). Thus, modulation of these levels is therefore unlikely to produce a detectable functional effect. In contrast, silencing MMP-9 in MMP-9-cells significantly decreased cell viability with respect to control siRNA-transfected cells, thus reverting the protective effect of MMP-9 on these cells (Figure 8F). These results clearly indicated that MMP-9 contributed to CLL cell resistance to ATO.

MMP-9 induces drug resistance by modulating the balance of anti- and pro-apoptotic proteins from the Bcl-2 family

To determine the molecular bases responsible for the observed drug-protecting effect of MMP-9, we analyzed whether the expression of prototype Bcl-2 family members was modulated by MMP-9. In initial experiments, Mock- and MMP-9-cells were treated with 5 μM ATO or vehicle and, after 24 h, lysed and analyzed by Western blotting. Figure 9A shows that upon ATO exposure, expression of the anti-apoptotic proteins Mcl-1 and Bcl-xL decreased in Mock-cells compared to their untreated counterpart, while Bcl-2 remained unchanged. In MMP-9-cells, however, all three proteins remained similar (Mcl-1) or were elevated (Bcl-xL, Bcl-2) with respect to untreated MMP-9-cells. Moreover, Mcl-1, Bcl-xL and Bcl-2 in ATO-treated MMP-9-cells were significantly upregulated compared to ATO-treated Mock-cells (Figure 9A). Similar analysis of selected pro-apoptotic proteins showed that Bax and Bim significantly increased in Mock-cells treated with ATO, compared to untreated cells, while Noxa

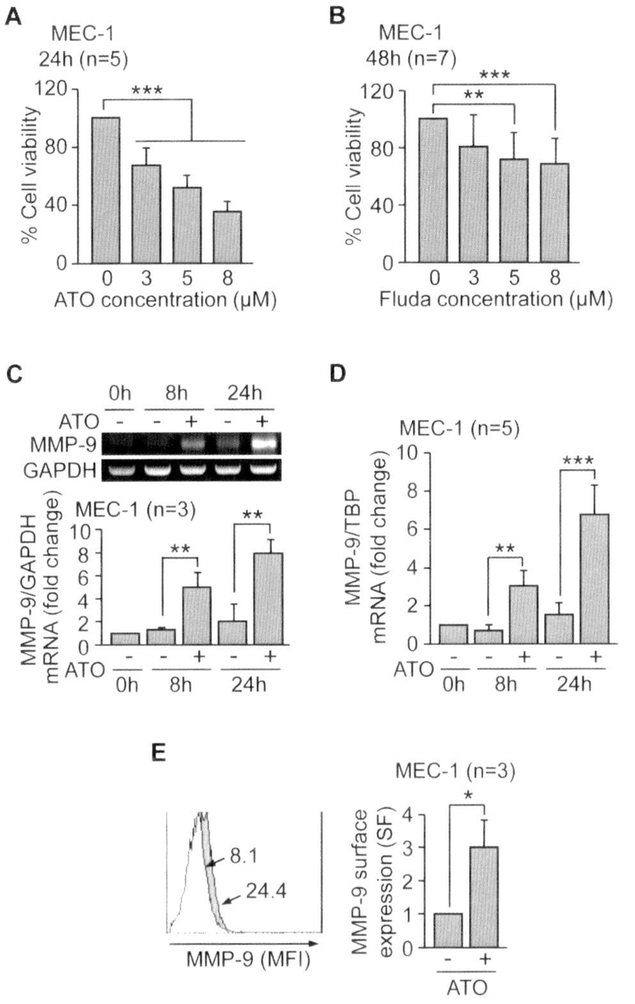

Figure 7. Effect of ATO and fludarabine on MEC-1 cells. (A, B) 7.5×10^4 MEC-1 cells in IMDM/0.1% FBS were treated or not with the indicated concentrations of ATO (A) or fludarabine (Fluda) (B). After 24 h (ATO) or 48 h (Fluda), cell viability was determined by the MTT assay. Control cell viability was normalized to 100 and average values are shown. (C,D) 5×10^6 MEC-1 cells were treated with 3 μM ATO for the indicated times and MMP-9 mRNA expression was analyzed by RT-PCR, using GAPDH as internal control (C) and qPCR, using TBP as internal control (D). Normalized average values (fold change) are shown. (E) 1.5×10^5 MEC-1 cells were treated or not with 3 μM ATO for 24 h and MMP-9 surface expression was analyzed by flow cytometry, using an anti-MMP-9 pAb or a control pAb. Histograms from a representative experiment and normalized average values for the three experiments performed are shown. White areas, control/untreated cells; grey areas, ATO-treated cells. Arrows indicate the specific fluorescence. *P≤0.05; **P≤0.01; ***P≤0.001.

expression was not significantly altered (Figure 9A). In contrast, the expression of Bax and Bim in MMP-9-cells treated with ATO was lower than in untreated MMP-9-cells. Moreover, Bax and Bim in ATO-treated MMP-9-cells were significantly lower than in ATO-treated Mock-cells (Figure 9A).

Since regulation of apoptosis/survival involves the balance of anti- and pro-apoptotic Bcl-2 family members, rather than individual levels [27], we also determined the ratios of these proteins in Mock and MMP-9-cells, before and after exposure to ATO. Figure 9B shows that, upon ATO treatment, the balance Mcl-1/Bim, Mcl-1/Noxa and Bcl-2/Bax, were all significantly increased in MMP-9-cells, compared to Mock-cells. These ratios were also significantly higher compared to untreated MMP-9-cells. However, these ratios were diminished in ATO-treated Mock-cells, compared to untreated Mock-cells (Figure 9B).

Mcl-1 is a critical molecule in CLL cell survival and exerts its function by sequestering BH3-only pro-apoptotic proteins such as Bim [28]. We therefore studied whether Mcl-1 and Bim were complexed in MMP-9 transfectants upon ATO exposure. Lysates of Mock or MMP-9-cells that had been treated or not with 5 μM ATO for 24 h, were immunoprecipitated with anti-Mcl-1 Abs and analyzed by Western blotting. Figure 9C shows that in untreated cells, similar amounts of Bim were pooled down by the anti-Mcl-1 Ab in both, Mock and MMP-9 transfectants. In contrast, upon ATO treatment, very little Bim co-immunoprecipitated with Mcl-1 in Mock-cells, while Bim remained bound to Mcl-1 and even increased in MMP-9 cells (Figure 9C).

Similar results were obtained for Mock- and MMP-9-cells treated with 5 μM fludarabine. As shown in Figure 10A, Mcl-1 and Bcl-xL were also significantly higher in MMP-9-cells compared to Mock-cells. Bcl-2 did not seem to play a role in this case, as its expression remained similar for both cell types, either in the absence or presence of fludarabine. As observed in the case of ATO, the ratios Mcl-1/Bim and Mcl-1/Noxa upon fludarabine treatment were significantly higher in MMP-9-cells than in Mock-cells, while the balance Bcl-2/Bax did not seem to play a role (Figure 10B).

MMP-9 regulates the balance of Bcl-2 family proteins in primary CLL cells treated with ATO

We next determined whether MMP-9 also modulated Bcl-2 family members in primary CLL cells. Cells from 3 different patients were cultured on BSA or MMP-9 for 1 h prior to adding 3 μM ATO. After 24 h, cells were lysed and lysates analyzed by Western blotting. Figure 11A shows that Mcl-1 was significantly upregulated, both in the absence or presence of ATO, in cells cultured on MMP-9 compared to cells cultured on BSA. Bcl-xL and Bcl-2 were also significantly increased on MMP-9-cultured CLL cells upon ATO treatment, compared to BSA-cultured cells. The ratios Mcl-1/Bim and Mcl-1/Noxa were also upregulated in MMP-9-cultured cells, both in the absence or presence of ATO, while the Bcl-2/Bax ratio was not modulated under these conditions (Figure 11B). Altogether these results indicated that MMP-9 induced drug resistance in CLL cells by regulating the expression and function of crucial anti-apoptotic and pro-apoptotic proteins of the Bcl-2 family.

Discussion

We have studied whether MMP-9 plays a role in CLL cell response to cytotoxic drugs, such as arsenic trioxide and fludarabine. We report for the first time the following findings: 1) upon an apoptotic stimulus, MMP-9 is transcriptionally upregulated and localizes to the surface of early apoptotic cells; 2) MMP-9 by itself or present in stroma induces CLL cell drug resistance; 3) MEC-1 cells stably transfected with MMP-9 show increased survival upon drug treatment; 4) the MMP-9 anti-apoptotic effect involves modulation of anti- and pro-apoptotic proteins from the Bcl-2 family.

Upregulation and membrane localization of MMP-9 was an early response to drug exposure that preceded detection of apoptosis and was necessarily associated to this process. Evidence for this comes from the fact that preventing cell death with the Z-VAD-FMK caspase inhibitor blocked MMP-9 mRNA induction and its cell surface localization upon ATO treatment. MMP-9

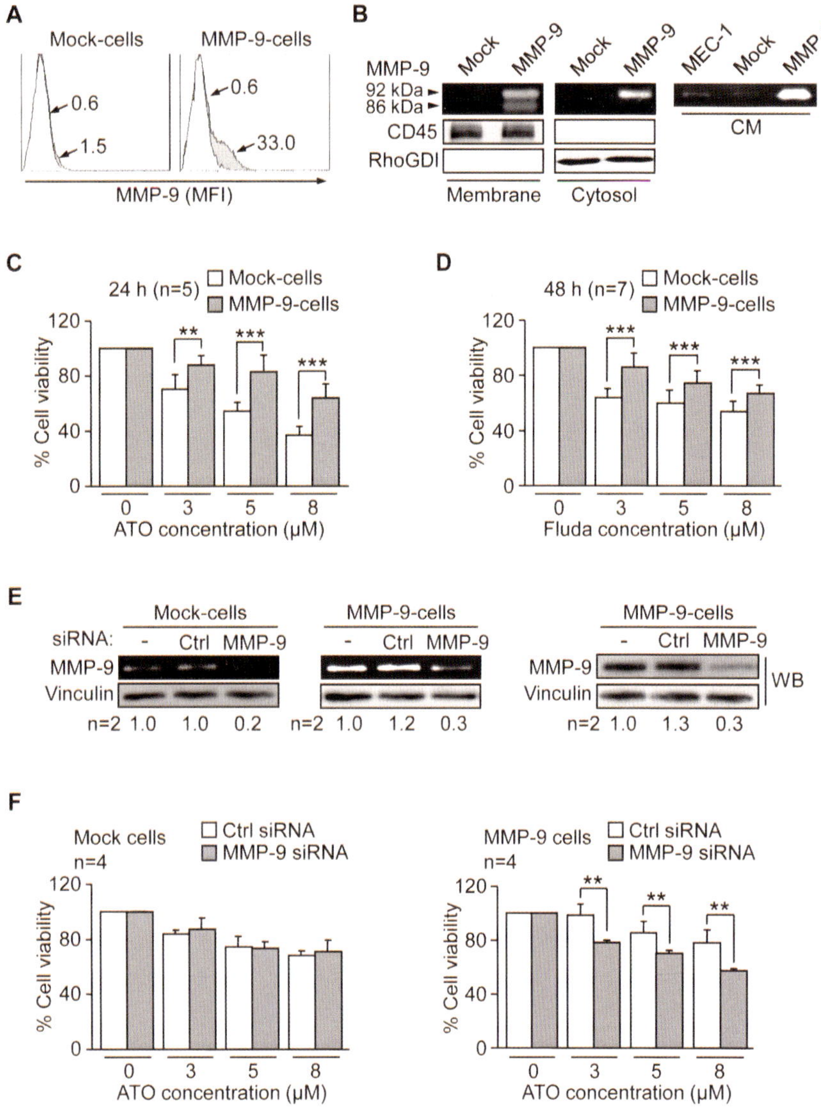

Figure 8. Effect of ATO and fludarabine on MEC-1 Mock-cells and MMP-9-cells. (A) 1.5×10^5 Mock- or MMP-9-cells were analysed by flow cytometry using an anti-MMP-9 pAb or a control pAb. Histograms for two representative experiments are shown. White areas: negative control; grey areas: MMP-9 surface expression. Arrows indicate the specific fluorescence (SF). (B) The membrane and cytosolic fractions from 5×10^6 Mock- or MMP-9-cells were separated and analyzed by gelatin zymography. RhoGDI and CD45 were visualized by Western blotting of the same lysates and used as controls for the procedure. The conditioned medium (CM) of the same cells was also analyzed by gelatin zymography. (C,D) 7.5×10^4 Mock- or MMP-9-cells in IMDM/0.1% FBS were treated or not with the indicated concentrations of ATO (C) or Fluda (D) and cell viability was determined after 24 h (ATO) or 48 h (Fluda) using the MTT assay. The viability in the absence of drugs was normalized to 100 and average values are shown. (E) 15×10^6 MEC-1 transfectants were nucleofected with MMP-9 or control siRNAs and analyzed after 24 h by gelatin zymography and Western blotting. Average quantitation of the MMP-9/vinculin ratios is also shown. (F) 7.5×10^4 siRNA-transfected Mock- or MMP-9-cells were treated or not with the indicated concentrations of ATO. After 24 h cell viability was determined by MTT. The viability in the absence of drugs was normalized to 100 and average values are shown. $^{**}P\leq0.01$, $^{***}P\leq0.001$.

membrane association was a specific event and involved interaction with α4β1 integrin and CD44, two reported MMP-9 receptors in CLL [16]. Additionally, the cell population with increased surface MMP-9 was coincident with that of early apoptotic cells, suggesting that MMP-9 remained mostly surface-bound to these cells upon secretion and modulated the apoptotic response. As MMP-9, as other MMPs, may play dual roles in apoptosis [18,19], one interpretation of our results could be that upregulation of MMP-9 facilitates the apoptotic process by targeting appropriate substrates or pathways. An alternative explanation is that MMP-9 antagonizes the apoptotic cell response to cytotoxic drugs, thus representing a survival compensatory mechanism. In support of this explanation, several previous studies have reported compensatory or survival response for MMP-9 in various cell systems. For example, in melanoma and breast carcinoma cells, apoptosis induced by TNF receptor ligands was clearly enhanced by inhibiting MMP-9 (or MMP-2) [29]. Similarly, blocking MMP-9 function sensitized colon adenocarcinoma cells to phorbol-esters [30] and glioma cells to Fas-induced apoptosis [31]. In another report using a xenograft model in mice, treatment of carcinoma cells with the chemotherapeutic agent paclitaxel increased MMP-9 expression and tumor cell metastasis, and this was also blocked with an MMP-9 inhibitor [32].

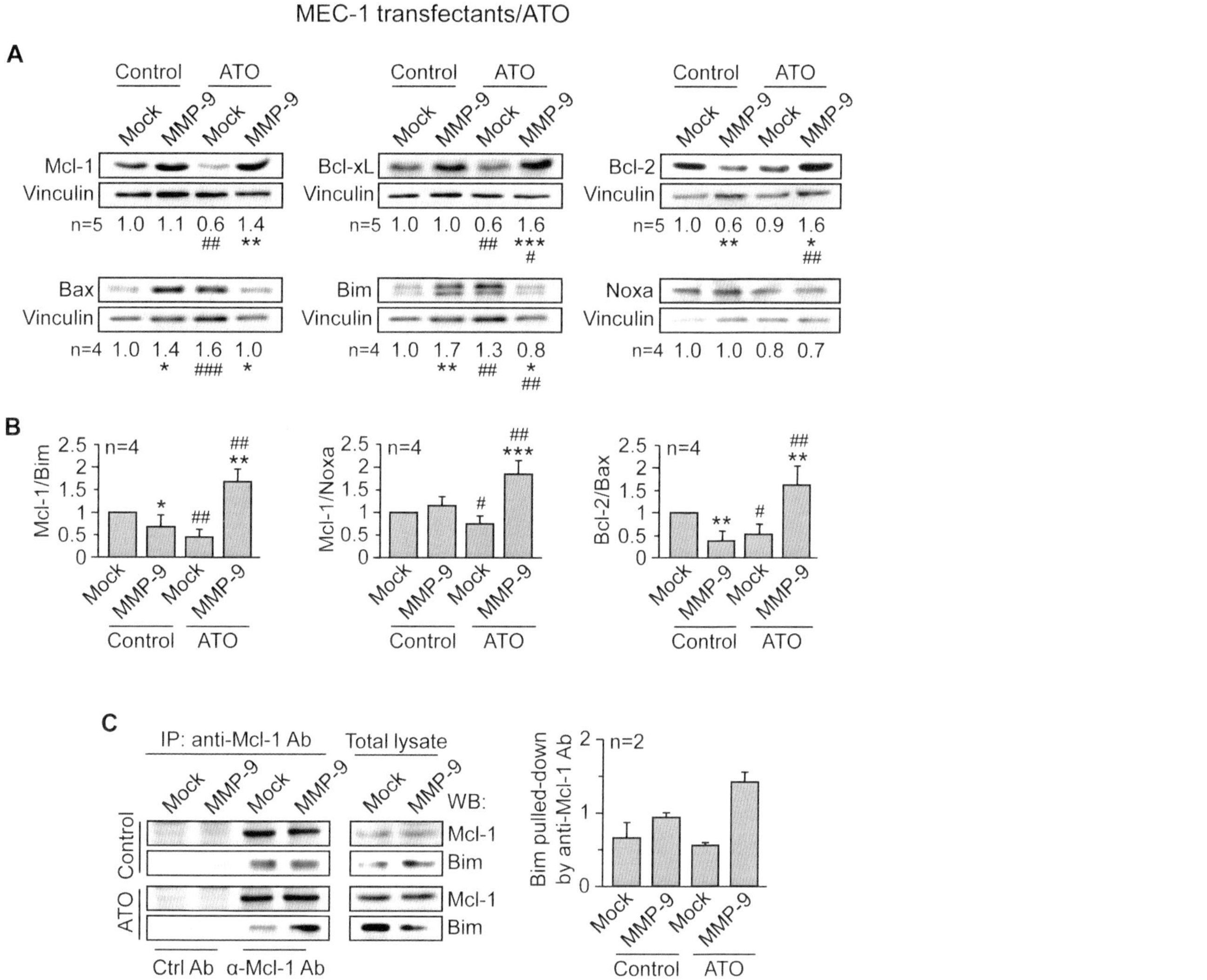

Figure 9. MMP-9 expression in MEC-1 cells prevents downregulation of anti-apoptotic Bcl-2 family proteins in response to ATO. (A) 5×10^6 Mock- or MMP-9-MEC-1 cells were treated or not with 5 μM ATO. After 24 h cells were lysed and the expression of the indicated proteins was analyzed by Western blotting, using vinculin as an internal control. A representative experiment is shown for each case and numbers indicate the average values from all experiments performed, after normalizing Mock control values to 1. (B) The indicated ratios of anti-apoptotic/pro-apoptotic proteins are shown. (C) 3×10^7 Mock- or MMP-9-cells were treated or not with 5 μM ATO for 24 h. Cells were lysed and lysates immunoprecipitated with anti-Mcl-1 or control Abs and analyzed by Western blotting. Values indicate the amount of Bim found in the Mcl-1 immunoprecipitates in both types of MEC-1 transfectants. * or $^{\#}$P≤0.05; ** or $^{\#\#}$P≤0.01; *** or $^{\#\#\#}$P≤0.001. Symbols are: *, Mock- vs MMP-9-cells; $^{\#}$, Mock- or MMP-9-cells treated with ATO compared to their respective untreated counterparts.

Using two different approaches we have obtained strong evidence to support an anti-apoptotic role for MMP-9 in the CLL cell response to ATO and fludarabine. First, the higher viability observed on cells cultured on MMP-9 during drug treatment compared to cells cultured on BSA. Notably, this anti-apoptotic role of MMP-9 was also observed in co-cultures of CLL and stromal cells, where blocking MMP-9 with antibodies completely reverted the stroma-induced drug resistance. We previously reported a role for MMP-9 in the protective effect of stroma against CLL cell spontaneous apoptosis in culture [17]. Other investigators have shown the involvement of several proteins (integrins, chemokines, Bcl-2 family proteins) in the resistance to certain therapeutic agents induced by stroma [33–35]. We now show for the first time that stromal cells induce CLL cell resistance to ATO and that MMP-9 has a prominent role in this resistance.

Further evidence for a survival role for MMP-9 in response to cytotoxic drugs comes from the fact that MEC-1-MMP-9 transfectants, representing an unambiguous system to identify MMP-9 functions, consistently showed higher viability in the presence of ATO or fludarabine than their corresponding MEC-1-Mock controls. Indeed, this effect was mediated by MMP-9 as silencing this protein reverted the survival advantage of the MMP-9 transfectants. Since our results show that MMP-9 is present in these transfectants as a cell-associated form as well as in the conditioned medium, it is possible that both fractions contribute to the increased survival of these cells. It is not known if the MMP-9 survival effect involves the same or different mechanisms as MMP-9 upregulation upon apoptotic stimuli, but the results of our study strongly support a compensatory survival role for MMP-9 in CLL.

We have addressed the molecular bases accounting for this drug-resistance effect of MMP-9 and have focused on molecules

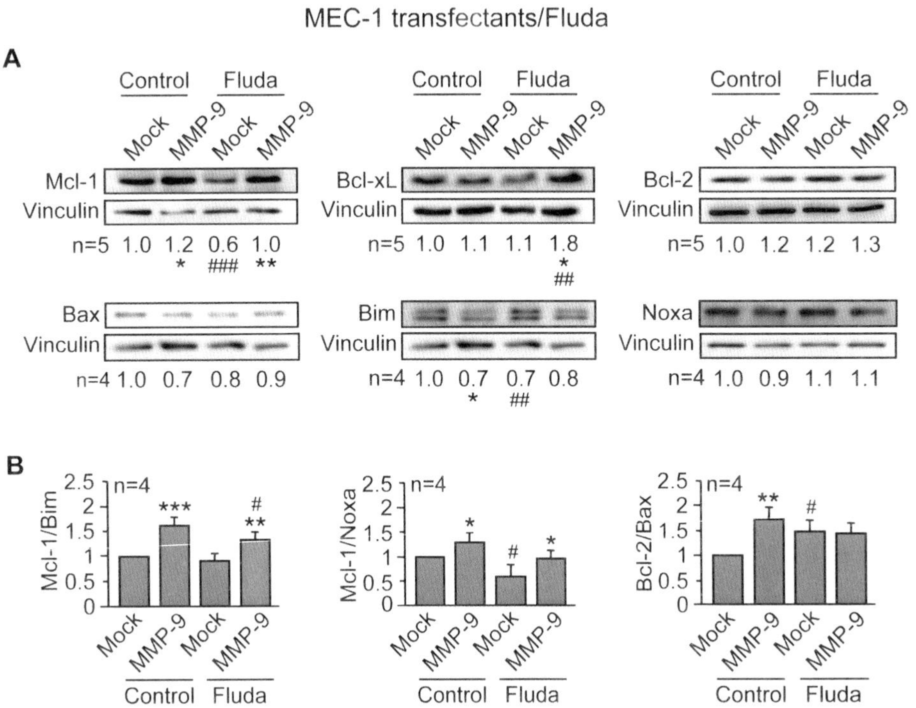

Figure 10. MMP-9 expression in MEC-1 cells prevents downregulation of anti-apoptotic Bcl-2 family proteins in response to fludarabine. (A,B) 5×10^6 Mock- or MMP-9-cells were treated or not with 5 μM fludarabine (Fluda). After 48 h cells were lysed and the indicated proteins (A) and ratios (B) analyzed as in Figure 9. * or #P≤0.05; ** or ##P≤0.01; *** or ###P≤0.001. Symbols are: *, Mock- vs MMP-9 cells; #, Mock- or MMP-9-cells treated with Fluda compared to their respective untreated counterparts.

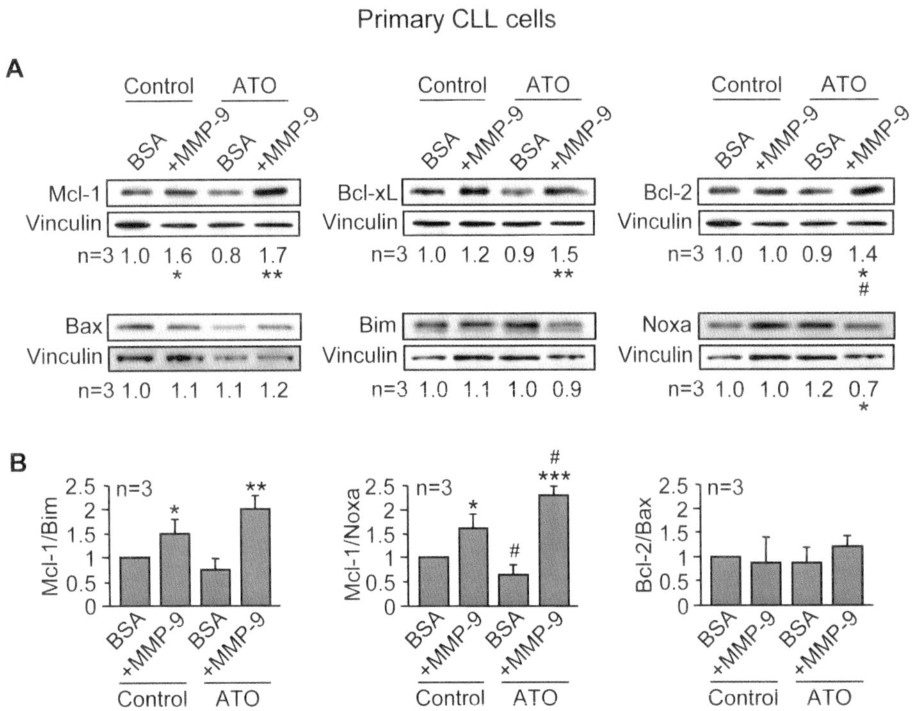

Figure 11. Culturing CLL cells on MMP-9 modulates Bcl-2 family proteins in response to ATO, preventing downregulation of Mcl-1, Bcl-xL and Bcl-2. (A,B) 10×10^6 primary CLL cells in RPMI/0.1% FBS were incubated on BSA- or 150 nM MMP-9-coated wells for 1 h prior to adding 3 μM ATO or vehicle. After 24 h, cell were lysed and the indicated proteins (A) and ratios (B) analyzed by Western blotting as explained. * or #P≤0.05; ** or ##P≤0.01; *** or ###P≤0.001. Symbols are: *, CLL cells on BSA vs CLL cells on MMP-9; #, ATO-treated cells compared to their respective untreated controls.

from the Bcl-2 family, well-known regulators of apoptosis [27]. The apoptotic action of ATO has been shown to involve downregulation of the anti-apoptotic protein Mcl-1 in several cell systems, including myeloma [36] and myeloid leukemia cells [37] and, in many cases, upregulation of the pro-apoptotic proteins Bax and/or Bim [36,38,39]. Indeed the balance Mcl-1/Bim was shown to be determinant in myeloma cell response to ATO [36] and in the resistance of acute and chronic leukemic cells to fludarabine [40]. Our present results clearly show that MMP-9, both in MEC-1 transfectants and in primary CLL cells, not only prevented downregulation of anti-apoptotic proteins (Mcl-1, Bcl-xL, Bcl-2) in response to ATO but also upregulated their levels with respect to basal expression. As this was accompanied by downregulation (or no alteration) of pro-apoptotic proteins (Bim, Bax), the anti-apoptotic/pro-apoptotic balance was clearly elevated in the presence of MMP-9, likely contributing to the MMP-9 survival effect. We previously reported that prevention of CLL cell spontaneous apoptosis by MMP-9 involved upregulation of Mcl-1 but not Bcl-xL or Bcl-2 [17]. We now show that, in the presence of ATO, MMP-9 seems to affect several of these proteins, perhaps to amplify the compensatory survival effect. In this regard, our results also indicate that Mcl-1, a crucial anti-apoptotic protein in CLL [28] was not dissociated from Bim upon ATO exposure on MMP-9-transfected cells, thus preventing Bim from causing mitochondrial damage and apoptosis. Our results further show that Mcl-1 and Bcl-xL were also upregulated by MMP-9 in response to fludarabine. This is in agreement with our previous report showing the involvement of these proteins in the fibronectin/α4β1 integrin-induced CLL cell resistance to fludarabine [41]. As in the case of ATO, the anti-apoptotic/pro-apoptotic protein ratio was elevated, suggesting that the protective effect of MMP-9 against apoptosis may be a general CLL cell response to cytotoxic drugs. In conclusion, our study is the first to establish that MMP-9 induces drug-resistance in CLL by modulating the balance of Bcl-2 family members. Targeting MMP-9 in combination with therapeutic agents may thus improve the CLL response to treatment.

Acknowledgments

We thank all the CLL patients who donated samples for this study, Guillermo Padilla for help with the statistical analyses, and Dr. Pedro Lastres for valuable help with the flow cytometry analyses.

Author Contributions

Conceived and designed the experiments: AGP IAJ EB. Performed the experiments: IAJ EB EUB NAM. Analyzed the data: AGP IAJ EB EUB NAM JAGM. Contributed reagents/materials/analysis tools: JAGM. Wrote the paper: AGP.

References

1. Zenz T, Mertens D, Küppers R, Döhner H, Stilgenbauer S (2010) From pathogenesis to treatment of chronic lymphocytic leukaemia. Nat Rev Cancer 10: 37–50.
2. Gaidano G, Foa, Dalla-Favera R (2012) Molecular pathogenesis of chronic lymphocytic leukemia. J Clin Invest 122: 3432–3438.
3. Pleyer L, Egle A, Hartmann TN, Greil R (2009) Molecular and cellular mechanisms of CLL: novel therapeutic approaches. Nat Rev Clin Oncol 6: 405–418.
4. Hallek M (2013) Chronic lymphocytic leukemia: 2013 update on diagnosis, risk stratification and treatment. Am J Hematol 88: 803–816.
5. Stephens DM, Byrd JC (2013) Improving the treatment outcome of patients with chronic lymphocytic leukemia through targeted antibody therapy. Hematol Oncol Clin North Am 27: 303–327.
6. Wang Z-Y, Chen Z (2008) Acute promyelocytic leukemia: from highly fatal to highly curable. Blood 111: 2505–2515.
7. Mi JQ, Li JM, Shen ZX, Chen SJ, Chen Z (2012) How to manage acute promyelocytic leukemia. Leukemia 26: 1743–1751.
8. Merkel O, Heyder C, Asslaber D, Hamacher F, Tinhofer I, et al. (2008) Arsenic trioxide induces apoptosis preferentially in B-CLL cells of patients with unfavourable prognostic factors including del17p13. J Mol Med 86: 511–552
9. Redondo-Muñoz J, Escobar-Díaz E, Hernández del Cerro M, Pandiella A, Terol MJ, et al. (2010) Induction of B-chronic lymphocytic leukemia cell apoptosis by arsenic trioxide involves suppression of the phosphoinositide 3-kinase/Akt survival pathway via c-jun-NH2 terminal kinase activation and PTEN upregulation. Clin Cancer Res 16: 4382–4391.
10. Burger JA (2012) Targeting the microenvironment in chronic lymphocytic leukemia is changing the therapeutic landscape. Curr Opin Oncol 24: 643–649.
11. Ramsay AD, Rodriguez-Justo M (2013) Chronic lymphocytic leukemia-the role of the microenvironment pathogenesis and therapy. Br J Haematol 162: 15–24.
12. Vandooren J, Van den Steen PE, Opdenakker G (2013) Biochemistry and molecular biology of gelatinase B or matrix metalloproteinase-9 (MMP-9): the next decade. Crit Rev Biochem Mol Biol 48: 222–272.
13. Bauvois B, Dumont J, Mathiot C, Kolb JP (2002) Production of matrix metalloproteinase-9 in early stage B-CLL: suppression by interferons. Leukemia 16: 791–798.
14. Redondo-Muñoz J, Escobar-Díaz E, Samaniego R, Terol MJ, García-Marco JA, et al. (2006) MMP-9 in B-cell chronic lymphocytic leukemia is up-regulated by alpha4beta1 integrin or CXCR4 engagement via distinct signaling pathways, localizes to podosomes, and is involved in cell invasion and migration. Blood 108: 3143–3151.
15. Redondo-Muñoz J, Terol MJ, García-Marco JA, García-Pardo A (2008) Matrix metalloproteinase-9 is up-regulated by CCL21/CCR7 interaction via extracellular signal-regulated kinase-1/2 signaling and is involved in CCL21-driven B-cell chronic lymphocytic leukemia cell invasion and migration. Blood 111: 383–386.
16. Redondo-Muñoz J, Ugarte-Berzal E, García-Marco JA, Hernández del Cerro M, Van den Steen PE, et al. (2008) α4β1 integrin and 190-kDa CD44v constitute a cell surface docking complex for gelatinase B/MMP-9 in chronic leukemic but not in normal B cells. Blood 112: 169–178.
17. Redondo-Muñoz J, Ugarte-Berzal E, Terol MJ, Van den Steen PE, Hernández del Cerro M, et al. (2010) Matrix Metalloproteinase-9 promotes chronic lymphocytic leukemia B cell survival through Its hemopexin domain. Cancer Cell 17: 160–172.
18. Egeblad M, Werb Z (2002) New functions for the matrix metalloproteinases in cancer progression. Nature Reviews Cancer 2: 161–174.
19. Mannello F, Luchetti E, Falcieri E, Papa S (2005) Multiple roles of matrix metalloproteinases during apoptosis. Apoptosis 10: 19–24.
20. Bailón E, Ugarte-Berzal E, Amigo-Jiménez I, Van den Steen P, Opdenakker G, et al. (2014) Overexpression of pro-gelatinase B/proMMP-9 affects migration regulatory pathways and impairs chronic lymphocytic leukemia cell homing to bone marrow and spleen. J Leuk Biol, in press.
21. Stacchini A, Aragno M, Vallario A, Alfarano A, Circosta P (1999) MEC1 and MEC2: two new cell lines derived from B-chronic lymphocytic leukaemia in prolymphocytoid transformation. Leuk Res 23: 127–136.
22. Morodomi T, Ogata Y, Sasaguri Y, Morimatsu M, Nagase H (1992) Purification and characterization of matrix metalloproteinase 9 from U937 monocytic leukaemia and HT1080 fibrosarcoma cells. Biochem J 285: 603–611.
23. Shooshtari P, Fortuno ES, Blimkie D, Yu M, Gupta A, et al. (2010) Correlation Analysis of Intracellular and Secreted Cytokines via the Generalized Integrated Mean Fluorescence Intensity (GiMFI). Cytometry A 77: 873–880.
24. Jayo A, Conde I, Lastres P, Martínez C, Rivera J, et al. (2010) L718P mutation in the membrane-proximal cytoplasmic tail of β3 promotes abnormal αIIβ3 clustering and lipid microdomain coalescence, and associates with a thrombasthenia-like phenotype. Haematologica 95: 1158–1166.
25. Van den Steen PE, Dubois B, Nelissen I, Rudd PM, Dwek RA (2002) Biochemistry and molecular biology of gelatinase B or matrix metalloproteinase-9 (MMP-9). Crit Rev Biochem Mol Biol 37: 375–536.
26. Burger JA, Gribben JG (2014) The microenvironment in chronic lymphocytic leukemia (CLL) and other B cell malignancies: insight into disease biology and new targeted therapies. Semin Cancer Biol 24:71–81.
27. Czabotar PE, Lessene G, Strasser A, Adams JM (2014) Control of apoptosis by the BCL-2 protein family: implications for physiology and therapy. Nat Rev Mol Cell Biol 15: 49–63.
28. Gandhi V, Balakrishnan K, Chen LS (2008) Mcl-1: the 1 in CLL. Blood 112: 3538–3540.
29. Nyormoi O, Mills L, Bar-Eli M (2003) An MMP-2/MMP-9 inhibitor, 5a, enhances apoptosis induced by ligands of the TNF receptor superfamily in cancer cells. Cell Death Differ 10: 558–569.
30. Meyer E, Vollmer JY, Boyer R, Stamenkovic (2005) Matrix metalloproteinases 9 and 10 inhibit protein kinase C-potentiated, p53-mediated apoptosis. Cancer Res 65: 4261–4272.
31. Chetty C, Lakka SS, Bhoopathi P, Gondi CS, Veeravalli KK (2010) Urokinase plasminogen activator receptor and/or matrix metalloproteinase-9 inhibition induces apoptosis signaling through lipid rafts in glioblastoma xenograft cells. Mol Cancer Ther 9: 2605–2617.
32. Gingis-Velitski S, Loven D, Benayoun L, Munster M, Bril R (2011) Host response to short-term, single-agent chemotherapy induces matrix metallopro-

teinase-9 expression and accelerates metastasis in mice. Cancer Research 71: 6986-6996.

33. Zeng Z, Samudio IJ, Munsell M, An J, Huang Z, et al. (2006) Inhibition of CXCR4 with the novel RCP168 peptide overcomes stroma-mediated chemoresistance in chronic and acute leukemias. Mol Cancer Ther 5: 3113-3121.
34. Balakrishnan K, Burger JA, Wierda WG, Gandhi V (2009) AT-101 induces apoptosis in CLL B cells and overcomes stromal cell mediated Mcl-1 induction and drug resistance. Blood 113: 149-153.
35. Buchner M, Baer C, Prinz G, Dierks C, Burger M, et al. (2010) Spleen tyrosine kinase inhibition prevents chemokine- and integrin-mediated stromal protective effects in chronic lymphocytic leukemia. Blood 115: 4497-4506.
36. Lunghi P, Giuliani N, Mazzera L, Lombardi G, Ricca M (2008) Targeting MEK/MAPK signal transduction module potentiates ATO-induced apoptosis in multiple myeloma cells through multiple signaling pathways. Blood 112: 2450-2460.
37. Wang R, Xia L, Gabrilove J, Waxman S, Jing Y (2013) Downregulation of Mcl-1 through GSK-3β activation contributes to arsenic trioxide-induced apoptosis in acute myeloid leukemia cells. Leukemia 27: 315-324.
38. Baysan A (2007) Arsenic trioxide induces apoptosis via the mitochondrial pathway by upregulating the expression of Bax and Bim in human B cells. Int J Oncol 30: 313-318.
39. Morales AA, Gutman D, Boise LH (2008) BH3-only proteins Noxa, Bmf, and Bim are necessary for arsenic trioxide-induced cell death in myeloma. Blood 111: 5152-5162.
40. Sharma A, Singh K, Mazumder S, Hill BT, Kalaycio M, et al. (2013) BECN1 and BIM interactions with MCL-1 determine fludarabine resistance in leukemic B cells. Cell Death Dis 4: e628.
41. de la Fuente MT, Casanova B, Moyano JV, Garcia-Gila M, Sanz L, et al. (2002) Engagement of alpha4beta1 integrin by fibronectin induces in vitro resistance of B chronic lymphocytic leukemia cells to fludarabine. J Leukoc Biol 71: 495-502.

15

The Role of Therapeutic Leukapheresis in Hyperleukocytotic AML

Friederike Pastore[1,3,4]*, Alessandro Pastore[1], Georg Wittmann[2], Wolfgang Hiddemann[1,3,4], Karsten Spiekermann[1,3,4]

1 Department of Internal Medicine III, University Hospital Munich, Ludwig-Maximilians-University Munich - Campus Großhadern, Munich, Germany, **2** Department of Transfusion Medicine, University Hospital Munich, Ludwig-Maximilians-University Munich - Campus Großhadern, Munich, Germany, **3** German Cancer Consortium (DKTK), Heidelberg, Germany, **4** German Cancer Research Center (DKFZ), Heidelberg, Germany

Abstract

Purpose: Hyperleukocytosis in AML with leukostasis is a serious life-threatening condition leading to a high early mortality which requires immediate cytoreductive therapy. Therapeutic leukapheresis is currently recommended by the American Society of Apheresis in patients with a WBC>100 G/l with signs of leukostasis, but the role of prophylactic leukapheresis before clinical signs of leukostasis occur is unclear.

Patients: We retrospectively analyzed the role of leukapheresis in 52 patients (median age 60 years) with hyperleukocytotic AML with and without clinical signs of leukostasis. Since leukapheresis was performed more frequently in patients with signs of leukostasis due to the therapeutic policy in our hospital, we developed a risk score for early death within seven days after start of therapy (ED_{d7}) to account for this selection bias and to independently measure the effect of leukapheresis on ED_{d7}.

Results: 20 patients received leukapheresis in combination to chemotherapy compared to 32 patients who received chemotherapy only. In a multivariate logistic regression model for the estimation of the probability of ED_{d7} thromboplastin time and creatinine remained as independent significant parameters and were combined to create an ED_{d7} risk score. The effect of leukapheresis on EDd7 was evaluated in a bivariate logistic regression together with the risk score. Leukapheresis did not significantly change early mortality in all patients with a WBC≥100 G/l.

Discussion: Prophylactic leukapheresis in hyperleukocytotic patients with and without leukostasis did not improve early mortality in our retrospective study. Larger and prospective clinical trials are needed to validate the risk score and to further explore the role of leukapheresis in AML with hyperleukocytosis.

Editor: Robert A. Winn, University of Colorado School of Medicine, United States of America

Funding: The authors have no support or funding to report.

Competing Interests: The authors have declared that no competing interests exist.

* E-mail: Friederike.Pastore@med.uni-muenchen.de

Introduction

Hyperleukocytosis is defined as white blood count (WBC)≥50–100 G/l and occurs in 5–18% of AML [1]. Hyperleukocytosis is often associated with the FAB subtypes M4/M5 and has been shown to be a risk factor for an adverse outcome, a high early death (ED) rate [2] and high relapse rate.

Critical hyperleukocytosis can cause leukostasis, a life-threatening condition with disturbance of microcirculation caused by occlusion of small vessels due to elevated WBC, endothelial adhesion of myeloid blasts and tissue infiltration [3].

Besides the high blood viscosity as a physical mechanism for the microcirculatory disturbances, blast cells have been shown to secrete cytokines (IL-1β and TNF-β) leading to an up-regulation of endothelial adhesion molecules (ICAM-1, VCAM 1, E-selectin) and thus a concomitant adhesion of blasts on the endothelium [3]. Elevated serum lactate levels might represent an early sign of microcirculatory failure [4].

Clinically, leukostasis syndrome most commonly affects the lungs in about 80%, the central nervous system and the kidneys in a rapid progressive often fatal course of disease [5,6]. As treatment of choice, a rapid reduction of the WBC is thought to be mandatory. Therefore chemotherapy is often combined with therapeutic leukapheresis, a physical method to reduce high WBC and blood viscosity.

Leukapheresis is known to be a generally safe procedure. Nevertheless, the placement of a large central venous catheters required for leukapheresis might bear an elevated risk of bleeding, especially since patients are often thrombocytopenic and suffer from coagulopathy [7].

Most authors agree, that leukapheresis does not seem to have an impact on long-term outcome in hyperleukocytotic AML patients with leukostasis [1,8,9]. Nevertheless, the role of leukapheresis on early mortality is contradictory in different studies [1,7–10] and has not been investigated in prospective clinical studies yet.

The aim of our study was to investigate the role of leukapheresis in hyperleukocytotic AML patients treated in our clinical center.

Materials and Methods

Patients

Between January 1999 and August 2012 we identified 69 previously treated or untreated AML patients older than 18 years with hyperleukocytosis (WBC≥100 G/l) admitted to our hospital by a laboratory screen (clinical chemistry data bank). Identified patients were cross-checked with medical records, discharge letters, diagnostics performed in our leukemia laboratory and the leukapheresis records in the department of transfusion medicine. Diagnoses included de novo AML, secondary and therapy-related AML.

Based on the number of 102 AML patients treated in our hospital from Januar 2012 until December 2013 and documented in the AML registry, we have treated about 727 AML patients in the period from January 1999 until August 2012.

Thus, the estimated rate of hyperleukocytotic AML in our center was 9.5%, which is in the range of published data.

The study was approved by our local institution (Internal medicine III, University Hospital LMU Munich). According to the European legislation no written consents are necessary for observational retrospective studies if data contain no personal identifiers and data are analyzed anonymously. Therefore, and because of the retrospective study design, informed consent was waived. All clinical investigations were conducted in accordance with the guidelines of the 2008 Declaration of Helsinki.

Diagnosis

AML diagnosis was established on the basis of standard morphologic and cytochemical examinations of peripheral blood and marrow smears according to the French-American-British (FAB) and the World Health Organization (WHO) criteria.

Furthermore cytogenetic analysis [11], FISH, immunophenotypic analysis of marrow aspirates was performed. Screening of established molecular markers e.g. mutations of *NPM1*, *FLT3-ITD*, *FLT3*-TKD and *MLL-PTD* was performed according standard protocols [12–17].

Statistics

Baseline comparisons between patients with and without therapeutic leukapheresis were calculated using the X^2 for dichotomous variables and the Mann Whitney U test for continuous parameters with SPSS version 20.0. Outcome parameters were calculated using logistic regression and Kaplan Meier plots. Median follow up was calculated using the reversed Kaplan Meier method.

For the assessment of the prognostic effect on ED each parameter was introduced in a univariate logistic regression. All significant univariate parameters (p-value <0.05) where tested pairwise in a bivariate logistic regression model. All significant parameters in bivariate analyses were introduced into a multivariate logistic regression model (p-value <0.05 required for inclusion in multivariate model). Multivariate logistic regression was performed with inclusion of all significant parameters without stepwise selection [18]. To account for the bias of small numbers, a bootstrap multivariate logistic regression model with 999 bootstrap replications was performed [19]. The covariates that remained independently significant in both multivariate models with a significance level of 5%, were used for the establishment of an ED risk score. Their regression coefficients were used for the calculation of the early mortality risk score [18]. For the estimation of the diagnostic quality of the risk score in terms of prediction of ED with a very high specificity and sensitivity and for the determination of the cutoff a receiver operating characteristic (ROC) curve analysis was performed. This area under the curve (AUC) illustrates the test performance reaching from 0.5 (= of no diagnostic value) to 1.0 (= best diagnostic value). For identification of the optimal cutoff between a low risk and a high risk group we defined to achieve a sensitivity and specificity of >75%.

Therapy

All intensively treated patients started with a chemotherapy with low dose cytarabine (100 mg/m^2 or 100 mg absolute) at the day of admission.

Depleting leukapheresis as initial therapeutic regime in hyperleukocytotic AML patients was performed additionally to chemotherapy in patients with laboratory signs of leukostasis e.g. elevated lactate level or elevated troponin since 2004. Between 1999 and 2003 institutional policy for the treatment of hyperleukocytosis did not involve leukapheresis as a routine treatment.

Endpoints

Primary endpoints of our retrospective investigation was mortality within 7 days, after 4 weeks and overall survival (OS), after diagnosis of hyperleukocytosis. Death within the first 7 days was defined as "early death" (ED_{d7}). Secondary endpoints were event-free survival (EFS) for all patients and cumulative incidence of relapse (CIR) for all patients in complete remission (CR). In patients who had undergone allogeneic transplantation OS, EFS and CIR were censored at the start of transplantation.

Furthermore we investigated the degree of blast clearance measured in the bone marrow one week after first induction treatment and the achievement of a complete remission.

Results

Patient characteristics

Fifty-two of 69 patients underwent intensive therapy in a curative intention. In the majority of patients (n = 43/52; 83%) hyperleukocytosis was present at first AML diagnosis. In 9 patients hyperleukocytosis occured at the time of relapse. Twenty patients

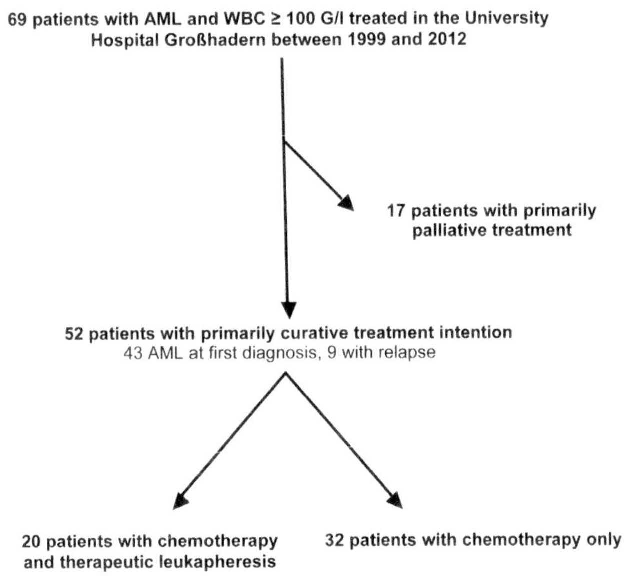

Figure 1. Overview of patient selection.

received chemotherapy and therapeutic leukapheresis, whereas 32 patients were treated with chemotherapy alone (**Figure 1**).

Seventeen patients who underwent primarily palliative treatment where excluded from further analyses. Reasons for palliative treatment at the time of first AML diagnosis included comorbidities (second advanced metastatic cancers e.g. coecum cancer, rectal cancer; severe heart insufficiency NYHA >III, terminal chronic renal failure), age >85 years and reduced baseline performance status according to the Eastern Cooperative Group (ECOG 4).

81% of the 52 intensively treated patients had de novo AML. Secondary AML arising from a myelodysplastic or myeloproliferative syndrome was diagnosed in 6% and therapy-related AML due to a chemotherapy or radio- therapy for a previous malignancy in 13% of patients.

Median age was 60 years, 58% were female. The majority of patients had an Eastern Cooperative Group (ECOG) performance status of 3 or 4 when admitted to the hospital (**Table 1**). Median WBC was 159 G/l and median bone marrow blasts 87%. 45% had an AML M4 or M5 according to the FAB classification of AML.

Pretreatment cytogenetic results were available for 49 patients (94%). By use of the cytogenetic classification of the ECOG [11] 4% had favorable, 84% had intermediate, and 12% had adverse-risk karyotypic abnormalities. According to the ELN classification, 66% of hyperleukocytotic patients belonged to the favorable and Intermediate-I-risk group [20]. 61% were cytogenetically normal. An overview of morphologic, cytogenetic and molecular abnormalities is provided in **Table 2.** Mutational analyses of both, *NPM1* and *FLT3-ITD*, were available in 79% of patients.

More than one third of patients showed clinical signs of leukostasis, such as dyspnea (44%), acute renal failure (25%) and neurologic symptoms (8%). Troponin and lactate levels were elevated in 65% and 23% of patients respectively (**Table 3**).

All patients started with a chemotherapy at the day of hospital admission. 23% received only cytarabine prephase (100 mg/m^2 or 100 mg absolute) since they died before the start of the first induction course, 33% received one induction course and 44% received double induction chemotherapy (**Table S1**). 33% of patients received allogeneic stem cell transplantation. 29% of patients were treated within clinical studies (AMLCG99 [NCT00266136] n = 5, AMLCG2004 [21] n = 4, AMLCG2008 [NCT01382147] n = 7).

Additional therapeutic leukapheresis procedures were performed in 20 of 52 patients. In 18/20 patients leukapheresis was performed once. One patient underwent two and one patient underwent three leukapheresis on a daily basis. In 18/20 patients

Table 1. Patient characteristics of all intensively treated patients with WBC≥100 G/l.

characteristic	n (n = 52)		%
Age (years)			
median		**60**	
range		**21–79**	
Female sex	**30**		**58**
ECOG 3/4	**37**		**84**
De novo AML	**42**		**81**
First diagnosis	**43**		**83**
WBC (G/l)			
median		**159**	
range		**100–322**	
Platelets (G/l)			
median		**45**	
range		**10–149**	
Hemoglobin level (g/dl)			
median		**9.5**	
range		**5.0–14.9**	
LDH level (U/l) n = 46			
median		**996**	
range		**444–7387**	
BM blasts (%) n = 40			
median		**87**	
range		**46–99**	
PB blasts (%) n = 47			
median		**84**	
range		**14*–99**	

Patients with hyperleukocytosis had a reduced ECOG performance status and highly elevated WBC, LDH level and blast counts.
Abbreviations: BM blasts; bone marrow blasts; EOCG, Eastern Cooperative Group; LDH, lactase dehydrogenase; PB blasts; blasts in the peripheral blood; WBC, white blood count.
*one patient with an AML M5A showed 14% of myeloblasts in the peripheral blood, not accounting for the 59% of monoblasts in AML M5.

Table 2. Morphologic, cytogenetic and molecular characteristics of patients with WBC≥100 G/l.

characteristic	n	%
FAB M4/M5	**23/51**	**45**
Cytogenetics		
Cytogenetically normal	**31/49**	**63**
PML-RARA	**2/49**	**4**
CBF-AML	**2/49**	**4**
***MLL*-rearrangements**	**5/49**	**10**
Complex karyotype	**4/49**	**8**
other	**5/49**	**10**
ELN risk		
ELN favorable	**10/45**	**22**
ELN intermediate-I	**20/45**	**44**
ELN intermediate-II	**9/45**	**20**
ELN adverse	**6/45**	**13**
Molecular genetics		
***NPM1*+**	**19/41**	**46**
***FLT3*-ITD+**	**20/46**	**44**
***FLT3*-TKD+**	**3/38**	**8**
***MLL*-PTD+**	**2/42**	**5**

Hyperleukocytotic patients commonly had AML FAB types M4/M5 or ELN favorable or intermediate-I risk.
Abbreviations: FAB, French-American-British classification of AML; ELN, European Leukemia Net classification of AML; *FLT3*-ITD, internal tandem duplication of the *FLT3* gene; *FLT3*-TKD, point mutation at D835 in the *FLT3*-tyrosine kinase domain of the *FLT3* gene; *MLL*-PTD, partial tandem duplication of the *MLL* gene; n, number; *NPM1*, nucleophosmin1.

Table 3. Clinical manifestations of hyperleukocytosis/leukostasis in all patients, patients with therapeutic leukapheresis plus chemotherapy and patients with chemotherapy only.

	All (n = 52)		LA/Chemo (n = 20)		Chemo (n = 32)		*P* LA/Chemo vs Chemo
characteristic	**n**	**%**	**n**	**%**	**n**	**%**	
Creatinine (mg/dl)							
median	1.2		1.2		1.1		n.s.
range	0.6–3.5		0.6–3.0		0.6–3.5		
Troponin (ng/ml) n = 23							
median	0.06		0.12		0.05		0.039
range	0.05–10.90		<0.05–10.90		<0.05–3.99		
Troponin (>0.05 ng/ml) n = 23	15	65	12/14	86	3/9	33	0.010
Lactate (mmol/l) n = 31							
median	1.4		1.7		1.2		n.s.
range	0.3–36.2		0.3–36.2		0.6–4.2		
Lactate (>2.4 mmol/l) n = 31	7	23	4/13	31	3/18	17	n.s.
PTT (sec) n = 51							
median	35		33		36		n.s.
range	20–141		20–141		24–59		
Thromboplastin time (%)							
median	60		51		63		0.005
range	6–85		6–80		39–85		
Fibrinogen (mg/dl) n = 35							
median	253		190		289		n.s.
range	52–577		52–484		71–577		
Antithrombin (%) n = 31							
median	89		73		95		0.002
range	11–129		11–113		58–129		
D-dimer (μg/ml) n = 15							
median	26.9		17.9		32.1		n.s.
range	0.0–40.0		1.7–40.0		0.0–40.0		
Dyspnea n = 46	20	44	14/20	70	6/26	23	0.001
Oxygen requirement n = 46							0.008
none	26	57	6/20	30	20/26	77	
nasal prongs (≤4l O2/min)	10	22	7/20	35	3/26	12	
oxygen mask (>5l O2/min)	7	15	4/20	20	3/26	12	
CPAP/ITN	3	6	3/20	15	0/26	0	
Neurologic derogation n = 50	4	8	4/20	20	0/30	0	0.011
Acute renal failure/HD/HF/Creatinine >1.5 mg/dl	13	25	7	35	6	19	n.s.

Patients receiving leukapheresis and chemotherapy showed significantly more clinical symptoms of leucostasis and a deregulated coagulation compared to the patients receiving chemotherapy only. This reflects the policy of leukapheresis in our hospital, since only patients with signs of leukocytosis underwent leukapheresis. Abbreviations: CPAP, continuous positive airway pressure; HD, hemodialysis; HF, hemofiltration; ITN, intubaton; LA, leukapheresis; PTT, partial thromboplastin time.

(90%) therapeutic leukapheresis was performed at day 0 or 1 after admission to the hospital, 2 patients underwent leukapheresis on day 2 and 4 respectively.

32 of 52 patients with hyperleukocytosis received chemotherapy without leukapheresis.

Median follow up for all patients was 14.9 months (95% confidence interval (CI): 6.3–23.4 months). Median overall survival (OS) was 8.8 months (95% CI: 5.4–12.3 months) in all patients uncensored for allogeneic transplantation and 7.4 months (95% CI: 4.1–10.6 months) when patients were censored at the time of allogeneic transplantation (**Figure 2A**). 8% of patients died within the first 24 hours and 17% within the first seven days after the diagnosis of hyperleukocytosis.

Comparison between patients with and without therapeutic leukapheresis

Since the policy in our hospital was to perform leukapheresis in patients with signs of leukocytosis, there were significant differences with regard to leukostasis parameters such as elevated troponin, dyspnea, oxygen need, neurologic disturbances at initial

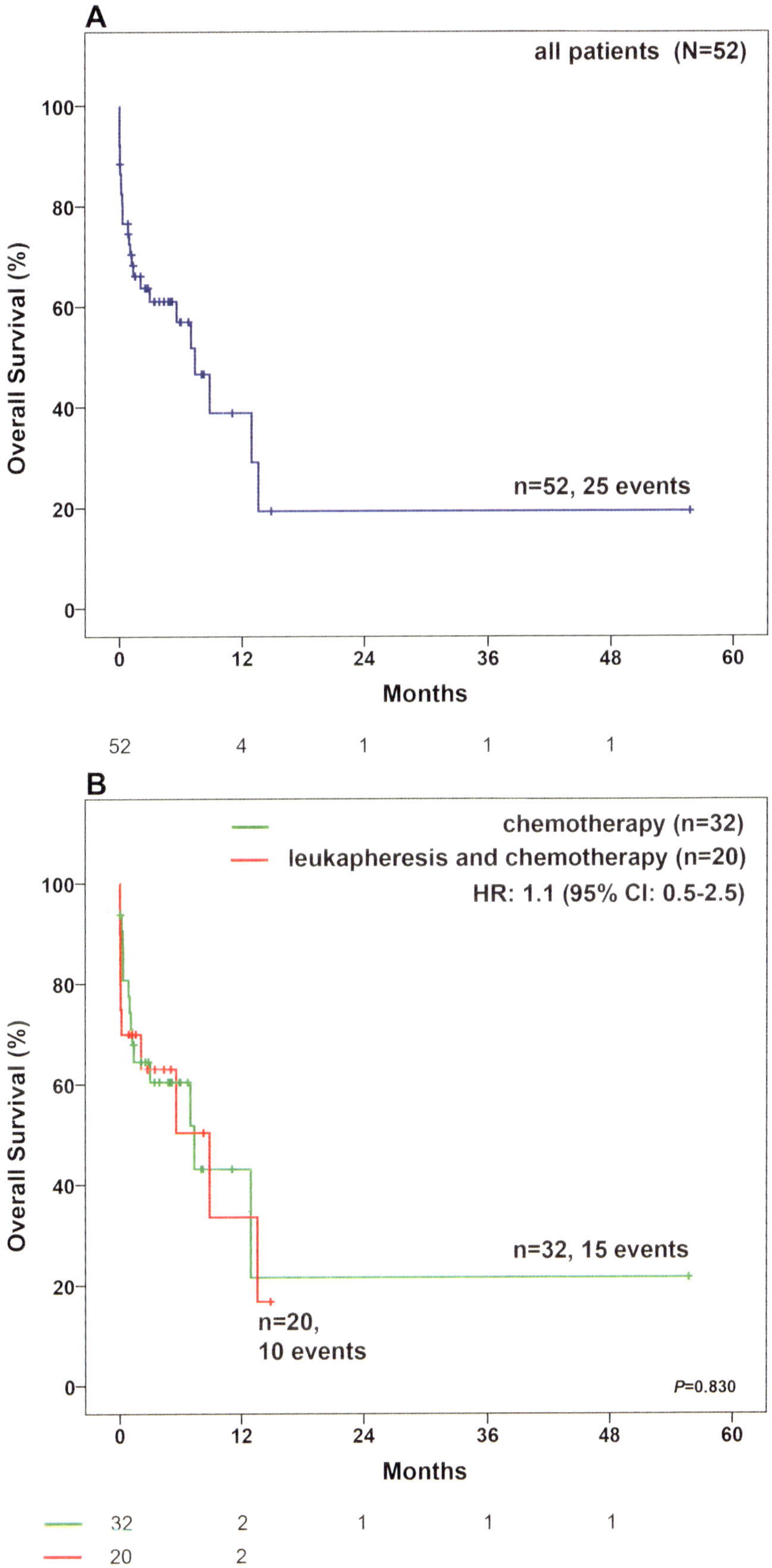

Figure 2. OS in patients with WBC≥100 G/l. (A) in all patients (B) in patients who received either chemotherapy only or chemotherapy combined with leukapheresis. Median OS was 7.4 months (95% CI: 4.1–10.6 months) in all patients, 7.4 months (95% CI: 1.3–13.4 months) in patients receiving chemotherapy only and 8.8 months (95% CI: 1.3–16.4 months) in patients with the combination of chemotherapy and leukapheresis. Abbreviations: CI, confidence interval; HR, Hazard Ratio, OS, Overall survival;

presentation between the 20 patients that were treated with leukapheresis and chemotherapy and the 32 patients with chemotherapy only (**Table 3**). Furthermore WBC (208 G/l vs. 142 G/l, $p = 0.023$) and LDH levels (1568 U/l vs. 845 U/l, $p = 0.030$) were significantly higher in the patients with leukapheresis illustrating the rapid turnover of immature cells. Coagulation was significantly disturbed in the leukapheresis group demonstrated by lower prothrombin time and antithrombin levels (**Table 3**).

There were no statistically significant differences in patients' performance status, sex or the type of AML (de novo AML, AML at first diagnosis, FAB type, cytogenetic risk group, ELN risk group or molecular characteristics). Also, median age in patients receiving leukapheresis combined with chemotherapy (62 years, range 21–79 years) and those receiving chemotherapy only (60 years, range 31–79 years), was not significant different ($p = 0.351$).

The number of induction cycles was significantly different between the two cohorts, especially in patients who did not receive a full induction cycle due to death or life threatening complications (40% in the leukapheresis group vs. 9% in the chemotherapy group).

Leukapheresis was a potent procedure to efficiently reduce WBC below 50 G/l significantly faster compared to chemotherapy alone (median 1 day [0–5 days] compared to 4 days [2–14 days] $p<0.001$) (**Figure S1, Figure 3**). Median reduction of the WBC after one leukapheresis was 77% (42%–90%).

Although patients that underwent therapeutic leukapheresis showed a significant faster reduction of WBC, they displayed a higher death rate within the first 24 hours and a trend to a higher early death rate compared to patients with chemotherapy alone (**Table 4**).

Achievement of an adequate early blast cell clearance or a complete remission as well as long term outcome (OS, EFS, CIR) were not different between the two cohorts (**Figure 2B, Figures S2 and S3**).

In both cohorts, older age was not a significant risk factor for a higher ED_{d7} rate or an impaired OS (data not shown).

Early Complications

Severe complications in the first seven days after the start of the treatment were mainly bleeding events or thromboembolic complications (**Table 5**).

Of all 52 patients, 5 experienced an intracerebral bleeding. Other major causes of bleeding events were located in the upper gastrointestinal tract ($n = 1$), bleeding in the pericard ($n = 1$), the pleura ($n = 1$) and the ascites ($n = 1$), makrohematuria ($n = 1$) and bleeding at central venous catheter puncture sites ($n = 2$). There was no statistical difference in the frequency of bleeding events between patients with and without leukapheresis.

Three patients developed thromboembolic complications such as pulmonary embolism, ischemic cerebral infarction as complication of a total occlusion of the carotid artery and splenic infarction.

In the two patients with the pulmonary embolism and the artery occlusion, the event occurred within 24 hours after leukapheresis.

The frequency of major thromboembolic complications showed a trend to occur more often in patients with leukapheresis.

Patients with ED_{d7} were in a significant worse performance status (ECOG 3/4 63% vs. 3%), showed higher LDH levels (1568 U/l vs. 926 U/l), more signs of leukostasis (dyspnea 78% vs. 35%; acute renal failure 67% vs. 2%) and a higher degree of coagulation disturbances (prothrombin time 40% vs. 60%; fibrinogen 73 mg/dl vs. 283 mg/dl) compared to patients that survived >7 days (**Table S2**).

Development of a risk score for Early Death

To address the question whether patients undergoing therapeutic leukapheresis have a higher early mortality because of the more aggressive disease itself and the adverse patient characteristics (higher ECOG performance status, more clinical signs of leukostasis e.g. dyspnea, neurological impairment, disturbed coagulation) or due to the procedure of leukapheresis itself we developed a risk score for ED_{d7}.

Therefore, we performed univariate logistic regression analyses with the endpoint ED_{d7} for all available clinical parameters (**Table S3**). We used a significance level of 5%.

Parameters with a univariate significant impact on ED_{d7} included a performance status $\geq$ ECOG 3/4, dyspnea vs. non dyspnea, prothrombin time, LDH level and creatinine. Age, sex, de novo AML, AML at first diagnosis, FAB type M4/M5, cytogenetic risk, ELN risk, normal karyotype, *NPM1* mutation status, *FLT3-ITD* mutation status, presence of a *FLT3*-TKD, presence of a *MLL*-PTD, WBC, platelet count, haemoglobin level,

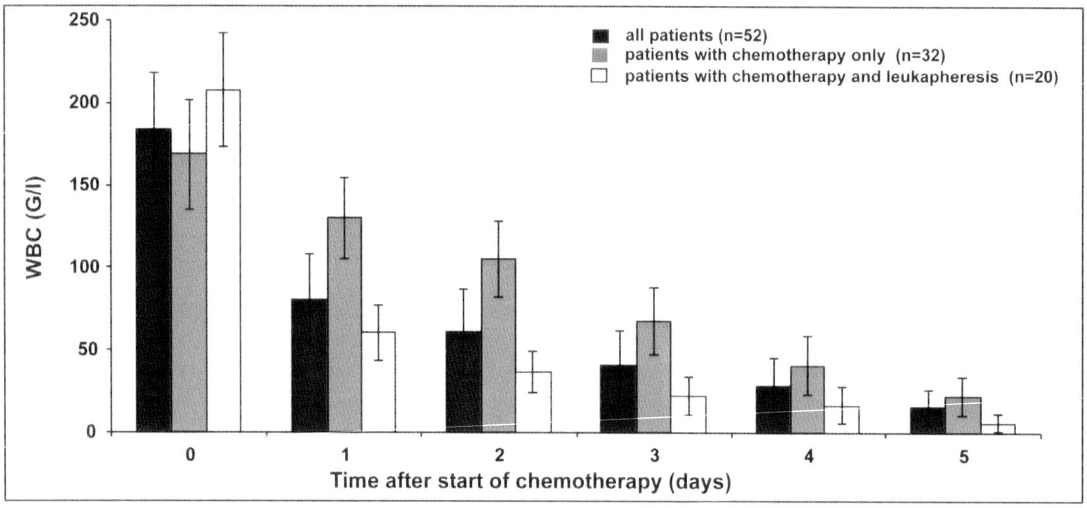

Figure 3. Efficacy of reduction of WBC with chemotherapy only and chemotherapy combined with leukapheresis. Abbreviations: WBC, white blood count.

Table 4. Outcome in all patients, patients with therapeutic leukapheresis plus chemotherapy and patients with chemotherapy only.

	All (n = 52)		LA/Chemo (n = 20)		Chemo (n = 32)		P LA/Chemo vs Chemo
endpoint	**n**	**%**	**n**	**%**	**n**	**%**	
Death							
≤24 hours	5	10	4	20	1	3	0.045
≤7 days	9	17	6	30	3	9	0.056
≤28 days	13	25	6	30	7	22	n.s.
≤100 days	19	37	7	35	12	38	n.s
≤ last follow up	25	48	10	50	15	47	n.s.
Adequate early blast clearance (n = 45)	28	62	9	56	19	66	n.s.
Complete remission (n = 47)	25	53	8	50	17	55	n.s.
Relapse (n = 25)	13	52	4	50	9	53	n.s.

Patients that were treated with leukapheresis and chemotherapy had a higher death rate in the first 24 hours and first 7 days compared to patients receiving chemotherapy only. Reasons for lack of evaluation for remission status in 5 patients were a) no diagnostic bone marrow biopsy due to patient desire (n = 1) b) loss of follow-up (n = 1), end of follow- up (n = 1), no complete induction therapy (n = 2).
Abbreviations: LA, leukapheresis, n, number.

bone marrow (BM) blasts and peripheral blood (PB) blasts, PTT, fibrinogen, antithrombin III, troponin, lactate levels, D-dimer and neurologic derogation displayed no significant effect on ED_{d7}.

In the next step, all univariate significant parameters were tested pairwise in bivariate logistic regression. In pairwise bivariate logistic regression only the prothrombin time, creatinine and the ECOG performance status retained their statistical significance with respect to ED_{d7}.

These three bivariate significant parameters were introduced in an inclusion multivariate logistic regression model with a significance level of 5% with and without 999 bootstrap replications, in which lower ECOG3/4, lower prothrombin time and higher creatinine kept their independent adverse prognostic impact on ED_{d7} (**Table 6**). Due to the incomplete documentation of the ECOG performance status, which was available in only 37/52 patients, and the lack of its significance in multivariate logistic regression with backward Wald stepwise selection, the risk score for ED_{d7} was calculated using the regression coefficients Beta from bivariate regression analysis of creatinine and thromboplastin time:

$$\text{Š } \mathbf{0.093} * \textbf{prothrombin time } (\%) \\ + \mathbf{0.968} * \textbf{creatinine (mg/dl)}$$

The median score was −4.47 (range: −6.84 to 1.68), and the median mortality risk within the first week was 6.7% (range: 0.4% to 99.0%). The risk score showed a highly significant univariate impact when applied into a logistic regression model on ED_{d7}, p = 0.002; Odds Ratio (OR): 2.7; 95% CI: 1.5–5.0).

As an internal control, the risk score was introduced with each parameter (age, gender, WBC, platelet count, hemoglobin level, peripheral blood blasts, bone marrow blasts, LDH, troponin, lactate, PTT, fibrinogen, antithrombin III, D-dimer, AML M4/M5, ELN risk group, cytogenetic risk group, cytogenetically normal AML vs. non cytogenetically normal AML, de novo AML, AML at first diagnosis vs. AML at relapse, *NPM1* mutation status, *FLT3-ITD* mutation status, presence of a *FLT3*-TKD, presence of a *MLL*-PTD, clinical parameters such as dyspnea vs. non dyspnea (oxygen requirement), neurologic derogation, shock and acute

Table 5. Complications within 7 days of treatment.

Complication	LA/Chemo (n = 20)		Chemo (n = 32)		*P*
	n	**%**	**n**	**%**	
Bleeding	7	35	5	16	n.s.
Cerebral bleeding	3	15	2	6	n.s.
Life threatening bleeding	2	10	2	6	n.s.
Thrombosis/Embolism	3	15	0	0	0.024
Without splenic infarction*	2	10	0	0	n.s.

There was a trend to more bleeding events and thromboembolic events within the patients receiving leukapheresis and chemotherapy.
*exact time point of the first manifestation splenic infarction is not clear; it was diagnosed in a CT scan performed after leukapheresis.
Abbreviations: LA, leukapheresis.

Vascular Endothelial Growth Factor A (*VEGFA*) Gene Polymorphisms Have an Impact on Survival in a Subgroup of Indolent Patients with Chronic Lymphocytic Leukemia

Carol Lozano-Santos[1], Jimena Martinez-Velasquez[3], Belen Fernandez-Cuevas[1], Natividad Polo[1], Belen Navarro[1], Isabel Millan[2], Jose Miguel Garcia[4], Rosa Collado[5], Pedro Sanchez-Godoy[6], Felix Carbonell[5], Jose Antonio Garcia-Vela[7], Jose Antonio Garcia-Marco[1¶], Natalia Gomez-Lozano[3*¶]

1 Department of Hematology, Hospital Universitario Puerta de Hierro Majadahonda & Instituto de Investigación Puerta de Hierro Majadahonda (IDIPHIM), Madrid, Spain, **2** Department of Statistics, Hospital Universitario Puerta de Hierro Majadahonda & Instituto de Investigación Puerta de Hierro Majadahonda (IDIPHIM), Madrid, Spain, **3** Group of Immunogenetics, Hospital Universitario Puerta de Hierro Majadahonda & Instituto de Investigación Puerta de Hierro Majadahonda (IDIPHIM), Madrid, Spain, **4** Group of Oncology, Hospital Universitario Puerta de Hierro Majadahonda & Instituto de Investigación Puerta de Hierro Majadahonda (IDIPHIM), Madrid, Spain, **5** Department of Hematology, Consorcio Hospital General Universitario de Valencia, Valencia, Spain, **6** Department of Hematology, Hospital Severo Ochoa de Madrid, Madrid, Spain, **7** Department of Hematology, Hospital Universitario Ramón y Cajal de Madrid, Madrid, Spain

Abstract

Vascular endothelial growth factor (VEGF)-mediated angiogenesis contributes to the pathogenesis of B-cell chronic lymphocytic leukaemia (CLL). We investigated the impact of *VEGFA* gene diversity on the clinical outcome of patients with this disease. A *VEGFA* haplotype conformed by positions rs699947 (–1540C>A), rs833061 (–460T>C) and rs2010963 (405C>G) and two additional single-nucleotide polymorphisms (SNPs), rs3025039 (936C>T) and rs25648 (1032C>T), were analysed in 239 patients at the time of their CLL diagnosis. Here, we showed that homozygosity for rs699947/rs833061/rs2010963 ACG haplotype ($ACG^{+/+}$ genotype) correlated with a reduced survival in CLL patients ($ACG^{+/+}$ vs other genotypes: HR = 2.3, p = 0.002; recessive model). In multivariate analysis, the $ACG^{+/+}$ genotype was identified as a novel independent prognostic factor (HR = 2.1, p = 0.005). Moreover, ACG homozygosity subdivided patients with CLL with otherwise indolent parameters into prognostic subgroups with different outcomes. Specifically, patients carrying the $ACG^{+/+}$ genotype with mutated IgV_H, very low and low-risk cytogenetics, initial clinical stage, CD38 negative status or early age at diagnosis showed a shorter survival ($ACG^{+/+}$ vs other genotypes: HR = 3.5, p = 0.035; HR = 3.4, p = 0.001; HR = 2.2, p = 0.035; HR = 3.4, p = 0.0001 and HR = 3.1, p = 0.009, respectively). In conclusion, *VEGFA* $ACG^{+/+}$ genotype confers an adverse effect in overall survival in CLL patients with an indolent course of the disease. These observations support the biological and prognostic implications of *VEGFA* genetics in CLL.

Editor: Masaru Katoh, National Cancer Center, Japan

Funding: This work was supported by Fundación para la Investigación Biomédica and Fondo de Investigación Sanitaria (FIS CP09-182), Instituto de Salud Carlos III. The authors were funded by the following institutions: NGL by a grant from programa Miguel Servet, Fondo de Investigación Sanitaria, Instituto de Salud Carlos III; CLS by a research grant from Roche Pharma and JMV by Fundación para la Investigación Biomédica Puerta de Hierro. The funders had no role in study design, data collection and analysis, decision to publish, or preparation of the manuscript.

Competing Interests: CLS received funding from Roche Farma for this work and has no other relationships, conditions or circumstances that present potential competing interests related with this work.

* Email: ngomez@idiphim.org

¶ These authors contributed equally to this work.

Introduction

A significant variability in the clinical course of B-cell chronic lymphocytic leukemia (CLL) exists as a result of multiple different pathogenic mechanisms. B cell receptor repertoire skewing and stereotypy and differences in the mutational status of the IgV_H gene demonstrate an antigen-driven process. Multiple genetic lesions associated with CLL (del13q14, trisomy 12, *TP53* deletion, *ATM* deletion, *NOTCH1* and *SF3B1* mutations and others) contribute to the initiation and progression of this leukemia. Recently, there has been a growing interest in determining the impact of microenvironmental interactions, such as angiogenesis, in the pathogenesis and progression of CLL.

Vascular endothelial growth factor (VEGF) is a pro-angiogenic factor with multiple roles in tumour formation that is involved in the pathophysiology of many hematologic disorders, including CLL. Several reports have shown an enhanced microvessel density in the bone marrow and lymph nodes in patients with CLL, as a result of a VEGF-dependent angiogenesis associated with an advanced stage of disease [1–3]. Furthermore, it has also been reported that the resistance to apoptosis of leukemic cells in CLL is mediated by VEGF-dependent autocrine and paracrine mechanisms of cell survival [4–7]. In addition to the angiogenic and antiapoptotic effects on CLL cells, VEGF regulates CLL cell motility [8,9] and the microenvironment-tumor interactions [10,11].

Considerable variation in VEGF expression exists among individuals. However, elevated VEGF levels in the serum or plasma of CLL patients positively correlate with disease progression [12] and such patients are more likely to progress rapidly to a more advanced stage of disease [13]. In addition, high levels of expression of one of its receptors, VEGFR2, correlate with shortened survival [14].

VEGFA is a gene comprised of eight coding exons and several alternative spliced forms that maps to chromosome region 6p1.2. Genetic polymorphisms have been identified outside of the coding region in the 5′ and 3′ flanking regions, and these polymorphisms seem to have an influence on gene expression. SNPs rs699947 (–1540C>A) and rs833061 (–460T>C) reside in the promoter region, rs2010963 (405C>G) and rs25648 (1032C>T) in the 5′UTR and rs3025029 (1689C>T) in the 3′UTR. These polymorphisms have been associated with a variation in the levels of VEGF protein [15–18] and predisposition to cancer development and progression [19–23].

Given the reported association of VEGF levels with certain clinical conditions in this leukemia, the present study evaluated whether an association exists between *VEGFA* genetic variability and its predictive value in determining the prognosis of CLL.

Materials and Methods

Study population

Two hundred and thirty-nine consecutive patients with newly diagnosed CLL from four Hospitals belonging to Grupo GLIMCE in Spain (Hospital Puerta de Hierro Majadahonda, Hospital de Getafe, Hospital Severo Ochoa [Madrid, Spain] and Hospital General [Valencia, Spain]) were enrolled in this retrospective study. Also, 183 age and gender-matched control individuals from the Blood Bank Department of Hospital Puerta de Hierro were analysed in order to evaluate the characteristic distribution of *VEGFA* single nucleotide polymorphisms (SNPs) in Spanish population from the same area. The diagnosis of CLL was based upon standard morphologic and immunophenotypic criteria. Written informed consent was given by participants for their clinical records to be used in this study. This project was approved by the Ethics Committee of Hospital Puerta de Hierro (Comité Ético de Investigación Clínica Hospital Puerta de Hierro Majadahonda). Progression of disease was defined according to NCI-Guidelines criteria [24].

The patient characteristics are summarised in Table 1. Genetic abnormalities were detected by conventional cytogenetics and FISH analysis and stratified as follows: very low-risk (deletion 13q), low-risk (trisomy 12and normal karyotype) and intermediate-risk (deletion 11q) and high-risk (*TP53* deletion) [25]. The mutational status of the IgV_H gene was analysed and classified according to ERIC recommendations [26]. CD38 and ZAP-70 expression was determined by flow cytometry.

Genotyping of *VEGFA* polymorphisms

DNA was extracted from peripheral blood cells using either DNAzol (MRC, Cincinnati, OH) or a Maxwell 16 Blood DNA purification kit (Promega Corp. Madison, CA). *VEGFA* rs699947 (–1540C>A), rs833061 (–460T>C), rs2010963 (405C>G), rs25648 (1032C>T) and rs3025039 (1689C>T) genotyping was performed using TaqMan MGB probes (Applied Biosystems, Foster City, CA). All reactions were performed in a 10 µL PCR reaction with 20 ng of genomic DNA. Allelic discrimination was determined using 7500 Real Time PCR (Applied Biosystems). To validate the genotyping method and haplotype estimation, selected informative samples were analysed by DNA sequencing in a 3130xl Genetic Analyzer Sequencer (Applied Biosystems). Polymorphic positions were named relative to the reference sequence [Genbank: NM_001171630,1].

Statistical Analysis

Individual haplotypes and their frequencies were estimated based upon a Bayesian algorithm using the Phase program (available at http://www.stat.washington.edu/stephens/phase.html[27]). Linkage disequilibrium (LD) analysis was performed using Haploview software. Pearson's χ^2 test was used to evaluate differences in the distribution of *VEGFA* SNPs alleles, haplotypes or genotypes between subgroups of patients based upon clinical or laboratory parameters.

Odds Ratio (OR) values (95% confidence interval) for the relative risks were calculated for alleles, genotypes and haplotypes. Additive, dominant (major homozygous plus heterozygous vs minor homozygous) and recessive (major homozygous vs heterozygous plus minor homozygous) models were applied to detect associations between genotypes and the clinical and molecular variables.

OS (overall survival) was defined as the interval between the date of diagnosis and the time of death due to CLL. The OS times of patients alive at last follow-up or lost to follow-up were censored. The association between the cumulative probability of OS among genotypes or haplotypes was calculated according to the Kaplan-Meier method, while significant differences between survival curves were evaluated with Mantel's log-rank test. Ten variables were screened by univariate analysis. Because some chromosomal aberrations resemble other molecular prognostic factors included as covariates (deletion 11q and deletion 17p corresponds to Δ*ATM* and Δ*TP53*, respectively), these were not included in the multivariate Cox model. CD38 and ZAP-70 were also excluded due to their elevated rate of missing values. All other variables were included in the adjusted analysis to verify their independent prognostic value. Statistical data analyses were performed using the Statistical Package for the Social Sciences (SPSS) software (SPSS 15, Chicago, IL, USA).

Results

Characteristics of *VEGFA* polymorphisms in the patient cohort

We analysed the genotypes of five SNPs of the *VEGFA* gene, rs699947 (–1540C>A), rs833061 (–460T>C) rs2010963 (405C>G), rs3025039 (936C>T) and rs25648 (1032C>T), on the basis of their previous description as genetic markers in other cancers and/or their potential effect on gene expression.

The cohort was comprised of 239 CLL patients with a mean age of 68±12 years and a male:female ratio of 1.32:1. Minor allele frequencies of *VEGFA* polymorphisms in our CLL cohort were > 5% and are summarized in Table 2. We investigated the linkage disequilibrium (LD) of the *VEGFA* polymorphisms in our study population. As the high LD of the four neighboring loci, rs699947, rs833061, rs2010963 and rs25648, was an evidence for shared segregation, we performed a haplotype analysis (data not shown). To perform an in-depth analysis, haplotypes were estimated from the genotypes defined by loci rs699947, rs833061 and rs2010963. The frequencies of the three main groups of haplotypes in the CLL

Table 1. Clinical and molecular characteristics of the CLL patients.

Variable		*N (%)*
Gender	Male	136 (56.9)
	Female	103 (43.1)
Age	<65	116 (48.5)
	>65	123 (51.5)
Binet stage	A	177 (74.1)
	B	51 (21.3)
	C	11 (4.6)
RAI stage	0	116 (48.5)
	I	54 (22.6)
	II	56 (23.4)
	III	6 (2.5)
	IV	7 (2.9)
Treatment	Yes	106 (44.4)
	No	132 (55.2)
	n.d.	1 (0.4)
Status	Dead	81 (33.9)
	Alive	158 (66.1)
Cause of death	Disease	73 (76.8)
	Other	8 (8.4)
Richter	Yes	16 (6.7)
	No	223 (93.3)
Molecular data		
Genetic lesions		
	Very low-risk (del13q)	67 (28.0)
	Low-Risk (NC, +12)	116 (48.5)
	Intermediate-risk (del11q)	20 (8.4)
	High-risk (Δ*TP53*)	36 (15.1)
CD38 expression	Negative	178 (74.5)
	Positive	32 (13.4)
	n.d.	29 (12.1)
ZAP-70	Negative	60 (25.1)
	Positive	50 (20.9)
	n.d.	129 (54.0)
IgV_H genes	M	98 (41)
	UM	124 (51.9)
	n.d.	17 (7.1)

NC: normal karyotype, n.d: not determined.

Table 2. Minor allele frequencies (MAF) of the *VEGF* polymorphisms studied in CLL patients.

Locus	**Alleles**	**Frequencies**
rs699947	C:A	0.45
rs833061	T:C	0.46
rs2010963	G:C	0.35
rs25648	C:T	0.15
rs3025039	C:T	0.13

cohort were ACG (0.39), CTC (0.38) and CTG (0.21), respectively.

All haplotypic and allelic frequencies were highly similar to those presented by a cohort of healthy blood donors from the same area (n = 183, data not shown). Moreover, because the majority of the participants of this study were of Spanish Caucasian origin, all frequencies fall in the same range of series reported in previous studies of other populations of white ethnicity [20,28,29].

VEGFA genotypes and CLL survival

We investigated the prognostic value of *VEGFA* variants in relation to patients' overall survival (OS). For this, we monitored the entire cohort of 239 patients diagnosed from January 1997 to December 2010, with a median follow-up of 63.2 months (1.4–179.4) and a five-year survival of 77.4%. In this cohort, we studied the prognostic value of the *VEGFA* rs699947/rs833061/rs2010963 and rs3025039 and rs25648 polymorphisms (Fig. 1).

Comparison of their genotypes in a recessive genetic model showed that patients with the homozygous rs699947/rs833061/rs2010963 ACG genotype ($ACG^{+/+}$) presented an increased mortality rate compared with patients with other genotypes (Fig. 1A). The median OS of patients with the $ACG^{+/+}$ genotype was 84.3 months compared with 173.1 months ($p = 0.001$) for patients with other genotypes ($ACG^{\times/-}$ = 1 copy ACG [$ACG^{+/-}$] + no copies ACG [$ACG^{-/-}$]). The adverse effect observed for the ACG haplotype appears to be recessive because patients with 1 copy of the risk haplotype ($ACG^{+/-}$ genotypes) and in the absence of the risk genotype ($ACG^{-/-}$ genotypes) behaved similarly, and no significant difference in median OS was observed between both groups (not reached vs 173.1 months, $p = 0.92$, Fig. 1B).

In addition to *VEGFA* genetics, other previously reported variables were also significant epidemiological, clinical and molecular risk factors in OS prediction in our cohort: clinical stage (Binet), IgV_H mutational status, *ATM* deletions, *TP53* disruptions, cytogenetic abnormalities, CD38 status and age at diagnosis (data not shown).

In the multivariate Cox regression model for OS, the conventional variables that showed an independent prognostic value were IgV_H mutational status, *ATM* deletions, *TP53* deletions and age of diagnosis. Additionally, the *VEGFA* $ACG^{+/+}$ genotype was identified as a novel prognostic parameter in OS, independent of other known factors (adjusted HR = 2.1, $p = 0.005$, Table 3).

Influence of VEGF genetic polymorphisms on clinical and molecular low-risk CLL subgroups

To identify protective or risk interactions, a review of the distribution of *VEGFA* variability in different subgroups of CLL was undertaken and revealed an asymmetric frequency of the $ACG^{+/+}$ genotypes in patients with different mutational status of the IgV_H genes (n = 222). The frequency of haplotype ACG defined by loci rs699947/rs833061/rs2010963 was 0.49 in the group of patients with poor prognosis (unmutated IgV_H genes; UM-CLL) and 0.38 in patients with favourable prognosis (mutated IgV_H genes; M-CLL). No asymmetries in the distribution of the haplotype ACG was found between groups defined by other epidemiological, clinical or molecular parameters.

Comparison in a recessive genetic model of the *VEGFA* rs699947/rs833061/rs2010963 genotypes (ACG+/+ vs ACG×/−) showed that homozygosity for the ACG haplotype was associated with forms of the disease with a worse prognosis. The $ACG^{+/+}$ genotype was 2.5 times more common among individuals with unfavourable prognosis (UM-CLL) relative to other genotypes (OR = 2.5, two-sided $p = 0.012$). These recessive genetic associations do not denote an allele-dose effect as frequencies of heterozygous genotypes are not increased in the UM-CLL group (see Table 4). No statistical associations were found between the $ACG^{+/+}$ genotype and other clinical or molecular variables analysed. Allele or genotype frequencies of polymorphisms rs3025039 and rs25648 also failed to associate with any of the analysed groups (data not shown).

As the aforementioned $ACG^{+/+}$ genotype was asymmetrically distributed in UM-CLL and M-CLL patients, we analysed the OS independently in the two groups. We did not observe any influence of the $ACG^{+/+}$ genotype on the OS of the UM-CLL group, but conversely, in the group of patients with a favourable outcome (M-CLL), this genotype significantly correlated with a shorter survival (median OS: $ACG^{+/+}$ = 105.5 months vs $ACG^{\times/-}$ = not reached; $p = 0.025$; Fig. 2). To further investigate a possible biological influence of this *VEGFA* genotype on the outcome of low-risk CLL, we performed the analysis within groups of patients defined by other markers of indolent course. We categorized our group of CLL patients by age at diagnosis, cytogenetic abnormalities, CD38 status or Binet stage (Fig. 2). Similarly to the subgroup with favourable $IgVH$ mutational status, in patients with very low or low-risk genetics (deletion 13q, trisomy 12, normal karyotype) a

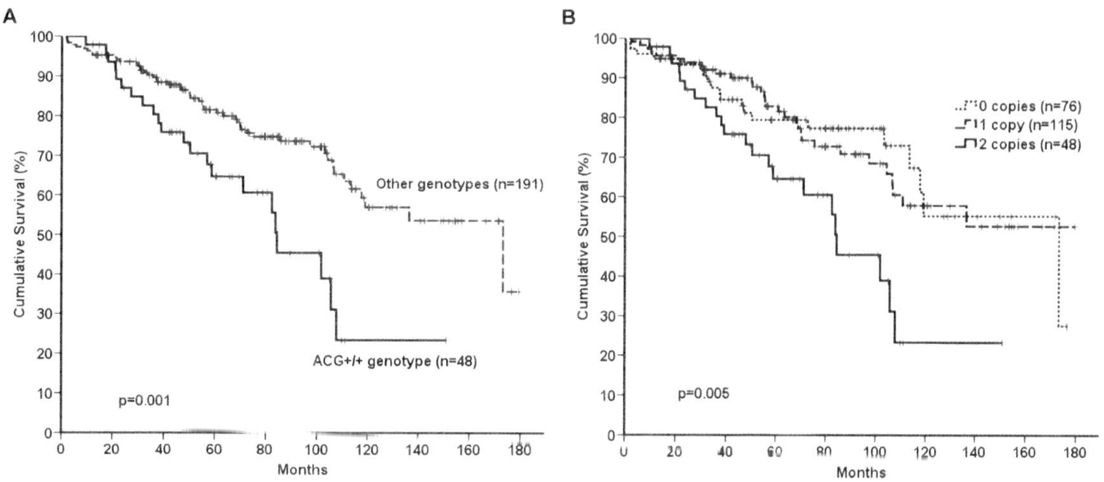

Figure 1. Association of *VEGFA* genotypes and OS of 239 CLL patients. Kaplan-Maier curves according to: (A) a recessive comparison of rs699947/rs833061/rs2010963 $ACG^{+/+}$ genotype and, (B) number of copies of ACG haplotype.

Table 3. Multivariate analysis of the associations between *VEGFA*rs699947/rs833061/rs2010963 genotypes and OS of CLL patients.

Variable	Comparison	HR (95% CI)	p-value
Age at diagnosis[a]	>65 vs <65	2.7 (1.7–4.4)	7×10^{-5}
Binet stage	B+C vs A	2.0 (1.2–3.4)	0.01
TP53 deletion	Yes vs No	3.8 (2.3–6.5)	5×10^{-7}
del11q	Yes vs No	1.9 (1.0–3.5)	0.051
IgVH genes	UM vs M	2.3 (1.3–4.3)	0.01
***VEGF*genotypes[b]**	**ACG$^{+/+}$ vs others**	**2.1 (1.2–3.5)**	**0.005**

[a]Patients aged 65 year have been classified >65.
[b]Haplotype rs699947/rs833061/rs2010963.
HR: hazard ratio, Pos: positive, Neg: negative.

decreased median OS from 173.1 to 101.7 months ($p = 1.3\times10^{-5}$) is associated with the presence of the ACG$^{+/+}$ genotype. Again, the ACG$^{+/+}$ genotype correlated with a reduction in the median OS from 173.1 to 105.5 months ($p = 0.031$) from 173.1 months to 82.3 months ($p = 3.8\times10^{-5}$) and from 173.1 to 84.3 ($p = 0.006$) in patients with an initial clinical stage (Binet A), negative expression of CD38 and age at diagnosis <65 years, respectively. In contrast, *VEGFA* genetics in the defined groups of poor outcome does not have any appreciable influence on the clinical course with the exception of the group of patients older than 65 years, in which the OS tended to be worse for those patients with the homozygous ACG$^{+/+}$ genotype.

Discussion

It has been extensively reported that angiogenesis mediated by the irregular expression of proangiogenic factors such VEGF by leukemic cells plays an important role in the pathogenesis of CLL. In this study, we analysed the contribution of *VEGFA* genetics in the clinical outcome of the leukaemia.

An analysis of the impact on disease progression of *VEGFA* SNPs in our population-based CLL cohort demonstrated that thers699947/rs833061/rs2010963 ACG genotype in homozygosity (ACG$^{+/+}$) is a strong independent predictor of OS. The reduced survival observed in these patients could be related to increased angiogenesis as a result of an enhanced gene expression described for *VEGFA* variants rs699947, rs833061 and rs2010963. This would constitute a potential biological rationalization to the genetic association described in this work. Nonetheless, the justification to our findings could be due to other VEGF-mediated mechanisms of the pathogenesis of CLL. High-expressor *VEGFA* genotypes could increase the resistance to apoptosis, the cell motility or influence the microenvironment to generate more aggressive tumoral cells and consequently contribute to the progression of the leukaemia.

A further analysis of *VEGFA* genetics in CLL subgroups defined by different clinical and molecular parameters assessed an association between the *VEGFA* ACG$^{+/+}$ genotype with a molecular marker of aggressive leukaemia: the unmutated status of the immunoglobulin variable gene segments (IgV_H). IgV_H mutation status parameter discriminates between leukaemia originating from B cells with an immunoglobulin gene submitted (mutated IgV_H) or not (unmutated IgV_H) to somatic hypermutation in the heavy chain variable region genes during ontogeny. Patients with a high number of mutations tend to have a better prognosis (M-CLL) than those with a low number (UM-CLL). Although the ACG$^{+/+}$ genotype is less frequent among M-CLL patients, it correlated with a shorter overall survival within this category. A

Table 4. Distribution of *VEGF* genotypes in B-CLL groups with different mutational status of theIgV_H genes.

Variant	Genotypes	M % (n) (N = 98)	UM %(n) (N = 124)	OR (95% IC)[b]	p-value
haplotype ACG[a]	X/X	35.7 (35)	29.0 (36)	1	
	ACG/X	52.0 (51)	45.2 (56)	1.1 (0.6–2.0)	0.83
	ACG/ACG	12.2 (12)	25.8 (32)	**2.5 (1.2–5.2)**	**0.012**
rs25648	C/C	72.4 (71)	70.2 (87)	1	
	C/T	26.5 (26)	29.0 (36)	0.9 (0.5–1.6)	0.69
	T/T	1.0 (1)	0.8 (1)	0.9 (0.5–1.6)	0.70
rs3025039	C/C	68.4 (67)	78.2 (97)	1	
	C/T	31.6 (31)	20.0 (26)	1.7 (0.9–3.2)	0.08
	T/T	0	0.8 (1)	1.7 (0.9–3)	0.1

M: patients with mutated IgV_H genes, UM: patients with unmutatedIgV_H genes.
OR: odds ratio; CI, confidence interval.
[a]Haplotype rs699947/rs833061/rs2010963. X genotype corresponds to n haplotypes other than ACG (CTC or CTG).
[b]The upper homozygous genotype of each variant is designated the reference with an arbitrary OR value of 1 upon which the OR of the other genotypes are based.
Significant risk factors are shown in bold.

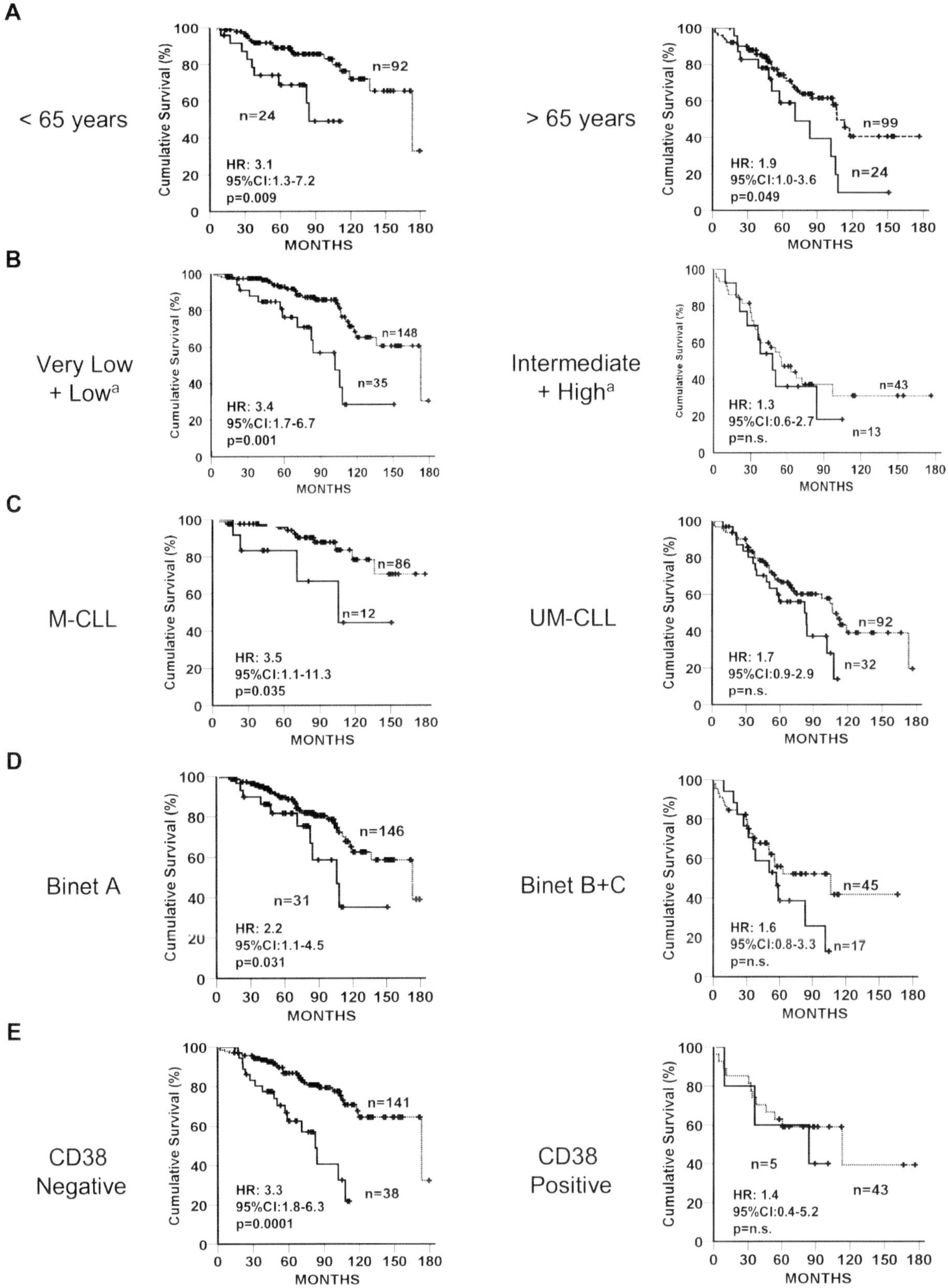

Figure 2. Association of *VEGFA* ACG+/+ genotype and OS of CLL patients with good prognostic features. Kaplan-Maier curves according to *VEGFA* ACG$^{+/+}$ genotype (solid line) and other genotypes (dotted line) in subgroups of patients divided by (A) age at diagnosis, (B) *IgVH* mutational status, (C) Binet stage, (D) CD38 status and, (E) genetic abnormalities. [a]Very low (del13q), low (normal karyotype), intermediate (Δ*ATM*) and high-risk (Δ*TP53*).

similar adverse effect of the $ACG^{+/+}$ genotype in disease progression was found when we stratified patients with good prognostic features such as genetic abnormalities of favourable prognosis, Binet stage A, negative expression of CD38 or early age at diagnosis. These results suggest a potential clinical utility of *VEGFA* genetics as predictors of reduced survival in patients with indolent leukaemia and would allow to further refine the classification of this group of CLL patients. Although our study did not find strong differences in survival associated to the $ACG^{+/+}$ genotype in patients with poor prognostic features, this observation might be perhaps more apparent than real. The large effect of other molecular factors in subgroups of poor outcome may be masking the differences in survival associated with *VEGFA* genotypes. Although we observed a large effect of *VEGFA* genotypes in the subgroup analyses, we were not able to analyse an independent cohort of CLL patients to confirm these differences in survival. In this manner, further studies in other CLL cohorts should be performed to validate these results and would be of relevant interest the analysis of *VEGFA* genetics and CLL in other ethnic groups. To date, exist few reports studying *VEGFA* polymorphisms as prognostic markers of CLL. A recent publication of a case-control study in a Polish CLL cohort [30], described an increased frequency of the rs3025039_allele T in patients with advanced stage (Rai III/IV) compared to healthy individuals.

A previous work by Pepper *et al* [31], found an anti-apoptotic over-expression of VEGF in CLL cells with high levels of CD38, which was associated to the reduced prognosis of the CD38-positive patients. However, we found a similar distribution of the *VEGFA* polymorphisms in patients with different CD38 expression levels indicating that the elevated VEGF expression of this subgroup is not a result of their *VEGFA* genetic background.

The *VEGFA* gene 5′-flanking region is highly variable and contains strongly linked polymorphisms. This increased diversity complicates the characterization of *VEGFA* haplotypes in the promoter region, but some of these linkages are consistently preserved and associated with disease and high *VEGFA* expression [18,23]. Alleles A of rs699947 and C of rs833061 are associated with an upstream 18-nucleotide insertion that could modify the binding of factors in the *VEGFA* promoter. It has therefore been hypothesized that it could be responsible for the enhanced expression of this gene [20]. It would be interesting to perform further studies analysing the *VEGFA* levels in serum, the vascularity in the bone marrow and/or the resistance to apoptosis of CLL cells of patients with the VEGFA ACG+/+ genotype in order to explore the implication of this genotype in the physiopathology of the leukemia. A previous report [1], described an increased vascularity in the UM-CLL subset establishing subsequently a relation of a progressive phenotype of the leukaemia with an enhanced or aggressive angiogenic environment. This observation could be the result of the association of the UM-CLL subgroup with the high-expressor *VEGFA* $ACG^{+/+}$ genotype that we have reported in this work.

The implication of the presence of increased vascularity in the bone marrow has been described in the outcome of various haematological diseases [32,33]. This led to the study of the clinical significance of *VEGFA* genetics in other hematologic malignancies. In acute myeloid leukaemia, the rs699947/rs833061/rs2010963 CTG haplotype and rs3025029 C/C genotype influence the leukaemia-free survival (LFS), event-free survival (EFS) and overall survival (OS) of patients [34]. In chronic myeloid leukaemia, the rs699947 A/A and rs833061 C/C genotypes correlate with progression to advanced disease [35]. *VEGFA* polymorphisms also associate with clinical parameters in non-Hodgkin's lymphoma (NHL). In these patients, rs699947 CA and CA + AA genotypes and rs3025039 TT genotypes, as well as, rs699947 A and rs3025039 T alleles are associated with decreased risk for invasion [36]. Furthermore, rs3025039 T allele was found more frequently in NHLs with worse prognosis (patients with International Prognostic Index (IPI)-3 and/or 4) [37].

Elevated serum levels of its receptor, VEGF-R2 were also associated with lymphocytosis, severe anaemia and shortened survival in CLL [14]. These results also support the role of the VEGF system in this leukaemia and suggest a potential benefit in evaluating polymorphisms in *VEGF-R2* that might have an impact on CLL outcome.

It has been shown that disruption of proangiogenic factors can inhibit tumour vessel density and growth, and the combination of anti-angiogenic agents with other drugs has certain synergetic effects in improving the OR rate in solid tumours. Although, results of the first clinical trials evaluating anti-VEGF therapy for patients with CLL indicate a lack of efficacy in patients with relapsed/refractory CLL [38], combining VEGF blocking with conventional treatments may be a potential therapeutic approach for patients with CLL. In addition to the hypothetical use of *VEGFA* SNPs to predict the clinical outcome for CLL, these polymorphisms could be used as markers of clinical efficacy for chemoimmunotherapy with novel agents targeting VEGF or its receptor (VEGFR) to prevent leukaemia progression [39].

In conclusion, *VEGFA* genetic diversity appears to influence the physiopathology of CLL. The genotyping of polymorphisms in this gene can be performed easily using a rapid PCR method and, together with other parameters, these genetic markers might be utilized both in clinical practice and in further studies of CLL to upgrade patients' prognosis and select target therapies.

Acknowledgments

We are indebted to all individuals who kindly donated blood samples and to the blood bank, Biobank staff and all technicians in the Molecular Cytogenetics laboratory of the Hospital Puerta de Hierro who helped with the sample collection and characterization. We are also grateful to Teresa Hernando and Jose Luis Bueno who helped with the epidemiologic aspects of the work.

Author Contributions

Conceived and designed the experiments: NGL. Performed the experiments: CLS JMV. Analyzed the data: JAGM NGL. Wrote the paper: NGL. Obtained the cytogenetic and molecular data: BFC NP RC JAGM. Provided clinical cases to the study: PSG FC JAGV BN JAGM. Performed the immunophenotyping analyses: JAGV. Reviewed the statistical analysis: IM JMG. Analysed the data: NGL JAGM CLS.

References

1. Maffei R, Martinelli S, Castelli I, Santachiara R, Zucchini P, et al (2010) Increased angiogenesis induced by chronic lymphocytic leukemia B cells is mediated by leukemia-derived Ang2 and VEGF. Leuk Res 34: 312–321. S0145-2126(09)00319-1 [pii];10.1016/j.leukres.2009.06.023 [doi].
2. Kini AR, Kay NE, Peterson LC (2000) Increased bone marrow angiogenesis in B cell chronic lymphocytic leukemia. Leukemia 14: 1414–1418.
3. Peterson L, Kini AR (2001) Angiogenesis is increased in B-cell chronic lymphocytic leukemia. Blood 97: 2529.
4. Farahani M, Treweeke AT, Toh CH, Till KJ, Harris RJ, et al (2005) Autocrine VEGF mediates the antiapoptotic effect of CD154 on CLL cells. Leukemia 19: 524–530. 2403631 [pii];10.1038/sj.leu.2403631 [doi].
5. Bairey O, Boycov O, Kaganovsky E, Zimra Y, Shaklai M, et al (2004) All three receptors for vascular endothelial growth factor (VEGF) are expressed on B-

chronic lymphocytic leukemia (CLL) cells. Leuk Res 28: 243 248. S014521260300256X [pii].
6. Lee YK, Bone ND, Strege AK, Shanafelt TD, Jelinek DF, et al (2004) VEGF receptor phosphorylation status and apoptosis is modulated by a green tea component, epigallocatechin-3-gallate (EGCG), in B-cell chronic lymphocytic leukemia. Blood 104: 788 794. 10.1182/blood-2003-08-2763 [doi];2003-08-2763 [pii].
7. Gehrke I, Gandhirajan RK, Poll-Wolbeck SJ, Hallek M, Kreuzer KA (2011) Bone marrow stromal cell-derived vascular endothelial growth factor (VEGF) rather than chronic lymphocytic leukemia (CLL) cell-derived VEGF is essential for the apoptotic resistance of cultured CLL cells. Mol Med 17: 619 627. molmed.2010.00210 [pii];10.2119/molmed.2010.00210 [doi].
8. Till KJ, Spiller DG, Harris RJ, Chen H, Zuzel M, et al (2005) CLL, but not normal, B cells are dependent on autocrine VEGF and alpha4beta1 integrin for chemokine-induced motility on and through endothelium. Blood 105: 4813 4819. 2004-10-4054 [pii];10.1182/blood-2004-10-4054 [doi].
9. Ugarte-Berzal E, Redondo-Munoz J, Eroles P, del Cerro MH, Garcia-Marco JA, et al (2010) VEGF/VEGFR2 interaction down-regulates matrix metallo-proteinase-9 via STAT1 activation and inhibits B chronic lymphocytic leukemia cell migration. Blood 115: 846 849. blood-2009-08-239426 [pii];10.1182/blood-2009-08-239426 [doi].
10. Edelmann J, Klein-Hitpass L, Carpinteiro A, Fuhrer A, Sellmann L, et al (2008) Bone marrow fibroblasts induce expression of PI3K/NF-kappaB pathway genes and a pro-angiogenic phenotype in CLL cells. Leuk Res 32: 1565 1572. S0145-2126(08)00126-4 [pii];10.1016/j.leukres.2008.03.003 [doi].
11. Ghosh AK, Secreto CR, Knox TR, Ding W, Mukhopadhyay D, et al (2010) Circulating microvesicles in B-cell chronic lymphocytic leukemia can stimulate marrow stromal cells: implications for disease progression. Blood 115: 1755 1764. blood-2009-09-242719 [pii];10.1182/blood-2009-09-242719 [doi].
12. Molica S, Vitelli G, Levato D, Gandolfo GM, Liso V (1999) Increased serum levels of vascular endothelial growth factor predict risk of progression in early B-cell chronic lymphocytic leukaemia. Br J Haematol 107: 605 610. bjh1752 [pii].
13. Gora-Tybor J, Blonski JZ, Robak T (2005) Circulating vascular endothelial growth factor (VEGF) and its soluble receptors in patients with chronic lymphocytic leukemia. Eur Cytokine Netw 16: 41 46.
14. Ferrajoli A, Manshouri T, Estrov Z, Keating MJ, O'Brien S, et al (2001) High levels of vascular endothelial growth factor receptor-2 correlate with shortened survival in chronic lymphocytic leukemia. Clin Cancer Res 7: 795 799.
15. Koukourakis MI, Papazoglou D, Giatromanolaki A, Bougioukas G, Maltezos E, et al (2004) VEGF gene sequence variation defines VEGF gene expression status and angiogenic activity in non-small cell lung cancer. Lung Cancer 46: 293 298. S0169500204002053 [pii];10.1016/j.lungcan.2004.04.037 [doi].
16. Prior SJ, Hagberg JM, Paton CM, Douglass LW, Brown MD, et al (2006) DNA sequence variation in the promoter region of the VEGF gene impacts VEGF gene expression and maximal oxygen consumption. Am J Physiol Heart Circ Physiol 290: H1848 H1855. 01033.2005 [pii];10.1152/ajpheart.01033.2005 [doi].
17. Renner W, Kotschan S, Hoffmann C, Obermayer-Pietsch B, Pilger E (2000) A common 936 C/T mutation in the gene for vascular endothelial growth factor is associated with vascular endothelial growth factor plasma levels. J Vasc Res 37: 443 448. 54076 [pii];54076 [doi].
18. Watson CJ, Webb NJ, Bottomley MJ, Brenchley PE (2000) Identification of polymorphisms within the vascular endothelial growth factor (VEGF) gene: correlation with variation in VEGF protein production. Cytokine 12: 1232 1235. 10.1006/cyto.2000.0692 [doi];S1043-4666(00)90692-6 [pii].
19. Awata T, Inoue K, Kurihara S, Ohkubo T, Watanabe M, et al (2002) A common polymorphism in the 5′-untranslated region of the VEGF gene is associated with diabetic retinopathy in type 2 diabetes. Diabetes 51: 1635 1639.
20. Brogan IJ, Khan N, Isaac K, Hutchinson JA, Pravica V, et al (1999) Novel polymorphisms in the promoter and 5′ UTR regions of the human vascular endothelial growth factor gene. Hum Immunol 60: 1245 1249. S0198-8859(99)00132-9 [pii].
21. Hansen TF, Spindler KL, Lorentzen KA, Olsen DA, Andersen RF, et al (2010) The importance of −460 C/T and +405 G/C single nucleotide polymorphisms to the function of vascular endothelial growth factor A in colorectal cancer. J Cancer Res Clin Oncol 136: 751 758. 10.1007/s00432-009-0714-1 [doi].
22. Jain L, Vargo CA, Danesi R, Sissung TM, Price DK, et al (2009) The role of vascular endothelial growth factor SNPs as predictive and prognostic markers for major solid tumors. Mol Cancer Ther 8: 2496 2508. 1535-7163.MCT-09-0302 [pii];10.1158/1535-7163. MCT-09-0302 [doi].
23. Stevens A, Soden J, Brenchley PE, Ralph S, Ray DW (2003) Haplotype analysis of the polymorphic human vascular endothelial growth factor gene promoter. Cancer Res 63: 812 816.
24. Cheson BD, Bennett JM, Grever M, Kay N, Keating MJ, et al (1996) National Cancer Institute-sponsored Working Group guidelines for chronic lymphocytic leukemia: revised guidelines for diagnosis and treatment. Blood 87: 4990 4997.
25. Rossi D, Rasi S, Spina V, Bruscaggin A, Monti S, et al (2013) Integrated mutational and cytogenetic analysis identifies new prognostic subgroups in chronic lymphocytic leukemia. Blood 121: 1403 1412. blood-2012-09-458265 [pii];10.1182/blood-2012-09-458265 [doi].
26. Ghia P, Stamatopoulos K, Belessi C, Moreno C, Stilgenbauer S, et al (2007) ERIC recommendations on IGHV gene mutational status analysis in chronic lymphocytic leukemia. Leukemia 21: 1 3. 2404457 [pii];10.1038/sj.leu.2404457 [doi].
27. Stephens M, Smith NJ, Donnelly P (2001) A new statistical method for haplotype reconstruction from population data. Am J Hum Genet 68: 978 989. S0002-9297(07)61424-4 [pii];10.1086/319501 [doi].
28. Freathy RM, Weedon MN, Shields B, Hitman GA, Walker M, et al (2006) Functional variation in VEGF is not associated with type 2 diabetes in a United Kingdom Caucasian population. JOP 7: 295 302. v07i03a05 [pii].
29. Girnita DM, Webber SA, Ferrell R, Burckart GJ, Brooks MM, et al (2006) Disparate distribution of 16 candidate single nucleotide polymorphisms among racial and ethnic groups of pediatric heart transplant patients. Transplantation 82: 1774 1780. 10.1097/01.tp.0000250656.33731.08 [doi];00007890 200612270 00046 [pii].
30. Wrobel T, Mazur G, Dzietczenia J, Gebura K, Kuliczkowski K, et al (2013) VEGF and bFGF gene polymorphisms in Polish patients with B-CLL. Med Oncol 30: 456. 10.1007/s12032-013-0456-4 [doi].
31. Pepper C, Ward R, Lin TT, Brennan P, Starczynski J, et al (2007) Highly purified CD38+ and. Leukemia 21: 687 696. 2404587 [pii];10.1038/sj.leu.2404587 [doi].
32. Aguayo A, Kantarjian H, Manshouri T, Gidel C, Estey E, et al (2000) Angiogenesis in acute and chronic leukemias and myelodysplastic syndromes. Blood 96: 2240 2245.
33. Hussong JW, Rodgers GM, Shami PJ (2000) Evidence of increased angiogenesis in patients with acute myeloid leukemia. Blood 95: 309 313.
34. Kim DH, Lee NY, Lee MH, Sohn SK, Do YR, et al (2008) Vascular endothelial growth factor (VEGF) gene (VEGFA) polymorphism can predict the prognosis in acute myeloid leukaemia patients. Br J Haematol 140: 71 79. BJH6887 [pii];10.1111/j.1365 2141.2007.06887. x [doi].
35. Kim DH, Xu W, Kamel-Reid S, Liu X, Jung CW, et al (2010) Clinical relevance of vascular endothelial growth factor (VEGFA) and VEGF receptor (VEGFR2) gene polymorphism on the treatment outcome following imatinib therapy. Ann Oncol 21: 1179 1188. mdp452 [pii];10.1093/annonc/mdp452 [doi].
36. Diao LP, Yu XM, Gao YH, Li Y, Liu HS, et al (2009) Association of VEGF genetic polymorphisms with the clinical characteristics of non-Hodgkin's lymphoma. J Cancer Res Clin Oncol 135: 1473 1481. 10.1007/s00432-009-0650-0 [doi].
37. Wrobel T, Mazu G, Dzietczenia J, Gebura K, Kuliczkowski K, et al (2013) VEGF and bFGF gene polymorphisms in patients with Non-Hodgkin's lymphoma. BioMed Research International 2013: 159813. 10.1155/2013/159813 [doi].
38. Shanafelt T, Zent C, Byrd J, Erlichman C, LaPlant B, et al (2010) Phase II trials of single-agent anti-VEGF therapy for patients with chronic lymphocytic leukemia. Leuk Lymphoma 51: 2222 2229. 10.3109/10428194.2010.524327 [doi].
39. Shanafelt TD, Byrd JC, LaPlant B, Zent CS, Call T, et al (2009) Pretreatment angiogenic cytokines predict response to chemoimmunotherapy in patients with chronic lymphocytic leukaemia. Br J Haematol 146: 660 664. BJH7811 [pii];10.1111/j.1365-2141.2009.07811.x [doi].

Inhibition of c-Myc Overcomes Cytotoxic Drug Resistance in Acute Myeloid Leukemia Cells by Promoting Differentiation

Xiao-Na Pan[1,2]ᵑ, Jia-Jie Chen[1,2]ᵑ, Le-Xun Wang[1,2], Ruo-Zhi Xiao[1,2], Ling-Ling Liu[1,2], Zhi-Gang Fang[1,2], Quentin Liu[1,2], Zi-Jie Long[1,2]*, Dong-Jun Lin[1,2]*

1 Department of Hematology, Third Affiliated Hospital, Sun Yat-sen University, Guangzhou, China, **2** Sun Yat-sen Institute of Hematology, Sun Yat-sen University, Guangzhou, China

Abstract

Nowadays, drug resistance still represents a major obstacle to successful acute myeloid leukemia (AML) treatment and the underlying mechanism is not fully elucidated. Here, we found that high expression of c-Myc was one of the cytogenetic characteristics in the drug-resistant leukemic cells. c-Myc over-expression in leukemic cells induced resistance to chemotherapeutic drugs, enhanced colony formation capacity and inhibited cell differentiation induced by all-trans retinoic acid (ATRA). Meanwhile, inhibition of c-Myc by shRNA or specific c-Myc inhibitor 10058-F4 rescued the sensitivity to cytotoxic drugs, restrained the colony formation ability and promoted differentiation. RT-PCR and western blotting analysis showed that down-regulation of C/EBPβ contributed to the poor differentiation state of leukemic cells induced by c-Myc over-expression. Importantly, over-expression of C/EBPβ could reverse c-Myc induced drug resistance. In primary AML cells, the *c-Myc* expression was negatively correlated with *C/EBPβ*. 10058-F4, displayed anti-proliferative activity and increased cellular differentiation with up-regulation of C/EBPβ in primary AML cells. Thus, our study indicated that c-Myc could be a novel target to overcome drug resistance, providing a new approach in AML therapy.

Editor: Wei-Guo Zhu, Peking University Health Science Center, China

Funding: This work was supported by the Science and Technology Project of Guangzhou (No. 2012J2200077 to Z.-J. Long), and the Fundamental Research Funds for the Central Universities (No. 11ykpy37 to Z.-J. Long). The funders had no role in study design, data collection and analysis, decision to publish, or preparation of the manuscript.

Competing Interests: The authors have declared that no competing interests exist.

* Email: longzij@mail.sysu.edu.cn (ZJL); lindj@mail.sysu.edu.cn (DJL)

ᵑ These authors contributed equally to this work.

Introduction

Acute myeloid leukemia (AML) is a kind of aberrant clonal hematopoietic malignancy originating from genetic mutations, or epigenetic aberrations in normal hematopoietic progenitors. Although chemotherapy results in clinical remission for AML, drug resistance still represents a huge challenge to achieve effective treatment, especially in relapsed or refractory AML patients [1,2]. Cytostatic drug resistance occurs through different mechanisms, including induction of drug detoxification [3], the over-expression of oncogene or inactivation of tumor suppressor gene [4,5], metabolic disturbance [6,7], as well as existence of leukemia stem cells [8]. Still, the exact mechanisms of drug resistance in leukemia have not been fully investigated. Elucidation of the intrinsic or acquired factors that mediate drug resistance remains of critical importance for the development of novel therapeutic strategies for relapsed or refractory AML patients.

The proto-oncogene *c-Myc* plays a pivotal role in cellular metabolism [9], apoptosis [10], differentiation [11], cell cycle progress [12], and tumorigenesis [13]. *c-Myc* encodes a basic helix-loop-helix leucine zipper transcription factor, which transcripts an array of downstream target genes [14]. c-Myc, as an attractive target for cancer therapy, is aberrantly expressed in a wide variety of human solid tumors [15] as well as leukemia [16]. Study reported that c-Myc over-expression was closely correlated to chemotherapy resistance in salivery carcinoma [17]. Inhibition of c-Myc overcame drug resistance in some cancers, such as Lewis lung carcinoma [18] and melanoma [19]. *c-Myc* antisense oligodeoxynucleotides increased cisplatin sensitivity in metastatic melanoma cell lines inherently resistant to cisplatin [20]. 10058-F4, a targeted inhibitor of c-Myc, was reported to be effective in anti-tumor treatment, such as hepatocellular carcinoma [21] and leukemia [22]. However, the precise role of c-Myc in drug resistance of leukemic cells has not yet been elucidated.

In this study, we identified the effects of c-Myc on drug resistance in leukemic cell lines and AML primary cells. We found that the up-regulated expression of c-Myc in leukemic cells promoted colony formation ability and maintained poor differentiation mediated by suppression of C/EBPβ, leading to drug resistance. Consistently, down-regulation of c-Myc abrogated colony formation capacity of leukemic cells and promoted cellular differentiation. Our study provided a new approach to overcome drug resistance by c-Myc inhibition in AML therapy.

Materials and Methods

Primary AML cell isolation

AML patient samples were obtained with the written informed consent in accordance with the Declaration of Helsinki and the approval by the Medical Ethical Committee of the Third Affiliated Hospital of Sun Yat-sen University. Bone marrow mononuclear cells (BMMCs) were enriched by Ficoll-Hypaque density gradient centrifugation. Refractory and relapsed (R) AML samples was included on the basis of the Chinese edition of NCCN Guidelines (Version 2011).

Cell culture

Primary leukemia BMMCs were resuspended in RPMI 1640 medium (Gibco, Grand Island, NY, USA) containing appropriate antibiotics and 10% fetal bovine serum (FBS, HyClone, Logan, UT, USA). K562 and U937 cell lines were purchased from American Type Culture Collection (ATCC, Manassas.VA, USA). NB4 and drug-resistant NB4-R2 cells were provided by Shanghai Institute of Hematology, Ruijin Hospital. Imatinib (Gleevec) resistant K562 cell line (K562/G) was the gift of Prof. Wen-Lin Huang, Cancer Center of Sun Yat-sen University.

Cell cytotoxicity Assay

Cell cytotoxicity was evaluated by MTT assay according to the manufacture's instruction. Briefly, leukemic cells or primary BMMCs were seeded in the 96-well U-bottomed plate. Subsequently, cells were treated with different drugs at different concentrations for indicated time. After MTT solution was added to each well, cells were incubated at 37°C for another 4 h and the absorbance was finally determined at 490 nm using the microplate reader (BioTek, Vermont, USA).

Colony formation assay

Cells with different drugs treatment were plated in 10% FBS medium with methylcellulose (R&D Systems, Minneapolis, MN, USA) for 6 days. The colony forming units (CFU) were counted using microscopy (IX81, Olympus, Japan), and the colony number was the sum of randomized forty visions.

Retroviral and lentiviral transduction

The MSCV 2.2 vector was kindly provided by Prof. Hua Huang (University of Colorado, Denver, USA). The *c-Myc* and *C/EBPβ* gene were cloned and inserted into the MSCV 2.2 vector. Retrovirus was produced from packaging cell line GP2-293 with the aid of pseudo-envelope vector. Lentiviral vector expressing short hairpins against human *c-Myc* (ShMYC) was constructed within the lentivirus plasmid vector pLL3.7 using the target sequence 5′-CCATAATGTAAACTGCCTCAA-3′. Lentiviral particles were produced by cotransfection of 293T cells with packaging vectors (pMD2.G and pPAX2). The virus supernatants were collected 48 h after transfection.

Cell morphology analysis

Cells were seeded into 6-well plates and incubated with specific drug for indicated time and collected for analysis. Cytospin slides were prepared, and the cells were counterstained with Wright-Giemsa. The morphology of cells was observed by microscopy (7×41, Olympus, Japan).

Western blotting analysis

Total cellular proteins were isolated with lysis buffer. Equal amounts of protein were subjected to SDS-PAGE and transferred to nitrocellulose membranes. The membranes were blocked and then incubated with c-Myc (Santa Cruz Biotechnology, Santa Cruz, CA, USA), C/EBPβ (Abcam, Cambridge, UK) and GAPDH antibody (Cell Signaling Technology Corp, Beverly, MA, USA). The protein bands were visualized using an enhanced chemiluminescence reagent (Sigma, St. Louis, MO, USA), according to the manufacturer's instruction.

Flow cytometry analysis

Analysis of CD11b expression was performed using the PE anti-human CD11b antibody (BD Biosciences, San Jose, CA, USA) for predicting the cellular differentiation.

Nitrotetrazolium blue chloride (NBT) reduction assay

The same amount of cells untreated or treated with ATRA for 72 h were incubated at 37°C for 1 h in RPMI 1640 medium containing 10% FBS and 0.1% NBT (Sigma-Aldrich, MO, USA). The cells were then centrifuged and dissolved in DMSO. The optical density was read at 570 nm.

RNA extraction and PCR analysis

RNA was isolated using Trizol reagent (Invitrogen, Grand Island, NY, USA), and reverse transcribed using M-MuLV reverse transcriptase (Fermentas, St Leon-Roth, Germany). Real-time PCR was performed using SYBR Green qPCR mix (Toyabo, Osaka, Japan) on Applied Biosystems 7500 Fast Real-Time PCR thermocycler (Applied Biosystems, Foster City, CA, USA) and quantified using ABI 7500 software.

Statistical analysis

Data were presented as mean ± SD. Statistical analysis was performed using SPSS v. 16.0 (SPSS, Inc.) and GraphPad Prism 6 (GraphPad Software, Inc.). A value of $p<0.05$ was considered statistically.

Results

c-Myc is high expressed in drug resistant leukemic cells

To find the cytogenetic characteristics in drug-resistant leukemic cells, two drug-resistant leukemic cell lines were applied for detecting the properties. NB4-R2 and K652/G were respectively resistant to all-trans-retinoic acid (ATRA) and imatinib, compared with their parental cell lines (NB4 and K562), as shown in Figure S1. The anti-proliferative effect of cytarabine (Ara-C), daunomycin (DNR) or doxorubicin (Doxo), clinical cytotoxic drugs for treating AML, was detected by MTT assay (Figure 1A). The IC50 values of Ara-C, DNR or Doxo at 48 h were 0.3900 μM, 0.2097 μg/ml or 0.0469 μg/ml respectively for NB4, 1.4770 μM, 0.4540 μg/ml or 0.0838 μg/ml for NB4-R2, 0.8010 μM, 0.3325 μg/ml or 0.0827 μg/ml for K562, and 6.0368 μM, 0.7375 μg/ml or 0.2063 μg/ml for K562/G. The result showed that NB4-R2 and K652/G were both resistant to Ara-C, DNR or Doxo, indicating that the two resistant leukemic cells had a broad-spectrum of resistance to clinical cytotoxic drugs. The colony number of NB4-R2 cells was more than that of NB4 cells under 6 days' culture (Figure 1B-a). Similar phenomenon was observed in K562/G cells compared to K562 cells (Figure 1B-b). The data indicated drug-resistant cell lines also displayed increased colony formation capacity. Chemotherapy resistance was closely correlated to *c-Myc* amplification, we thus testify whether c-Myc over-expression was involved in the drug-resistant leukemic cells. Western blotting assay revealed that the expression level of c-Myc was higher in drug-resistant cells (NB4-R2 and K562/G) than in the control cells (Figure 1C), suggesting that high c-Myc expression was correlated with enhanced drug-resistance and colony formation capacity in leukemic cells.

c-Myc over-expression contributes to drug resistance and high colony formation capacity in leukemic cells

In order to identify the effect of c-Myc on drug resistance and colony formation in leukemia, we constructed the stable leukemic cell line with c-Myc over-expression or knock-down for colony formation assay and drug sensitivity test. The stable leukemic cell line with c-Myc over-expression (NB4/MYC) was derived from the drug-sensitive NB4 cells infected with MSCV retrovirus with *c-Myc* gene while NB4 cells with MSCV-GFP vector was used as the control (NB4/GFP). Lentiviral vector expressing short hairpins against human *c-Myc* (ShMYC) was used to reduce c-Myc expression in drug-resistant cell line NB4-R2 (NB4-R2 ShMYC), while lentiviral virus with the non-target ShRNA acted as the control (NB4-R2 Con). Western blotting showed that c-Myc expression was increased in NB4/MYC cells, while decreased in NB4-R2 ShMYC (Figure 2A). Next, the colony formation assay showed that c-Myc over-expression enhanced the colony formation ability in NB4 cells, and that reduced c-Myc expression restrained the colony formation in drug-resistant cells NB4-R2, as shown in Figure 2B. Drug sensitivity test based on MTT assay was performed to testify the cytotoxic effect with Ara-C, DNR or Doxo treatment when up- or down-regulation of c-Myc in leukemic cells. Cells were treated with Ara-C (0.1 μM), DNR (0.2 μg/ml) or Doxo (0.04 μg/ml) for 48 h. The rate of cell viability of NB4/GFP vs NB4/MYC in treatment with the indicated concentration of Ara-C, DNR or Doxo was 61.38%±3.26% vs 70.86%±3.75%, 59.82%±4.51% vs 68.37%±4.13%, or 60.85%±4.85% vs 80.64%±3.83% respectively, while the rate of NB4-R2 Con vs NB4-R2 ShMYC was 69.57%±2.12% vs 47.41%±1.74%, 80.89%±2.38% vs 67.19%±2.14%, or 80.70%±2.32% vs 60.21%±2.37% respectively, as shown in Figure 2C. Thus, increased c-Myc expression in NB4 cells promoted drug resistance to Ara-C, DNR or Doxo. In contrast, decreased c-Myc expression in drug-resistant cells NB4-R2 rescued the sensitivity to the cytotoxic drugs. Similar phemonemon was also observed in U937 cells (Figure S2A–2C).

c-Myc inhibits cell differentiation induced by ATRA

c-Myc acted as a key transcriptional regulator to maintain stemness in cancer stem like cells [23,24]. c-Myc was also proposed to play a role in the transition from proliferation to differentiation in oligodendrocyte progenitor cells [25]. To explain the mechanism that high c-Myc expression induced drug resistance and promoted colony formation capacity in leukemic cells, we used the cell differentiation model of NB4 cells induced by ATRA. The result showed that the percentage of CD11b-positive cells induced by ATRA was significantly decreased from 35.8%±4.0% to 7.4%±2.0% after c-Myc over-expression in NB4 cells (Figure 3A). As well, NB4/GFP cells treated with ATRA represented nucleolus disappearance and obvious nuclear segmentation by Wright-Giemsa staining. However, this phenotype was reversed in NB4/MYC cells (Figure 3B). The retard of maturation resulting from c-Myc over-expression was also detected by NBT reduction assay (Figure 3C). Consistantly, c-Myc over-expression also inhibited U937 cells differentiation induced by ATRA (Figure S2D–2F). Contrarily, NB4-R2 ShMYC cells with reduced expression of c-Myc showed more CD11b-positive cells after ATRA treatment than the control cells (Figure 3D). The result was consistent with morphologic observation and NBT reduction assay (Figure 3E, 3F). Thus, the drug resistant cells were inclined to maintain poorly differentiated state resulting from elevated expression of c-Myc.

Over-expression of C/EBPβ reverses c-Myc induced drug resistance

C/EBPβ was essential in the process of granulocytic differentiation. The DNA binding capacity and protein expression level of C/EBPβ were increased evidently in ATRA-induced differentiation of APL cells [26]. Here, we assessed whether high colony formation ability and dedifferentiation state of drug resistant leukemic cells induced by c-Myc was through manipulating C/EBPβ. RT-PCR and western blotting analysis were performed to further validate the expression of C/EBPβ. C/EBPβ was increased after ATRA treatment in NB4/GFP cells, but high c-myc expression inhibited the up-regulation of C/EBPβ in both mRNA and protein levels (35KD and 38KD isoforms) after ATRA treatment (Figure 4A). The data suggested that C/EBPβ was especially down-regulated by c-Myc in ATRA-induced differentiation. To testify the effect of C/EBPβ in drug resistance, C/EBPβ was over-expressed in NB4/MYC cells (NB4/MYC C/EBPβ) by transient retrovirus transduction (Figure 4B-a). MTT assay was carried out to detect the drug sensitivity of NB4/MYC C/EBPβ cells treated with Ara-C (0.1 μM), DNR (0.2 μg/ml) or Doxo (0.04 μg/ml). Result showed that C/EBPβ could rescue drug sensitiviy in NB4/MYC cells (Figure 4B-b, c, d), futher indiating that down-regulation of C/EBPβ was involved in drug resistance induced by c-Myc.

c-Myc inhibitor 10058-F4 restrains drug resistance and colony formation ability induced by c-Myc over-expression

c-Myc was reported to dimerize with Max to play a part in gene transcription. 10058-F4, a small-molecule c-Myc inhibitor, specifically disrupts the c-Myc/Max heterodimerization, resulting in inhibiting the transcriptional function of c-Myc [27]. To clarify the effect of 10058-F4 on drug-resistant leukemic cells, MTT assay was performed to detect the anti-proliferative effect of 10058-F4. Result showed that the drug-resistant cell lines (NB4-R2 and NB4/MYC) were more sensitive to 10058-F4 than the drug-sensitive cell lines (NB4 and NB4/GFP) in both dose- and time-dependent manners (Figure 5A). We also found that the colony formation capacity of both drug-resistant and -sensitive cells were completely impeded by 10058-F4 (Figure 5B). In addition, 10058-F4 promoted the sensitivity of drug resistant cells responsing to Doxo treatment (Figure 5C). The data suggested that 10058-F4 could act as a new targeted therapeutic drug to improve the efficacy of chemotherapy in drug resistant leukemic cells.

Inhibition of c-Myc suppresses proliferation and induces differentiation in primary AML cells

To futher investigate the relation between c-Myc and C/EBPβ in primary AML cells, BMMCs from AML patients were collected, which contained 5 refractory and relapsed (R) AML patients and 4 newly diagnosed (N) AML patients. RT-PCR analysis showed that the expression of *c-Myc* was higher in refractory and relapsed patients than in newly diagnosed patients (Figure 6A-a). Meanwhile, *C/EBPβ* expression was significantly lower in refractory and relapsed patients (Figure 6A-b). Besides, the inverse correlation between *c-Myc* and *C/EBPβ* mRNA level was observed in primary AML cells (Figure 6A-c). Next, BMMCs from 5 AML patients were treated with 10058-F4, and flow

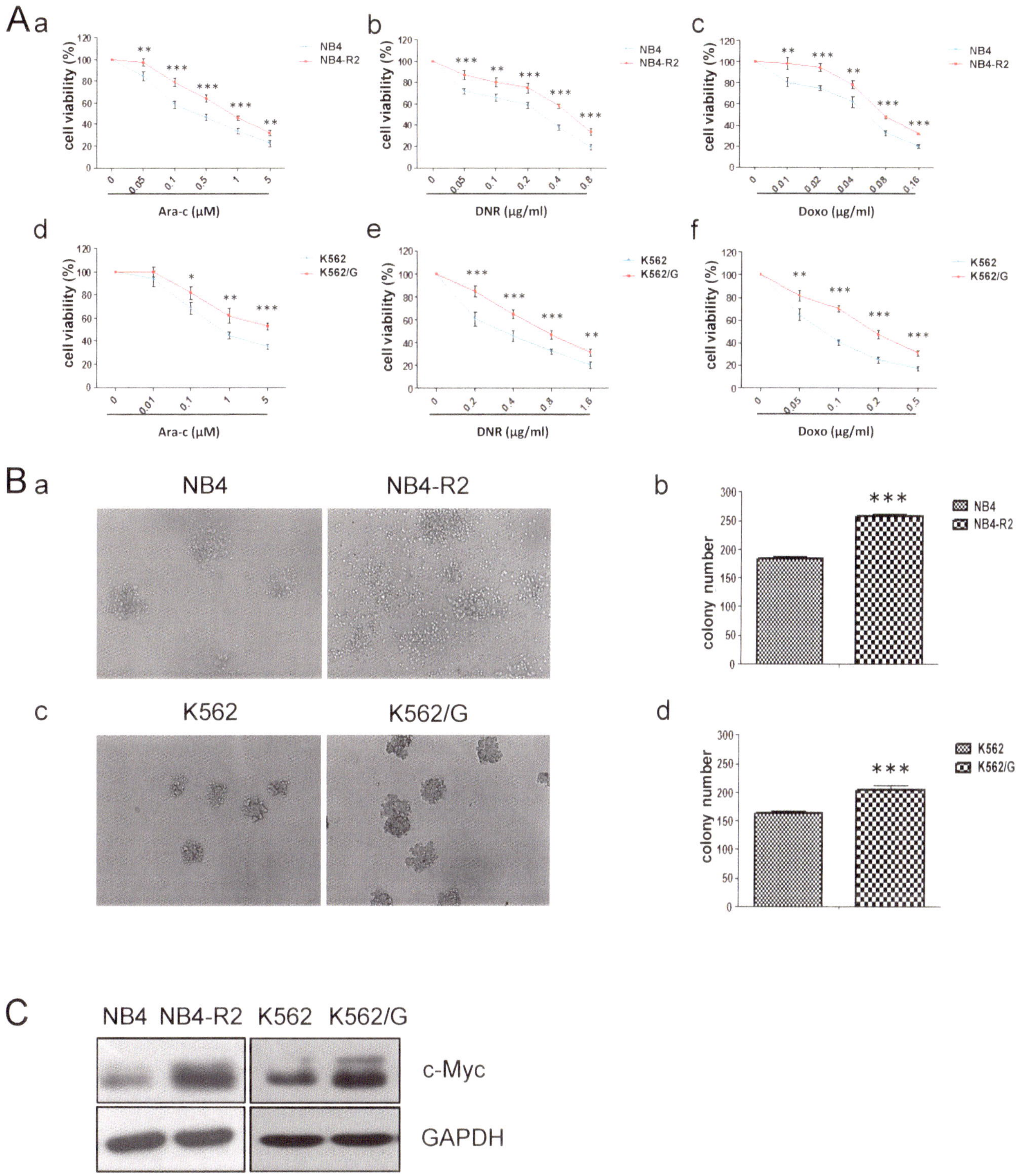

Figure 1. c-Myc is high expressed in drug resistant leukemic cells. (A) Drug-resistant cells (NB4-R2 and K562/G) and drug-sensitive cells (NB4 and K562) were treated with various concentrations of Ara-C, DNR or Doxo for 48 h and subjected to MTT assay. (B) The colony formation images of drug-resistant and -sensitive cells were obtained using a light microscope (magnification, ×200) under 6 days' culture (a,c), and the statistical data were followed (b,d). (C) Western blotting was performed to analyze c-Myc expression. Cell lysates were incubated with antibodies against c-Myc and GAPDH as indicated. Data summarized three independent experiments. *$p<0.05$, **$p<0.01$, ***$p<0.001$, Student's t test.

cytometry was used to detect the differentiation state of primary AML cells. Our data showed that the percentage of CD11b-positive cells was increased after 10058-F4 treatment, illustrating that inhibition of c-Myc expression promoted the primary AML cells to differentiate to mature cells (Figure 6B). In the meantime, the cytotoxic effect of 10058-F4 was detected by MTT assay, and

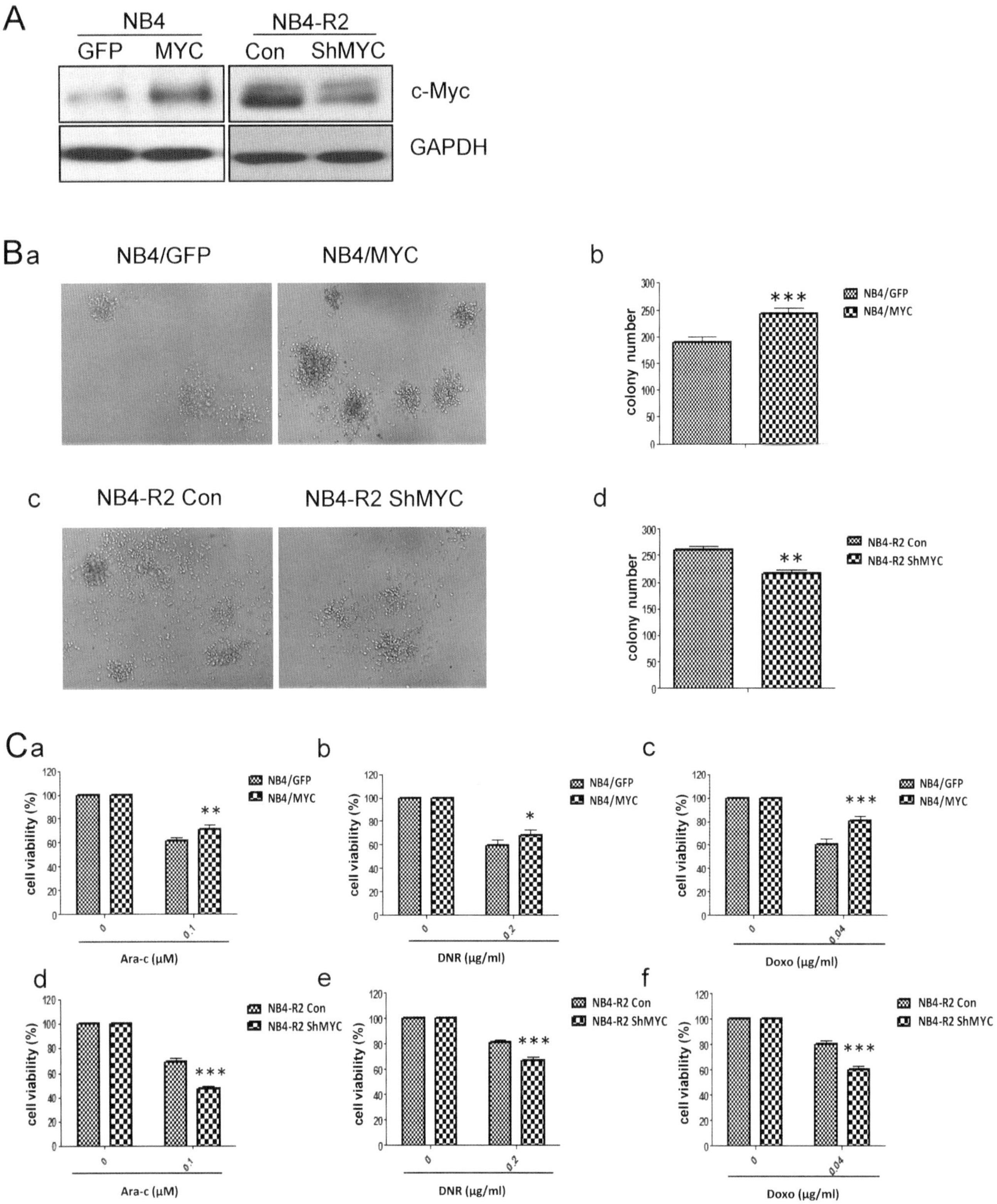

Figure 2. c-Myc over-expression contributes to drug resistance and high colony formation capacity in leukemic cells. (A) c-Myc was over-expressed in NB4 cells (NB4/MYC), and was knocked down in NB4-R2 cells (NB4-R2 ShMYC). Cell lysates were subjected to western blotting analysis. (B) The colonies were photographed under the light microscope (magnification, ×200; a,c), and the statistical results were shown (b,d). (C) The stable leukemic cell lines with up- or down-expression of c-Myc were treated with Ara-C (0.1 μM), DNR (0.2 μg/ml) or Doxo (0.04 μg/ml) for 48 h. Drug sensitivity was testified by MTT assay. Data summarized three independent experiments. *p<0.05, **p<0.01, ***p<0.001, Student's t test.

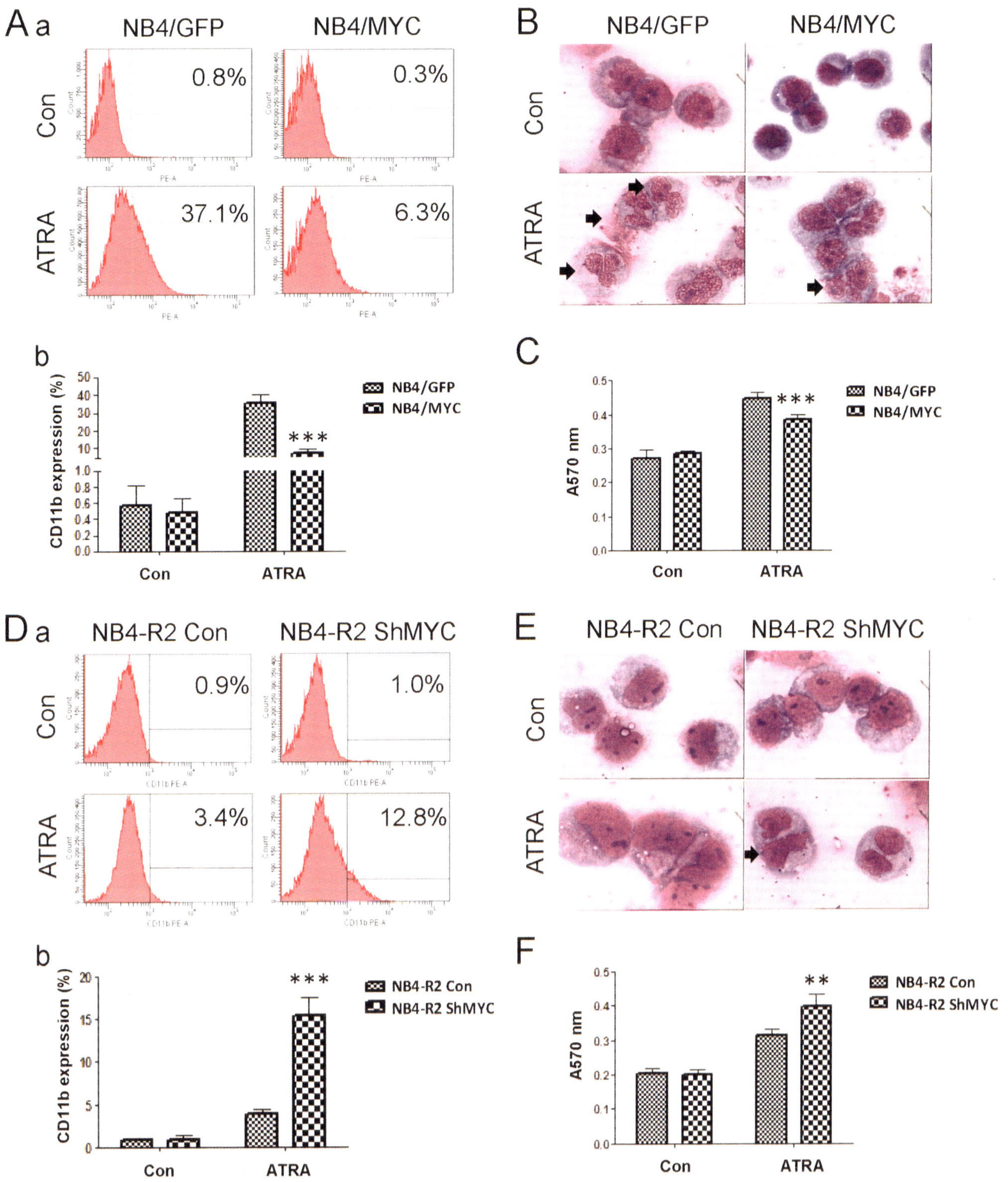

Figure 3. c-Myc inhibits cell differentiation induced by ATRA. NB4/GFP and NB4/MYC, as well as NB4-R2 Con and NB4-R2 ShMYC, were treated with 1 μM ATRA for 72 h. (A, D) Cells were then subjected to flow cytometry to determine the expression of CD11b (a), and the percentages of CD11b positive cells were under census (b). (B, E) Wright-Giemsa staining images of cells were captured by oil immersion lens (magnification, ×1 000). Segmented cells after 72 h of ATRA incubation were annotated by black arrows. (C, F) NBT reduction assay was performed to clarify the differentiation state. $^{**}p<0.01$, $^{***}p<0.001$, Student's t test.

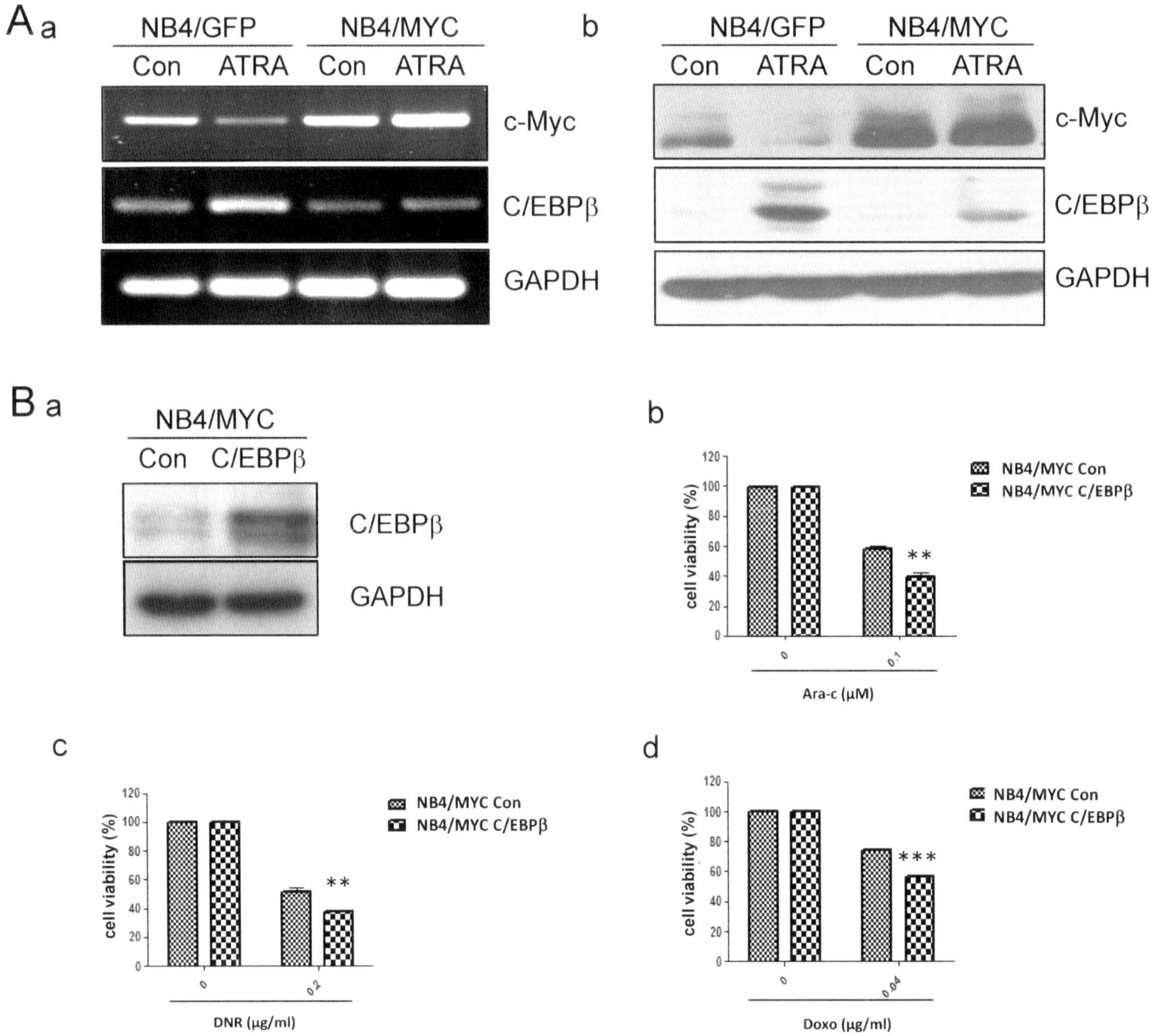

Figure 4. Over-expression of C/EBPβ reverses c-Myc induced drug resistance. (A) NB4/GFP and NB4/MYC cells were treated with 1 μM ATRA for 72 h. Expression of c-Myc, C/EBPβ was tested by RT-PCR and Western blot assay. GAPDH was used as an internal control. (B) C/EBPβ was over-expressed in NB4/MYC cells (NB4/MYC C/EBPβ). Western blotting analysis was performed to detect expression of C/EBPβ (a). NB4/MYC C/EBPβ cells were treated with Ara-C (0.1 μM), DNR (0.2 μg/ml) or Doxo (0.04 μg/ml) for 48 h. Drug sensitivity was testified by MTT assay (b–d). Data summarized three independent experiments. **$p<0.01$, ***$p<0.001$, Student's t test.

cell viability was reduced to 49.94%±8.99% after treatment (Figure 6C). In addition, *C/EBPβ* was up-regulated in primary AML cells treated with 10058-F4 (Figure 6D). Therefore, 10058-F4 could induce differentiation and retard the proliferation in primary AML cells.

Discussion

Here, we addressed that up-regulation of c-Myc expression was one of cytogenetic characteristics in the drug-resistant leukemic cells with increased colony formation capacity (Figure 1). Over-expression of c-Myc in NB4 cells reduced the drug sensitivity to Ara-C, DNR or Doxo, and enhanced the capacity of colony formation (Figure 2). Inversely, inhibition of c-Myc by shRNA or specific c-Myc inhibitor 10058-F4 rescued the sensitivity to Ara-C, DNR or Doxo treatment in drug resistant cells and reduced the colony formation (Figure 2, 5). In the ATRA-induced differentiation model, c-Myc over-expression reduced CD11b expression, and exhibited a decreased reduction of NBT to formazan (Figure 3), which was associated with C/EBPβ down-regulation (Figure 4). Importantly, in primary AML BMMCs, the expression of *c-Myc* and *C/EBPβ* displayed a strong negative correlation. 10058-F4 showed anti-proliferative activity and increased cellular differentiation with up-regulation of C/EBPβ expression (Figure 6). These results clearly indicated an important role of c-Myc in the drug resistance of AML and demonstrated that c-Myc inhibition could overcome drug resistance in AML treatment.

Several studies reported that high c-Myc expression promoted tumor formation and development *in vitro* and *in vivo* while its down-regulation caused tumor cell growth arrest, enhanced

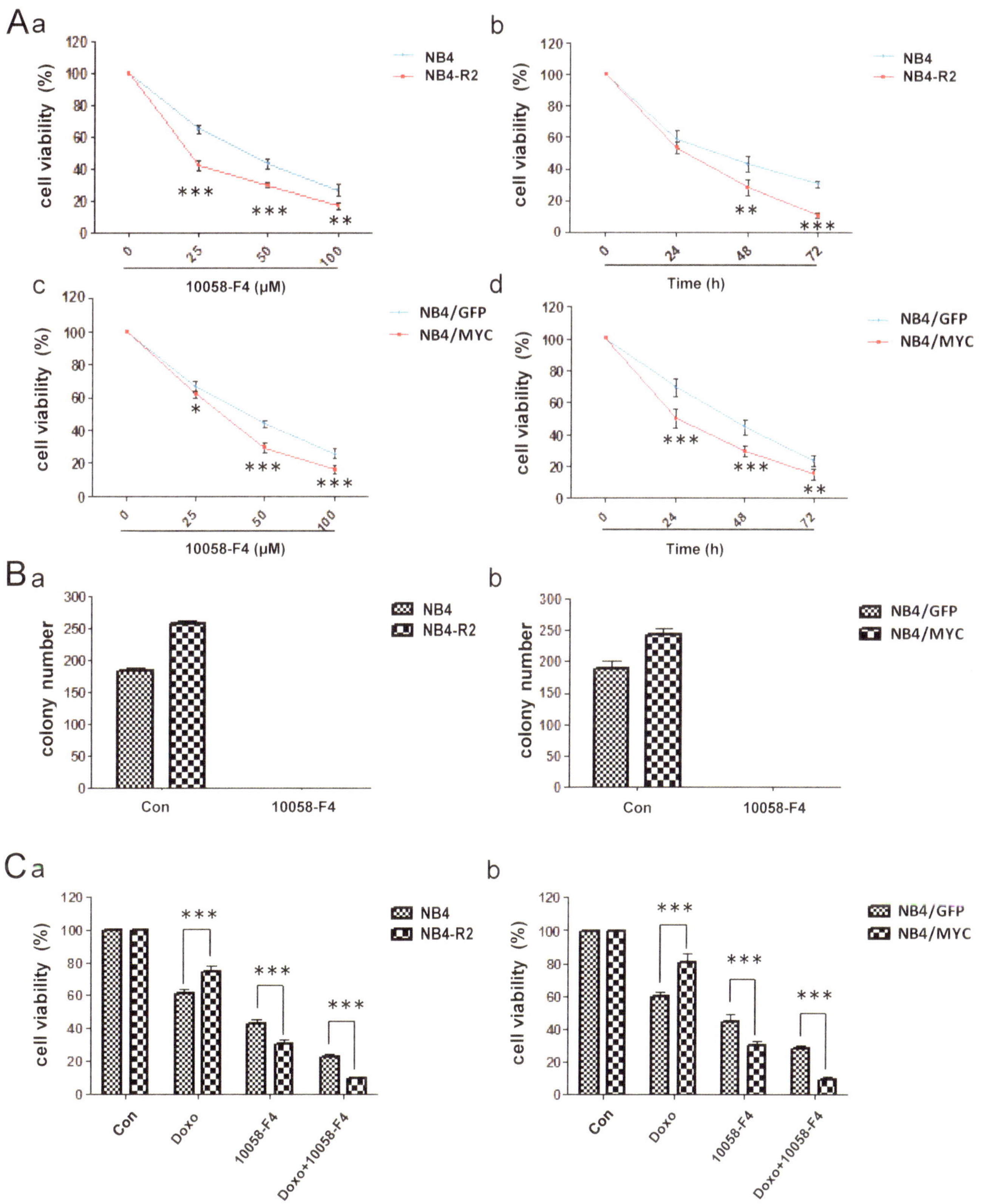

Figure 5. c-Myc inhibitor 10058-F4 restrains drug resistance and colony formation ability induced by c-myc over-expression. (A) High c-Myc expression cells (NB4-R2 and NB4/MYC) and the control cells (NB4 and NB4/GFP) were exposed to various concentrations of 10058-F4 for various times, and cell viability was determined by MTT assay. (B) The colony number of cells was noted by the column diagram. (C) The two group of cells were exposed to Doxo (0.04 μg/ml) and 10058 (50 μM) alone or combination. MTT assay was performed to testify the cell viability. Data summarized three independent experiments. *$p<0.05$, **$p<0.01$, ***$p<0.001$, Student's t test.

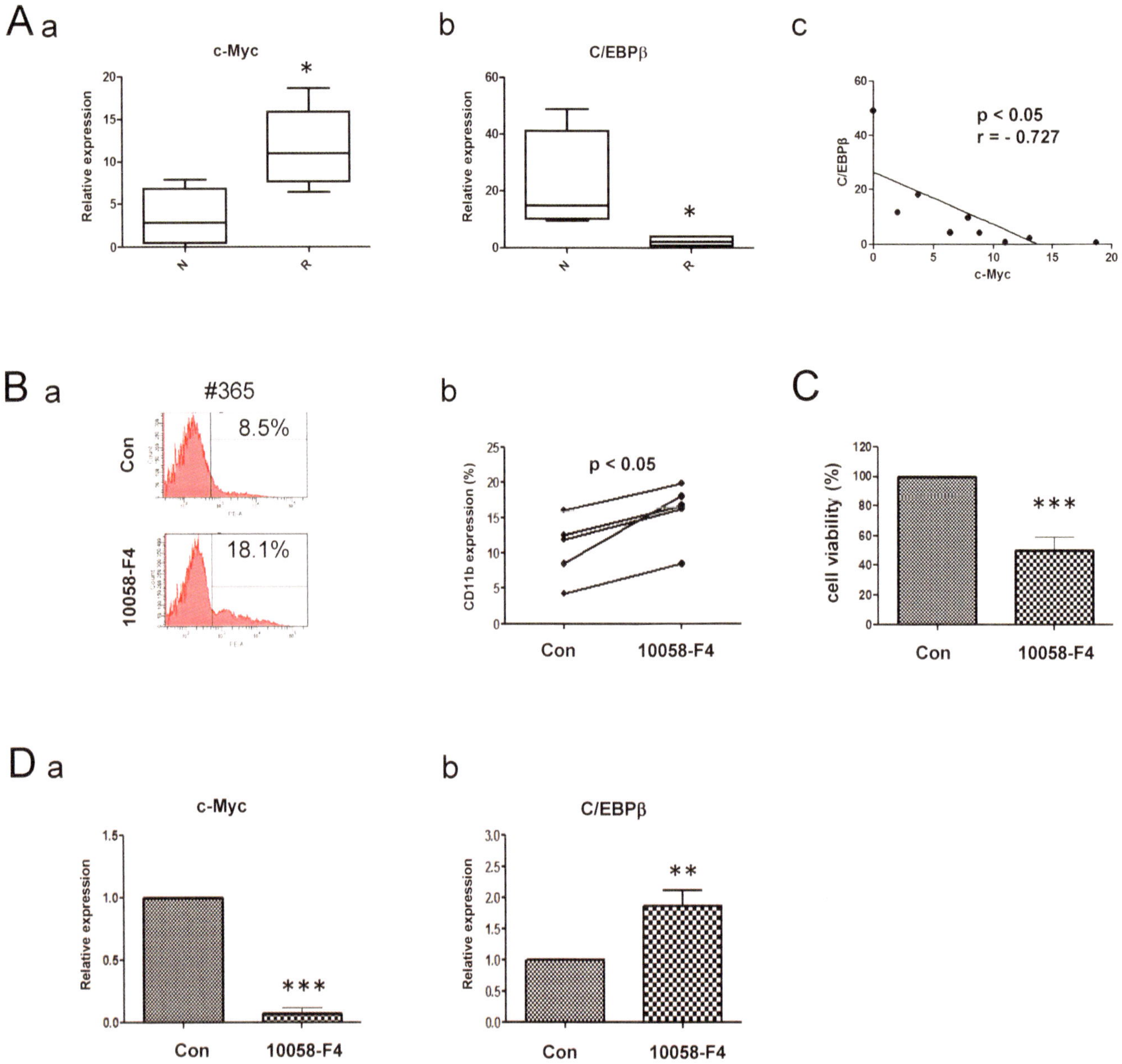

Figure 6. Inhibition of c-Myc suppresses proliferation and induces differentiation in primary AML cells. (A) BMMCs were collected from AML patients, which contained 5 refractory and relapsed (R) AML patients and 4 newly diagnosed (N) AML patients. Real time-PCR analysis was performed to clarify the mRNA expression of *c-Myc* (a) and *C/EBPβ* (b). The relative expression values from different patients were presented in a box plot graph. The horizontal line within each box represented the median value. The correlation between *c-Myc* and *C/EBPβ* expression was shown as (c). (B) BMMCs from five newly diagnosed AML patients were treated with 100 μM 10058-F4 for 48 h. The CD11b-positive cells was analyzed by flow cytometry (a), and the percentages of CD11b expression were under census (n = 5; b). (C) The anti-proliferation of 10058-F4 to BMMCs was detected by MTT assay. (D) The expression of *c-Myc* and *C/EBPβ* in BMMCs treated with 10058-F4 was detected by Real-time PCR. *p<0.05, **p<0.01, ***p<0.001, Student's t test.

apoptosis, senescence, or differentiation [28]. Importantly, c-Myc expression contributed to leukemogenesis and promoted the leukemia disease progress [13]. c-Myc inhibition prevented leukemia initiation and impaired the growth of relapsed pediatric T-ALL cells [29]. Clinical studies reported that AML patients had significantly higher c-Myc expression than health controls [16]. Our finding showed that the drug-resistant leukemic cells displayed high c-Myc expression with increased colony formation capacity, as shown in Figure 1, which suggested that high level of c-Myc expression might predict poor prognosis. c-Myc over-expression reduced the sensitivity of NB4 cells to Ara-C, DNR or Doxo, and increased cell colony formation ability, while c-Myc inhibition in NB4-R2 cells restored the sensitivity to Ara-C, DNR or Doxo treatment and reduced the colony formation capacity (Figure 2). Thus, c-Myc expression was positively correlated with drug resistance of leukemic cells, and could act as a significant clinical biomarker for AML prognosis.

As a key transcriptional factor, c-Myc decides the cell fate through regulation of a series of downstream genes. c-Myc regulates 15% of all genes expression through binding on

Enhancer Box sequences (E-boxes) and recruiting histone acetyltransferases (HATs) [30,31]. Previous study showed that c-Myc determined transcriptional profiles of ATP-binding cassette (ABC) transporter genes in CML CD34+ hematopoietic progenitor cells, leading to drug efflux and resistance [32]. As well, c-Myc regulated multiple microRNAs, including induction of microRNAs with oncogenic properties and repression of microRNAs with tumor suppressor function. c-Myc increased miR-144/451 expression, contributing to the acquired imatinib resistance in K562 cells [33]. In addition, c-Myc antagonized the differentiation induced by imatinib in CML cells [11]. Of importance, low stage of cell differentiation was associated with poor outcome in tumors [34]. Using the ATRA-induced differentiation model, c-Myc over-expression in NB4 cells maintained poor differentiation, as presenting with decrease of CD11b expression and NBT reduction (Figure 3). Moreover, c-Myc inhibitor 10058-F4 increased CD11b expression in the AML patient BMMCs (Figure 6). These results indicated that c-Myc expression was associated with drug resistance of AML cells through maintaining the state of poor differentiation.

With the characterization of the interplay between c-Myc and downstream targets, the mechanism of c-Myc maintains cell immature state still needs to clarify. Myc down-regulated C/EBP transcription factors was reported previously [35]. It has been shown that c-Myc repressed C/EBPα [36], and interacted with Max and Miz1 to suppress C/EBPδ promoter activity and gene expression [37]. In our study, we found that c-Myc over-expression inhibited the expression of C/EBPβ induced by ATRA treatment. C/EBPβ over-expression could reverse c-Myc induced drug resistance (Figure 4). Importantly, the expression of *c-Myc* was negatively correlated with *C/EBPβ* in primary AML cells (Figure 6). Thus, AML cells might maintain immature or poorly differentiated state to prevent cytotoxicity through C/EBPβ repression by c-Myc. Inhibition of c-Myc in AML could help to reverse the drug resistance of leukemic cells and enhance the treatment efficacy.

The main reason for the poor five-year survival rate in AML patients was that leukemic cells displayed drug resistance to the current drugs, leading to disease relapse. Thus, new approach in AML treatment with specific inhibitor targeting drug resistance related genes was required to reduce AML relapse. Previous reports showed that c-Myc inhibition sensitized the chemotherapeutic agents against different types of tumors, including liver cancer [21], Lewis lung carcinoma [18] and melanoma [38]. In our study, c-Myc inhibitor 10058-F4 promoted AML cells differentiation through increasing the rate of CD11b positive section and restored cell sensitivity to Ara-C, DNR or Doxo (Figure 5, 6), indicating that inhibition of c-Myc activity could suppress the drug resistance to chemotherapeutics in AML cells by promoting cell differentiation. Currently, CX-3453 targeting c-Myc was now in phase II clinical trials (NCT00780663) for neuroendocrine carcinoma. With the wide use of c-Myc inhibitor for different cancers in clinical trials, it should be considerate to apply c-Myc inhibitor in combination therapies to overcome drug resistance, reducing disease relapse.

In conclusion, we found that c-Myc over-expression in AML cells reduced the sensitivity to chemotherapeutic drugs. Inhibition of c-Myc could rescue drug sensitivity by increasing C/EBPβ expression. Taken together, c-Myc inhibition provided a novel strategy to overcome drug resistance in AML treatment.

Supporting Information

Figure S1 NB4-R2 and K562/G cells are respectively resistant to ATRA and imatinib. (A) NB4 and NB4-R2 cells were treated with various concentrations of ATRA for 72 h, and MTT assay was performed. (B) K562 and K562/G were exposed to various concentrations of imatinib for 48 h, and the cell viability was also tested by MTT assay. ***$p<0.001$, Student's t test.

Figure S2 c-Myc over-expression induces drug resistance and high colony formation capacity in U937 cells. (A) c-Myc was over-expressed in U937 cells (U937/MYC). Cell lysates were subjected to western blotting analysis. (B) The statistical result of colony formation number was shown. (C) U937/GFP and U937/MYC cells were treated with Ara-C (0.1 μM), DNR (0.2 μg/ml) or Doxo (0.04 μg/ml) for 48 h. Drug sensitivity was testified by MTT assay (a–c). (D)U937/GFP and U937/MYC cells were treated with 1 μM ATRA for 72 h. Flow cytometry was performed to determine the expression of CD11b (a), and the percentages of CD11b positive cells were under census (b). (E) Wright-Giemsa staining images of cells were captured by oil immersion lens (magnification, ×1 000). Segmented cells after 72 h of ATRA incubation were annotated by black arrows. (F) NBT reduction assay was performed to clarify the differentiation state. Data summarized three independent experiments. *$p<0.05$, **$p<0.01$, ***$p<0.001$, Student's t test.

Acknowledgments

We thank the members of Quentin Liu lab and Medical Research Center, Third Affiliated Hospital, Sun Yat-sen University for their critical comments. We also thank Wen-Xing Lai for his technical support.

Author Contributions

Conceived and designed the experiments: ZJL DJL. Performed the experiments: XNP JJC LXW RZX LLL ZGF. Analyzed the data: XNP JJC ZJL. Contributed reagents/materials/analysis tools: ZJL DJL QL. Contributed to the writing of the manuscript: XNP JJC ZJL.

References

1. Funato T, Harigae H, Abe S, Sasaki T (2004) Assessment of drug resistance in acute myeloid leukemia. Expert Rev Mol Diagn 4: 705–713.
2. Estey EH (2013) Acute myeloid leukemia: 2013 update on risk-stratification and management. Am J Hematol 88: 318–327.
3. Nielsen DL (2004) Mechanisms and functional aspects of multidrug resistance in Ehrlich ascites tumour cells. Dan Med Bull 51: 393–414.
4. Negoro E, Yamauchi T, Urasaki Y, Nishi R, Hori H, et al. (2011) Characterization of cytarabine-resistant leukemic cell lines established from five different blood cell lineages using gene expression and proteomic analyses. Int J Oncol 38: 911–919.
5. Zeng DF, Zhang J, Zhu LD, Kong PY, Li JP, et al. (2014) Analysis of drug resistance-associated proteins expressions of patients with the recurrent of acute leukemia via protein microarray technology. Eur Rev Med Pharmacol Sci 18: 537–543.
6. Liu LL, Long ZJ, Wang LX, Zheng FM, Fang ZG, et al. (2013) Inhibition of mTOR pathway sensitizes acute myeloid leukemia cells to aurora inhibitors by suppression of glycolytic metabolism. Mol Cancer Res 11: 1326–1336.
7. Long Y, Tsai WB, Wangpaichitr M, Tsukamoto T, Savaraj N, et al. (2013) Arginine deiminase resistance in melanoma cells is associated with metabolic reprogramming, glucose dependence, and glutamine addiction. Mol Cancer Ther 12: 2581–2590.
8. Wong RS, Cheong SK (2012) Leukaemic stem cells: drug resistance, metastasis and therapeutic implications. Malays J Pathol 34: 77–88.
9. Masui K, Tanaka K, Akhavan D, Babic I, Gini B, et al. (2013) mTOR complex 2 controls glycolytic metabolism in glioblastoma through FoxO acetylation and upregulation of c-Myc. Cell Metab 18: 726–739.
10. Sheth A, Escobar-Alvarez S, Gardner J, Ran L, Heaney ML, et al. (2014) Inhibition of human mitochondrial peptide deformylase causes apoptosis in c-myc-overexpressing hematopoietic cancers. Cell Death Dis 5: e1152.

11. Gomez-Casares MT, Garcia-Alegria E, Lopez-Jorge CE, Ferrandiz N, Blanco R, et al. (2013) MYC antagonizes the differentiation induced by imatinib in chronic myeloid leukemia cells through downregulation of p27(KIP1.). Oncogene 32: 2239-2246.
12. Singh AM, Dalton S (2009) The cell cycle and Myc intersect with mechanisms that regulate pluripotency and reprogramming. Cell Stem Cell 5: 141-149.
13. Hoffman B, Amanullah A, Shafarenko M, Liebermann DA (2002) The proto-oncogene c-myc in hematopoietic development and leukemogenesis. Oncogene 21: 3414-3421.
14. Dang CV, O'Donnell KA, Zeller KI, Nguyen T, Osthus RC, et al. (2006) The c-Myc target gene network. Semin Cancer Biol 16: 253-264.
15. Field JK, Spandidos DA (1990) The role of ras and myc oncogenes in human solid tumours and their relevance in diagnosis and prognosis (review). Anticancer Res 10: 1-22.
16. Delgado MD, Albajar M, Gomez-Casares MT, Batlle A, Leon J (2013) MYC oncogene in myeloid neoplasias. Clin Transl Oncol 15: 87-94.
17. Walker TL, White JD, Esdale WJ, Burton MA, DeCruz EE (1996) Tumour cells surviving in vivo cisplatin chemotherapy display elevated c-myc expression. Br J Cancer 73: 610-614.
18. Knapp DC, Mata JE, Reddy MT, Devi GR, Iversen PL (2003) Resistance to chemotherapeutic drugs overcome by c-Myc inhibition in a Lewis lung carcinoma murine model. Anticancer Drugs 14: 39-47.
19. Tsai WB, Aiba I, Long Y, Lin HK, Feun L, et al. (2012) Activation of Ras/PI3K/ERK pathway induces c-Myc stabilization to upregulate argininosuccinate synthetase, leading to arginine deiminase resistance in melanoma cells. Cancer Res 72: 2622-2633.
20. Leonetti C, Biroccio A, Candiloro A, Citro G, Fornari C, et al. (1999) Increase of cisplatin sensitivity by c-myc antisense oligodeoxynucleotides in a human metastatic melanoma inherently resistant to cisplatin. Clin Cancer Res 5: 2588-2595.
21. Lin CP, Liu JD, Chow JM, Liu CR, Liu HE (2007) Small-molecule c-Myc inhibitor, 10058-F4, inhibits proliferation, downregulates human telomerase reverse transcriptase and enhances chemosensitivity in human hepatocellular carcinoma cells. Anticancer Drugs 18: 161-170.
22. Huang MJ, Cheng YC, Liu CR, Lin S, Liu HE (2006) A small-molecule c-Myc inhibitor, 10058-F4, induces cell-cycle arrest, apoptosis, and myeloid differentiation of human acute myeloid leukemia. Exp Hematol 34: 1480-1489.
23. Civenni G, Malek A, Albino D, Garcia-Escudero R, Napoli S, et al. (2013) RNAi-mediated silencing of Myc transcription inhibits stem-like cell maintenance and tumorigenicity in prostate cancer. Cancer Res 73: 6816-6827.
24. Nair R, Roden DL, Teo WS, McFarland A, Junankar S, et al. (2013) c-Myc and Her2 cooperate to drive a stem-like phenotype with poor prognosis in breast cancer. Oncogene.
25. Magri L, Gacias M, Wu M, Swiss VA, Janssen WG, et al. (2014) c-Myc-dependent transcriptional regulation of cell cycle and nucleosomal histones during oligodendrocyte differentiation. Neuroscience.
26. Yu L, Zhang YD, Zhou J, Yao DM, Li X (2013) Identification of target genes of transcription factor CEBPB in acute promyelocytic leukemia cells induced by all-trans retinoic acid. Asian Pac J Trop Med 6: 473-480.
27. Follis AV, Hammoudeh DI, Daab AT, Metallo SJ (2009) Small-molecule perturbation of competing interactions between c-Myc and Max. Bioorg Med Chem Lett 19: 807-810.
28. Soucek L, Evan GI (2010) The ups and downs of Myc biology. Curr Opin Genet Dev 20: 91-95.
29. Roderick JE, Tesell J, Shultz LD, Brehm MA, Greiner DL, et al. (2014) c-Myc inhibition prevents leukemia initiation in mice and impairs the growth of relapsed and induction failure pediatric T-ALL cells. Blood 123: 1040-1050.
30. Haggerty TJ, Zeller KI, Osthus RC, Wonsey DR, Dang CV (2003) A strategy for identifying transcription factor binding sites reveals two classes of genomic c-Myc target sites. Proc Natl Acad Sci U S A 100: 5313-5318.
31. Frank SR, Parisi T, Taubert S, Fernandez P, Fuchs M, et al. (2003) MYC recruits the TIP60 histone acetyltransferase complex to chromatin. EMBO Rep 4: 575-580.
32. Porro A, Iraci N, Soverini S, Diolaiti D, Gherardi S, et al. (2011) c-MYC oncoprotein dictates transcriptional profiles of ATP-binding cassette transporter genes in chronic myelogenous leukemia CD34+ hematopoietic progenitor cells. Mol Cancer Res 9: 1054-1066.
33. Liu L, Wang S, Chen R, Wu Y, Zhang B, et al. (2012) Myc induced miR-144/451 contributes to the acquired imatinib resistance in chronic myelogenous leukemia cell K562. Biochem Biophys Res Commun 425: 368-373.
34. Fredlund E, Ringner M, Maris JM, Pahlman S (2008) High Myc pathway activity and low stage of neuronal differentiation associate with poor outcome in neuroblastoma. Proc Natl Acad Sci U S A 105: 14094-14099.
35. Mink S, Mutschler B, Weiskirchen R, Bister K, Klempnauer KH (1996) A novel function for Myc: inhibition of C/EBP-dependent gene activation. Proc Natl Acad Sci U S A 93: 6635-6640.
36. Li LH, Nerlov C, Prendergast G, MacGregor D, Ziff EB (1994) c-Myc represses transcription in vivo by a novel mechanism dependent on the initiator element and Myc box II. EMBO J 13: 4070-4079.
37. Si J, Yu X, Zhang Y, DeWille JW (2010) Myc interacts with Max and Miz1 to repress C/EBPdelta promoter activity and gene expression. Mol Cancer 9: 92.
38. Citro G, D'Agnano I, Leonetti C, Perini R, Bucci B, et al. (1998) c-myc antisense oligodeoxynucleotides enhance the efficacy of cisplatin in melanoma chemotherapy in vitro and in nude mice. Cancer Res 58: 283-289.

Early versus Deferred Treatment for Smoldering Multiple Myeloma: A Meta-Analysis of Randomized, Controlled Trials

Minjie Gao[1 ❡], Guang Yang[1 ❡], Van S. Tompkins[2], Lu Gao[1], Xiaosong Wu[1], Yi Tao[1], Xiaojing Hu[1], Jun Hou[1], Ying Han[1], Hongwei Xu[3], Fenghuang Zhan[3]*, Jumei Shi[1]*

1 Department of Hematology, Shanghai Tenth People's Hospital, Tongji University School of Medicine, Shanghai, China, **2** Department of Pathology, University of Iowa Carver College of Medicine, Iowa City, Iowa, United States of America, **3** Department of Internal Medicine, University of Iowa Carver College of Medicine, Iowa City, Iowa, United States of America

Abstract

Purpose: Whether patients with smoldering multiple myeloma (SMM) needed to receive early interventional treatment remains controversial. Herein, we conducted a meta-analysis comparing the efficacy and safety of early treatment over deferred treatment for patients with SMM.

Methods: MEDLINE and Cochrane Library were searched to May 2014 for randomized controlled trials (RCTs) that assessed the effect of early treatment over deferred treatment. Primary outcome measure was mortality, and secondary outcome measures were progression, response rate, and adverse events.

Results: Overall, 5 trials including 449 patients were identified. There was a markedly reduced risk of disease progression with early treatment (Odds Ratio [OR] = 0.13, 95% confidence interval [CI] = 0.07 to 0.24). There were no significant differences in mortality and response rate (OR = 0.85, 95% CI = 0.45 to 1.60, and OR = 0.63, 95% CI = 0.32 to 1.23, respectively). More patients in the early treatment arm experienced gastrointestinal toxicities (OR = 10.02, 95%CI = 4.32 to 23.23), constipation (OR = 8.58, 95%CI = 3.20 to 23.00) and fatigue or asthenia (OR = 2.72, 95%CI = 1.30 to 5.67). No significant differences were seen with the development of acute leukemia (OR = 2.80, 95%CI = 0.42 to 18.81), hematologic cancer (OR = 2.07, 95%CI = 0.43 to 10.01), second primary tumors (OR = 3.45, 95%CI = 0.81 to 14.68), nor vertebral compression (OR = 0.18, 95%CI = 0.02 to 1.59).

Conclusions: Early treatment delayed disease progression but increased the risk of gastrointestinal toxicities, constipation and fatigue or asthenia. The differences on vertebral compression, acute leukemia, hematological cancer and second primary tumors were not statistically significant. Based on the current evidence, early treatment didn't significantly affect mortality and response rate. However, further much larger trials were needed to provide more evidence.

Editor: Zhenyu Li, University of Kentucky, United States of America

Funding: This study was supported by grants from the National Natural Science Foundation of China (No. 81372391, 81071856 to J.S., 81000199 to X.H., 81250110552 to T.V., and 81228016 to F.Z.), Shanghai Science and Technology Program (No. 12410705100 to J.S.), Shanghai Tenth People's Hospital Funds (No. 040113015 to J.S.). The funders conceived and designed the experiments, contributed reagents/materials/analysis tools, drafted the paper, and read and approved the final paper.

Competing Interests: The authors have declared that no competing interests exist.

* Email: shijumei@hotmail.com (JMS); fenghuang-zhan@uiowa.edu (FHZ)

❡ These authors contributed equally to this work.

Introduction

Multiple myeloma (MM) is a cancer of plasma cells that accumulate in the bone marrow and produce a monoclonal protein [1]. It is the second most common hematologic cancer, accounting for 15–20% of deaths from hematologic cancer and about 2% of deaths from cancer [1,2]. Advances in the basic understanding of MM and the introduction of novel agents including thalidomide, lenalidomide and bortezomib, have delayed progression and prolonged patients' survival. Despite these advances, unfortunately there is still no cure for MM, and the goal of therapy is to prolong survival [3,4]. Prognosis of patients with MM depends mainly on the stage of the disease [5].

According to the International Myeloma Working Group guidelines, MM-related neoplastic conditions have been categorized into monoclonal gammopathy of undetermined significance (MGUS), smoldering (asymptomatic) myeloma (SMM), solitary plasmacytoma of bone, and symptomatic multiple myeloma [6]. Diagnosed symptomatic multiple myeloma falls into one of three stages, IB, II, or IIIA/B, whereas SMM is identified as stage IA myeloma as determined by Durie/Salmon staging [6]. SMM patients are at high risk of progressing to symptomatic myeloma, with a median time to progression of approximately 1–2 years [7]. This intermediate condition is characterized by monoclonal protein concentrations of more than or equal to 3 g/dL and/or bone marrow plasma cells that are more than or equal to 10% without myeloma related organ or tissue impairment [8–10]. 54% of SMM patients will progress to frank multiple myeloma 5 years after initial diagnosis. This value exceeds 70% 15 years post-diagnosis [11,12].

Historically, the majority of patients with SMM are followed without therapy until symptoms developed [13,14]. The main reason for this conservative approach was that previous options for MM therapy were limited and toxic and unable to improve survival benefit [5,15] based on the conclusions from three small, randomized controlled trials prior to 2003 [16–18]. These trials compared early treatment with melphalan and prednisone with observation and demonstrated a significant delay in time to progression. However, this did not translate into better overall survival. Because all the trials included in the He et al. meta-analysis [5] used non-targeted agents (melphalan and prednisone) and had small sample sizes, the treatment of SMM remained controversial [12]. A better understanding of the biology of MM has led to a wealth of novel agents to treat it, providing for the possibility that at least some of these new agents may be used to effectively intervene at early stages of MM. Investigators have since begun to carry out clinical trials to evaluate novel drugs and new combinations of existing treatments in SMM. From the year 2003 onwards, two phase randomized, controlled trials (RCTs) have been completed [19,20] and one phase III RCT with 370 SMM patients is ongoing. Immuno-modulatory agents (IMiDs) were used in each of these three more recent RCTs.

To gain a better, more complete and current understanding of the efficacy and safety of early treatment over deferred treatment for SMM patients, we conducted a meta-analysis based on data from the five completed phase III RCTs. Our analysis includes the three trials [16–18] previously used by He et al. [5] but also include the two more recent trials that used IMiDs [19,20]. In performing our meta-analysis we address whether early treatment of SMM with the newer, targeted agents (IMiDs) have improved clinical benefit over the non-targeted agents (melphalan and prednisone), and whether increasing the sample size provides more reliable data for early treatment regardless of agent type.

Methods

Search strategy

We used MEDLINE and Cochrane Library to locate all relevant studies published up to May 2014. The search criterion was listed in Table S1 and Table S2. We used 'the related articles' function in PubMed to identify other potentially relevant articles. Further, we searched the ClinicalTrials.gov registry. We also checked all the references of retrieved articles and asked for additional data and explanations when key information relevant to the meta-analysis was missing. The data was collected only from published, peer-reviewed papers.

Selection criteria

Studies included in our analyses were required to be RCTs that compared early versus deferred treatment for SMM. The treatment strategy and the criteria used for selecting patients also needed to be reported. Further, every RCT must have either reported clinical outcomes or safety of the treatments. The eligibility of each study was assessed independently by two investigators.

Data extraction and methodological quality assessment

The quality of trials was evaluated by two independent reviewers by examining the adequacy of the allocation randomization, allocation concealment, blinding, data analysis, withdrawals and dropouts and power analysis. Two reviewers performed data extraction independently based on selection criteria. If a disagreement arose, agreement was achieved through consultation with a third reviewer.

Outcomes Assessments

Our primary outcome for this meta-analysis was mortality. Secondary outcomes included progression, response rate and adverse events. Mortality was defined as time from randomization to death from any cause. Progression was defined as time from randomization to documentation of progression. Safety outcomes included the incidence of adverse events, specifically gastrointestinal toxicities, constipation, fatigue or asthenia, vertebral compression, acute leukemia, hematological cancer and second primary tumor.

Statistical analysis

The effect of treatment for each study was expressed as Odds Ratio [OR] of the early treatment arm over deferred treatment arm, with 95% confidence interval [CI]. A random-effect model was obtained to conduct a meta-analysis of all the relevant RCTs to get a conservative conclusion. Heterogeneity was assessed by both chi-squared test and I^2 statistics. Statistically significant heterogeneity was defined as p-value <0.10 or I^2 statistic$>50\%$. Revman software (5.2) was used to perform all calculations.

Results

1 Selection of the trials

Our initial search yielded 279 potentially relevant studies, of which 90 studies were duplicated and 176 studies were deemed ineligible after screening titles and abstracts (Figure 1). The full text of the remaining 13 studies was reviewed in full, of which five randomized controlled trials fully met the inclusion criteria [16–20]. Excluded full-text studies, with the reasons for exclusion, were listed in Table S3.

2 Description of trials

An outline of the five trials is provided in Table 1. The trial results were published between 1993 and 2013. A total of 449 patients with SMM were included. Three of the trials used melphalan and prednisone as early treatment agents [16–18]. Two of the trials used IMiDs as early treatment agents [19–20]. The methodological quality of the 5 trials is summarized in Table 2. Two trials described the methods of randomization and allocation concealment [17,18]. Three trials used an intention-to-treat analysis [16,19,20]. None of the five trials described power analysis and reported double blinding of the participants and outcome assessors. All trials described withdrawls and dropouts [16–20].

3 Mortality

In the early treatment and deferred treatment arms, 223 and 226 patients were evaluable for mortality, respectively. In total, there were 77 deaths in the early treatment arm and 81 deaths in the deferred treatment arm. As shown in Figure 2, no statistically

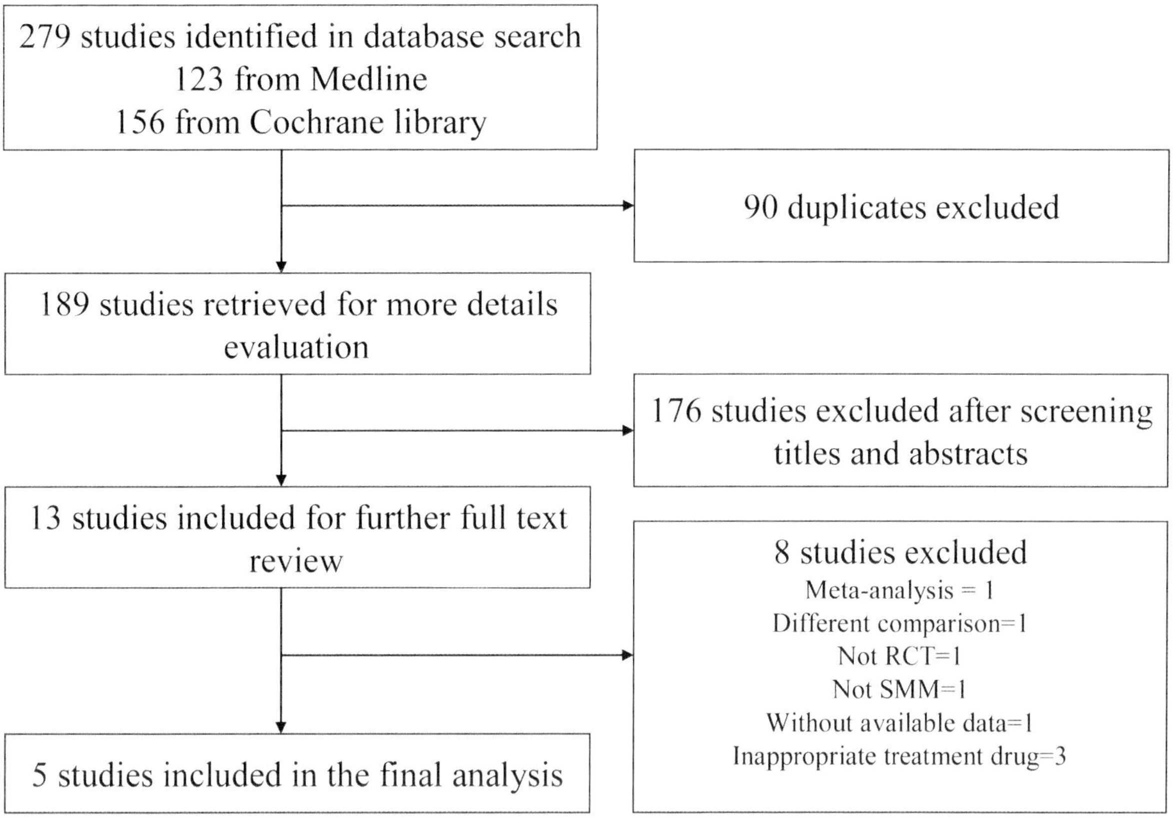

Figure 1. Flowchart of the selection of studies.

significant heterogeneity was observed ($p = 0.10$, $I^2 = 49\%$), and there was no significant difference in overall mortality between the two arms (pooled OR = 0.85, 95%CI = 0.45 to 1.60). When stratifying the data according to treatment type, neither alkylators nor IMiDs had a significantly reduced mortality. There was evidence of significant heterogeneity in the IMiDs group ($I^2 = 52\%$).

4 Progression

In the early and deferred treatment arms, 198 and 201 patients were evaluable for disease progression, respectively. Twenty-seven (27) patients progressed to MM in the early treatment arm compared to 108 in the deferred treatment arm. As shown in Figure 3, there was a markedly reduced risk of disease progression with early treatment (pooled OR = 0.13, 95%CI = 0.07 to 0.24).

Table 1. Characteristics of studies fulfilling inclusion criteria in the meta-analysis.

Author [year]	Disease	Early treatment defined as	Deferred treatment defined as	No. of enrolled/ analyzed patients	Intervention
Hjorth [1993]	SMM	Immediate treatment on diagnosis/randomization	Observation until symptomatic disease progression	E: 25/25 D: 25/25	M: 0.25 mg/kg P: 2 mg/kg d1-4 of 6 w intervals
Riccardi [1994]	SMM	Immediate treatment on diagnosis/randomization	Observation until symptomatic disease progression	E:38/34 D:40/40	M: 0.21 mg/kg d1-4 of 6 w intervals P: 0.5 mg/kg d1-10 of 6 w intervals
Riccardi [2000]	SMM	Immediate treatment on diagnosis/randomization	Observation until symptomatic disease progression	E:75/72 D:70/66	M: 0.21 mg/kg d1-4 of 6 w intervals P: 0.5 mg/kg d1-10 of 6 w intervals
Witzig [2013]	SMM	Immediate treatment on diagnosis/randomization	Observation until symptomatic disease progression	E:35/35 D:33/33	ZLD: 4 mg/d Thal: 200 mg/d a 28 d cycle
Mateos [2013]	High-risk SMM	Immediate treatment on diagnosis/randomization	Observation until symptomatic disease progression	E:57/57 D:62/62	Induction (L: 25 mg/d d1-21 Dex: 20 mg/d d1-4,12–15 4 w intervals, 9 cycles) Maintenance (L: 10 mg/d d1-21, a 28 d cycle, 2 y)

MM: multiple myeloma; SMM: smouldering myeloma; M: melphalan; P: prednisone; ZLD: zoledronic acid; Thal: thalidomide; L: lenalidomide; Dex: dexamethasone; E: early treatment arm; D: deferred treatment arm; d: day; w: week; y: year.

Table 2. Methodological quality assessment of included trial.

Author [year]	Allocation generation	Allocation concealment	Double blinding	ITT	Withdrawls and dropouts described	Power analysis described
Hjorth [1993]	Unclear	Unclear	No	Yes	Yes	No
Riccardi [1994]	Computer generated	Adequate	No	No	Yes	No
Riccardi [2000]	Computer generated	Adequate	No	No	Yes	No
Witzig [2013]	Unclear	Unclear	No	Yes	Yes	No
Mateos [2013]	Unclear	Unclear	No	Yes	Yes	No

ITT: intention-to-treat.

No statistically significant heterogeneity was observed ($p = 0.23$, $I^2 = 31\%$). When divided by the treatment type, early treatment with either alkylators or IMiDs significantly delayed disease progression. There was evidence of significant heterogeneity in the alkylators group ($I^2 = 69\%$).

5 Response Rate

In the early and deferred treatment arms, 100 and 56 patients were evaluable for response rate, respectively. There were 43 responses in the early treatment arm and 31 responses in the deferred treatment arm. As shown in Figure 4, no heterogeneity was observed ($p = 0.45$, $I^2 = 0\%$). There was no significant difference in response rate between the two arms (pooled OR = 0.63, 95%CI = 0.32 to 1.23).

6 Adverse events

6.1 Acute leukemia. Acute leukemia was reported in three trials. 4 of 131 patients in the early treatment arm and 1 of 131 patients in the deferred arm developed acute leukemia. No heterogeneity was observed ($p = 0.59$, $I^2 = 0\%$). The incidence of acute leukemia in the early treatment arm did not differ significantly from that in the deferred treatment arm (pooled OR = 2.80, 95%CI = 0.42 to 18.81) (Figure 5).

6.2 Hematologic cancer. Hematologic cancer was reported in four studies. 5 of 188 patients in the early treatment arm and 2 of 193 patients in the deferred arm developed hematologic cancer. No heterogeneity was observed ($p = 0.74$, $I^2 = 0\%$). The incidence of hematologic cancer in the early treatment arm did not significantly differ from that in the deferred treatment arm (pooled OR = 2.07, 95%CI = 0.43 to 10.01) (Figure. 5).

6.3 Second primary tumors. Second primary tumors were reported in four studies. 8 of 188 patients in the early treatment arm and 2 of 193 patients in the deferred arm developed second primary tumors. No heterogeneity was observed ($p = 0.82$, $I^2 = 0\%$). The incidence of second primary tumors did not significantly differ between the early and deferred treatment arms (pooled OR = 3.45, 95%CI = 0.81 to 14.68) (Figure 5).

6.4 Vertebral compression. Vertebral compression was reported in two trials. None of the 97 patients in the early treatment arm, but 4 of 91 patients in the deferred treatment arm

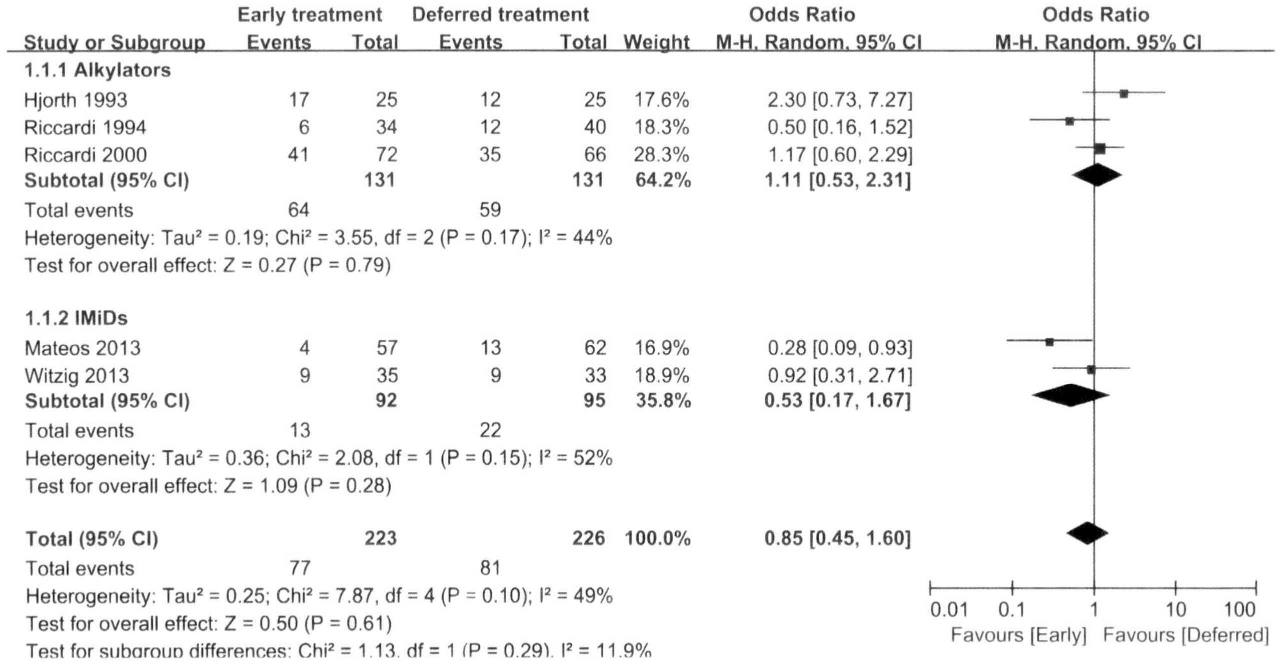

Figure 2. Mortality odds ratios of early treatment versus deferred treatment. The 95% CIs are shown. Squares represent the odds ratios and 95% CI for alkylators or IMiDs and finally for the overall estimate. CIs, confidence intervals; IMiDs, immuno-modulatory agents.

Study or Subgroup	Early treatment Events	Early treatment Total	Deferred treatment Events	Deferred treatment Total	Weight	Odds Ratio M-H, Random, 95% CI
1.2.1 Alkylators						
Riccardi 1994	4	34	12	40	19.6%	0.31 [0.09, 1.08]
Riccardi 2000	5	72	34	66	25.8%	0.07 [0.03, 0.20]
Subtotal (95% CI)		**106**		**106**	**45.4%**	**0.14 [0.03, 0.61]**
Total events	9		46			
Heterogeneity: Tau² = 0.77; Chi² = 3.27, df = 1 (P = 0.07); I² = 69%						
Test for overall effect: Z = 2.63 (P = 0.009)						
1.2.2 IMiDs						
Mateos 2013	13	57	47	62	33.0%	0.09 [0.04, 0.22]
Witzig 2013	5	35	15	33	21.5%	0.20 [0.06, 0.64]
Subtotal (95% CI)		**92**		**95**	**54.6%**	**0.12 [0.06, 0.25]**
Total events	18		62			
Heterogeneity: Tau² = 0.01; Chi² = 1.04, df = 1 (P = 0.31); I² = 4%						
Test for overall effect: Z = 5.84 (P < 0.00001)						
Total (95% CI)		**198**		**201**	**100.0%**	**0.13 [0.07, 0.24]**
Total events	27		108			
Heterogeneity: Tau² = 0.13; Chi² = 4.32, df = 3 (P = 0.23); I² = 31%						
Test for overall effect: Z = 6.33 (P < 0.00001)						
Test for subgroup differences: Chi² = 0.03, df = 1 (P = 0.86), I² = 0%						

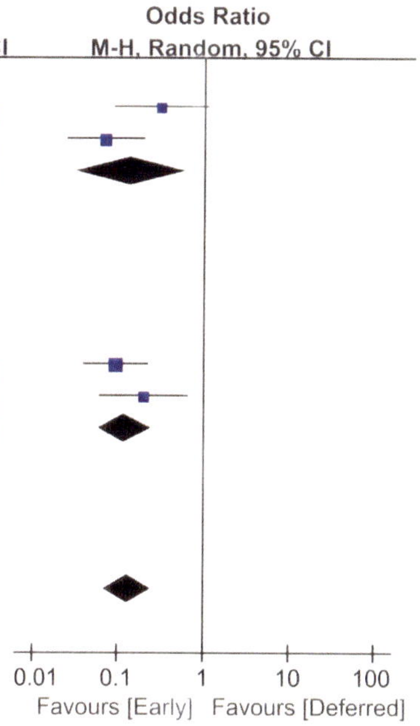

Figure 3. Progression rate odds ratios of early treatment versus deferred treatment. The 95% CIs are shown. Squares represent the odds ratios and 95% CI for alkylators or IMiDs and finally for the overall estimate. CIs, confidence intervals; IMiDs, immuno-modulatory agents.

suffered from vertebral compression. No heterogeneity was observed ($p = 0.99$, $I^2 = 0\%$). The incidence of vertebral compression in the early treatment arm did not significantly differ from that in the deferred treatment arm (pooled OR = 0.18, 95%CI = 0.02 to 1.59) (Figure 5).

6.5 Gastrointestinal toxicities. Gastrointestinal toxicities, including both constipation and diarrhea, were reported in only two the trials. Both studies reported the incidence of constipation, but only one reported the incidence of diarrhea. Forty-six (46) of 92 patients in the early treatment arm and 9 of 95 patients in the deferred treatment arm suffered from gastrointestinal toxicities. No heterogeneity was observed ($p = 0.46$, $I^2 = 0\%$). Patients in the early treatment arm experienced a greater incidence of gastrointestinal toxicities (pooled OR = 10.02, 95%CI = 4.32 to 23.23) (Figure 5).

6.6 Constipation. 32 of 92 patients in the early treatment arm and 7 of 95 patients in the deferred treatment arm suffered from constipation when only constipation among gastrointestinal toxicities was evaluated. No heterogeneity was observed ($p = 0.65$, $I^2 = 0\%$). We found significant differences between the two arms, with more patients in early treatment arm experiencing greater incidence of constipation (pooled OR = 8.58, 95%CI = 3.20 to 23.00) (Figure 5), but all the cases were grade 1 or 2.

6.7 Fatigue or asthenia. Fatigue or asthenia was reported in two trials. 42 of 92 patients in the early treatment arm and 26 of 95 patients in the deferred treatment arm experienced fatigue or asthenia. No heterogeneity was observed ($p = 0.58$, $I^2 = 0\%$). We found significant differences between the two arms, with a greater incidence of fatigue or asthenia in the early versus deferred treatment arms (pooled OR = 2.72, 95%CI = 1.30 to 5.67) (Figure 5). Fatigue or asthenia at grade 1 or 2 was reported in 37 of 92 patients in the early treatment arm and 23 of 95 patients in the deferred treatment arm. Higher grade fatigue or asthenia (3 or 4) was reported in 5 of 92 patients in the early treatment arm and 3 of 95 patients in the deferred treatment arm.

Discussion

The meta-analysis by He et al. in 2003 [5] evaluated three RCTs that used melphalan and prednisone to treat patients with SMM. Researchers have since questioned whether their conclusion that early treatment did not decrease mortality was actually a false-negative result. This was based on the fact that they only had

Study or Subgroup	Early treatment Events	Early treatment Total	Deferred treatment Events	Deferred treatment Total	Weight	Odds Ratio M-H, Random, 95% CI
Hjorth 1993	13	25	12	22	33.7%	0.90 [0.29, 2.85]
Riccardi 2000	30	75	19	34	66.3%	0.53 [0.23, 1.19]
Total (95% CI)		**100**		**56**	**100.0%**	**0.63 [0.32, 1.23]**
Total events	43		31			
Heterogeneity: Tau² = 0.00; Chi² = 0.56, df = 1 (P = 0.45); I² = 0%						
Test for overall effect: Z = 1.35 (P = 0.18)						

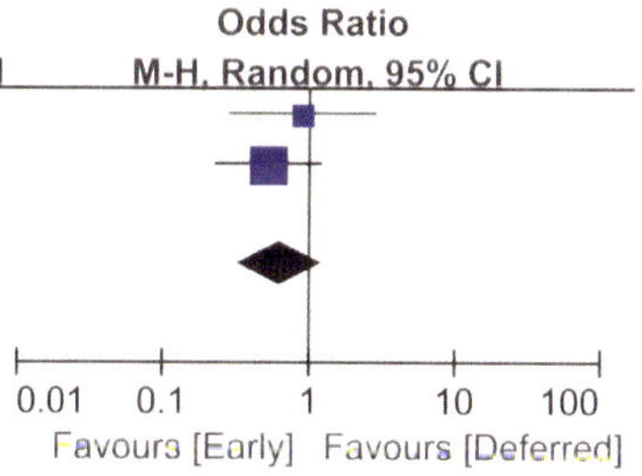

Figure 4. Response rate odds ratios of early treatment versus deferred treatment. Squares on the odds ratios plot are proportional to the weight of each study, which is based on the M-H method. Odds ratios are presents with 95% CIs. CIs, confidence intervals.

Study or Subgroup	Early treatment Events	Early treatment Total	Deferred treatment Events	Deferred treatment Total	Weight	Odds Ratio M-H, Random, 95% CI
1.3.1 Acute leukemia						
Riccardi 1994	0	34	0	40		Not estimable
Hjorth 1993	2	25	0	25	38.1%	5.43 [0.25, 118.96]
Riccardi 2000	2	72	1	66	61.9%	1.86 [0.16, 20.97]
Subtotal (95% CI)		**131**		**131**	**100.0%**	**2.80 [0.42, 18.81]**
Total events	4		1			
Heterogeneity: Tau² = 0.00; Chi² = 0.29, df = 1 (P = 0.59); I² = 0%						
Test for overall effect: Z = 1.06 (P = 0.29)						
1.3.2 Hematologic cancer						
Mateos 2013	0	34	0	40		Not estimable
Hjorth 1993	2	25	0	25	26.0%	5.43 [0.25, 118.96]
Riccardi 2000	1	57	1	62	31.8%	1.09 [0.07, 17.83]
Riccardi 1994	2	72	1	66	42.2%	1.86 [0.16, 20.97]
Subtotal (95% CI)		**188**		**193**	**100.0%**	**2.07 [0.43, 10.01]**
Total events	5		2			
Heterogeneity: Tau² = 0.00; Chi² = 0.59, df = 2 (P = 0.74); I² = 0%						
Test for overall effect: Z = 0.91 (P = 0.36)						
1.3.3 Second primary tumors						
Riccardi 1994	0	34	0	40		Not estimable
Hjorth 1993	2	25	0	25	22.0%	5.43 [0.25, 118.96]
Riccardi 2000	2	72	1	66	35.6%	1.86 [0.16, 20.97]
Mateos 2013	4	57	1	62	42.4%	4.60 [0.50, 42.47]
Subtotal (95% CI)		**188**		**193**	**100.0%**	**3.45 [0.81, 14.68]**
Total events	8		2			
Heterogeneity: Tau² = 0.00; Chi² = 0.40, df = 2 (P = 0.82); I² = 0%						
Test for overall effect: Z = 1.68 (P = 0.09)						
1.3.4 Vertebral compression						
Hjorth 1993	0	25	2	25	49.5%	0.18 [0.01, 4.04]
Riccardi 2000	0	72	2	66	50.5%	0.18 [0.01, 3.78]
Subtotal (95% CI)		**97**		**91**	**100.0%**	**0.18 [0.02, 1.59]**
Total events	0		4			
Heterogeneity: Tau² = 0.00; Chi² = 0.00, df = 1 (P = 0.99); I² = 0%						
Test for overall effect: Z = 1.54 (P = 0.12)						
1.3.5 Gastrointestinal toxicity						
Mateos 2013	24	57	3	62	43.6%	14.30 [4.00, 51.11]
Witzig 2013	22	35	6	33	56.4%	7.62 [2.49, 23.32]
Subtotal (95% CI)		**92**		**95**	**100.0%**	**10.02 [4.32, 23.23]**
Total events	46		9			
Heterogeneity: Tau² = 0.00; Chi² = 0.54, df = 1 (P = 0.46); I² = 0%						
Test for overall effect: Z = 5.37 (P < 0.00001)						
1.3.6 Constipation						
Mateos 2013	10	57	1	62	22.3%	12.98 [1.60, 104.99]
Witzig 2013	22	35	6	33	77.7%	7.62 [2.49, 23.32]
Subtotal (95% CI)		**92**		**95**	**100.0%**	**8.58 [3.20, 23.00]**
Total events	32		7			
Heterogeneity: Tau² = 0.00; Chi² = 0.20, df = 1 (P = 0.65); I² = 0%						
Test for overall effect: Z = 4.27 (P < 0.0001)						
1.3.7 Fatigue or Asthenia						
Witzig 2013	27	35	20	33	48.8%	2.19 [0.76, 6.29]
Mateos 2013	15	57	6	62	51.2%	3.33 [1.19, 9.32]
Subtotal (95% CI)		**92**		**95**	**100.0%**	**2.72 [1.30, 5.67]**
Total events	42		26			
Heterogeneity: Tau² = 0.00; Chi² = 0.31, df = 1 (P = 0.58); I² = 0%						
Test for overall effect: Z = 2.66 (P = 0.008)						

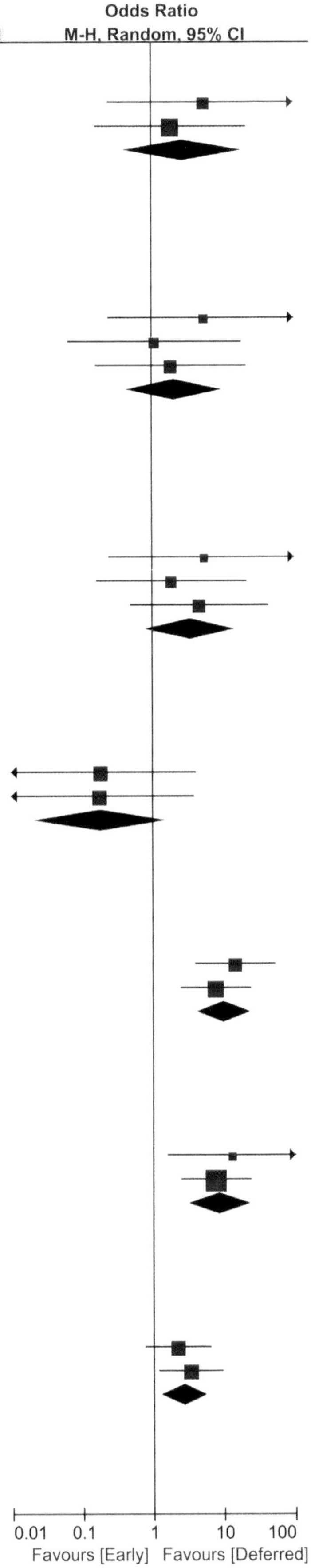

Figure 5. Adverse events rate odds ratios of early treatment versus deferred treatment. Squares on the odds ratios plot are proportional to the weight of each study, which is based on the M-H method. Odds ratios are presents with 95% CIs. CIs, confidence intervals.

262 patients in their analysis, which was only 70% of the requisite 350 patients or more that were needed to reliably detect 15% mortality difference based on the Pogue and Yusuf formula they used. In our analysis, 449 patients were included, providing us more statistical power to evaluate this difference. However, even with a greater number of patients, there was no survival benefit in treating SMM patients early. This held true when the data were combined or when we analyzed the trials by treatment group, alkylators and IMiDs, respectively. Notably, doing this puts us under the same criticism of the work by He et al. because of the reduced number of patients in each group. More large-scale trials with IMiDs and newly emerging therapies are needed to provide more evidence.

Mhaskar et al. [20] performed a meta-analysis of 10 RCTs comparing efficacy of early versus late first-line treatments for cancer. They conducted subgroup analysis based on cancer type, including MM. Their subgroup analyses for MM showed no difference in survival and response rate. But there was statistically significant difference in progression-free-survival. These results were consistent with ours. But they did not compare safety of early versus late first-line treatments for MM, which is one important part in our analysis.

Only the Mateos trial [21], among all trials included here, showed that mortality was significantly lower in the early treatment arm compared to that of the deferred treatment arm (7% versus 21%; OR = 0.28, 95%CI = 0.09 to 0.93). Interestingly, although all the patients included in all the trials we analyzed had SMM, the patients in the Mateos trial included a large number of high risk SMM. The addition of the high risk SMM patients could contribute to the different clinical outcomes. This is, however, confounded because there has not been a consistent definition for high risk SMM [22–24], and none of the other trials selected patients with high risk SMM, so we could not address this question. Moving forward, it will be important not only to evaluate early treatment for patients with high-risk SMM, but also to consistently define high-risk SMM.

Along with no reduction in mortality, we also found that early treatment with alkylators did not significantly improve response rates. Notably, these data were available for only two trials. Since the response rate of the deferred treatment arm in these trials with IMiDs were not reported, we were not sure whether early treatment with IMiDs could improve response rates, comparatively.

Despite there being no difference in mortality or response rates between the early and deferred treatment arms, our meta-analysis demonstrated that early treatment decreased the risk of disease progression. This also held true when we stratified the trials by treatment with either alkylators or IMiDs. The fact that overall mortality is not reduced but progression is delayed indicates that the early treatment group survives for a shorter amount of time than the deferred treatment group once the disease has progressed. This suggests that early treatment might actually predispose toward a more aggressive, more difficult to treat MM disease once it has progressed. The addition of molecular analyses at both diagnosis and progression may help to explain this phenomenon.

In addition to efficacy, safety is an equally important consideration for whether to subject patients to early treatment. Only vertebral compression and acute leukemia were analyzed in the meta-analysis of 2003. Apart from these adverse events, we also extracted data on gastrointestinal toxicity, hematological cancer, second primary tumor, and fatigue or asthenia. Other adverse events, such as neuropathy, anemia, rash and infection were not consistently reported, and were not considered in this analysis. Although there was a trend for increased incidence of acute leukemia, hematologic cancer, second primary tumors and vertebral compression, our meta-analysis revealed that there was no statistically significant difference between the early and deferred treatment arms. There were few cases that reported these adverse events and follow-up time was limited. Therefore, our findings should be further verified with more RCTs and longer follow-up times. Analyses of gastrointestinal toxicities showed that early treatment with IMiDs was associated with an increased incidence. When only constipation was evaluated, we found an increased incidence for the early IMiD treatment group, but all the cases were moderate. Data on gastrointestinal toxicities were not available for trials that used alkylators. Data were integrated regarding fatigue and asthenia because they were frequently reported together. Early treatment with IMiDs appeared to increase the incidence of fatigue or asthenia, but most cases were moderate. Such data were not available for studies that used alkylators. Our findings call attention to gastrointestinal toxicities and fatigue or asthenia as the predominant safety concerns associated with treating SMM patients with IMiDs.

There were a number of limitations of this meta-analysis. First, all individual studies used in our analyses had small sample sizes and did not have predetermined power analyses. Due to the small sample sizes, the data on vertebral compression, acute leukemia, hematological cancer and second primary tumor were not interpretable. Second, only two of the included studies reported an adequate method for randomized allocation and allocation concealment. Third, sample sizes were also too small for reliable subgroup analyses for IMiDs versus alkylators. Fourth, separate subgroup analysis was not possible on low- versus high-risk SMM. Finally, statistically significant heterogeneity was seen in subgroup of progression ($I^2 = 69\%$) and in subgroup of mortality ($I^2 = 52\%$). This might be derived largely from potential differences in the proportion of different SMM risk stratification, non-uniform reporting of clinical parameters, and variability in clinical factors.

Despite these limitations, our meta-analysis demonstrated that early treatment did indeed delay disease progression, but delaying progression did not translate into an improved response rate or decreasing mortality. However, further RCTs were needed to determine if early treatment of SMM with the newer, targeted agents and/or patients characteristics were more likely to improve response rate and overall survival. Early treatment also resulted in an increased risk of gastrointestinal toxicities and fatigue or asthenia.

Supporting Information

Table S1 Search criterion of Medline (via Pubmed, from inception to May 16, 2014).

Table S2 Search criterion of Cochrane Library (from inception to May 17, 2014).

Table S3 Characteristics of excluded full-text studies.

Checklist S1 PRISMA checklist.

Author Contributions

Conceived and designed the experiments: JmS FhZ MjG. Performed the experiments: MjG GY. Analyzed the data: MjG GY. Contributed reagents/materials/analysis tools: VST LG XsW YT XjH JH YH HwX. Wrote the manuscript: JmS FhZ MjG GY. Obtaining funding: JmS FhZ XjH VST. Read and approved the final paper: MjG GY VST LG XsW YT XjH JH YH HwX JmS FhZ.

References

1. Raab MS, Podar K, Breitkreutz I, Richardson PG, Anderson KC (2009) Multiple myeloma. Lancet 374: 324–339.
2. Smith D, Yong K (2013) Multiple myeloma. BMJ 346: f3863.
3. Dolloff NG, Talamo G (2013) Targeted therapy of multiple myeloma. Adv Exp Med Biol 779: 197–221.
4. Harousseau JL (2010) Optimising patient outcomes in myeloma. Cancer Treat Rev 36 Suppl 2: S33–S35.
5. He Y, Wheatley K, Clark O, Glasmacher A, Ross H, et al. (2003) Early versus deferred treatment for early stage multiple myeloma. Cochrane Database Syst Rev D4023.
6. Palumbo A, Sezer O, Kyle R, Miguel JS, Orlowski RZ et al. (2009) International Myeloma Working Group guidelines for the management of multiple myeloma patients ineligible for standard high-dose chemotherapy with autologous stem cell transplantation. Leukemia 23: 1716–1730.
7. Rajkumar SV, Gertz MA, Lacy MQ, Dispenzieri A, Fonseca R, et al.(2003) Thalidomide as initial therapy for early-stage myeloma. Leukemia 17: 775–779.
8. Fouquet G, Guidez S, Herbaux C, Demarquette H, Leleu X (2013) [Smoldering multiple myeloma.]. Rev Med Interne.
9. Waxman AJ, Kuehl M, Balakumaran A, Weiss B, Landgren O (2010) Smoldering (asymptomatic) multiple myeloma: revisiting the clinical dilemma and looking into the future. Clin Lymphoma Myeloma Leuk 10: 248–257.
10. Kyle RA, Rajkumar SV (2007) Monoclonal gammopathy of undetermined significance and smouldering multiple myeloma: emphasis on risk factors for progression. Br J Haematol 139: 730–743.
11. Kyle RA, Remstein ED, Therneau TM, Dispenzieri A, Kurtin PJ, et al. (2007) Clinical course and prognosis of smoldering (asymptomatic) multiple myeloma. N Engl J Med 356: 2582–2590.
12. Ghobrial IM (2013) Revisiting treatment paradigms in high-risk smoldering multiple myeloma: out with the old, in with the new? Leuk Lymphoma 54: 2328–2330.
13. Korde N, Kristinsson SY, Landgren O (2011) Monoclonal gammopathy of undetermined significance (MGUS) and smoldering multiple myeloma (SMM): novel biological insights and development of early treatment strategies. Blood 117: 5573–5581.
14. Blade J, Dimopoulos M, Rosinol L, Rajkumar SV, Kyle RA (2010) Smoldering (asymptomatic) multiple myeloma: current diagnostic criteria, new predictors of outcome, and follow-up recommendations. J Clin Oncol 28: 690–697.
15. Rajkumar SV (2012) Preventive strategies in monoclonal gammopathy of undetermined significance and smoldering multiple myeloma. Am J Hematol 87: 453–454.
16. Hjorth M, Hellquist L, Holmberg E, Magnusson B, Rodjer S, et al. (1993) Initial versus deferred melphalan-prednisone therapy for asymptomatic multiple myeloma stage I–a randomized study. Myeloma Group of Western Sweden. Eur J Haematol 50: 95–102.
17. Riccardi A, Ucci G, Luoni R, Brugnatelli S, Mora O, et al. (1994) Treatment of multiple myeloma according to the extension of the disease: a prospective, randomised study comparing a less with a more aggressive cystostatic policy. Cooperative Group of Study and Treatment of Multiple Myeloma. Br J Cancer 70: 1203–1210.
18. Riccardi A, Mora O, Tinelli C, Vanlentini D, Brugnatelli S, et al. (2000) Long-term survival of stage I multiple myeloma given chemotherapy just after diagnosis or at progression of the disease: a multicentre randomized study. Cooperative Group of Study and Treatment of Multiple Myeloma. Br J Cancer 82: 1254–1260.
19. Witzig TE, Laumann KM, Lacy MQ, Hayman SR, Dispenzieri A et al. (2013) A phase III randomized trial of thalidomide plus zoledronic acid versus zoledronic acid alone in patients with asymptomatic multiple myeloma. Leukemia 27: 220–225.
20. Mhaskar AR, Quinn G, Vadaparampil S, Djulbegovic B, Gwede CK, et al. (2010) Timing of first-line cancer treatments - early versus late - a systematic review of phase III randomized trials. Cancer Treat Rev 36: 621–628.
21. Mateos MV, Hernandez MT, Giraldo P, de la Rubia J, de Arriba F, et al. (2013) Lenalidomide plus dexamethasone for high-risk smoldering multiple myeloma. N Engl J Med 369: 438–447.
22. Rajkumar SV, Larson D, Kyle RA (2011) Diagnosis of smoldering multiple myeloma. N Engl J Med 365: 474–475.
23. Larsen JT, Kumar SK, Dispenzieri A, Kyle RA, Katzmann JA, et al. (2013) Serum free light chain ratio as a biomarker for high-risk smoldering multiple myeloma. Leukemia 27: 941–946.
24. Bianchi G, Kyle RA, Larson DR, Witzig TE, Kumar S, et al. (2013) High levels of peripheral blood circulating plasma cells as a specific risk factor for progression of smoldering multiple myeloma. Leukemia 27: 680–685.

Distance to High-Voltage Power Lines and Risk of Childhood Leukemia – an Analysis of Confounding by and Interaction with Other Potential Risk Factors

Camilla Pedersen[1]*, Elvira V. Bräuner[1,2], Naja H. Rod[3], Vanna Albieri[1], Claus E. Andersen[4], Kaare Ulbak[5], Ole Hertel[6,7], Christoffer Johansen[1,8], Joachim Schüz[9], Ole Raaschou-Nielsen[1]

1 Danish Cancer Society Research Center, Copenhagen Ø, Denmark, **2** Danish Building Research Institute, Aalborg University, Construction and Health, Copenhagen SV, Denmark, **3** Social Medicine Section, Department of Public Health, University of Copenhagen, Copenhagen K, Denmark, **4** Risø National Laboratory for Sustainable Energy, Radiation Research Division, Technical University of Denmark, Roskilde, Denmark, **5** National Institute of Radiation Protection, Herlev, Denmark, **6** Department of Environmental Science, Aarhus University, Roskilde, Denmark, **7** Department for Environmental, Social and Spatial Change (ENSPAC), Roskilde University, Roskilde, Denmark, **8** Oncology Clinic, Finsen Centre, Rigshospitalet 5073, University of Copenhagen, Copenhagen Ø, Denmark, **9** International Agency for Research on Cancer (IARC), Section of Environment and Radiation, Lyon, France

Abstract

We investigated whether there is an interaction between distance from residence at birth to nearest power line and domestic radon and traffic-related air pollution, respectively, in relation to childhood leukemia risk. Further, we investigated whether adjusting for potential confounders alters the association between distance to nearest power line and childhood leukemia. We included 1024 cases aged <15, diagnosed with leukemia during 1968–1991, from the Danish Cancer Registry and 2048 controls randomly selected from the Danish childhood population and individually matched by gender and year of birth. We used geographical information systems to determine the distance between residence at birth and the nearest 132–400 kV overhead power line. Concentrations of domestic radon and traffic-related air pollution (NO_x at the front door) were estimated using validated models. We found a statistically significant interaction between distance to nearest power line and domestic radon regarding risk of childhood leukemia ($p = 0.01$) when using the median radon level as cut-off point but not when using the 75th percentile ($p = 0.90$). We found no evidence of an interaction between distance to nearest power line and traffic-related air pollution ($p = 0.73$). We found almost no change in the estimated association between distance to power line and risk of childhood leukemia when adjusting for socioeconomic status of the municipality, urbanization, maternal age, birth order, domestic radon and traffic-related air pollution. The statistically significant interaction between distance to nearest power line and domestic radon was based on few exposed cases and controls and sensitive to the choice of exposure categorization and might, therefore, be due to chance.

Editor: Ramiro Garzon, The Ohio State University, United States of America

Funding: This work was supported by a grant by the foundation Children with Cancer UK (formerly Children with Leukaemia) http://www.childrenwithcancer.org.uk/, by Danish Energy Association for provision on data on power lines, and by the Danish Cancer Society. The funders had no role in study design and analysis, decision to publish, or preparation of the manuscript. Danish Energy have provided data on power lines.

Competing Interests: Regarding the financial disclosure statement the authors can confirm that Danish Energy is the Danish Energy Association, which is a commercial and professional organization for Danish energy companies. The Danish Energy Association has not supported the research project financially but the transmission companies have provided data on power lines for the project.

* Email: camped@cancer.dk

Introduction

In 2001 a working group at the International Agency for Research on Cancer (IARC) classified exposure to extremely low-frequency magnetic fields (ELF-MF) as 'possibly carcinogenic to humans' and exposure to extremely low-frequency electric fields were grouped as 'not classifiable as to its carcinogenicity to humans' [1]. The classification of ELF-MF was primarily based on epidemiological findings, showing an association between residential exposure to ELF-MF and childhood leukemia [2]. There is no known biological explanation for this association and the epidemiological findings have not been supported by animal studies [3]. Therefore, it is not known whether the observed association reflects a causal relationship or is due to bias, confounding or chance [2,3].

In 2005 a large-scale case-control study from Great Britain [4] showed an association between proximity of residence at birth to high-voltage power lines and the risk of childhood leukemia. The association extended beyond distances where the 'power line'-induced ELF-MF exceed background levels, which suggests that the association was not explained by the magnetic field but perhaps by some other risk factor. Several studies have looked for potential confounders which could explain the observed association between ELF-MF and childhood leukemia [5–18] including socioeconomic status, residential mobility, residence type, viral contacts, environmental tobacco smoke, dietary agents, and traffic density; but none of them appear to explain the association [19]. Little is known about the etiology of childhood leukemia and there are only few established causes of childhood leukemia including exposure to ionizing radiation (X-rays and gamma rays) and certain genetic diseases such as Down's syndrome [20,21]. The limited knowledge of the etiology of childhood leukemia makes it difficult to exclude the possibility of some yet unknown risk factor or of the combination of a number of risk factors, which could confound the analysis between ELF-MF and childhood leukemia [19].

The lack of an accepted biological explanation for the observed association between ELF-MF and childhood leukemia have raised doubt about the causality of the association. Several mechanisms of how extremely low-frequency electric and magnetic fields can cause cancer have, however, been proposed [3]. One hypothesis is that the electric field from power lines interacts with airborne pollutant particles and thereby increases the harmful effect of these particles [22–25]. Airborne particles such as tobacco smoke, radon decay products, chemical pollutants, spores, bacteria and viruses might all affect health. These particles can be deposited on the skin or in the airways by inhalation [3,25]. In 1999 Fews et al. [23] found a higher deposition of pollutant aerosols on the body under high-voltage power lines, which they argued was due to the oscillation of charged particles in the electric field from the power line. Further, Fews et al. [24] suggested that the electric field from high-voltage power lines can cause electrical breakdown of the air resulting in emission of clouds of positive and negative ions, which can charge particles that pass through them. Since charged particles are more likely than uncharged particles to be deposited when close to the walls of the respiratory airways or to the skin, this could increase the exposure and thereby the adverse health effect of such particles.

The major objective of our study was, therefore, to investigate possible interactions between distance from residence to nearest power line and domestic radon and traffic-related air pollution, respectively, in relation to childhood leukemia risk; to our knowledge this has not previously been investigated. Additionally, we investigated whether adjusting for potential confounding factors alters the association between distance from residence at birth to nearest power line and childhood leukemia. We adjusted for factors observed to be associated with childhood leukemia risk in other studies, specifically socioeconomic status of the municipality, urbanization, maternal age, birth order, domestic radon and traffic-related air pollution [20,21,26,27], which might also be related to distance from residence to nearest power line. The main effect of distance to nearest power line and childhood leukemia risk has been reported in a previous paper [28].

Materials and Methods

Ethics statement

The Danish Data Protection Agency (2007-41-0239) approved the study. In accordance with Danish law written consent was not obtained as the study was entirely register-based and did not involve biological samples from, or contact with study participants.

Cases and controls

We identified all children in Denmark diagnosed with leukemia (all types) before the age of 15 years during the period 1968–1991 (inclusively) through the virtually complete nationwide Danish Cancer Registry [29]. Children with a previous cancer diagnosis were excluded. Two controls for each case were individually matched by gender and year of birth and were selected by incidence density sampling from the Danish Civil Registration System. All children born in Denmark, who were alive, without cancer and living in Denmark at the time of diagnosis of their matched case were eligible to become a control in the study.

We identified 1024 cases diagnosed with leukemia and selected 2048 matched controls, constituting a population of 3072 children (Figure S1).

Distance to nearest power line

The addresses of cases and controls at birth were obtained from the Danish Civil Registration System and we identified geographical coordinates by linkage to the Danish Address Database. The geographical coordinates refer to the front door of each residence (for apartments the main entrance door) and are precise within a few meters. We collected data on existing and historical 132–400 kV overhead power lines with alternating current from the seven Danish transmission companies. The mapped grid includes 4336 km of current and historical power lines (23.1% 400 kV, 0.9% 220 kV, 46.3% 150 kV, 29.8% 132 kV). In addition information on the date when the line was put into and out of operation was collected. For the lines for which we only had information on the year of operation (77.5%), we set the date of operation to 31 December and the date when the line was put out of operation was set to 1 January. This restrictive approach was applied to avoid assigning exposure to unexposed individuals. The distance from residence at birth to the nearest power line that existed at the date of birth was calculated in ArcGIS 9.3. We successfully calculated distance for 2797 (91.0%) of the addresses at birth. Distance could not be calculated due to missing information in the address for 100 (9.8%) cases and 175 (8.5%) controls (Figure S1). Distance was categorized into three groups: 0–199 meters, 200–599 meters and ≥600 meters, in accordance with the categorization used by Draper et al. [4].

Domestic radon

Domestic radon concentration at address at birth was estimated using a validated regression model constructed to predict radon concentrations in Danish dwellings on the basis of register data including geographical region, soil type, and house characteristics such as type of house, floor, basement, and building materials. Details on the model are given in previous papers [30,31].

Exposure to domestic radon at address at birth was successfully estimated for 2904 (94.5%) addresses. We could not estimate domestic radon exposure for 62 (6.1%) cases and 106 (5.2%) controls (Figure S1).

Traffic-related air pollution

We used the sum of nitrogen oxide gasses, NO_x (nitrogen monoxide (NO) + nitrogen dioxide (NO_2)), as an indicator for air pollution from traffic because NO_x correlates strongly with other traffic-related pollutants in Danish streets, especially ultrafine PM (Particulate matter): $r = 0.93$ for total particle number concentration (size, 10–700 nm) and $r = 0.70$ for PM_{10} (mass of particles with an aerodynamic diameter less than 10 μm) [32,33]. The average concentration of NO_x at the front door of the address at birth was estimated by use of the Operational Street Pollution Model taking into account both the street-level pollution as well as the background pollution [34,35,36,37]. In short the model was used to estimate the air pollution level from street information (such as width of the street, the height of the buildings, the distance between building and street sections with no buildings), the traffic density on the street, the proportion of vehicles weighing more than 3,500 kg, the average speed in combination with information on emission factors for the Danish car fleet, meteorological variables (wind speed, temperature and solar radiation) and background level of air pollution at the front door.

Exposure to traffic-related air pollution at the birth address was successfully estimated for 2942 (95.8%) addresses and could not be estimated for 45 (4.4%) cases and 85 (4.2%) controls (Figure S1).

Potential confounders

Socioeconomic status of the municipality (the average gross income of the municipality) has been described in detail previously [27], where it was estimated for children born in the period 1976–1991. Children born in the period 1953–1975 were assigned the municipality income level based on data in 1976. Definition of rural and urban area was based on the official Danish classification. Information on maternal age and birth order was provided by linkage with the Danish Civil Registration System using the personal identification number. We also adjusted the analyses for domestic radon and traffic-related air pollution.

We had no information on socio-economic status of the municipality for 6 cases and 12 controls, on urbanization for 100 cases and 175 controls, on maternal age for 43 cases and 77 controls and on birth order for 43 cases and 78 controls (Figure S1).

Statistical analysis

Because of the nested case-control design of the study, with equal follow-up time for a case and the matched controls, the rate ratios [38] (hereafter denoted relative risks (RR)) for childhood cancer and 95% confidence intervals (CIs) were estimated by conditional logistic regression models with the "PROC PHREG" procedure in SAS 9.2.

We analyzed the association between distance to nearest power line and risk of childhood leukemia both with and without adjustment for potential confounders. The potential confounders included socio-economic status of the municipality (categorical; < 10 pct., 10–90 pct., >90 pct.), urbanization (categorical; countryside, urban area), maternal age at time of birth (categorical; <30y, ≥30y), birth order (categorical; 1, ≥2), domestic radon (categorical; <50 pct., 50–90 pct., >90 pct.) and traffic-related air pollution (categorical; <50 pct., 50–90 pct., >90 pct.).

We analyzed possible interactions between distance to power lines and domestic radon and traffic-related air pollution, respectively. Since there is no known biological relevant cut-off point for radon or NO_x, we dichotomized domestic radon and traffic-related air pollution using the median value as cut-off; in sensitivity analyses we used the 75th percentile as cut-off point. In an additional sensitivity analysis we divided radon and NO_x into tertiles in order to investigate a potential dose-response association. All interaction analyses were adjusted for the potential confounders: socioeconomic status of the municipality, urbanization, maternal age at time of birth, birth order and domestic radon and traffic-related air pollution, respectively. From the former study on radon [31] we had information on radon for cases and controls until 1994 and therefore we conducted an additional sensitivity analysis (unadjusted) of the interaction between power lines and radon to maximize the power. Furthermore, the interaction was analyzed including radon as a continuous variable. The p-value for the interaction was obtained by comparing and testing the model with the interaction term against the model with only the main effect by means of the likelihood ratio test.

Due to small samples in some of the categories in the analysis of the interaction between distance to power line and radon, exact methods for logistic regression were also applied using LogXact. It was only possible to compute models without adjustment for confounding factors.

Results

We excluded 139 (13.6%) cases and 248 (12.1%) controls due to missing data on distance to power line or any of the potential confounding factors: domestic radon, traffic-related air pollution, socioeconomic status of the municipality, urbanization, maternal age or birth order. Further, we excluded 6 cases and 179 controls since they no longer had a matched control or case, leaving 879 (85.8%) cases and 1621 (79.2%) controls for the analyses (Figure S1).

In Table 1 the distribution of potential confounders by case-controls status and by distance to nearest power line is shown. Cases were more likely than controls to be living in a municipality with a lower socioeconomic status at time of birth, to have a mother at the age of 30 or older at time of birth, and to have at least one older sibling. Cases and controls were similar regarding exposure to domestic radon and traffic-related air pollution at address at birth and regarding whether they were living in a town or at the countryside at the time of birth. Children living close to power lines tended to live in the countryside, to be exposed to higher concentrations of domestic radon, and to be exposed to smaller concentrations of air pollution than children living further away. Children living close to power lines were similar to children living far away regarding socioeconomic status of the municipality, maternal age and birth order.

Table 2 presents the crude and adjusted associations between distance to power lines and childhood leukemia. Adjusting for potential confounders had virtually no effect on the estimated association between distance to nearest power line and childhood leukemia.

Table 3 shows the respective joint effects of distance to nearest power line and domestic radon and air pollution on leukemia. We found a statistically significant interaction between distance to nearest power line and domestic radon ($p = 0.01$). The RR for children living 0–199 meters of a power line and being exposed to domestic radon ≥42 Bq/m^3 was 2.88 (95% CI: 1.01–8.27) compared to children living ≥600 meters from a power line and exposed to domestic radon <42 Bq/m^3. Children living 200–599 meters from a power line and being exposed to domestic radon < 42 Bq/m^3 had a lower risk with an RR of 0.24 (95% CI: 0.07–0.83) compared to children living ≥600 meters from a power lines and exposed to domestic radon <42 Bq/m^3. There was no evidence of interaction between distance to nearest power line and traffic-related air pollution ($p = 0.73$). The sensitivity analysis including domestic radon and traffic-related air pollution with a cut-off at the 75th percentile showed no significant interaction with domestic radon ($p = 0.90$) or air pollution ($p = 0.59$) (Tables S1) and there was no dose-response association when radon and air pollution were divided into tertiles (Table S2). The interaction between power lines and radon remained statistically significant in the sensitivity analysis including radon until 1994, however, the RR for children exposed to radon concentrations of ≥42 Bq/m^3 and living within 200 meters of a power line was no longer statistically significant (RR = 2.62 (95% CI: 0.97–7.07)) (Table S3). When radon was included as a continuous variable the interaction between distance to power line and radon was not statistically significant ($p = 0.37$) (data not shown). The result of the interaction analysis using exact methods was similar to the result of the unadjusted analysis using asymptotic methods (both presented in Table S4). The RR for children living within 200 m of a power line and exposed to radon concentrations of ≥42 Bq/m^3 was still elevated but not statistically significant.

Table 1. Potential confounders by case-control status and distance to nearest power line.

	Case-control status				P-value (χ^2-test)	Distance to nearest power line (meters)						P-value (χ^2-test)
	Cases		Controls			0–199		200–599		≥600		
	N	(%)	N	(%)		N	(%)	N	(%)	N	(%)	
Socioeconomic status					0.02							0.15
10% most poor	46	(5.2)	52	(3.2)		0	(0.0)	1	(0.9)	97	(4.1)	
80% middle group	739	(84.1)	1362	(84.0)		19	(86.4)	86	(81.1)	1996	(84.2)	
10% most rich	94	(10.7)	207	(12.8)		3	(13.6)	19	(17.9)	279	(11.8)	
Urbanization					0.63							0.01
Town	639	(72.7)	1193	(73.6)		15	(68.2)	65	(61.3)	1752	(73.9)	
Country side	240	(27.3)	428	(26.4)		7	(31.8)	41	(38.7)	620	(26.1)	
Maternal age (years)					0.01							0.89
<30	644	(73.3)	1260	(77.7)		16	(72.7)	82	(77.4)	1806	(76.1)	
≥30	235	(26.7)	361	(22.3)		6	(27.3)	24	(22.6)	566	(23.9)	
Birth order					0.02							0.62
1	363	(41.3)	746	(46.0)		8	(36.4)	44	(41.5)	1057	(44.6)	
>1	516	(58.7)	875	(54.0)		14	(63.6)	62	(58.5)	1315	(55.4)	
Domestic radon (Bq/m^3)[1]					0.77							<0.01
<42	432	(49.2)	818	(50.5)		7	(31.8)	26	(24.5)	1217	(51.3)	
42–101	360	(41.0)	640	(39.5)		13	(59.1)	62	(58.5)	925	(39.0)	
≥102	87	(9.9)	163	(10.1)		2	(9.1)	18	(17.0)	230	(9.7)	
NO_x at the front door (ppb)[1]					0.21							0.04
<9	460	(52.3)	790	(48.7)		13	(59.1)	62	(58.5)	1175	(49.5)	
9–20	338	(38.5)	662	(40.8)		8	(36.4)	42	(39.6)	950	(40.1)	
≥21	81	(9.2)	169	(10.4)		1	(4.6)	2	(1.9)	247	(10.4)	
Total	879	(100.0)	1621	(100.0)		22	(100.0)	106	(100.0)	2372	(100.0)	

[1]Cut-point is the 50th and 90th percentile.

Table 2. Crude and adjusted RRs for leukemia in association with distance to nearest power line.

Distance to nearest power line (meters)	Cases	Controls	Total	Model 1[a]		Model 2[b]		Model 3[c]		Model 4[d]	
	N (%)	N (%)		RR (CI)	P-value	RR (CI)	P-value	RR (CI)	P-value	RR (CI)	P-value
0–199	10 (1.1)	12 (0.7)	22	1.65 (0.71–3.83)		1.77 (0.76–4.11)		1.73 (0.74–4.02)		1.68 (0.72–3.92)	
200–599	29 (3.3)	77 (4.8)	106	0.68 (0.44–1.05)		0.69 (0.45–1.07)		0.70 (0.45–1.09)		0.70 (0.45–1.09)	
≥600	840 (95.6)	1532 (94.5)	2372	1.00	0.11	1.00	0.11	1.00	0.13	1.00	0.13
Total	879 (100.0)	1621 (100.0)	2500								

[a] The crude model.
[b] Adjusted for socioeconomic status and urbanization.
[c] Adjusted for the same as model 2 and for maternal age and birth order.
[d] Adjusted for the same as model 3 and for domestic radon and air pollution

Discussion

We found a statistically significant interaction between distance to nearest power line and domestic radon regarding risk of childhood leukemia when using the median radon level as cut-off point but not when using the 75th percentile of radon exposure as cut-off point. We found no evidence of an interaction between distance to nearest power line and traffic-related air pollution. We found almost no change in the estimated association between distance to power lines and risk of childhood leukemia when adjusting for socioeconomic status of the municipality, urbanization, maternal age, birth order, domestic radon and traffic-related air pollution.

Strengths and limitations

Our study was a register-based case-control study covering the entire population of Denmark. Cases were identified in a virtually complete national cancer registry, and the Central Population Registry provided an excellent basis for an unbiased sampling of controls. The potential for selection bias in our study is, therefore, minimal. We identified around 90% of current as well as historical power lines with ≥132 kV and according to two of the transmission companies (covering approximately 25% of all power lines) the data on power lines had a precision of 3–5 meters. The geographical coordinates used to identify the front door at the address at birth had a precision of few meters. For apartments the main entrance door was identified, which for the majority of apartments is within 5 meters, however, for some types of apartments a larger deviation may be expected.

Distance to nearest power line, domestic radon and air pollution was estimated for the address at birth, although exposure accumulated over all childhood addresses might be more relevant [31]. However, since interactions were in focus in the present study, we included the exposures at birth addresses only to ensure that the exposure to power lines (distance from residence) and exposure to domestic radon and traffic-related air pollution was present at the same address, which is essential for the analysis of interaction.

It is a limitation of the study that the analyses of interaction were based on few cases and controls for some of the cells of table 3. Data on air pollution was available from a previous study for children diagnosed during the period 1968–1991. It was not feasible to collect data for an extended period, though it would have contributed with more cases and controls and thereby more power in the analyses.

Exposure to domestic radon and traffic-related air pollution at the birth address were both modeled using successfully validated prediction models which have been applied in previous studies [31,39–41]. Radon values predicted by the model have previously been validated against measured values: Some non-differential misclassification occurs, but 80% of the lowest exposures (<50 Bq/m^3) were correctly classified and 60% of the highest exposures (>100 Bq/m^3) were correctly classified [31]. The internationally widely used [36] Operational Street Pollution Model used to predict the NO_x concentration at the front door has been validated by comparing the calculated nitrogen dioxide (NO_2) values with measured values at 204 locations in Denmark with an R^2 value of 0.82 [42]. Even though more precise estimates for exposure may be obtained with measured values, modeled estimates make it possible to avoid participation bias and to obtain a larger amount of participants than would be possible with measurement in each house.

Table 3. The joint effects of distance to nearest power line and domestic radon and air pollution, respectively, on leukemia.

	Adjusted			
	RR (95% CI)	(N cases; N controls)		P-value for interaction
	Distance (meters)			
	0–199	200–599	≥600	
Domestic radon (Bq/m^3)[1, 2]				
<42	0.33 (0.04–2.80)	0.24 (0.07–0.83)	1.00	0.01
	(1; 6)	(3; 23)	(428; 789)	
≥42	2.88 (1.01–8.27)	0.85 (0.52–1.39)	0.95 (0.79–1.16)	
	(9; 6)	(26; 54)	(412; 743)	
NO_x at the front door (ppb)[1, 3]				
<9	2.21 (0.73–6.64)	0.68 (0.38–1.21)	1.00	0.73
	(7; 6)	(17; 45)	(436; 739)	
≥9	1.02 (0.25–4.17)	0.67 (0.34–1.33)	0.92 (0.76–1.11)	
	(3; 6)	(12; 32)	(404; 793)	

[1]Cut-point is the median.
[2]The adjusted analysis includes following potential confounders: socioeconomic status, urbanization, maternal age, birth order and air pollution.
[3]The adjusted analysis includes following potential confounders: socioeconomic status, urbanization, maternal age, birth order and domestic radon.

Comparison with other studies and interpretation

In a previous study, where we included all children diagnosed with leukemia before the age of 15 years during the period 1968–2006, we report a OR of 0.76 (95% CI: 0.40–1.45) for children who lived 0–199 meters from the nearest power line compared with children who lived ≥600 meters away [28]. In the present study we report an RR of 1.68 (95% CI: 0.72–3.92) when living 0–199 meters from the nearest power line compared to those living ≥600 from the nearest power line. The 95% CIs of the two estimates widely overlap and none of the estimates are statistically significant, which indicate that the different estimates are due to chance and are two versions of the same null-result.

We found a statistically significant interaction between distance from residence to nearest power line and domestic radon but no interaction between distance and traffic-related air pollution. The interaction with radon showed a higher risk of childhood leukemia if living close to power lines and being exposed to high radon concentrations. This is in line with the hypothesis by Fews et al. [24] that ions of positive and negative charge emitted from power lines increases the proportion of charged radon particles and thereby increases the deposition of radon decay products on the skin or in the airways. Thus, the hypothesis by Fews et al. could explain the interaction observed in the present study. On the other hand the effect of the ions-clouds is expected to have the highest impact on particles arising outdoors whilst the exposure to radon is highest indoor where it can concentrate. According to an independent Advisory Group on Non-Ionising Radiation, advising The National Radiological Protection Board (NRPB) in UK, some of the ions are expected to enter the houses but the effect of the ion-clouds must be lower inside the house, since some of the ions would be deposited on the walls where entering the houses [3,25]. There could also be other explanations for an interaction between power lines and domestic radon in relation to childhood leukemia; for instance if the exposure to power lines makes the child more vulnerable to exposure to radon, or vice versa.

The interpretation of the observed interaction is not straightforward since it is not only based on a statistically significant higher risk among those exposed to high radon and living close to a power line but also a statistically significant lower risk among those being exposed to low domestic radon and living 200–599 meters from a power line, which is not easy to explain. The observed interaction might be due to chance because of few cases and controls in several cells. The finding of no statistically significant interaction when the 75th percentile was used as cut-off also suggests that the interaction found when using the median as cut-off might be due to chance. Even if the interaction between power lines and radon in relation to childhood leukemia is true, the potential effect in terms of absolute risk would be very small.

We found almost no change in the estimated association between distance to power lines and risk of childhood leukemia when adjusting for socioeconomic status of the municipality, urbanization, maternal age, birth order, domestic radon and traffic-related air pollution. This is in line with other studies investigating the association between ELF-MF and childhood leukemia, where the inclusion of potential confounders had no substantial effect on the estimates [5–18].

Conclusion

The statistically significant interaction observed between power lines and radon might be due to chance since numbers were small and the interaction was no longer significant when changing the cut-point for radon exposure. We found no support for an interaction between power lines and traffic-related air pollution and no change in the estimated association between distance to power lines and the risk of childhood leukemia by adjustment for potential confounding factors.

Supporting Information

Figure S1 Number of cases and controls in the study.

Table S1 The joint effects of distance to nearest power line and domestic radon and air pollution, respectively, on leukemia.

Table S2 The joint effects of distance to nearest power line and domestic radon and air pollution, respectively, on leukemia.

Table S3 The joint effects of distance to nearest power line and domestic radon on leukemia for the period 1968–1994.

Table S4 The joint effects of distance to nearest power line and domestic radon on leukemia risk with exact methods and with asymptotic methods.

Author Contributions

Conceived and designed the experiments: ORN JS CJ CP. Performed the experiments: CP. Analyzed the data: CP EVB NHR VA ORN. Contributed reagents/materials/analysis tools: CEA KU OH. Wrote the paper: CP.

References

1. IARC Working Group on the Evaluation of Carcinogenic Risks to Humans (2002) Non-ionizing radiation, Part 1: Static and extremely low-frequency (ELF) electric and magnetic fields. In: IARC Monographs on the Evaluation of Carcinogenic Risks to Humans volume 80. Lyon: IARCPress.
2. Schüz J, Ahlbom A (2008) Exposure to electromagnetic fields and the risk of childhood leukaemia: a review. Radiat Prot Dosimetry 132: 202–211. doi:10.1093/rpd/ncn270.
3. WHO (2007) Extremely low frequency fields. Geneva: World Health Organization. (Environmental health criteria 238).
4. Draper G, Vincent T, Kroll ME, Swanson J (2005) Childhood cancer in relation to distance from high voltage power lines in England and Wales: a case-control study. BMJ 330: 1290–1292.
5. Wünsch-Filho V, Pelissari DM, Barbieri FE, Sant'Anna L, de Oliveira CT, et al. (2011) Exposure to magnetic fields and childhood acute lymphocytic leukemia in São Paulo, Brazil. Cancer Epidemiol 35: 534–539. doi:10.1016/j.canep.2011.05.008.
6. Kroll ME, Swanson J, Vincent TJ, Draper GJ (2010) Childhood cancer and magnetic fields from high-voltage power lines in England and Wales: a case-control study. Br J Cancer 103: 1122–1127. doi:10.1038/sj.bjc.6605795.
7. Schüz J, Grigat JP, Brinkmann K, Michaelis J (2001) Residential magnetic fields as a risk factor for childhood acute leukaemia: results from a German population-based case-control study. Int J Cancer 91: 728–735.
8. Ahlbom A, Day N, Feychting M, Roman E, Skinner J, et al. (2000) A pooled analysis of magnetic fields and childhood leukaemia. Br J Cancer 83: 692–698.
9. UK Childhood Cancer Study Investigators (2000) Childhood cancer and residential proximity to power lines. Br J Cancer 83: 1573–1580.
10. UK Childhood Cancer Study Investigators (1999) Exposure to power-frequency magnetic fields and the risk of childhood cancer. Lancet 354: 1925–1931.
11. McBride ML, Gallagher RP, Thériault G, Armstrong BG, Tamaro S, et al. (1999) Power-frequency electric and magnetic fields and risk of childhood leukemia in Canada. Am J Epidemiol 149: 831–842.
12. Green LM, Miller AB, Villeneuve PJ, Agnew DA, Greenberg ML, et al. (1999) A case-control study of childhood leukemia in southern Ontario, Canada, and exposure to magnetic fields in residences. Int J Cancer 82: 161–170.
13. Green LM, Miller AB, Agnew DA, Greenberg ML, Li J, et al. (1999) Childhood leukemia and personal monitoring of residential exposures to electric and magnetic fields in Ontario, Canada. Cancer Causes Control 10: 233–243.
14. Linet MS, Hatch EE, Kleinerman RA, Robison LL, Kaune WT, et al. (1997) Residential exposure to magnetic fields and acute lymphoblastic leukemia in children. N Engl J Med 337: 1–7.
15. Michaelis J, Schüz J, Meinert R, Menger M, Grigat JP, et al. (1997) Childhood leukemia and electromagnetic fields: results of a population-based case-control study in Germany. Cancer Causes Control 8: 167–174.
16. Petridou E, Trichopoulos D, Kravaritis A, Pourtsidis A, Dessypris N, et al. (1997) Electrical power lines and childhood leukemia: a study from Greece. Int J Cancer 73: 345–348.
17. London SJ, Thomas DC, Bowman JD, Sobel E, Cheng TC, et al. (1991) Exposure to residential electric and magnetic fields and risk of childhood leukemia. Am J Epidemiol 134: 923–937.
18. Savitz DA, Wachtel H, Barnes FA, John EM, Tvrdik JG (1988) Case-control study of childhood cancer and exposure to 60-Hz magnetic fields. Am J Epidemiol 128: 21–38.
19. Kheifets L, Shimkhada R (2005) Childhood leukemia and EMF: review of the epidemiologic evidence. Bioelectromagnetics 26(Suppl 7): S51–S59.
20. Little J (1999) Epidemiology of Childhood Cancer. IARC scientific publications 149. Lyon: International Agency for Research on Cancer.
21. Rossig C, Juergens H (2008) Aetiology of childhood acute leukaemias: current status of knowledge. Radiat Prot Dosimetry 132: 114–118. doi:10.1093/rpd/ncn269.
22. Henshaw DL, Ross AN, Fews AP, Preece AW (1996) Enhanced deposition of radon daughter nuclei in the vicinity of power frequency electromagnetic fields. Int J Radiat Biol 69: 25–38.
23. Fews AP, Henshaw DL, Keitch PA, Close JJ, Wilding RJ (1999) Increased exposure to pollutant aerosols under high voltage power lines. Int J Radiat Biol: 75: 1505–1521.
24. Fews AP, Henshaw DL, Wilding RJ, Keitch PA (1999) Corona ions from powerlines and increased exposure to pollutant aerosols. Int J Radiat Biol 75: 1523–1531.
25. AGNIR - Advisory Group on Non-Ionising Radiation (2004) Particle deposition in the vicinity of power lines and possible effects on health. Chilton: National Radiological Protection Board, (Documents of the NRPB, Vol. 15, No. 1).
26. Eden T (2010) Aetiology of childhood leukaemia. Cancer Treat Rev 36: 286–297. doi:10.1016/j.ctrv.2010.02.004.
27. Raaschou-Nielsen O, Obel J, Dalton S, Tjønneland A, Hansen J (2004) Socioeconomic status and risk of childhood leukaemia in Denmark. Scand J Public Health 32: 279–286.
28. Pedersen C, Raaschou-Nielsen O, Rod NH, Frei P, Poulsen AH, et al. (2013). Distance from residence to power line and risk of childhood leukemia: a population-based case-control study in Denmark. Cancer Causes Control. doi:10.1007/s10552-013-0319-5.
29. Gjerstorff ML (2011) The Danish cancer registry. Scand J Public Health 39(7 Suppl): 42–45. doi:10.1177/1403494810393562.
30. Andersen CE, Raaschou-Nielsen O, Andersen HP, Lind M, Gravesen P, et al. (2007) Prediction of 222Rn in Danish dwellings using geology and house construction information from central databases. Radiat Prot Dosimetry 123: 83–94.
31. Raaschou-Nielsen O, Andersen CE, Andersen HP, Gravesen P, Lind M, et al. (2008) Domestic radon and childhood cancer in Denmark. Epidemiology 19: 536–543. doi:10.1097/EDE.0b013e318176bfcd.
32. Hertel O, Solvang S, Andersen HV, Palmgren F, Wåhlin P, et al. (2001) Human exposure to traffic pollution. Experience from Danish studies. Pure Appl Chem 73: 137–145.
33. Ketzel M, Wåhlin P, Berkowicz R, Palmgren F (2003) Particle and trace gas emission factors under urban driving conditions in Copenhagen based on street and roof-level observations. Atmos Environ 37: 2735–2749.
34. Raaschou-Nielsen O, Hertel O, Vignati E, Berkowicz R, Jensen SS, et al. (2000) An air pollution model for use in epidemiological studies: evaluation with measured levels of nitrogen dioxide and benzene. J Expo Anal Environ Epidemiol 10: 4–14.
35. Berkowicz R (2000) OSPM - a parametrised street pollution model. Environ Monit Assess 65: 323–331.
36. Kakosimos KE, Hertel O, Ketzel M, Berkowicz R (2010) Operational Street Pollution Model (OSPM) – a review of performed application and validation studies, and future prospects. Environ Chem 7: 485–503. doi:10.1071/EN10070.
37. Jensen SS, Berkowicz R, Hansen HS, Hertel O (2001) A Danish decision-support GIS tool for management of urban air quality and human exposures. Transportation Res. Part D: Transport and Environment, 6: 229–241.
38. Prentice RL, Breslow NE (1978) Retrospective studies and failure time models. Biometrika 65: 153–158.
39. Bräuner EV, Andersen ZJ, Andersen CE, Pedersen C, Gravesen P, et al. (2013) Residential radon and brain tumour incidence in a Danish cohort. PLoS One 8: e74435. doi:10.1371/journal.pone.0074435.
40. Bräuner EV, Andersen CE, Sørensen M, Andersen ZJ, Gravesen P, et al. (2012) Residential radon and lung cancer incidence in a Danish cohort. Environ Res 118: 130–136. doi:10.1016/j.envres.2012.05.012.
41. Bräuner EV, Andersen CE, Andersen HP, Gravesen P, Lind M, et al. (2010) Is there any interaction between domestic radon exposure and air pollution from traffic in relation to childhood leukemia risk? Cancer Causes Control 21: 1961–1964. doi:10.1007/s10552-010-9608-4.
42. Ketzel M, Berkowicz R, Hvidberg M, Jensen SS (2011) Evaluation of AirGIS: a GIS-based air pollution and human exposure modelling system. Int J Environment and Pollution 47: 226–238.

20

The Gene Expression Response of Chronic Lymphocytic Leukemia Cells to IL-4 Is Specific, Depends on ZAP-70 Status and Is Differentially Affected by an NFκB Inhibitor

Natalia Ruiz-Lafuente[1,6¶], María-José Alcaraz-García[1,6¶], Silvia Sebastián-Ruiz[1,6], Joaquín Gómez-Espuch[2,6], Consuelo Funes[2,6], José-María Moraleda[2,4,6], María-Carmen García-Garay[3], Natividad Montes-Barqueros[1,6], Alfredo Minguela[1,5,6], María-Rocío Álvarez-López[1,5,6], Antonio Parrado[1,6*]

1 Servicio de Inmunología, Hospital Clínico Universitario Virgen de la Arrixaca, Murcia, Spain, **2** Servicio de Hematología y Hemoterapia, Hospital Clínico Universitario Virgen de la Arrixaca, Murcia, Spain, **3** Servicio de Hematología y Hemoterapia, Hospital General Universitario Santa Lucía, Cartagena, Spain, **4** Universidad de Murcia, Murcia, Spain, **5** Centro de Investigación Biomédica en Red de enfermedades hepáticas y digestivas, Murcia, Spain, **6** Instituto Murciano de Investigación Biosanitaria Virgen de la Arrixaca (IMIB-Arrixaca), Murcia, Spain

Abstract

Interleukin 4 (IL-4), an essential mediator of B cell development, plays a role in survival of chronic lymphocytic leukemia (CLL) cells. To obtain new insights into the function of the IL-4 pathway in CLL, we analyzed the gene expression response to IL-4 in CLL and in normal B cells (NBC) by oligonucleotide microarrays, resulting in the identification of 232 non-redundant entities in CLL and 146 in NBC (95 common, 283 altogether), of which 189 were well-defined genes in CLL and 123 in NBC (83 common, 229 altogether) ($p<0.05$, 2-fold cut-off). To the best of our knowledge, most of them were novel IL-4 targets for CLL (98%), B cells of any source (83%), or any cell type (70%). Responses were significantly higher for 54 and 11 genes in CLL and NBC compared to each other, respectively. In CLL, ZAP-70 status had an impact on IL-4 response, since different sets of IL-4 targets correlated positively or negatively with baseline expression of ZAP-70. In addition, the NFκB inhibitor 6-Amino-4-(4-phenoxyphenethylamino)quinazoline, which reversed the anti-apoptotic effect of IL-4, preferentially blocked the response of genes positively correlated with ZAP-70 (e.g. CCR2, SUSD2), but enhanced the response of genes negatively correlated with ZAP-70 (e.g. AUH, BCL6, LY75, NFIL3). Dissection of the gene expression response to IL-4 in CLL and NBC contributes to the understanding of the anti-apoptotic response. Initial evidence of a connection between ZAP-70 and NFκB supports further exploration of targeting NFκB in the context of the assessment of inhibition of the IL-4 pathway as a therapeutic strategy in CLL, especially in patients expressing bad prognostic markers.

Editor: Ken Mills, Queen's University Belfast, United Kingdom

Funding: This work was supported by grants from Plan Nacional de I+D+I 2004-2007, Programa de Promoción de la Investigación Biomédica y en Ciencias de la Salud del Ministerio de Sanidad y Consumo (PI07/0135 to AP) and Plan Nacional de I+D+I 2008-2011, Acción Estratégica en Salud (PI10/01226 to AP) (Instituto de Salud Carlos III (ISCIII) co-financed with European Regional Development Funds, "Una manera de hacer Europa"), II PCTRM 2007–2010, Fundación Séneca, Agencia de Ciencia y Tecnología de la Región de Murcia (08721/PI/08 to AP, and 04487/GERM/06 to MRAL), ISCIII Spanish Cell Therapy Network (Tercel; RD06/0010/0023 to JMM), and the CIBERehd scientific program to MRAL. The funders had no role in study design, data collection and analysis, decision to publish, or preparation of the manuscript.

Competing Interests: The authors have declared that no competing interests exist.

* Email: antonio.parrado@carm.es

¶ These authors contributed equally to this work.

Introduction

Chronic lymphocytic leukemia (CLL) is a malignant disease characterized by the proliferation of CD5+CD23+ B cells. The clinical course is heterogeneous in CLL. About half of patients live for decades and never require treatment, while the other half become symptomatic or progress to late stages of the disease and require chemotherapy. Low rate of mutation of the IGHV sequence, and high levels of expression of ZAP-70, CD38, and CD49d/ITGA4, are prognostic risk markers [1]. Despite this heterogeneity, gene expression profiles (GEP) in CLL are relatively homogeneous, considering that specific CLL signatures clearly discriminate CLL cells from B cells of other related pathologic entities and from normal B cells [2–8], whereas specific signatures for CLL prognostic groups are based on more subtle differences [9–12]. CLL cells spontaneously and rapidly die *in vitro*, because they lack essential signals provided by the natural microenvironment [13]. CLL cells interact with bone marrow stromal cells, and with T cells, antigen-presenting cells and dendritic cells within the lymph node proliferation centers (or pseudofollicles). Cytokines, chemokines, integrins, and other ligands and receptors play key roles in proliferation and survival within these cellular niches [14].

Interleukin-4 (IL-4) is a cytokine secreted by activated T cells, NK-T cells, basophils, eosinophils and mast cells. Paracrine stimulation through the IL-4 membrane receptor (IL-4R) induces signaling cascades leading to maturation of B-cell precursors into immunoglobulin-secreting cells and antigen presenting cells, proliferation of activated B cells, and induction of isotype switching toward IgE [15]. The activated IL-4R phosphorylates JAK1 and JAK3. JAK1 phosphorylates STAT6 which homodimerizes and enter the nucleus to regulate gene expression. JAK1 and JAK3 lead to anti-apoptotic signaling through PI3K/AKT and the mitochondrial pathway, and through the Ras/MAPK pathway and NFκB activation [16]. NFκB activation is anti-apoptotic in CLL [17,18]. In B cells, IL-4 induces preferentially the non-canonical NFκB pathway [19]. IL-4 induces efficient STAT6 phosphorylation and activation in CLL [20]. However, binding of NFκB to the promoter of IGHE, CD86 and MHCII is necessary for STAT6 binding and transcription [19,21,22].

IL-4 efficiently protects CLL cells from spontaneous apoptosis or killing with agents such as fludarabine and chlorambucil [13,24,25]. CLL cells have been reported to be more prone than normal B cells (NBC) to spontaneous apoptosis [13], and those expressing good prognostic markers more than those expressing bad prognostic markers [23]. IL-4 acts in a paracrine rather than autocrine manner in CLL [26]. GEPs in follicular lymphoma suggest that a connection dependent on IL-4 between T cells and the malignant B cells sustains tumorigenesis [27]. Similarly, IL-4 could play a role in CLL pathogenesis and progression. Several studies have focused on identifying the IL-4 targets in mouse B splenocytes [28], some lymphoma subtypes [29], and other non B cell types (see additional references in Table S5). However, the gene expression response to IL-4 in CLL is poorly known.

We report here the first study aimed at identifying the IL-4 targets in CLL. We found sets of genes differentially regulated by IL-4 in CLL and NBC, and within CLL, depending on ZAP-70 expression, suggesting that the gene expression response to IL-4 may be relevant in CLL pathogenesis and prognosis. Finally, we found evidence for a dual mechanism which links the gene expression response to IL-4, NFκB activity, and ZAP-70 expression, based on the observation that a proportion of the IL-4 targets have a higher response in ZAP-70 positive patients which can be blocked by an NFκB inhibitor, and another group of IL-4 targets have a higher response in ZAP-70 negative patients which can be further induced by the NFκB inhibitor.

Methods

Sample collection

Peripheral blood samples from 38 chronic lymphocytic leukemia (CLL) patients and 13 controls with normal lymphopoiesis were obtained. The study was approved by the Review Board of Hospital Clínico Universitario Virgen de la Arrixaca, and the participants provided their written informed consent. All the patients had leukocytosis and did not receive treatment during the prior 3 months to sample collection. From the 38 CLL patients, 23 were studied by microarray and 15 were included later to increase the statistical significance of validations (Table S1).

Cell isolation

Samples were processed to isolate the B cells by negative selection procedures which were based on cocktails containing CD2, CD16, CD36 and CD235a antibodies for depletion of T

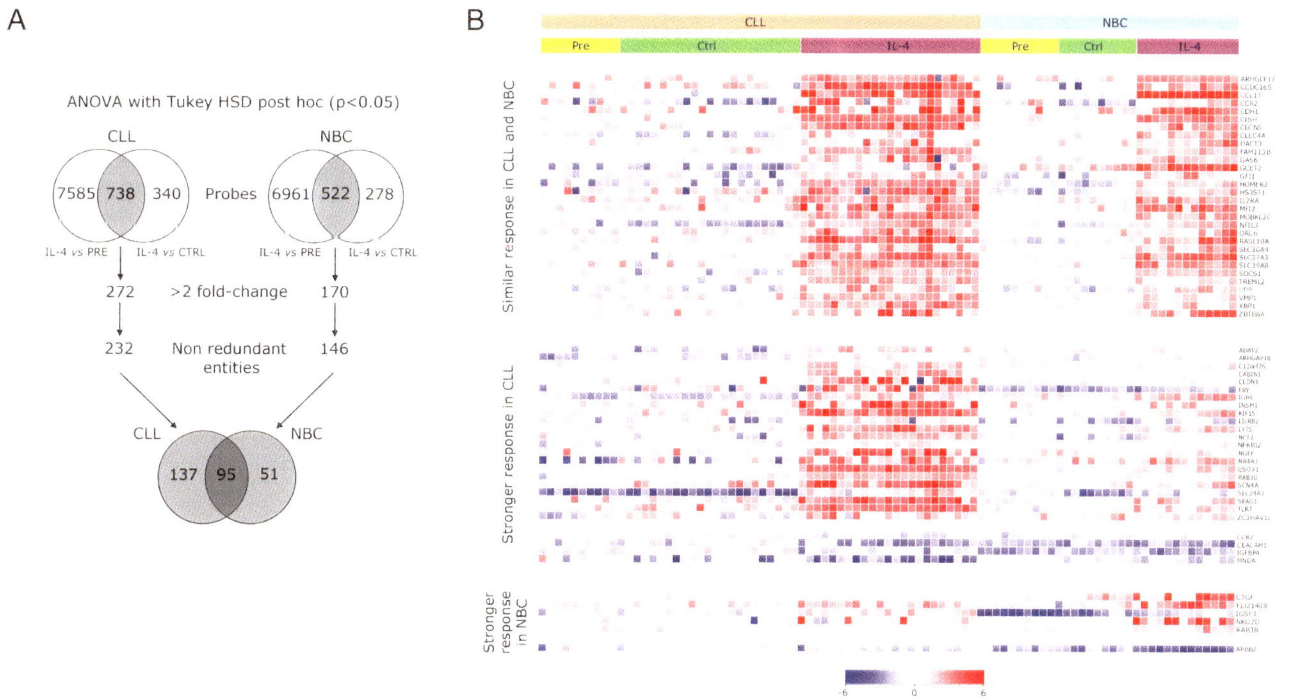

Figure 1. Identification of the IL-4 targets in CLL and in NBC. (A) Scheme of the strategy used to identify the IL-4 targets in patients and in controls. (B) Heat maps for expression of IL-4 targets which had: *top panel*, similar changes in CLL and NBC and above 3-fold change for both; *center panel*, significantly higher changes in CLL and above 3-fold change in CLL; *bottom panel*, significantly higher changes in NBC and above 3-fold change in NBC. IL-4 targets are ordered alphabetically. In the event that several probes represent the same gene, only one is shown. Relative expression levels are depicted according to the shown $\log_2$ color scale.

Table 1. Top 50 IL4 targets in CLL and NBC.

CLL		NBC	
Gene Symbol	**Fold Change**[†]	**Gene Symbol**	**Fold Change**[†]
SLC24A3	61.79	CCL17	24.37
CCR2	34.08	CCR2	17.79
NFIL3	30.62	**NKG2D**	16.18
CCL17	19.82	NFIL3	15.33
HOMER2	18.72	CLEC4A	10.87
QSOX1	16.83	HOMER2	10.45
SOCS1	14.21	CCDC165	8.26
NCF2	13.85	CISH	7.65
RASL10A	13.56	HS3ST1	7.62
CLCN5	12.98	RASL10A	7.55
SLC39A8	12.29	SLC37A3	6.94
SLC37A3	12.00	QSOX1	6.92
NGEF	11.18	VDR	6.59
CISH	10.98	MFI2	6.51
NR4A3	10.08	SLC30A4	6.41
XBP1	9.47	PEG10	6.41
SPAG1	8.97	ENPP1	6.09
KIF15	7.57	**TMEM71**	6.06
BCL6	7.10	SLC39A8	5.91
IGHE	7.09	CLCN5	5.77
CCDC165	6.83	ZBTB8A	5.31
CLEC4A	6.65	**CTGF**	5.19
SUSD2	6.33	MOBKL2C	4.98
TLR7	6.23	NETO1	4.89
SCN4A	6.23	CDH1	4.83
MOBKL2C	6.03	GCET2	4.82
INSM1	5.90	MACROD2	4.76
ADAP2	5.89	**RAB3B**	4.60
RNF19A	5.82	FAM126A	4.33
CARD9	5.63	IL2RA	4.29
CDH1	5.62	GNG8	4.29
TREML2	5.56	IL4I1	4.25
TBC1D8	5.50	ARHGEF17	4.09
FCRL2	5.46	GAS6	4.00
CLDN1	5.45	ZNF443	3.96
LY75	5.40	**IGSF3**	3.94
SLC30A4	5.36	APOL6	3.93
AUH	5.11	PALLD	3.83
MFI2	5.08	SPINT2	3.81
GFI1	5.08	**FLJ21408**	3.79
SLC47A1	4.90	TREML2	3.76
VMP1	4.58	SOCS1	3.74
FAM126A	4.55	GFI1	3.61
CHSY1	4.53	PHF20L1	3.57
HS3ST1	4.46	KMO	3.43
GCET2	4.38	C16orf87	3.36
ZC3HAV1L	4.31	IGHE	3.31
RNF125	4.16	IL4R	3.30

Table 1. Cont.

CLL		NBC	
Gene Symbol	**Fold Change**†	**Gene Symbol**	**Fold Change**†
MNDA	−4.39	**APBB2**	−3.51
CCR7	−4.48	SLC2A5	−4.07

(†) Mean fold change for comparison IL-4 vs Ctrl.
Genes in **bold** characters: significantly higher in CLL or NBC for both comparisons (IL-4 vs Pre and IL-4 vs Ctrl).

cells, NK cells, monocytes, macrophages, and erythrocytes. The RossetteSep Human B Cell Enrichment Cocktail kit (StemCell Technologies, Vancouver, Canada) was suitable for CLL samples, since these are rich in malignant B cells. Small volumes of peripheral blood (10 mL) were collected from patients, and B cell isolation was directly performed during Ficoll centrifugation, following the manufacturer's instructions. The Dynabeads Untouched Human B cells kit (Invitrogen, Carlsbad, CA) was a suitable choice for normal B cells (NBC) due to the low content of B cells in the peripheral blood of normal subjects (usually less than 10% of the lymphocytes). Larger volumes of peripheral blood were collected (500 mL), PBMC were isolated by centrifugation over Ficoll 1.077 g/mL, and NBC isolated using the kit, following the manufacturer's instructions. Enrichment was determined by labelling with CD19-FITC, CD3-PE, and CD5-PE-Cy7 ((BD Biosciences), followed by acquisition in a FACScalibur flow cytometer (BD Biosciences), and analysis using the CellQuest software. Purity of CD19+ cells was 93.5±1.41% (mean ±s.e.m.) in NBC and 97.54±0.34% in CLL, including 0.56±0.17% of CD19+CD5- potential normal B cells within the CLL fractions (range 0–1.98%). The percentage of ZAP-70 positive cells within the CD19+CD5+ fraction of CLL was determined from aliquots of peripheral blood subjected to red cell lysis, permeabilization with the Cytofix/Cytoperm kit, and labelling with CD19-FITC, ZAP70-PE, CD5-PE-Cy7, and CD3-APC (BD Biosciences).

Cell culture and determination of apoptosis

Following purification, three fractions of the purified CLL and NBC were processed: a) at time zero ("Pre"); b) after being cultured for 18 hours in RPMI-1640 medium supplemented with 10% fetal calf serum (Cambrex, East Rutherford, NJ) ("Ctrl"); and c) as b, but with adding 10 ng/mL of human recombinant IL-4 (BD Biosciences, San Diego, CA) ("IL-4"). In the absence of sufficient material, the Ctrl culture was not carried out in 3 NBC (NBC06, NBC07, and NBC08). In selected patients, additional fractions were treated with IL-4 plus InSolution NF-kB activation inhibitor [6-Amino-4-(4-phenoxyphenylethylamino)quinazoline] (Merck, Nottingham, UK) at 1 µM and 10 µM. Apoptosis of the cultured cells was determined by dual labelling with annexin V and propidium iodide (BD Biosciences), and flow cytometry analysis.

RNA isolation

Total RNA was isolated using the miRNeasy Mini Kit (Qiagen, Hilden, Germany). RNA samples were quantitated in a NanoDrop 2000 (Thermo Fisher Scientific, Whaltham, MA). RNA quality was examined in an Agilent 2100 Bioanalyzer (Agilent Technologies, Palo Alto, CA). Only samples with R.I.N. (RNA Integrity Number) >7.0 were further studied.

Microarray analysis

From each RNA sample, 250 ng were labeled with cyanine 5-CTP (Cy5) using Agilent Two Color Quick Amp Labeling and RNA Spike-In kits, according to the manufacturer's protocol. A pooled sample composed of equimolar amounts of RNA from Pre samples of 4 CLL and 4 NBC (reference), was labelled with cyanine 3-CTP (Cy3). The labeled cRNAs were mixed together and hybridized onto Agilent Whole Human Genome Microarrays (4×44 k) targeting 19,596 Entrez Gene RNAs, using the Agilent Gene Expression Hybridization kit. After hybridization, the microarray slides were washed and scanned in an Agilent G2565CA DNA Microarray Scanner. Images were analyzed with the Agilent Feature Extraction software to automatically generate the datasets. Log_{10} ratios (test vs reference) were computed after normalization correction performed by linear and Lowess methods. The datasets were statistically analyzed and visualized using the GeneSpring GX software (Agilent), using the one-way ANOVA test ($p<0.05$) between samples Pre, Ctrl, and IL-4, with post hoc Tukey HSD analysis (Figure 1A). The computation of p-values was performed using the Benjamini-Hochberg FDR correction. CLL and NBC were analyzed independently for each cell type. Those entities that passed the analysis with increases or decreases above 2-fold for comparisons IL-4 vs Pre, and IL-4 vs Ctrl concurrently and with the same direction of change were considered IL-4 targets. Similarly, entities that passed the ANOVA test with post hoc analysis with increases or decreases above 2-fold for comparisons Pre vs Ctrl, and IL-4 vs Ctrl concurrently and with the same direction of change, excluding some genes that were among the IL-4 targets, represented genes whose expression was altered by cell culture but remained stable under culture with IL-4. Finally, entities that passed the ANOVA test with post hoc analysis with increases or decreases above 2-fold for comparisons Pre vs Ctrl, and Pre vs IL-4 concurrently and with the same direction of change, excluding some genes that were in the previous two lists, represented genes whose expression was altered by cell culture and not stabilized by IL-4. Our initial analysis performed with the first 10 patients and controls showed an elevated number of entities with significant changes induced by cell culture and not stabilized by IL-4, indicating that our approach of subtracting sample Ctrl was essential to identify changes specifically induced by IL-4. However, most changes identified for comparisons IL-4 vs Ctrl were also significant for comparison IL-4 vs Pre. For this reason, comparison IL-4 vs Pre was judged as dispensable from that time. Thus, our final microarray analysis was based on 23 CLL patients (10 Pre, 23 Ctrl, and 23 IL-4), and 13 NBC samples (10 Pre, 10 Ctrl, and 13 IL-4). Cells from patient CLL01 treated with IL-4 plus NFκB inhibitor was also studied by microarray. Datasets were deposited at the Gene Expression Omnibus database under accession number GSE55288. After defining the IL-4 targets, to determine whether they had responses of different magnitude

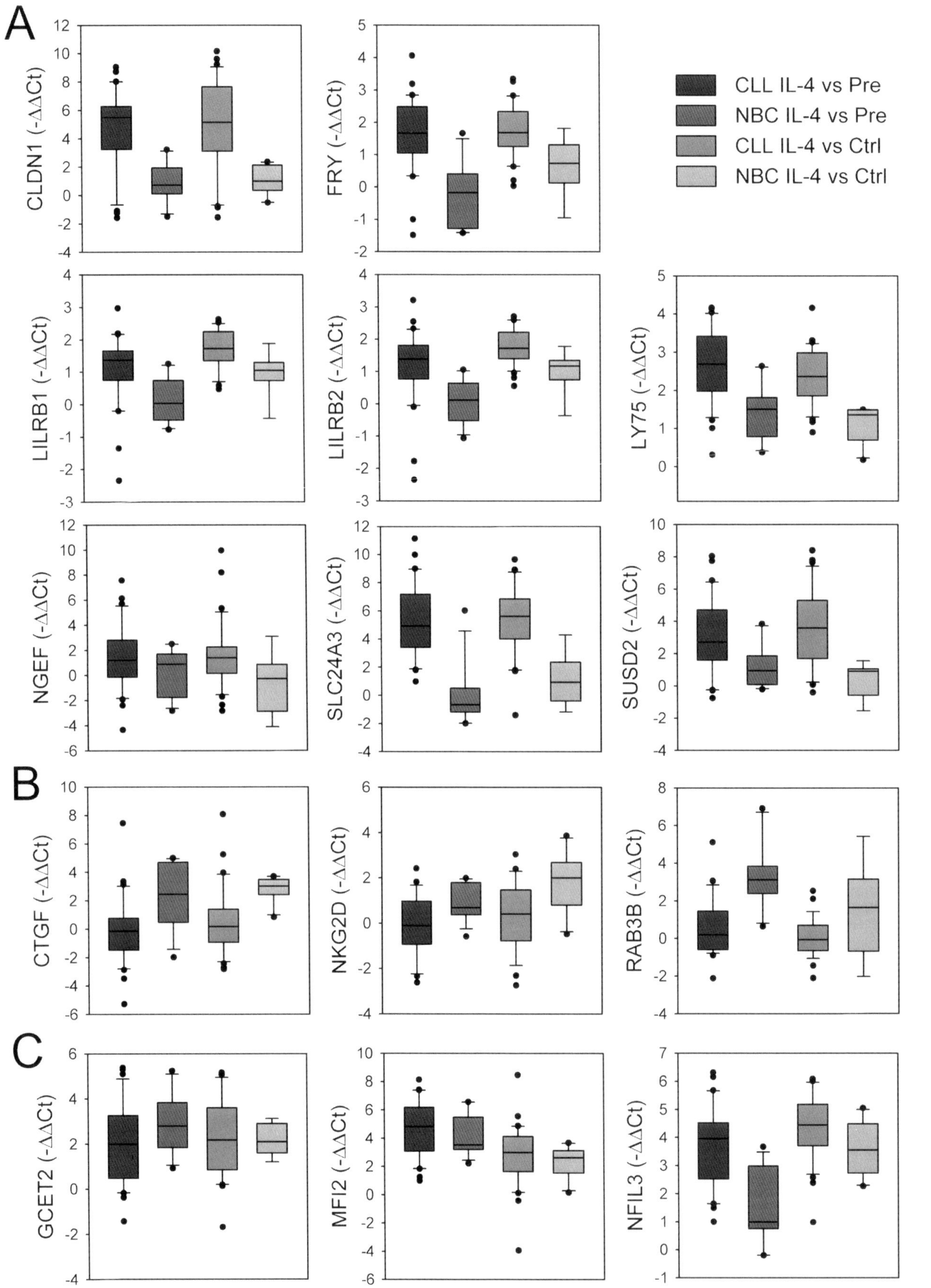
A
B
C
CLL IL-4 vs Pre
NBC IL-4 vs Pre
CLL IL-4 vs Ctrl
NBC IL-4 vs Ctrl
CLDN1 (-ΔΔCt)
FRY (-ΔΔCt)
LILRB1 (-ΔΔCt)
LILRB2 (-ΔΔCt)
LY75 (-ΔΔCt)
NGEF (-ΔΔCt)
SLC24A3 (-ΔΔCt)
SUSD2 (-ΔΔCt)
CTGF (-ΔΔCt)
NKG2D (-ΔΔCt)
RAB3B (-ΔΔCt)
GCET2 (-ΔΔCt)
MFI2 (-ΔΔCt)
NFIL3 (-ΔΔCt)

Figure 2. Validation of IL-4 targets in CLL and NBC by qPCR. Box whiskers representations of qPCR validations of 14 IL-4 targets representative of (A) restricted to CLL; (B) restricted to NBC; and (C) common to CLL and NBC. QPCR data are expressed as −ΔΔCt. IL-4 targets are ordered alphabetically.

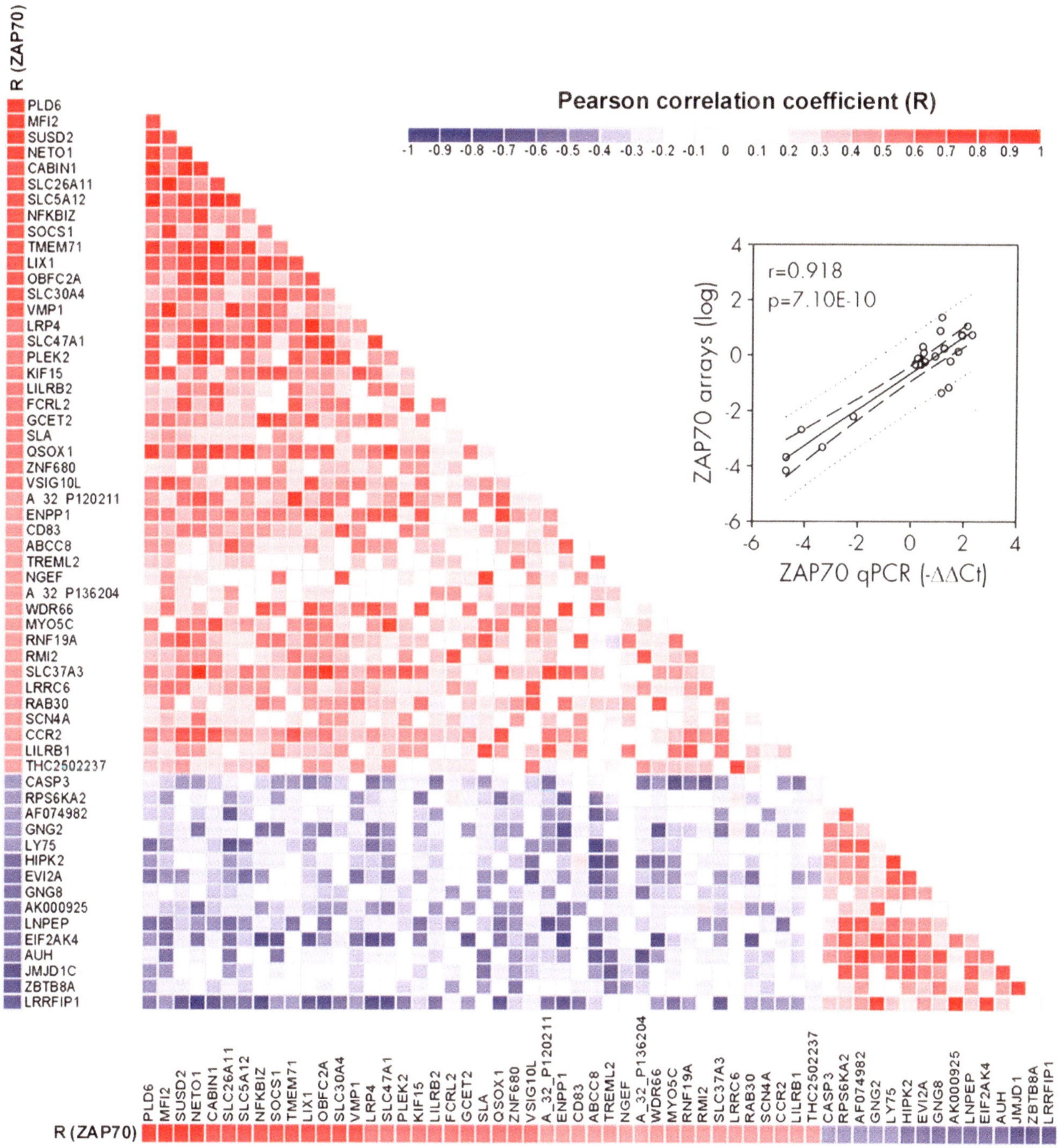

Figure 3. Pearson correlation analysis of the IL-4 upregulated targets compared between themselves and with ZAP-70. Triangular heat map representing the pairwise correlation coefficients (R) of the IL-4 upregulated targets between themselves. The IL-4 targets are ordered according to their correlation coefficients with ZAP-70, which are represented at the left and bottom sides. Cut-off values for positive or negative correlations with ZAP-70 were set at 0.4 and −0.4, respectively. In the event that several probes represent the same gene, only one is shown. Correlation coefficients are depicted according to the shown color scale. Inset shows Pearson correlation analysis between ZAP-70 levels by microarray (expressed as log_2 ratios) and by qPCR (expressed as −ΔΔCt ratios).

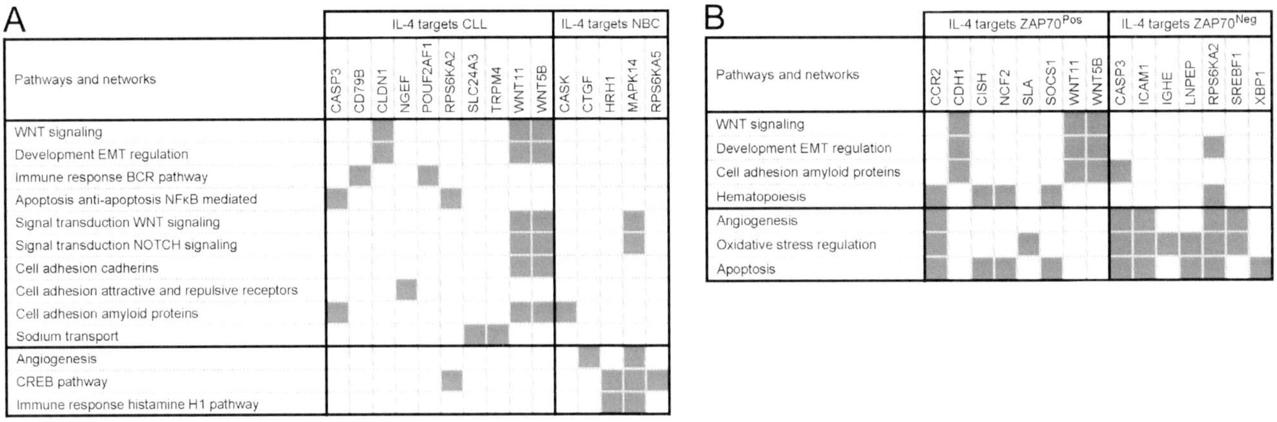

Figure 4. Pathways and networks differently affected according to MetaCore analysis of IL-4 targets. (A) Pathways and networks differently affected in CLL and NBC. (B) Pathways and networks differently affected in ZAP-70 positive and negative patients. Relevant genes for these functions within each group are specified.

between CLL and NBC, the extent of changes in each individual (expressed as $\log_2$ ratios for IL-4 vs Ctrl) was compared by the Student t test using the SigmaStat statistical analysis package (Systat Software Inc, San Jose, CA). In addition, the behavior of the different IL-4 targets was compared between patients by Pearson correlation analysis using SigmaStat, and by hierarchical clustering analysis using the Ward's linkage method on euclidean distances. Predictions for molecular interactions, activation state of trascription factors, biological functions, canonical pathways, and process networks, interpreted from the sets of genes differentially expressed, were performed using the MetaCore software (Thomsom Reuters Systems Biology, New York City, NY).

Quantitative PCR (qPCR)

RNA samples were subjected to retrotranscription with the iScript cDNA Synthesis Kit (Bio-Rad, Hercules, CA), following the manufacturer's instructions. QPCR was performed with the SYBR Premix Ex Taq (Takara Bio, Mountain View, CA) in an ABI Prism 7000 Sequence Detection System. QuantiTect primer assays (Qiagen) specific for the following genes were used: AUH, BCL6, CCR2, CDH1, CLDN1, CTGF, FRY, GAPDH, GCET2, INSM1, LILRB1, LILRB2, LY75, MFI2, NFIL3, NGEF, NKG2D, RAB3B, SLC24A3, SUSD2, and ZAP-70. ZAP-70 mRNA quantification via qPCR is a strong surrogate marker of IGHV mutational status and a powerful prognostic factor [30]. This method can be applied to purified B cells, and does not require an internal control (T cells) to evaluate the positivity limit. Both qPCR and microarray measures of ZAP-70 expression were used for analysis of correlations with GEPs. GAPDH was used as reference for all the qPCR assays. Measures were performed in duplicate. Analysis with the 7000 System SDS software provided the cycle threshold (Ct) values. The average Ct values for GAPDH were subtracted from the average Ct values for IL-4 target genes, resulting in the ΔCt values. Next, the ΔCt value for the reference sample was subtracted from all the others including itself, resulting in the ΔΔCt values. Finally, the relative expression values, expressed as fold change compared to the reference, were generated using the formula $2^{-\Delta\Delta Ct}$. For validation of microarray data, the fold changes obtained by microarray, expressed as $\log_2$, and the −ΔΔCt values obtained by qPCR were compared by the Student t test, and by Pearson correlation analysis, using SigmaStat.

Results

Basal GEPs of CLL and NBC

To obtain an indication that our methodological approach was reliable, the baseline GEPs of CLL and NBC were compared by the Student t test, and the genes differentially expressed were contrasted with the literature [2–12]. Many of the genes significantly overexpressed (e.g. ABCA6, FMOD, IGFBP4, IGSF3, LEF1, RASGRF1, RHOC, ROR1, WNT3), or underexpressed (e.g. EBF1, HIF1A, IQSEC1, KLF3, MS4A1, SIPA1, TRIB2, TUBB1, VAV3, ZBTB16) in CLL, were concordant with previous studies, thereby providing proof of the validity of our microarray study. The complete list (cut-off 2-fold, $p<0.05$ (Table S2)), and a heat map representation of the most significant (cut-off 3-fold, $p<0.001$ (Figure S1)), are provided. Of note, no significant difference for IL4R expression was found between CLL and NBC.

Identification of IL-4 targets in CLL and NBC

Microarray analysis identified 232 non-redundant entities in CLL (188 upregulated, 44 downregulated; Table S3), and 146 non-redundant entities in NBC (133 up, 13 down; Table S4) as IL-4 targets (cut-off 2-fold, $p<0.05$), being 95 common to both groups (90 up, 5 down), 137 restricted to CLL (98 up, 39 down), and 51 restricted to NBC (43 up, 8 down). Because an incubation period of 18 h allows regulation of direct and indirect IL-4 targets, we assume that the genes with the highest levels of change would probably be direct targets. The 50 IL-4 targets with the highest levels of change in CLL and NBC are shown in Table 1. From the 283 non-redundant entities identified as IL-4 targets in CLL and NBC altogether, 229 were well-defined genes (189 in CLL, 129 in NBC, 89 common), and the remaining corresponded to sequences not fully defined. To the best of our knowledge, 186 out of the 189 genes (98.5%) were novel IL-4 targets for CLL, 191 out of the 229 genes (83%) were novel IL-4 targets for B cells of any source, and 160 out of the 229 genes (70%), were novel IL-4 targets for any cell type (Table S5). Therefore, the vast majority of the genes identified in our study were novel IL-4 targets. The search for genes differentially regulated between CLL and NBC was refined by comparing the intensity of their changes by the Student t test ($p<0.05$). As a result, 54 genes (38 up, 16 down) had higher responses in CLL, and 11 genes (9 up, 2 down) had higher responses in NBC

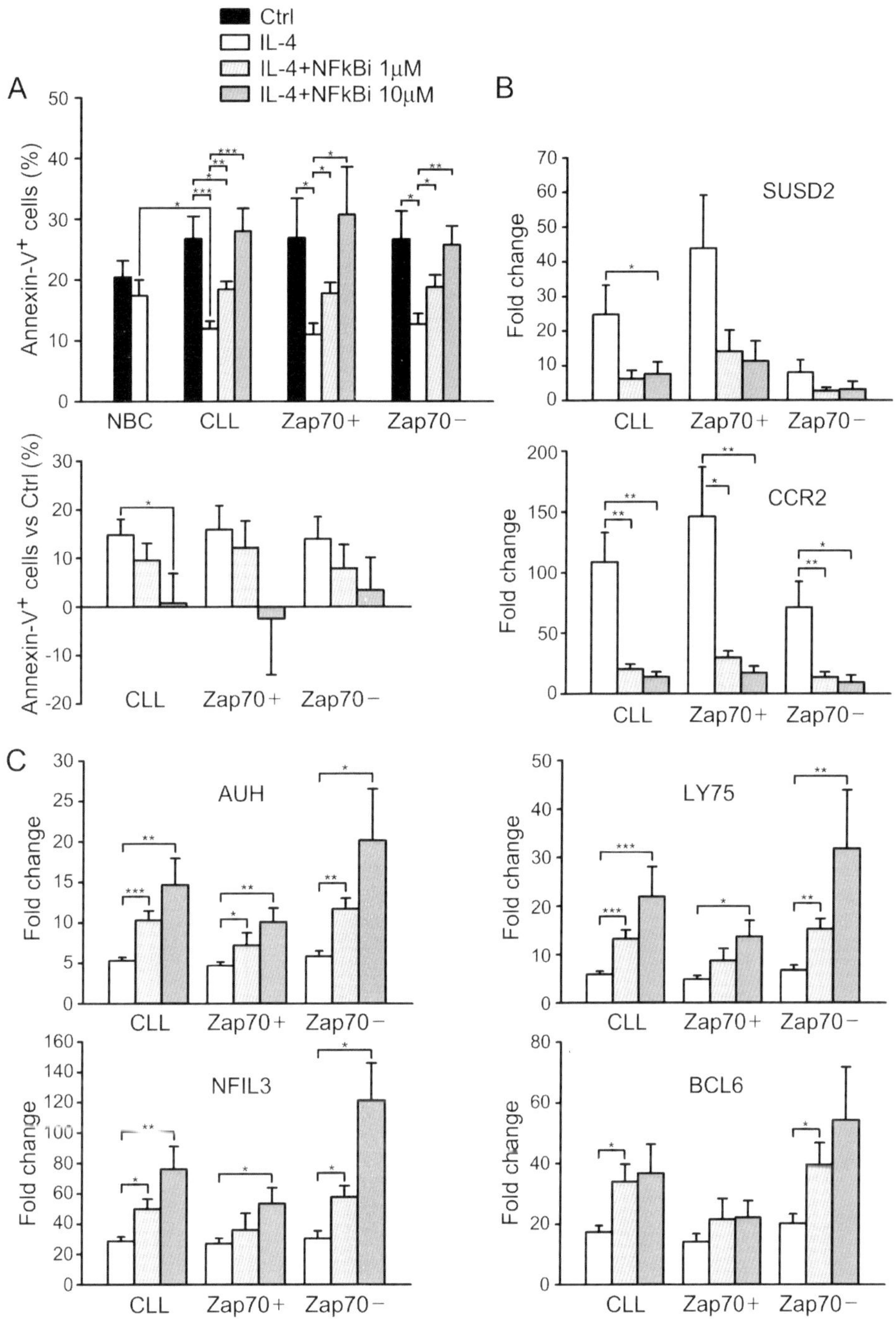

Figure 5. Effect of an NFκB inhibitor on apoptosis and gene expression response to IL-4 in CLL. (A) Apoptosis of NBC and CLL cells cultured for 18 h in the absence or presence of IL-4, and CLL cells cultured with IL-4 plus an NFκB activation inhibitor (NFκBi) at 1 μM and 10 μM. CLL are represented together and also separated in ZAP-70 positive and negative. Apoptosis was measured as the percentage of cells labelled with Annexin V (*top panel*). The *bottom panel* represents results in CLL patients after subtracting the percentage of apoptotic cells of the Ctrl samples to the IL-4, IL-4 plus 1 μM NFκBi, and IL-4 plus 10 μM NFκBi samples. T tests were used to compare the levels of apoptosis between cell types and conditions. When differences were significant the p-values are indicated as follows: *, $p<0.05$; **, $p<0.01$; ***, $p<0.001$. (B) Expression of the ZAP-70^{Pos} IL-4 targets SUSD2 and CCR2, and (C) of the ZAP-70^{Neg} IL-4 targets AUH, LY75, NFIL3, and BCL6), measured by qPCR, in 7 ZAP-70 positive and 8 ZAP-70 negative patients. The ratios for expression of IL-4 targets following treatment with IL-4 alone, IL-4 plus NFκBi at 1 μM, and IL-4 plus NFκBi at 10 μM, compared to Ctrl, are represented. P-values are depicted as in A.

(Table S3, Table S4, and Figure 1B centre and bottom showing a selection of those that changed above 3-fold). These findings suggest that IL-4 probably induces divergent pathways in CLL and NBC.

Validation of microarray analysis

To validate microarray experiments, representative IL-4 targets, restricted to CLL or NBC, or unrestricted, were assayed by qPCR (Figure 2). In most cases, comparison using the Student's t test validated microarray data. For most genes, both techniques

Table 2. IL-4 targets correlated with protection by IL-4 in CLL.

Gene Symbol	Fold change[†]	R-coefficient	p-value
HOMER2	18.72	0.579	3.80E-02
BCL6	7.10	0.598	3.08E-02
CLEC4A	6.65	0.657	1.47E-02
FCRL2	5.46	0.813	7.29E-04
CABIN1	4.09	0.600	3.03E-02
RMI2	3.90	0.660	1.41E-02
LILRB2	3.86	0.665	1.32E-02
FRY	3.62	0.568	4.28E-02
GIT2	2.70	0.633	2.01E-02
TMEM71	2.66	0.735	4.22E-03
BDH2	2.65	0.668	1.25E-02
PLEK2	2.59	0.579	3.80E-02
ZNF107	2.14	0.721	5.42E-03
GADD45B	-2.89	-0.564	4.48E-02

(†) Mean fold change for comparison IL-4 vs Ctrl.

correlated significantly ($p<0.05$, Figure S2). At the protein level, other authors and ourselves have provided, in previous reports, validation for several IL-4 targets detected in this study, such as CYSLTR1 [31], IGHE [32] and NFIL3 [33] in B cells, or for DOCK10 in CLL and NBC cells [34].

Correlations between IL-4 targets, and with basal expression of ZAP-70

To determine whether the gene expression response to IL-4 was homogeneous between patients, a correlation analysis between changes of every pair of genes, and between changes of each gene and the basal levels of expression of ZAP-70, CD38, and ITGA4 (whose levels did not significantly change under culture or treatment with IL-4) were performed. The numbers of non-redundant entities correlated positively or negatively with ZAP-70 were 42 and 20, respectively, setting the cut-off values of R-coefficient at ±0.4 (Figure 3; the R-coefficients for all the IL-4 targets are shown in Table S10). Expression of ZAP-70 determined by microarray and qPCR were correlated (Figure 3 inset). This analysis indicates that specific sets of genes were preferentially induced in the ZAP-70 positive or negative patients. According to this criterion, the IL-4 targets were categorized as ZAP-70^{Pos} or ZAP-70^{Neg}, respectively. These conclusions were validated by hierarchical clustering analysis of these sets of genes using their fold changes, resulting in segregation of patients into two clusters, one containing the ZAP-70 positive patients and the other the ZAP-70 negative patients (Figure S3). Expression of ZAP-70, CD38, and ITGA4 significantly correlated in CLL ($R=0.512$ for ZAP-70 and CD38, $R=0.509$ for ZAP-70 and ITGA4, and $R=0.393$ for CD38 and ITGA4); and in general, also correlated similarly with the IL-4 targets (e.g., positive correlations with SUSD2, CABIN1, OBFC2A, SLC5A12, SLC37A3, PLD6, or negative correlations with EVI2A), though the number of IL-4 targets significantly correlated with ZAP-70 was higher than with CD38 or ITGA4 (Table S10). Analysis of the gene response to IL-4 according to cytogenetic characteristics of patients or between untreated and previously treated patients did not result in significant findings, possibly due to the low number of cases within some of the groups compared. Therefore, the gene response to IL-4 is related to the expression of CLL prognostic markers, especially ZAP-70.

Functional interpretation of the IL-4 target data sets using the MetaCore database and analysis tools

Based on upregulation of specific genes, MetaCore analysis of the CLL data set suggested activation of Wnt signaling and cell adhesion, whereas analysis of the NBC data set suggested activation of Creb signaling and angiogenesis (Fig. 4A). Analysis of the ZAP-70^{Pos} data set suggested activation of Wnt signaling, regulation of epithelial to mesenchymal transition, and cell adhesion, whereas analysis of the ZAP-70^{Neg} data set suggested activation of oxidative stress regulation, and angiogenesis (Figure 4B). Taken together, MetaCore functional analyses support that IL-4 may transduce specific pathways in CLL and NBC, and according to ZAP-70 expression in CLL.

Correlations between IL-4 targets and apoptosis

Apoptosis was studied by flow cytometry analysis of annexin V positive cells. IL-4 significantly reduced spontaneous apoptosis of CLL cells, but not of NBC cells in this time period (Figure 5A). Therefore, CLL cells were more prone to spontaneous apoptosis but also better protected by IL-4 than NBC, in agreement with previous studies [13]. Differential basal expression between CLL and NBC of apoptosis-related genes, such as Bcl2 family members, and/or changes of expression during culture, might account for the different sensitivity to spontaneous apoptosis. Within the Bcl2 family, we observed significant basal overexpression of pro-apoptotic BBC3 and BMF in CLL, but also underexpression of pro-apoptotic BCL2L11/BIM (Table S2). According to MetaCore analysis, additional 86 apoptosis-related genes had different basal levels (data not shown), being some of them more than 10-fold underexpressed in CLL (GNG11, IL6, FHL2, NGFRAP1, and ITGB3). Cell culture induced changes of an elevated number of genes that persisted in the presence of IL-4 in CLL (Table S6) and in NBC (Table S7). Of them, FOS, FOSB, DUSP1, CEBPD, and ITGB2 were more than 5-fold downregulated in both cell types, GZMA and JUN had stronger downregulation in CLL (indeed, JUN was one of the IL-4 targets (Table S3)), and MYLK,

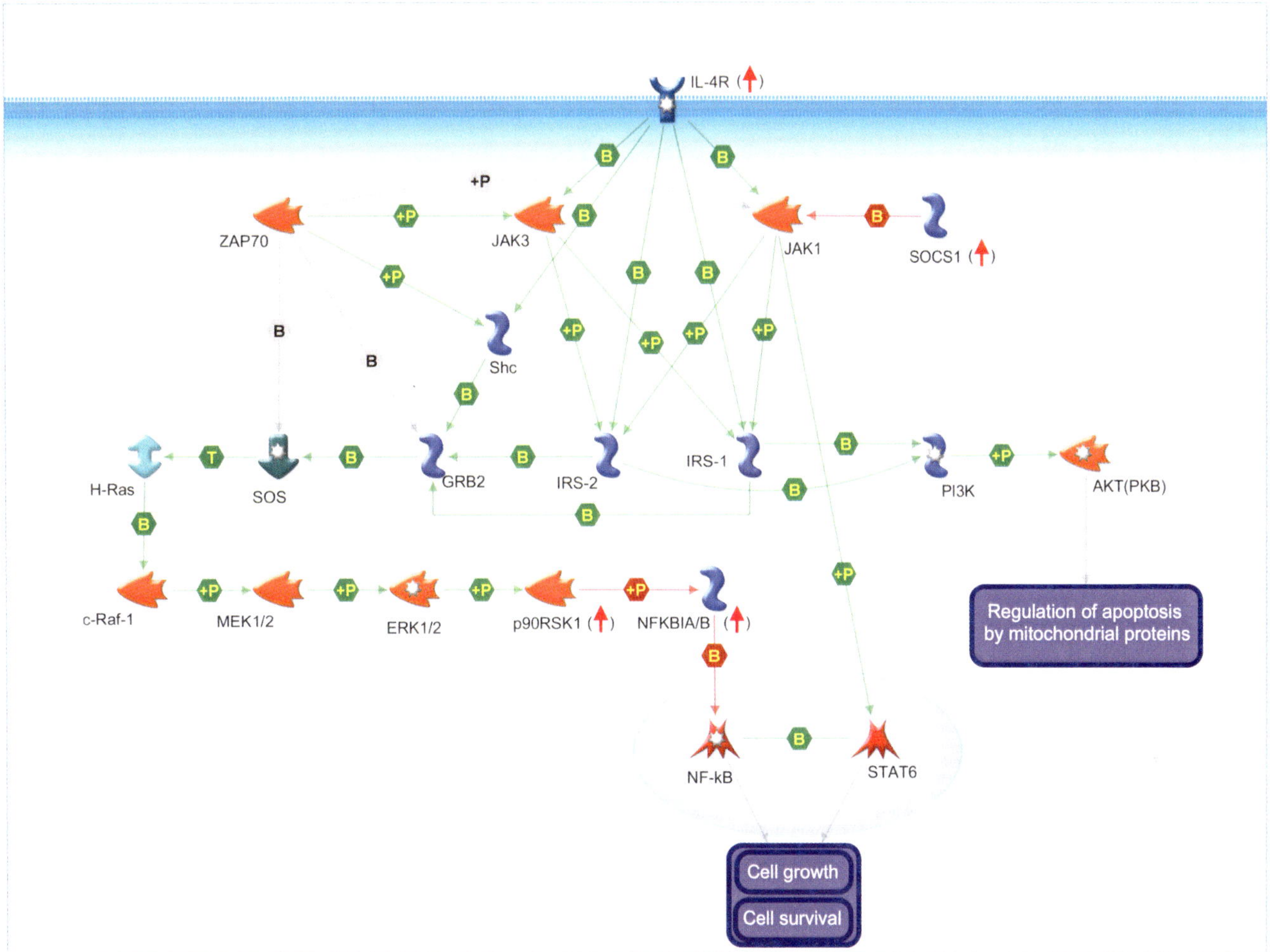

Figure 6. Map of the IL-4 signaling pathway and the potential role of ZAP-70. Adaptation of the pathway map entitled "Immune response_IL-4 – anti-apoptotic action" from MetaCore from Thomson Reuters. The map has been simplified leaving the minimal elements for activation of transcription factors essential in regulation of gene expression. ZAP-70 and its interactions with members of the pathway reported in the MetaCore database have been added to suggest its potential involvement in the pathway, and a link has been added for the reported interaction between NFκB and STAT6 [21]. Red arrows indicate that IL4R, SOCS1, RPS6AK2, and NFKBIZ are components of the pathway identified as IL-4 upregulated targets in this study. Other genes of the pathway were significantly regulated by cell culture, such as AKT3 (up) and GRB2 (down).

PRKAR2B, SELP, FHL2, JUND, SMPD3, and CLDN5, in NBC. Within the Bcl2 family, BCLAF1 was downregulated by cell culture similarly in CLL and NBC, and BMF was upregulated by cell culture only in NBC. With regards to the differential anti-apoptotic effect of IL-4, MetaCore analysis identified, as related to apoptosis, the IL-4 upregulated targets CASP3, CCR2, CISH, GFI1, ICAM1, LNPEP, NCF2, NFKBIZ, RPS6KA2, SOCS1, and XBP1, and the IL-4 downregulated target GADD45B, in CLL (Table S3), but only CCR2, CISH, SOCS1, and XBP1, in NBC (Table S4). In addition, CAMKK1 and ESR2 were upregulated by cell culture but recovered their baseline levels by IL-4 in CLL (Table S8), and GNG4 and HRK were upregulated, and JAK2 was downregulated by cell culture, but their levels were stabilized by IL-4 in NBC (Table S9). Therefore, many genes may contribute to the increased response of CLL to IL-4. In addition, we compared the percentages of protection and the levels of change of the IL-4 targets in CLL, and found significant correlations, pointing out new potential anti-apoptotic players, of which HOMER2 and BCL6 had the highest increases (Table 2). No significant differences were observed in the levels of spontaneous apoptosis or protection by IL-4 between ZAP-70 positive and negative patients (Figure 5A), despite the fact that levels of some apoptosis-related IL-4 targets suffered significantly higher increases in ZAP-70 positive patients (SOCS1, NFKBIZ) or in ZAP-70 negative patients (LNPEP, RPS6KA2).

Effects of an NFκB activation inhibitor on the gene expression response to IL-4

To investigate the role of NFκB on the gene expression response to IL-4 in CLL, we used a quinazoline that inhibits the transactivation capacity of NFκB [35], in a ZAP-70 positive patient (CLL01). We found that the NFκB inhibitor preferentially downregulated the response of the ZAP-70^{Pos} genes, and upregulated the response of the ZAP-70^{Neg} genes (Table S10). The NFκB activation inhibitor counteracted the anti-apoptotic effect of IL-4 in CLL in a dose-dependent manner, especially in ZAP-70 positive patients at 10 μM (Figure 5A). The response of selected ZAP-70^{Pos} targets (SUSD2, and CCR2 (Figure 5B)), and ZAP-70^{Neg} targets (AUH, LY75, NFIL3, and BCL6 (Figure 5C) to IL-4 plus NFκB activation inhibitor was confirmed by qPCR in 7 ZAP-70 positive and 8 ZAP-70 negative patients. Upregulation of the ZAP-70^{Neg} targets by the NFκB inhibitor was higher in ZAP-70 negative patients.

Discussion

The study of the changes in the GEPs induced by microenvironmental factors may help to understand the underlying mechanisms sustaining CLL pathogenesis. Despite the fact that IL-4 has been recognized as a key survival factor in CLL for a long time, the GEPs induced by IL-4 in CLL are poorly known. Here, we identified 229 well-defined genes as IL-4 targets in CLL and NBC altogether, most of which were novel IL-4 targets for CLL, B cells of diverse origin, lymphocytes, or other cell types. The previously known IL-4 targets that were also identified in our study provided a proof of validity for our microarray study. An additional validation was obtained by qPCR analysis on a significant set of genes. The introduction of two reference samples helped to define accurately the IL-4 targets by exclusion of those genes modulated by cell culture, but in general, comparison IL-4 vs Ctrl was necessary and sufficient.

In our analysis, the number of IL-4 targets was higher in CLL than in NBC. This outcome has two alternative (non-exclusive) explanations. First, that the different size of patient and control populations favors an increased detection of statistically significant targets with relatively heterogeneous response in CLL. Second, that indeed CLL have a stronger gene expression response. A substantial part of the gene response was common to CLL and NBC, qualitatively and quantitatively. However, sets of 54 and 11 genes with differential responses (most of them specific) were found in CLL and NBC, respectively. Previous studies had reported increased expression of the IL-4 receptor in CLL, at the protein [13], and the mRNA level by microarray [5], but in another study differences were not found [36]. In our study, as in the latter, no significant differences were observed between the basal levels of IL4R mRNA in CLL and NBC. The first two studies were performed with lower number of samples and/or used B cell samples of different source (tonsil). Furthermore, in our study the IL4R gene was induced similarly by IL-4 in CLL and NBC, suggesting that the differential response arises downstream of IL4R.

Correlations with useful prognostic markers may help to reveal new altered pathways and alternative therapeutic targets. We observed that two sets of IL-4 targets had changes correlated positively and negatively with the basal levels of ZAP-70. ZAP-70 has not been previously related to the IL-4 pathway, but several interactions with components of this pathway had been reported (Figure 6). Differentially regulated genes play essential roles in developmental and survival pathways, such as Wnt signaling and cell adhesion in the ZAP-70^{Pos} set (CDH1, WNT5B, WNT11). CDH1 expression was reported to be repressed epigenetically in CLL [37], and our data suggest that IL-4 overcomes this repression, especially in ZAP-70 positive patients (and also in patients expressing the adhesion protein ITGA4). These data may be related with recent evidence that ZAP-70 positive CLL cells exhibit higher adhesion capacity to stromal cells in response to CD40L+IL-4 [38]. Previous studies have detected increased levels of the anti-apoptotic proteins BCL2, using IL-4 [24], or MCL1, BCL2L1, BCL2A1, or XIAP, using the CD40L/IL-4 system [39,40], without correlation at the mRNA level, and our study using IL-4 alone did not detect significant changes of expression of their transcripts either. However, our study contributes several candidate genes for the anti-apoptotic mechanism of IL-4 in CLL, for the higher sensitivity of CLL cells to cell culture, and for the higher protective effect of IL-4 in CLL cells compared to NBC.

Some of the IL-4 targets, and some of the genes whose levels were altered by culture but stabilized by IL-4, were previously related to apoptosis, and their responses were often stronger in CLL (e.g. CASP3, GFI1, ICAM1, LNPEP, NCF2, NFKBIZ, RPS6KA2, GADD45B). In addition, several IL-4 targets, some of which had not been previously related to apoptosis, correlated to the levels of cytoprotection. The most upregulated genes of this list, HOMER2 and BCL6, also had significant stronger responses in CLL (HOMER2 for comparison IL-4 vs Pre, and BCL6 for comparison IL-4 vs Ctrl, Table S3). HOMER2 belongs to a family of scaffolding proteins that prevent neuronal apoptosis through PI3K and the glutamate receptor [41], and regulate T cell activation by binding to NFAT [42], but its role in B cells remains largely unknown. BCL6 is a repressor transcription factor associated to worse prognosis in CLL [43]. The identification of these genes provides a starting point for future studies aimed at defining precisely the survival mechanism of IL-4. In contrast to the study of Coscia and co-workers [23] which reports lower sensitivity to spontaneous apoptosis of CLL cells expressing poor prognosis markers, we did not observe significant differences in sensitivity of ZAP-70 positive and negative patients, despite differential regulation of several apoptosis-related IL-4 targets (SOCS1, NFKBIZ, LNPEP, RPS6KA2). However, we did observe differential cytoprotection following treatment with IL-4 and an NFκB inhibitor (see below).

NFκB and ZAP-70 are effectors of the BCR signalling pathway. NFκB expression is induced following BCR signalling, and associates to cell survival and expression of ZAP-70 in CLL [44]. ZAP-70 enhances the BCR signalling responses in CLL [45,46]. NFκB inhibitors induce apoptosis of CLL cells, and ZAP-70 positive patients have higher NFκB activity and increased sensitivity [47,48]. We show that an NFκB inhibitor counteracted the anti-apoptotic effect of IL-4, especially in ZAP-70 positive patients, and the gene expression response of a great part of IL-4 targets, especially the ZAP-70^{Pos} targets which, therefore, would depend on NFκB for IL-4 responsiveness. However, the inhibitor potentiated the response of a collection of genes, especially the ZAP-70^{Neg} targets, suggesting a novel mechanism by which ZAP-70 and NFκB could work together to diminish responsiveness to IL-4 of this gene set. Examples of genes of both groups were confirmed by qPCR, such as CCR2, the chemokine receptor of CCL2, involved in CLL survival [49], NFIL3, a pro-survival transcription factor in B cells [50], and BCL6. Revealing the existence of this dual mechanism has been made possible by performing transcriptome-wide studies. The search for a molecular explanation, including the role played by ZAP-70, will be the goal of future studies. JAK3 has also been targeted with promising results in CLL using the specific inhibitor PF-956980 [25]. Our preliminary data indicate that PF-956980, similarly to the NFκB inhibitor, counteracts protection by IL-4, but abrogates completely the gene expression response both of ZAP-70^{Pos} and ZAP-70^{Neg} targets (data not shown), suggesting that targeting this step, which blocks STAT6 activation, fully abolishes the pathway.

In summary, the present study identifies sets of new genes that respond differentially to IL-4 in CLL depending on ZAP-70 expression and NFκB activation, contributing to the understanding of the anti-apoptotic response to IL-4 of CLL. In the context of evaluating inhibition of the IL-4 pathway as a therapeutic strategy in CLL, several steps may be targeted. Because inhibition of NFκB counteracts cytoprotection by IL-4, and is associated to an attenuated response of a set of IL-4 targets, NFκB targeting should be further explored especially in CLL patients expressing bad prognostic markers.

Supporting Information

Figure S1 Comparison of baseline GEPs of CLL and NBC. Heatmap representation of genes basally underexpressed (A) and overexpressed (B) in CLL compared to NBC, above a cut-off value of 3-fold change, and p values of less than 0.001, at time zero after purification of B cells. In the event that several probes represent the same gene, only one is shown. The relative level of gene expression is depicted according to the shown color scale.

Figure S2 Validation of microarray analysis by qPCR. Pearson correlation analysis between microarray and qPCR for 16 IL-4 targets. Microarray data were expressed as log fold change ratios, and qPCR data as $-\Delta\Delta Ct$ ratios. The CLL and NBC samples are represented together. Correlation coefficients (r) and p-values are indicated. The IL-4 targets were ordered alphabetically.

Figure S3 Hierarchical clustering analysis for IL-4 upregulated targets correlated with ZAP70. (A) Hierarchical clustering analysis using the $ZAP70^{Pos}$ IL-4 targets. (B) Hierarchical clustering analysis using the $ZAP70^{Neg}$ IL-4 targets. In order to make groups of similar size, we selected, among the 23 patients studied by microarray, the 5 patients with the lowest levels of ZAP70, the 5 patients with the highest levels of ZAP70 and other 6 patients with intermediate values. Both analyses were able to separate CLL into two clusters containing the 5 positive and 5 negative patients. In the event that several probes represent the same gene, only one is shown. Fold changes for the IL-4 targets, or relative levels for basal expression of ZAP70 by microarray, are depicted according to the shown $\log_2$ color scale.

Table S1 Characteristics of CLL patients.

Table S2 Differential basal gene expression levels between CLL and NBC.

Table S3 IL-4 targets in CLL and comparison of their responses with those in NBC.

Table S4 IL-4 targets in NBC and comparison of their responses with those in CLL.

Table S5 Novel and previously known IL-4 targets in diverse cell types (with references) among the IL-4 targets identified in CLL and NBC in the present study.

Table S6 Gene expression changes induced by culture not counteracted by IL-4 in CLL.

Table S7 Gene expression changes induced by culture not counteracted by IL-4 in NBC.

Table S8 Gene expression changes induced by culture counteracted by IL-4 in CLL.

Table S9 Genes expression changes induced by culture counteracted by IL-4 in NBC.

Table S10 Effects of an NFκB activation inhibitor on the response of the IL-4 upregulated targets in a CLL patient (CLL01, Zap70 positive).

Acknowledgments

We thank Dr. Christine Chomienne and Dr. Rose Ann Padua for helpful comments.

Author Contributions

Conceived and designed the experiments: NRL MJAG AP. Performed the experiments: NRL MJAG SSR NMB AM AP. Analyzed the data: NRL MJAG AP. Contributed reagents/materials/analysis tools: JGE CF MCGG JMM MRAL. Wrote the paper: AP.

References

1. Chiorazzi N (2012) Implications of new prognostic markers in chronic lymphocytic leukemia. Hematology Am Soc Hematol Educ Program 2012: 76–87.
2. Klein U, Tu Y, Stolovitzky GA, Mattioli M, Cattoretti G, et al. (2001) Gene expression profiling of B cell chronic lymphocytic leukemia reveals a homogeneous phenotype related to memory B cells. J Exp Med 194: 1625–1638.
3. Rosenwald A, Alizadeh AA, Widhopf G, Simon R, Davis RE, et al. (2001) Relation of gene expression phenotype to immunoglobulin mutation genotype in B cell chronic lymphocytic leukemia. J Exp Med 194: 1639–1647.
4. Stratowa C, Löffler G, Lichter P, Stilgenbauer S, Haberl P, et al. (2001) CDNA microarray gene expression analysis of B-cell chronic lymphocytic leukemia proposes potential new prognostic markers involved in lymphocyte trafficking. Int J Cancer 91: 474–480.
5. Zheng Z, Venkatapathy S, Rao G, Harrington CA (2002) Expression profiling of B cell chronic lymphocytic leukemia suggests deficient CD1-mediated immunity, polarized cytokine response, altered adhesion and increased intracellular protein transport and processing of leukemic cells. Leukemia 16: 2429–2437.
6. Jelinek DF, Tschumper RC, Stolovitzky GA, Iturria SJ, Tu Y, et al. (2003) Identification of a global gene expression signature of B-chronic lymphocytic leukemia. Mol Cancer Res 1: 346–361.
7. Wang J, Coombes KR, Highsmith WE, Keating MJ, Abruzzo LV (2004) Differences in gene expression between B-cell chronic lymphocytic leukemia and normal B cells: a meta-analysis of three microarray studies. Bioinformatics 20: 3166–3178.
8. Dürig J, Nückel H, Hüttmann A, Kruse E, Hölter T, et al. (2003) Expression of ribosomal and translation-associated genes is correlated with a favorable clinical course in chronic lymphocytic leukemia. Blood 101: 2748–2755.
9. Wiestner A, Rosenwald A, Barry TS, Wright G, Davis RE, et al. (2003) ZAP-70 expression identifies a chronic lymphocytic leukemia subtype with unmutated immunoglobulin genes, inferior clinical outcome, and distinct gene expression profile. Blood 101: 4944–4951.
10. Stankovic T, Hubank M, Cronin D, Stewart GS, Fletcher D, et al. (2004) Microarray analysis reveals that TP53- and ATM-mutant B-CLLs share a defect in activating proapoptotic responses after DNA damage but are distinguished by major differences in activating prosurvival responses. Blood 103: 291–300.
11. Rodríguez A, Villuendas R, Yáñez L, Gómez ME, Díaz R, et al. (2007) Molecular heterogeneity in chronic lymphocytic leukemia is dependent on BCR signaling: clinical correlation. Leukemia 21: 1984–1991.
12. Seifert M, Sellmann L, Bloehdorn J, Wein F, Stilgenbauer S, et al. (2012) Cellular origin and pathophysiology of chronic lymphocytic leukemia. J Exp Med 209: 2183–2198.
13. Douglas RS, Capocasale RJ, Lamb RJ, Nowell PC, Moore JS (1997) Chronic lymphocytic leukemia B cells are resistant to the apoptotic effects of Transforming Growth Factor-β. Blood 89: 941–947.
14. Burger JA, Montserrat E (2013) Coming full circle: 70 years of chronic lymphocytic leukemia cell redistribution, from glucocorticoids to inhibitors of B-cell receptor signaling. Blood 121: 1501–1509.
15. Okada H, Banchereau J, Lotze MT (2003) Interleukin-4. In Thompson AW, Lotze MT, editors. The Cytokine Handbook, Vol. I. London: Academic Press. pp 227–262
16. Zamorano J, Mora AL, Boothby M, Keegan AD (2001) NF-kappa B activation plays an important role in the IL-4-induced protection from apoptosis. Int Immunol 13: 1479–1487.

17. Furman RR, Asgary Z, Mascarenhas JO, Liou HC, Schattner EJ (2000) Modulation of NF-kappa B activity and apoptosis in chronic lymphocytic leukemia B cells. J Immunol 164: 2200-2206.
18. Cuní S, Pérez-Aciego P, Pérez-Chacón G, Vargas JA, Sánchez A, et al. (2004) A sustained activation of PI3K/NF-kappaB pathway is critical for the survival of chronic lymphocytic leukemia B cells. Leukemia 18: 1391-1400.
19. Thieu VT, Nguyen ET, McCarthy BP, Bruns HA, Kapur R, et al. (2007) IL-4-stimulated NF-kappaB activity is required for Stat6 DNA binding. J Leukoc Biol 82: 370-379.
20. Bhattacharya N, Reichenzeller M, Caudron-Herger M, Haebe S, Brady N, et al. (2014) Loss of cooperativity of secreted CD40L and increased dose-response to IL4 on CLL cell viability correlates with enhanced activation of NF-kB and STAT6. Int J Cancer. doi: 10.1002/ijc.28974. [Epub ahead of print].
21. Shen CH, Stavnezer J (1998) Interaction of stat6 and NF-kappaB: direct association and synergistic activation of interleukin-4-induced transcription. Mol Cell Biol 18: 3395-3404.
22. Messner B, Stütz AM, Albrecht B, Peiritsch S, Woisetschläger M (1997) Cooperation of binding sites for STAT6 and NF kappa B/rel in the IL-4-induced up-regulation of the human IgE germline promoter. J Immunol 159: 3330-3337.
23. Coscia M, Pantaleoni F, Riganti C, Vitale C, Rigoni M, et al. (2011) IGHV unmutated CLL B cells are more prone to spontaneous apoptosis and subject to environmental prosurvival signals than mutated CLL B cells. Leukemia 25: 828-837.
24. Dancescu M, Rubio-Trujillo M, Biron G, Bron D, Delespesse G, et al. (1992) Interleukin 4 protects chronic lymphocytic leukemic B cells from death by apoptosis and upregulates Bcl-2 expression. J Exp Med 176: 1319-1326.
25. Steele AJ, Prentice AG, Cwynarski K, Hoffbrand AV, Hart SM, et al. (2010) The JAK3-selective inhibitor PF-956980 reverses the resistance to cytotoxic agents induced by interleukin-4 treatment of chronic lymphocytic leukemia cells: potential for reversal of cytoprotection by the microenvironment. Blood 116: 4569-4577.
26. Mainou-Fowler T, Proctor SJ, Miller S, Dickinson AM (2001) Expression and production of interleukin 4 in B-cell chronic lymphocytic leukaemia. Leuk Lymphoma 42: 689-698.
27. Pangault C, Amé-Thomas P, Ruminy P, Rossille D, Caron G, et al. (2010) Follicular lymphoma cell niche: identification of a preeminent IL-4-dependent T(FH)-B cell axis. Leukemia 24: 2080-2089.
28. Schroder AJ, Pavlidis P, Arimura A, Capece D, Rothman PB (2002) Cutting edge: STAT6 serves as a positive and negative regulator of gene expression in IL-4-stimulated B lymphocytes. J Immunol 168: 996-1000.
29. Lu X, Nechushtan H, Ding F, Rosado MF, Singal R, et al. (2005) Distinct IL-4-induced gene expression, proliferation, and intracellular signaling in germinal center B-cell-like and activated B-cell-like diffuse large-cell lymphomas. Blood 105: 2924-2932.
30. Stamatopoulos B, Meuleman N, De Bruyn C, Pieters K, Anthoine G, et al. (2010) A molecular score by quantitative PCR as a new prognostic tool at diagnosis for chronic lymphocytic leukemia patients. PLoS ONE 5: 12780.
31. Early SB, Barekzi E, Negri J, Hise K, Borish L, et al. (2007) Concordant modulation of cysteinyl leukotriene receptor expression by IL-4 and IFN-gamma on peripheral immune cells. Am J Respir Cell Mol Biol 36: 715-720.
32. Finkelman FD, Katona IM, Urban JF Jr, Snapper CM, Ohara J, et al. (1986) Suppression of in vivo polyclonal IgE responses by monoclonal antibody to the lymphokine B-cell stimulatory factor 1. Proc Natl Acad Sci USA 83: 9675-9678.
33. Kashiwada M, Levy DM, McKeag L, Murray K, Schröder AJ, et al. (2010) IL-4-induced transcription factor NFIL3/E4BP4 controls IgE class switching. Proc Natl Acad Sci USA 107: 821-826.
34. Alcaraz-García MJ, Ruiz-Lafuente N, Sebastián-Ruiz S, Majado MJ, González-García C, et al. (2011) Human and mouse DOCK10 splicing isoforms with alternative first coding exon usage are differentially expressed in T and B lymphocytes. Hum Immunol 72: 531-537.
35. Tobe M, Isobe Y, Tomizawa H, Nagasaki T, Takahashi H, et al. (2003) A novel structural class of potent inhibitors of NF-kappa B activation: structure-activity relationships and biological effects of 6-aminoquinazoline derivatives. Bioorg Med Chem 11: 3869-3878.
36. Kaminski A, Demaine A, Prentice A (1998) Cytoplasmic interleukin-4 (IL-4) and surface IL-4 receptor expression in patients with B-cell lymphocytic leukemia. Blood 92: 2188-2189.
37. Moskalev EA, Luckert K, Vorobjev IA, Mastitsky SE, Gladkikh AA, et al. (2012) Concurrent epigenetic silencing of wnt/β-catenin pathway inhibitor genes in B cell chronic lymphocytic leukaemia. BMC Cancer 2012; 12: 213.
38. Lafarge ST, Johnston JB, Gibson SB, Marshall AJ (2014) Adhesion of ZAP-70+ chronic lymphocytic leukemia cells to stromal cells is enhanced by cytokines and blocked by inhibitors of the PI3-kinase pathway. Leuk Res 38: 109-115.
39. Willimott S, Baou M, Naresh K, Wagner SD (2007) CD154 induces a switch in pro-survival Bcl-2 family members in chronic lymphocytic leukaemia. Br J Haematol 138: 721-732.
40. Cosimo E, McCaig AM, Carter-Brzezinski LJM, Wheadon H, Leach MT, et al. (2013) Inhibition of NF-kB-mediated signaling by the cyclin-dependent kinase inhibitor CR8 overcomes prosurvival stimuli to induce apoptosis in chronic lymphocytic leukemia cells. Clin Cancer Res 19: 2393-2405.
41. Rong R, Ahn JY, Huang H, Nagata E, Kalman D, et al. (2003) PI3 kinase enhancer-Homer complex couples mGluRI to PI3 kinase, preventing neuronal apoptosis. Nat Neurosci 6: 1153-1161.
42. Huang GN, Huso DL, Bouyain S, Tu J, McCorkell KA, et al. (2008) NFAT binding and regulation of T cell activation by the cytoplasmic scaffolding Homer proteins. Science 319: 476-481.
43. Jantus Lewintre E, Reinoso Martín C, García Ballesteros C, Pendas J, Benet Campos C, et al. (2009) BCL6: somatic mutations and expression in early-stage chronic lymphocytic leukemia. Leuk Lymphoma 50: 773-780.
44. López-Guerra M, Roué G, Pérez-Galán P, Alonso R, Villamor N, et al. (2009) p65 activity and ZAP-70 status predict the sensitivity of chronic lymphocytic leukemia cells to the selective IkappaB kinase inhibitor BMS-345541. Clin Cancer Res 15: 2767-2776.
45. Chen L, Huynh L, Apgar J, Tang L, Rassenti L, et al. (2008) ZAP-70 enhances IgM signaling independent of its kinase activity in chronic lymphocytic leukemia. Blood 111: 2685-2692.
46. Calpe E, Codony C, Baptista MJ, Abrisqueta P, Carpio C, et al. (2011) ZAP-70 enhances migration of malignant B lymphocytes toward CCL21 by inducing CCR7 expression via IgM-ERK1/2 activation. Blood 118: 4401-4410.
47. Pickering BM, de Mel S, Lee M, Howell M, Habens F, et al. (2007) Pharmacological inhibitors of NF-kappaB accelerate apoptosis in chronic lymphocytic leukaemia cells. Oncogene 26: 1166-1177.
48. Hewamana S, Alghazal S, Lin TT, Clement M, Jenkins C, et al. (2008) The NF-kappaB subunit Rel A is associated with in vitro survival and clinical disease progression in chronic lymphocytic leukemia and represents a promising therapeutic target. Blood 111: 4681-4689.
49. Burgess M, Cheung C, Chambers L, Ravindranath K, Minhas G, et al. (2012) CCL2 and CXCL2 enhance survival of primary chronic lymphocytic leukemia cells in vitro. Leuk Lymphoma 53: 1988-1998.
50. Ikushima S, Inukai T, Inaba T, Nimer SD, Cleveland JL, et al. (1997) Pivotal role for the NFIL3/E4BP4 transcription factor in interleukin 3-mediated survival of pro-B lymphocytes. Proc Natl Acad Sci U S A 94: 2609-2614.

Optimal Chemotherapy for Leukemia: A Model-Based Strategy for Individualized Treatment

Devaraj Jayachandran[1], Ann E. Rundell[2], Robert E. Hannemann[1,2], Terry A. Vik[3], Doraiswami Ramkrishna[1]*

1 School of Chemical Engineering, Purdue University, West Lafayette, Indiana, United States of America, 2 Weldon School of Biomedical Engineering, Purdue University, West Lafayette, Indiana, United States of America, 3 Riley Hospital for Children, Indianapolis, Indiana, United States of America

Abstract

Acute Lymphoblastic Leukemia, commonly known as ALL, is a predominant form of cancer during childhood. With the advent of modern healthcare support, the 5-year survival rate has been impressive in the recent past. However, long-term ALL survivors embattle several treatment-related medical and socio-economic complications due to excessive and inordinate chemotherapy doses received during treatment. In this work, we present a model-based approach to personalize 6-Mercaptopurine (6-MP) treatment for childhood ALL with a provision for incorporating the pharmacogenomic variations among patients. Semi-mechanistic mathematical models were developed and validated for i) 6-MP metabolism, ii) red blood cell mean corpuscular volume (MCV) dynamics, a surrogate marker for treatment efficacy, and iii) leukopenia, a major side-effect. With the constraint of getting limited data from clinics, a global sensitivity analysis based model reduction technique was employed to reduce the parameter space arising from semi-mechanistic models. The reduced, sensitive parameters were used to individualize the average patient model to a specific patient so as to minimize the model uncertainty. Models fit the data well and mimic diverse behavior observed among patients with minimum parameters. The model was validated with real patient data obtained from literature and Riley Hospital for Children in Indianapolis. Patient models were used to optimize the dose for an individual patient through nonlinear model predictive control. The implementation of our approach in clinical practice is realizable with routinely measured complete blood counts (CBC) and a few additional metabolite measurements. The proposed approach promises to achieve model-based individualized treatment to a specific patient, as opposed to a standard-dose-for-all, and to prescribe an optimal dose for a desired outcome with minimum side-effects.

Editor: Francesco Pappalardo, University of Catania, Italy

Funding: This work was supported by an NSF CAREER Award and funded under the American Recovery and Reinvestment Act of 2009 (ARRA) under the grant ECCS-0846572. D.J. would like to acknowledge the Lynn Fellowship for computational life sciences. The funders had no role in study design, data collection and analysis, decision to publish, or preparation of the manuscript.

Competing Interests: The authors have declared that no competing interests exist.

* Email: ramkrish@purdue.edu

Introduction

1.1. Background on ALL & Maintenance Therapy

Acute Lymphoblastic Leukemia (ALL) is a malignant state of the bone marrow characterized by an abnormal and uncontrolled proliferation of lymphoblasts. In the U.S., yearly incidence of ALL is more than 5,000 [1] and is the leading class of cancer among children. Treatment for ALL comprises three phases. Newly diagnosed patients undergo remission-induction treatment using a combination of chemotherapeutics to bring down the tumor burden to less than 1% of the initial leukemic cells [2]. This is followed by consolidation therapy using high-dose of drugs to target specific locations of usual leukemic cell migration. The final phase of the treatment is maintenance therapy (MT) which utilizes relatively mild doses of drug over a period of 2–3 years to eradicate residual leukemic cells. Common acute side-effects during ALL treatment include but are not limited to myelosuppression, gastro-intestinal intolerance, hepatotoxicity, pancreatitis and neuropathy.

Having accomplished a high 5-year event-free-survival (EFS) rate of ~85%, the next obvious focus is on minimizing acute and chronic treatment-related side-effects. This may include: i) identifying patient subgroups that are non-responsive and/or are prone to excessive side-effects and ii) choosing optimal dosage for each subgroup/patient. Though the 5-year EFS is obviously significant, and deceptively so in some sense, two thirds of the long-term survivors embattle treatment related late effects [3–5]. Recurrent ALL, secondary neoplasm and other multiple chronic medical conditions are prevalent among the survivors. They also encounter psychosocial issues, impaired quality of life and enjoy lower rate of socioeconomic advantages [3]. Clinical studies show that the administration of high dose of chemotherapeutic agents poses a significant risk towards long-term survival and quality-of-life among childhood cancer survivors [3,6–9].

1.2. Importance and Issues of Maintenance Therapy

Maintenance therapy forms an important and indispensable part of the overall ALL treatment program. About 40% of the patients have minimal residual disease (MRD) at the end of consolidation; MRD is highly correlated with relapse rate [10]. Hence, a carefully designed and administered MT protocol is important to eradicate the residual disease. Patient self-adminis-

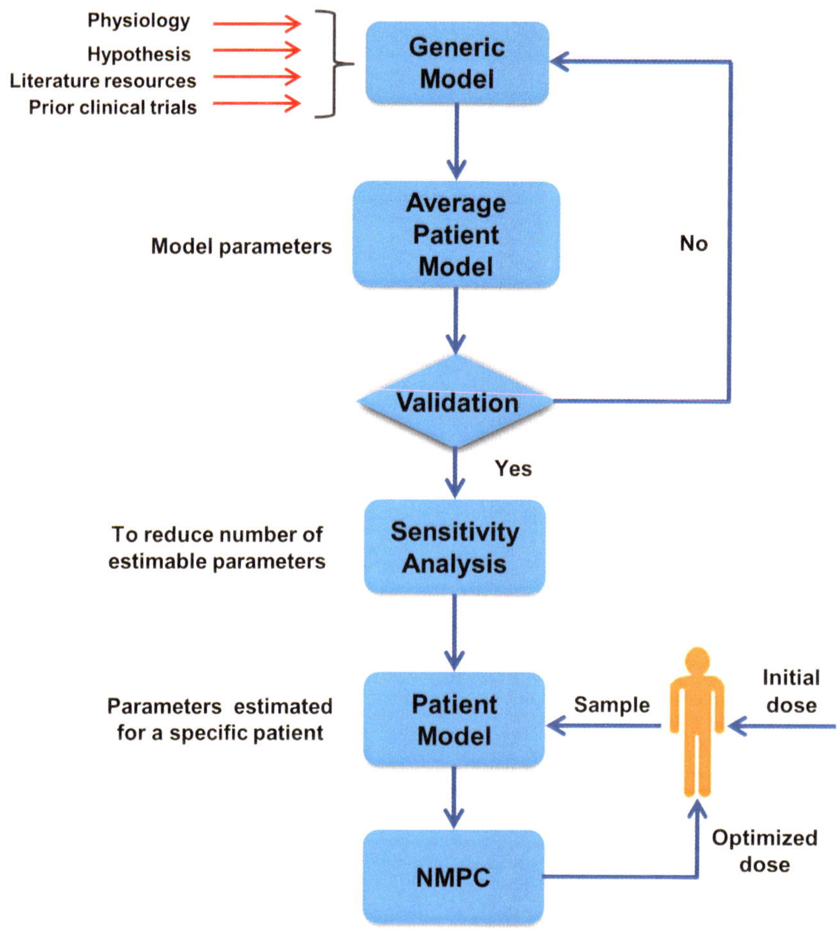

Figure 1. A generalized approach for model-based prediction and optimization of treatment outcome. A model representing the underlying physiology is formulated and average patient parameters are estimated using data from literature and past clinical trials. GSA is used to reduce the parameter space and identify most sensitive parameters with sparse clinical data. Following nominal initial dose, few measurements are taken from an individual patient in order to adapt the model to the patient. Patient-specific model is used to predict the treatment outcome and subsequent doses are optimized based on NMPC prediction.

tered oral combination of 6-Mercaptopurine (6-MP) and Methotrexate (MTX) is shown to improve the overall treatment outcome [10–12]. Clinical studies show that inadequate maintenance therapy leads to recurrent ALL whereas aggressive treatment results in acute side-effects and secondary malignancies, thus calling for the optimization and individualization of MT [13–17]. Hence, it is very important to monitor and optimize the treatment intensity during MT.

There are, among others, two major challenges encountered during MT of childhood ALL. First is the genetic polymorphism exhibited in the enzyme activity of Thiopurine Methyl-transferase (TPMT), an enzyme that plays a major role in conversion of 6-MP into various metabolites [18]. TPMT genetic polymorphism is directly correlated with treatment outcome and hence it is adopted as a companion diagnostic tool in many 6-MP protocols [14,19,20]. 6-MP is a pro-drug which undergoes intracellular metabolism involving two competing metabolic pathways [21]. The desired pathway leading to 6-thioguanine nucleotide (6-TGN) is catalyzed by an enzyme HGPRT. The catabolic pathways are catalyzed by TPMT which leads to the formation of various methyl-mercaptopurines (MeMP). The relative activities of HGPRT and TPMT are genetically transcribed and regulated for a given patient and dictates the net concentration of the active metabolite 6-TGN and hence the treatment outcome. For instance, in patients with high TPMT activity, 6-TGN pathway is suppressed, resulting in low 6-TGN concentration and hence treatment failure. On the other hand, in patients with low TPMT activity, encounter life-threatening myelotoxicity and treatment interruptions. Hence, it is prudent to utilize the TPMT genotype/phenotype as a basis to guide the treatment protocol for an individual patient [22].

Second is the inability to evaluate the treatment progression during MT due to the residual nature of the disease. Measurement of residual leukemic cells during MT remains elusive given the milder treatment condition and low turn-over rate of leukemia cells. During MT, bone marrow cell populations are exposed to 6-MP; when the cells move to the periphery, they retain the metabolized products. Thus, the concentration of 6-TGN in peripheral red blood cells (RBCs) is shown to indicate the systemic exposure to the chemotherapy agent and hence correlated to the treatment efficacy and toxicity [23]. Clinical studies show that the mean corpuscular volume (MCV) of the peripheral RBCs increases significantly due to the exposure to 6-TGN and provides an opportunity to be utilized as a surrogate marker for treatment

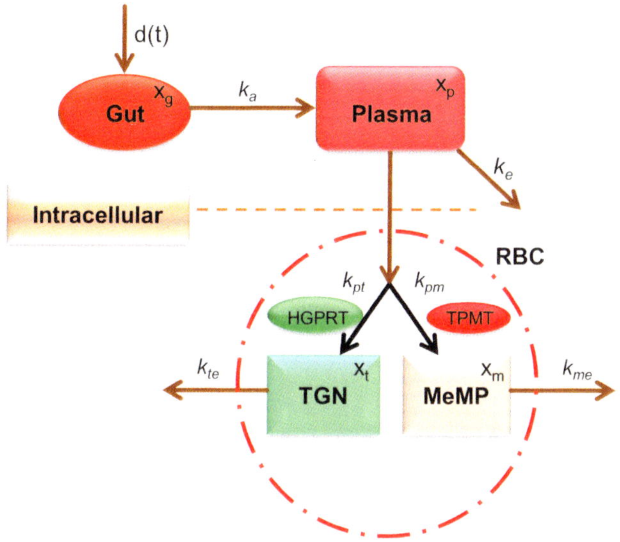

Figure 2. Schematic representation of 6-MP metabolism. Following oral intake to the gut, 6-MP is absorbed into the plasma from where it is eliminated through various routes. From plasma, 6-MP diffuses into the cells and enzymatically converted to 6-TGN and MeMP, which in turn are eliminated from the cells at a constant rate.

monitoring [23–25]. Currently, in ALL MT, patients are initially treated with doses based on body surface area and are titrated to target neutrophil range of 1000–2000/μL. However, it is not possible to precisely judge the nadir of neutrophil level.

1.3. Importance of Individualized Treatment

Though mathematical models and optimal control theory have been utilized in almost all fields of science and engineering for over a century with tremendous contributions, they are not utilized to their fullest potential in medical applications [26]. Application of Mathematical approaches have shown excellent utilities in understanding and solving several issues in HIV, diabetes [27,28]. Several aspects of cancer dynamics have also been studied through mathematical models [29–31]. Mathematical models, suitably empowered by systems theoretic methodology, derive their strength from their potential to quantitatively evaluate known or conjectured mechanisms of physiological processes. Clinical studies on childhood ALL show that some treatment regimens perform better than others [17,32,33]. A Pediatric Oncology Group study concluded that compared to twice-daily regimen, daily dosing regimen resulted in significantly higher metabolites of 6-MP [32]. In a recent study on Brazilian childhood ALL patients during MT [33], significantly higher 5-year EFS and overall survival rates were observed in intermittent treatment group. These results suggest that since one dose regimen performs better than the other, there exists an optimal regimen that performs better than many other regimens. Unfortunately, it is not possible to explore all possible combinations of regimens in a clinical trial.

We recently developed a semi-mechanistic model for indirect measurement of treatment efficacy using MCV of the RBCs as a surrogate marker [25]. The model considered a given concentration of active metabolite 6-TGN in RBCs and predicts dynamic changes of MCV in response to 6-TGN. Metabolism of 6-MP into 6-TGN and side-effects were not considered in that work. The present study aims to extend the model by explicitly incorporating the metabolism of 6-MP to 6-TGN and the major side-effect (leukopenia) during treatment. In addition, a simple and effective model-reduction technique based on global sensitivity analysis (GSA) is introduced to reduce the parameter space. This is important because personalization requires model adaptation to an individual patient through effective identification of parameters with sparse clinical data. The proposed modeling and sensitivity based approach will take into account the pharmacogenetic variation, through TPMT enzyme activity, to estimate the initial

Table 1. Glossary of state variables and parameters for 6-MP model.

Model variables	Description		Units
x_g	Amount of 6-MP in Gut		pmol
x_p	Amount of 6-MP in Plasma		pmol
x_t	Concentration of 6-TGN in RBCs		pmol/8 $\times 10^8$ RBCs
x_m	Concentration of MeMP in RBCs		pmol/8 $\times 10^8$ RBCs
Parameters	**Description**	**Units**	**Values**
k_a	6-MP Absorption Rate from Gut	per day	4.8
k_e	6-MP Elimination Rate from Plasma	per day	5.0
k_{pt}	6-MP to 6-TGN Conversion Rate	pmol 6-MP converted per day	29.8
K_t	MM Constant for 6-TGN	pmol	4.04×10^5
k_{pm}	6-MP to MeMP Conversion Rate	pmol 6-MP converted per day	655.8
K_m	MM Constant for MeMP	pmol	3.28×10^5
k_{te}	6-TGN Elimination Rate from RBCs	per day	0.0714
k_{me}	MeMP Elimination Rate from RBCs	per day	0.06
e	Actual TPMT Activity	Units per ml RBC	13
e^{max}	Maximum TPMT Activity	Units per ml RBC	26
ν_{pt}	Stoichiometric coefficient for 6-TGN Conversion	pmol 6-TGN produced per pmol 6-MP/8 $\times 10^8$ RBCs	1
ν_{pm}	Stoichiometric coefficient for MeMP Conversion	pmol MeMP produced per pmol 6-MP/8 $\times 10^8$ RBCs	1

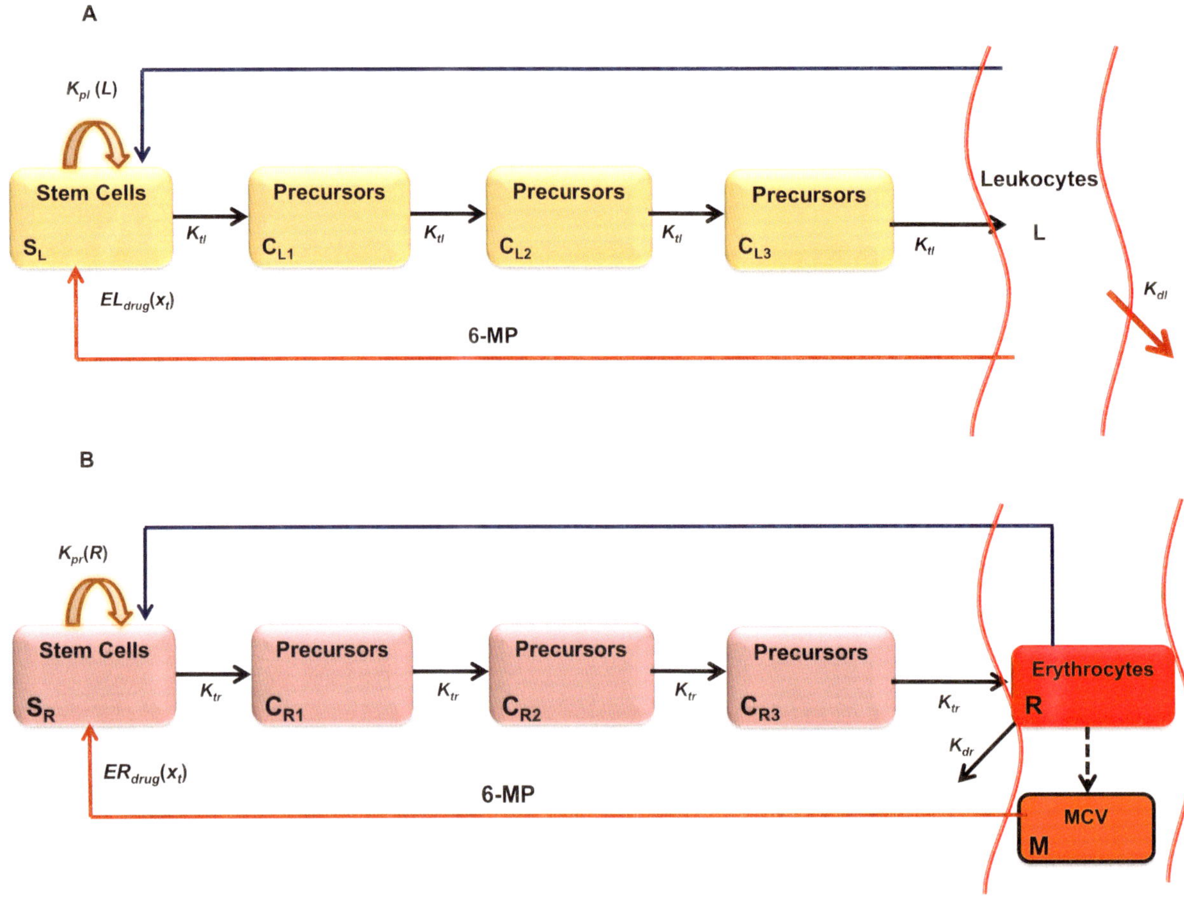

Figure 3. Simplified schematics of the leukopoiesis and erythropoiesis model. Stem cells reside in the bone marrow, proliferate, mature and enter the circulation as fully functional leukocytes. Stem cells receive biochemical feedback for proliferation from the circulating blood. On treatment initiation, 6-MP enters the bone marrow and imparts cytotoxicity to the stem cells. Leukocytes and RBC MCV in the circulating blood are routinely measured and used as a dose-limiting parameter. A. Leukopoiesis, B. Erythropoiesis. Additional compartment for MCV was added to account for the dynamic changes following 6-MP treatment. Solid arrows represent cellular movement; dashed arrow represents property changes.

Table 2. Glossary of state variables and parameters for leukopoiesis model.

Model variables	Description		Units
S_L	No. of proliferating progenitors		cells per kg
C_{L1}	No. of maturing leukocyte precursors		cells per kg
C_{L2}	No. of maturing leukocyte precursors		cells per kg
C_{L2}	No. of maturing leukocyte precursors		cells per kg
L	No. of circulating leukocytes		cells per liter blood
Parameters	**Description**	**Units**	**Values**
k_{pl}^{max}	Maximum proliferation rate	per day	0.3287
ρ	Feedback parameter	cells per liter blood	8.2×10^9
γ_l	Steepness parameter for feedback	none	0.4368
EL_{max}	Maximum effect of drug on L	per day	0.0782
ECL_{50}	Saturation constant for drug on L	pmol/8×10^8 RBCs	84
k_{tl}	Inter-compartmental transfer rate	per day	0.1207
k_{dl}	Clearance rate of leukocytes	per day	0.5346

Table 3. Glossary of state variables and parameters for MCV model.

Model variables	**Description**		**Units**
S_R	No. of proliferating erythrocyte progenitors		cells per kg
C_{R1}	No. of maturing erythroid precursors		cells per kg
C_{R2}	No. of maturing erythroid precursors		cells per kg
C_{R3}	No. of maturing erythroid precursors		cells per kg
R	No. of circulating erythrocytes		cells per kg
M	MCV of circulating erythrocytes		femto liter (fL)
Parameters	**Description**	**Units**	**Values**
k_{pr}^{max}	Maximum proliferation rate	per day	1.4
ψ	Feedback parameter	cells per kg	4.02×10^{11}
γ_r	Steepness parameter for feedback	none	0.1
ER_{max}	Maximum effect of drug on L	per day	0.0022
ECR_{50}	Saturation constant for drug on L	pmol/8$\times10^8$ RBCs	82.2
k_{tr}	Inter-compartmental transfer rate	per day	0.702
k_{dr}	Clearance rate of circulating leukocytes	per day	0.0085
α	Empiric coefficient for 6-TGN effect on MCV	fL/pmol/8$\times10^8$ RBCs	0.055
$M0$	Baseline MCV	fL	85

dose based on established therapeutic window. Once measurements (6-TGN, MCV and Leukocyte levels) are available following initial dose, patient specific sensitive parameters are identified. Once individual patient model is available, we used nonlinear model predictive control (NMPC) to optimize the dosage subject to a minimum level of WBC. The uncertainty in the patient-specific parameters associated with the treatment response models can be minimized by adaptively changing them according to the frequently available CBC data. The model is simple enough to be implemented in the clinical settings and requires few measurements of metabolites concentration and routinely measured CBC data to be able to adapt to individual patients. Although not modeled explicitly, implementation of such approach may help to improve the long-term EFS and quality-of-life among childhood ALL patients as they are the resultants of inappropriate dosing. The overall strategy is depicted in Fig.1. In section 2, we detail the methodologies utilized in this work including models to describe 6-MP metabolism, leukopoiesis and MCV dynamics. In section 3, we show some of the important results of this work with the simulation of virtual patients' response to 6-MP treatment. In sections 4, we discuss the results and implications of this work.

Models and Methods

Let a generic dynamic model for any given drug and patient be given by a system of ordinary differential equations with the following form,

$$\frac{d\boldsymbol{x}(t)}{dt}=f(\boldsymbol{x}(t),\boldsymbol{\theta},\boldsymbol{u}(t)); \quad \boldsymbol{x}(0)=\boldsymbol{c} \quad \boldsymbol{y}(t)=g(\boldsymbol{x}(t),\boldsymbol{\theta},\boldsymbol{u}(t)) \qquad (1)$$

where $x(t)\in\Re^n$:state variables, $\theta\in\Re^p$:model parameters, $u(t)\in\Re^q$: drug input, $c\in\Re^n$:initial conditions, $y(t)\in\Re^l$:model output. In most circumstances $f(\boldsymbol{x}(t),\boldsymbol{\theta},\boldsymbol{u}(t))$ will be a nonlinear function and a numerical solution is readily available. For the purpose of this study, the parameter space $\theta\in\Re^p$ is divided into redundant parameters, $\tilde{\theta}\in\Re^r$ and sensitive parameters $\hat{\theta}\in\Re^s=\Re^{p-r}$. Sensitive parameters are identified for each patient whereas redundant parameters are fixed for all patients at average value.

2.1. Modeling 6-MP Metabolism

Although the TPMT pharmacogenomics and the metabolism of 6-MP is one of the extensively studied systems in clinical pharmacology literature, mathematical models are limited. We are only aware of the works of Hawwa et al. [34] where TPMT genotype was considered as one of the covariates to describe the inter-individual variations. However, many studies show that TPMT phenotype is a better marker than the TPMT genotype because there is a huge variation of TPMT enzyme activity within a specific genotype. A simplified schematic of the 6-MP metabolism accounting for two major metabolites is shown in Fig. 2. Following oral intake to the gut, 6-MP is absorbed at the rate of k_a into the plasma where it undergoes first-pass elimination at the rate of k_e. From plasma, 6-MP gets into RBCs followed by intracellular metabolism. There is a negligible concentration of 6-MP reported inside RBCs [35]; hence, we assume that 6-MP gets metabolized as soon as it enters RBC. 6-MP undergoes metabolism through two major pathways driven by HGPRT and TPMT leading to 6-TGN (active) and MeMP (inactive), respectively. Though there are several forms of MeMP produced, for modeling purpose, they are lumped into a single component collectively catalyzed by TPMT. 6-TGN and MeMP are eliminated from RBCs at the rates of k_{te} and k_{me} respectively. v_{pt} and v_{pm} are included for unit consistency across equations.

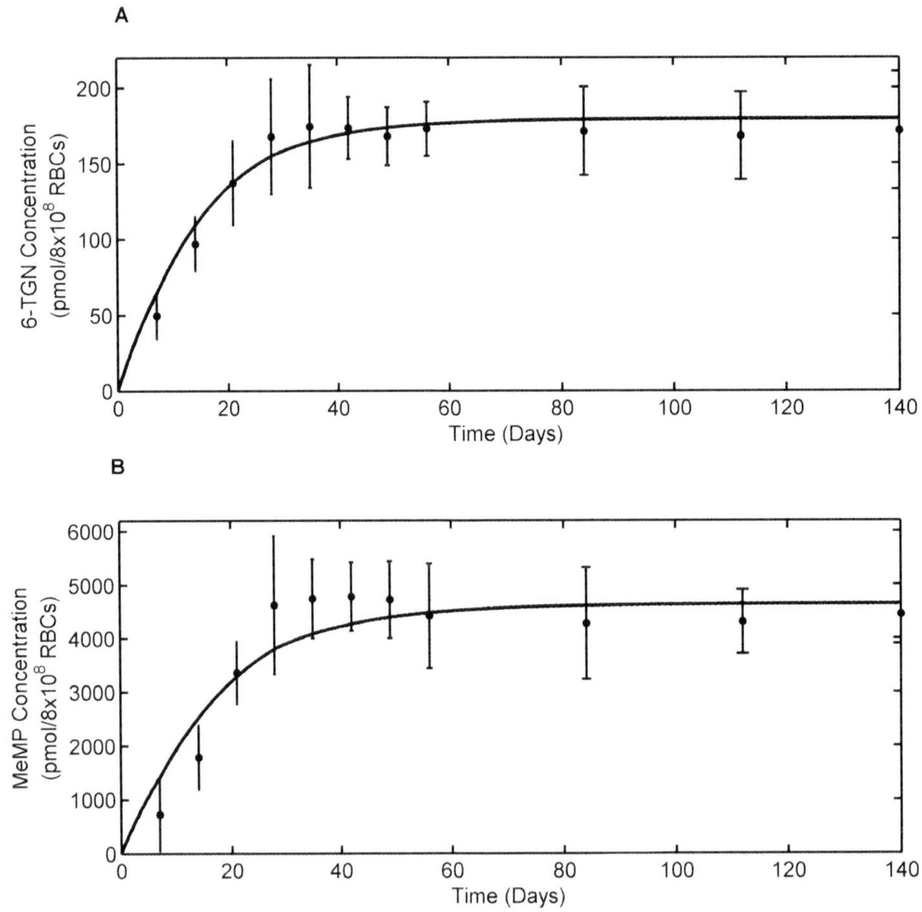

Figure 4. Average patient 6-MP model fit to literature data. A. Model fit to RBC 6-TGN concentration data. B. Model fit to RBC MeMP concentration data. Solid dots represent data points and curves represent 6-MP model (Eqn. 2) fit. Error bars represent standard error.

$$\begin{aligned}
\frac{dx_g}{dt} &= -k_a x_g + d(t) \\
\frac{dx_p}{dt} &= k_a x_g - k_e x_p - \frac{k_{pt}(1-e_{rel})x_p}{K_t + x_p} - \frac{k_{pm} e_{rel} x_p}{K_m + x_p} \\
\frac{dx_t}{dt} &= \frac{v_{pt} k_{pt}(1-e_{rel})x_p}{K_t + x_p} - k_{te} x_t \\
\frac{dx_m}{dt} &= \frac{v_{pm} k_{pm} e_{rel} x_p}{K_m + x_p} - k_{me} x_m
\end{aligned} \tag{2}$$

The model equations for 6-MP metabolism based on mass-action kinetics are shown in Eqn. 2. The description and units of all the state variables and parameters are listed in Table 1. The conversion of 6-MP into 6-TGN and MeMP is modeled using Michaelis–Menten (M-M) kinetics. Patient specific TPMT enzyme activity is represented as a relative activity level to their maximum level. Thus,

$$e_{rel} = \frac{e}{e_{max}} \tag{3}$$

where e denotes TPMT enzyme activity. It is observed in the clinical studies that the production of 6-TGN is not limited by the

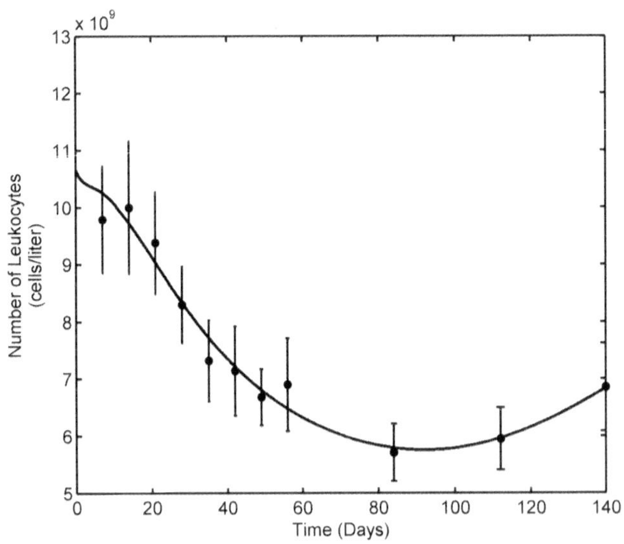

Figure 5. Leukopoiesis model fit to average patient data. Solid dots represent average patient data and curve represent leukocyte model (Eqn. 4) fit. The model mimics the clinical observation during 6-MP treatment; Depletion of leukocytes following 6-MP dosing has been countered by the body's feed-back mechanism. Error bars represent standard error.

HGPRT activity but is negatively correlated with TPMT activity [36]. Hence, it is assumed that a fraction (e_{rel}) of 6-MP is converted to methylated metabolites based on the enzyme activity observed in a specific patient and the rest ($1-e_{rel}$) is converted to active 6-TGN.

2.2. Modeling Treatment Response

In humans, blood cells (RBCs, WBCs, platelets etc.) are one of the most dynamic and vital population of cells with high turnover rates. Since most of the cytotoxic drugs, such as 6-MP, are designed to target fast-renewing cells, they invariably destroy bone marrow cells. Consequently, monitoring of peripheral blood count has become an integral part during chemotherapy to assess the bone marrow toxicity. However, this is a reactive rather than a proactive approach as the bulk of the damage is done to the immature, bone marrow cells instead of the peripheral cells. Since the maturation takes about 5–12 days, there will be a marked delay in the realization of the effects in the periphery. Thus, the prediction of the cellular dynamics during 6-MP treatment would help to forecast the oncoming decline in the cell population and adopt corrective measures before the patient contracts the side-effect. Mathematical models are in use to describe many facets of the hematopoiesis processes [37,38]. Although mechanistic models are rich in physiology and are able to display diverse system behavior, they come with the price of several parameters. With the constraint on data, semi-mechanistic models of specific behavior within the exhaustive overall process would be of much use.

2.2.1. Modeling Leukopoiesis. The model to study the effect of chemotherapy on leukocytes was inspired by [39]. The schematic diagram of the leukopoiesis is depicted in Fig. 3A. The stem cells and early proliferating progenitors are depicted as compartment S_L. During early stages of stem cell differentiation, cells have the potential to proliferate. As they mature, they expel their nucleus and loose their proliferating potential [40]. 6-MP's cytotoxicity is due to incorporation of 6-TGN as false nucleotides into the DNA. Hence, 6-MP will have no influence on cells in the later stages lacking nuclei. Consequently, it is assumed that the cells in this compartment are the sole casualties of the cytotoxic drugs. Proliferation rate of the cells in this compartment is a function of leukocytes in the circulating system i.e. $k_{pl}=k_{pl}(L)$. This feedback mechanism is mediated by a cytokine known as granulocyte-colony stimulating factor (G-CSF). The next three compartments, viz. C_{L1}, C_{L2} and C_{L3}, cater for the maturation process. Cells in these compartments are not susceptible to cytotoxic drugs as they are not proliferating. The fully matured, functional leukocytes enter the circulation, perform their functions for a specified period and die at a constant rate.

$$\begin{aligned}
\frac{dS_L}{dt} &= k_{pl}(L)S_L - EL_{drug}(x_t)S_L - k_{tl}S_L\\
\frac{dC_{L1}}{dt} &= k_{tl}S_L - k_{tl}C_{L1}\\
\frac{dC_{L2}}{dt} &= k_{tl}C_{L1} - k_{tl}C_{L2}\\
\frac{dC_{L3}}{dt} &= k_{tl}C_{L2} - k_{tl}C_{L3}\\
\frac{dL}{dt} &= k_{tl}C_{L3} - k_{dl}L
\end{aligned} \tag{4}$$

The equations for leukopoiesis model are given in Eqn. 4. The description and units for all the state variables and parameters for the leukopoiesis model are listed in Table 2. In the stem cell compartment, positive feedback for proliferation with amplitude modulated negatively by L is represented using the following structure:

$$k_{pl}(L) = k_{pl}^{max}\frac{\rho^{\gamma l}}{\rho^{\gamma l}+L^{\gamma l}} \tag{5}$$

Although the feedback is mediated by biochemical messenger G-CSF, the concentration of G-CSF is inversely proportional to circulating leukocytes as G-CSF is mainly cleared by the receptors on the leukocytes [41]. Unlike the term used in [39], which is a monotonically increasing function of leukocytes, Eqn. 5 has a saturating nature which derives its basis from receptor theory [42–44]. 6-MP effect in this compartment assumes the following Hill type kinetics.

$$EL_{drug} = \frac{EL_{max}x_t}{ECL_{50}+x_t} \tag{6}$$

where x_t is the 6-TGN concentration obtained from 6-MP model. The cells are transferred to the maturing compartments at the rate of k_{tl}. The matured cells enter the circulation at the rate of k_{tl} and die at the rate of k_{dl}.

2.2.2. Modeling MCV Dynamics. Erythropoiesis, similar to leukopoiesis, is a process through which the body generates erythrocytes and hence assumes a similar model structure. The schematic diagram of erythropoiesis and MCV dynamics is shown in Fig. 3B. The proliferating fraction of the erythroid stem cells and early progenitors are represented as S_R. Cells in this compartment are assumed to be vulnerable to 6-MP. Proliferation rate of these cells is regulated by the number of RBCs R. This feedback mechanism is mediated by a cytokine known as

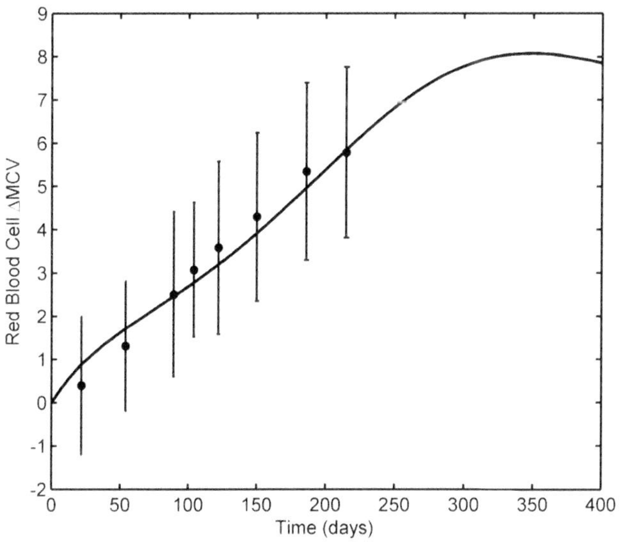

Figure 6. MCV model fit to average patient MCV data. Solid dots represent the data from literature and the solid line shows the model (Eqn. 7) fit with 6-TGN concentration of 158 pmol/8×10^8 RBCs. The model fits the data well; it reaches the steady state and stays at ΔMCV of ~8 fL, which is typically observed during 6-MP treatment at Riley Hospital for Children. Error bars represent standard error.

Table 4. List of parameters identified for individualization through GSA (in bold letters) together with other fixed parameters.

Parameters	$P\left\{\delta(\tilde{\theta}_{i,0})<(.)\right\}\geq 0.95$	% error(actual/ maximum)
6-MP Model (Variable for GSA: x_t)		
$\mathbf{k_{pt}}$	**84.61**	**100**
$\mathbf{k_{te}}$	**46.36**	**54.8**
K_t	0.0003	3.5×10^{-4}
k_e	0.0002	2.4×10^{-4}
k_a	4.0×10^{-5}	4.7×10^{-5}
k_{pm}	2.1×10^{-9}	2.5×10^{-9}
K_m	2.1×10^{-9}	2.5×10^{-9}
$\mathbf{k_{me}}$	0	0
Leukopoiesis Model (Variable for GSA: L)		
$\mathbf{k_{tl}}$	**65.54**	**100**
k_{pl}^{max}	**49.12**	**74.9**
$\mathbf{k_{dl}}$	**39.02**	**59.5**
γ_l	**22.61**	**34.5**
$\mathbf{EL_{max}}$	**17.60**	**26.9**
θ	2.18	3.32
ECL_{50}	0.25	0.38
MCV Model (Variable for GSA: M)		
$\mathbf{k_{tr}}$	**76.48**	**100**
k_{pr}^{max}	**50.09**	**65.5**
$\mathbf{k_{dr}}$	**20.71**	**27.1**
α	**11.00**	**14.4**
$\mathbf{ER_{max}}$	**10.49**	**13.7**
γ_r	2.48	3.24
ψ	0.71	0.93
ECR_{50}	0.0034	0.004

erythropoietin (EPO). C_{R1},C_{R2} and C_{R3} represent the maturing erythroid precursors. Fully functional RBCs enter the periphery, circulate for ~120 days and die at a constant rate. MCV, which is the total volume of RBCs divided by the number of RBCs, in compartment M increases due to two phenomena: 1) inflow of new cells from the bone marrow (RBCs are larger when they enter the circulation and loose about 15% of the volume during their lifetime), 2) due to the administration of 6-MP. MCV decreases due to the death of RBCs which depends on the current MCV. When $\boldsymbol{x_t=0}$, the only influence on MCV would be the imbalance in RBC production. At steady state (and without 6-MP), the two terms on the right hand side will cancel each other.

$$\begin{aligned}
\frac{dS_R}{dt} &= k_{pr}(R)S_R - ER_{drug}(x_t)S_R - k_{tr}S_R \\
\frac{dC_{R1}}{dt} &= k_{tr}S_R - k_{tr}C_{R1} \\
\frac{dC_{R2}}{dt} &= k_{tr}C_{R1} - k_{tr}C_{R2} \\
\frac{dC_{R3}}{dt} &= k_{tr}C_{R2} - k_{tr}C_{R3} \\
\frac{dR}{dt} &= k_{tr}C_{R3} - k_{dr}R \\
\frac{dM}{dt} &= [(\alpha x_t + M_0)k_{tr}C_{R3} - k_{dr}MR]/R
\end{aligned} \tag{7}$$

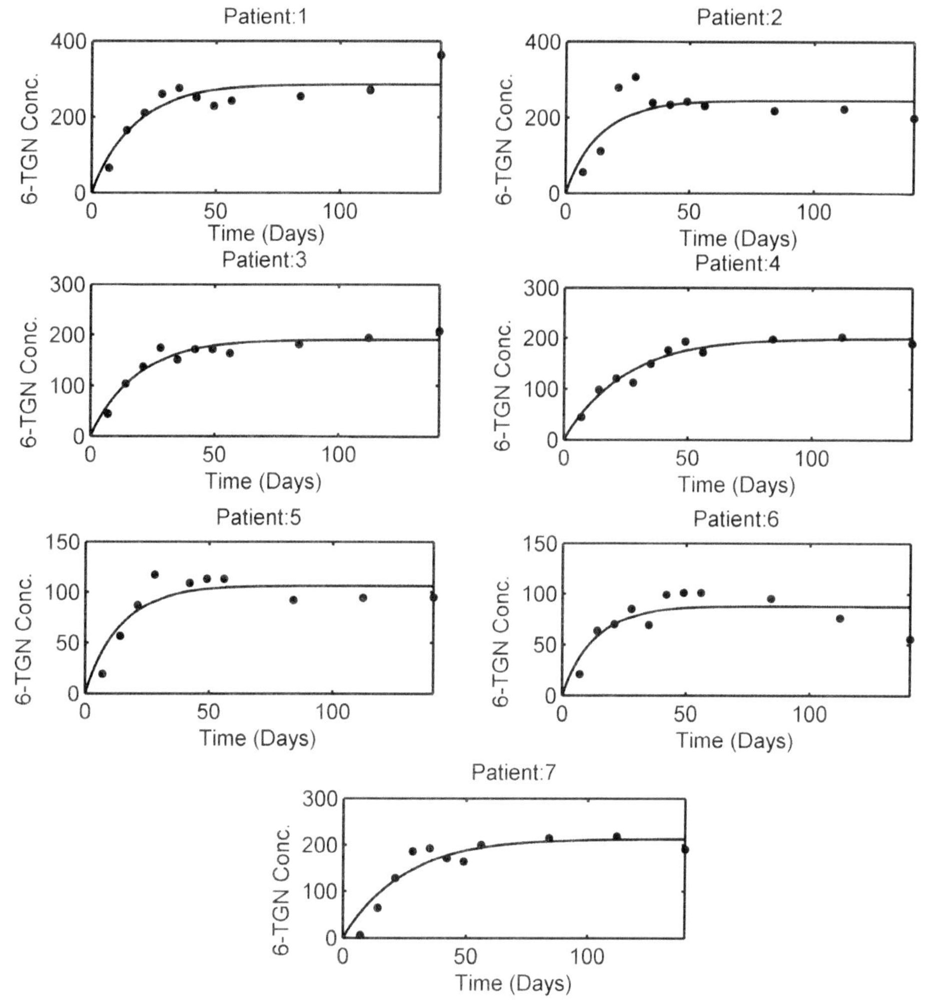

Figure 7. 6-MP model fit to individual patient data obtained from literature. Solid dots indicate the individual patient 6-TGN concentration and the solid line represents the model fit. Patient # 8 was omitted from analysis as it is observed that the dosing was discontinued or substantially lowered. The estimated patient-specific parameters are provided in Table 5.

The model equations for erythropoiesis and MCV dynamics are given in Eqn.7. The feedback for proliferation amplification in stem cell compartment, was approximated by the inverse proportion of the circulating RBCs as follows,

$$k_{pr}(R) = k_{pr}^{max}\frac{\psi^{\gamma_r}}{\psi^{\gamma_r}+R^{\gamma_r}} \qquad (8)$$

The effect of 6-MP treatment on this cell population is modeled using Hill type kinetics.

$$ER_{drug} = \frac{ER_{max}x_t}{ECR_{50}+x_t} \qquad (9)$$

A linear relationship, with coefficient α, was assumed for the effect of drug on the MCV [23]. The loss of MCV was attributed to the death of the RBCs. The resulting total volume was normalized by the total number of RBCs. ΔMCV is calculated as the change in MCV from the baseline (untreated MCV) when 6-MP is administered. The description and units for all the state variables and parameters for the MCV model are listed in Table 3.

2.3 Parameter Estimation

Model parameters were estimated through minimization of sum of squared errors between model predicted values and the experimental data with the following cost function

$$\underset{\theta}{argmin}\left(\sum_{j=1}^{l}\sum_{i=1}^{n_{exp}}\left[\frac{y_j(t_i|\theta)-\hat{y}_j(t_i)}{w_j}\right]^2\right) \qquad (10)$$

where n_{exp} represents the number of experimental data points, $\hat{y}_j$ is the experimental data. When more than one variable is measured, appropriate weight, w_j is used to normalize the cost function. Hybrid genetic algorithm is used as an optimization routine to perform the error minimization step and implemented using Matlab functions 'ga' and 'fmincon' [45]. Parameter bounds for optimization algorithm were chosen from feasible physiological ranges available in the literature.

Table 5. Patient-specific parameters estimated for 6-MP, leukopoiesis and MCV models.

6-MP Model					
Pat. No.	k_{pt}	k_{te}			
1	38.4	0.0646			
2	41.4	0.0815			
3	23.9	0.0604			
4	18.76	0.0453			
5	17.4	0.0788			
6	15.83	0.0867			
7	20.04	0.0452			
Mean	25.1	0.0661			
SD	10.45	0.017			
Min	15.83	0.0452			
Max	41.4	0.0867			
Leukopoiesis Model					
Pat. No.	k_{pl}^{max}	γ_l	EL_{max}	k_{tl}	k_{dl}
i	0.338	0.45	0.06	0.123	0.3653
ii	0.322	0.465	0.068	0.12	0.661
iii	0.434	0.3445	0.081	0.1852	0.6637
iv	0.3943	0.9154	0.2075	0.0926	0.525
v	0.392	0.1786	0.093	0.1411	0.5145
vi	0.3735	1.8	0.2513	0.0858	0.5711
vii	0.447	0.9012	0.1664	0.1305	0.679
viii	0.8	0.4818	0.2506	0.2663	1.2261
Mean	0.4376	0.6921	0.1472	0.1431	0.6507
SD	0.1525	0.5155	0.0817	0.0584	0.2546
Min	0.322	0.1786	0.06	0.0858	0.3653
Max	0.8	1.8	0.2513	0.2663	1.2261
MCV Model					
Pat. No.	k_{pr}^{max}	k_{tr}	ER_{max}	k_{dr}	α
a	1.682	0.862	0.004	0.0131	0.095
b	1.284	0.657	0.0085	0.0126	0.038
c	0.871	0.444	0.0075	0.0074	0.0375
d	1.4243	0.735	0.0037	0.014	0.0527
e	2.204	1.131	0.002	0.0198	0.105
f	1.6631	0.847	0.016	0.0155	0.0544
g	1.55	0.787	0.0058	0.0122	0.0393
h	1.94	0.992	0.0044	0.0156	0.047
i	1.594	0.811	0.0088	0.0123	0.0509
j	1.92	0.981	0.0179	0.0202	0.0456
Mean	1.6132	0.8247	0.0079	0.0143	0.0565
SD	0.3736	0.1917	0.0053	0.0038	0.0238
Min	0.871	0.444	0.002	0.0074	0.0375
Max	2.204	1.131	0.0179	0.0202	0.105

2.4 Model Reduction through Global Sensitivity Analysis

Due to a large inter-patient variability in treatment response, the models developed here have to be adapted to individual patients' characteristics through parameters. Since clinical data are generally sparse, it is not possible to uniquely identify all the parameters as the system is underdetermined. This quandary can be addressed through model reduction using sensitivity analysis (SA) to identify redundant parameters in the model [46]. SA aims to distribute, either quantitatively or qualitatively, the variation in the model output to variation in the model inputs, e.g. parameters.

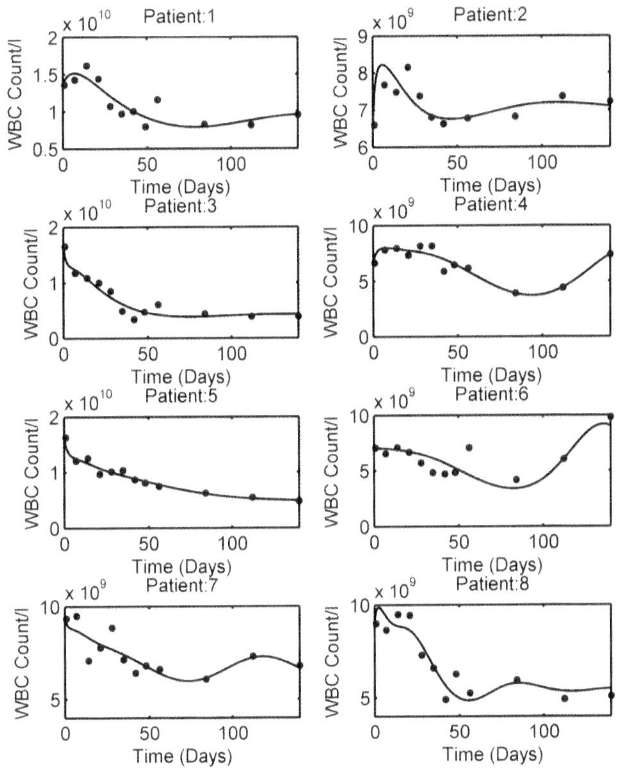

Figure 8. Leukopoiesis model fit to individual patient data obtained from literature. Solid dots indicate the individual patient WBC count and solid lines represent the model fit. The estimated patient-specific parameters are provided in Table 5. The model mimics diverse behavior observed during 6-MP treatment.

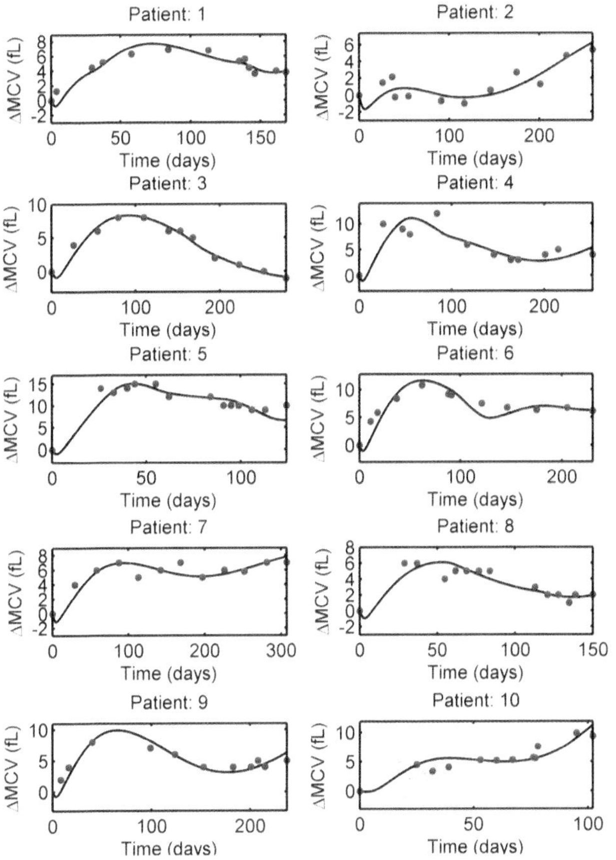

Figure 9. MCV model fit to individual patient data obtained from Riley Hospital for Children. Solid dots indicate ΔMCV of individual patient undergoing 6-MP treatment and solid lines represent the model fit. The estimated patient-specific parameters are provided in Table 5.

Although it is reasonable to assume that the changes in the model input affect the model output, not all inputs influence the model identically. Thus, SA sheds light on the important model parameters that drive the model outputs. Since the model parameters vary widely among patients, we employ global sensitivity analysis (GSA). Soboĺ technique was used to estimate the total sensitivity indices [47]. Lower and upper bounds were chosen at 50% and 200% of the mean respectively. 1000 sets of parameter were sampled through sparse-grid technique. Although redundant parameters have little influence over the variable of our interest, they impart indirect effect through other auxiliary variables. Hence, redundant parameters are fixed at a nominal value (equal to that for an average patient) instead of being eliminated. Since any uncertainty in the estimation of the highly sensitive parameters will influence the model prediction greatly, it is prudent to estimate the most sensitive parameters as accurately as possible with the limited data available and be less concerned about the least sensitive ones. The error involved in such an approximation can be estimated as follows [47].

Let the set of parameters be $\mathbf{\theta} \equiv \left(\hat{\mathbf{\theta}}, \tilde{\mathbf{\theta}}\right)$ in which $\tilde{\mathbf{\theta}} \equiv \left(\tilde{\theta}_1, \tilde{\theta}_2, \ldots, \tilde{\theta}_r\right) \in \Re^r$ represents the r redundant parameters and $\hat{\mathbf{\theta}}$ comprises the sensitive parameters. Further let f_o represent f with $\mathbf{\theta} - \left(\hat{\mathbf{\theta}}, \tilde{\mathbf{\theta}}_{\mathbf{o}}\right)$ where $\tilde{\mathbf{\theta}}_{\mathbf{o}}$ denotes the redundant parameters fixed at nominal value. For any redundant parameter $\tilde{\theta}_i$, if $S^{tot}_{\tilde{\theta}_i} < < 1$, then the error of approximating f with f_0, $\delta(\tilde{\theta}_{i,0})$, by fixing $\tilde{\theta}_i$ at a nominal value $\tilde{\theta}_{i,0}$ can be estimated by

$$P\left\{\delta(\tilde{\theta}_{i,0}) < \left(1 + \frac{1}{\varepsilon}\right) S^{tot}_{\tilde{\theta}_i}\right\} \geq 1 - \varepsilon; \qquad where \quad 0 < \varepsilon \leq 1 (11)$$

where $S^{tot}_{\tilde{\theta}_i}$ is the total sensitivity index of the model output corresponding to parameter $\tilde{\theta}_i$. For an arbitrary value of $\varepsilon = 1/3$, the probability of getting $\delta(\tilde{\theta}_{i,0}) < 4S^{tot}_{\tilde{\theta}_i}$ is more than 2/3.

2.5 Optimal Treatment Planning through NMPC

The final step in model-based individualized dosing is the determination of optimal dosage using patient-specific models. In this work, we utilize NMPC to optimize the dose due to its inherent nature of calculating the input based on the predicted system behavior subject to the state and input constraints as well as the optimization of a given cost function [48,49]. In general, based on the measurement obtained at time τ, the controller predicts the evolution of treatment response over a prediction horizon T and estimates the dosing profile that optimizes the predetermined clinical objective function. To account for disturbances and model-patient mismatch, the optimization problem is solved for *finite* horizon but only the first dosing action is prescribed. The remaining samples are discarded and a new optimization problem is solved based on $y_{\tau+1}$ at the next clinical visit $(\tau + 1)$. For the case of regulating the system in Eq. 1 to the predetermined

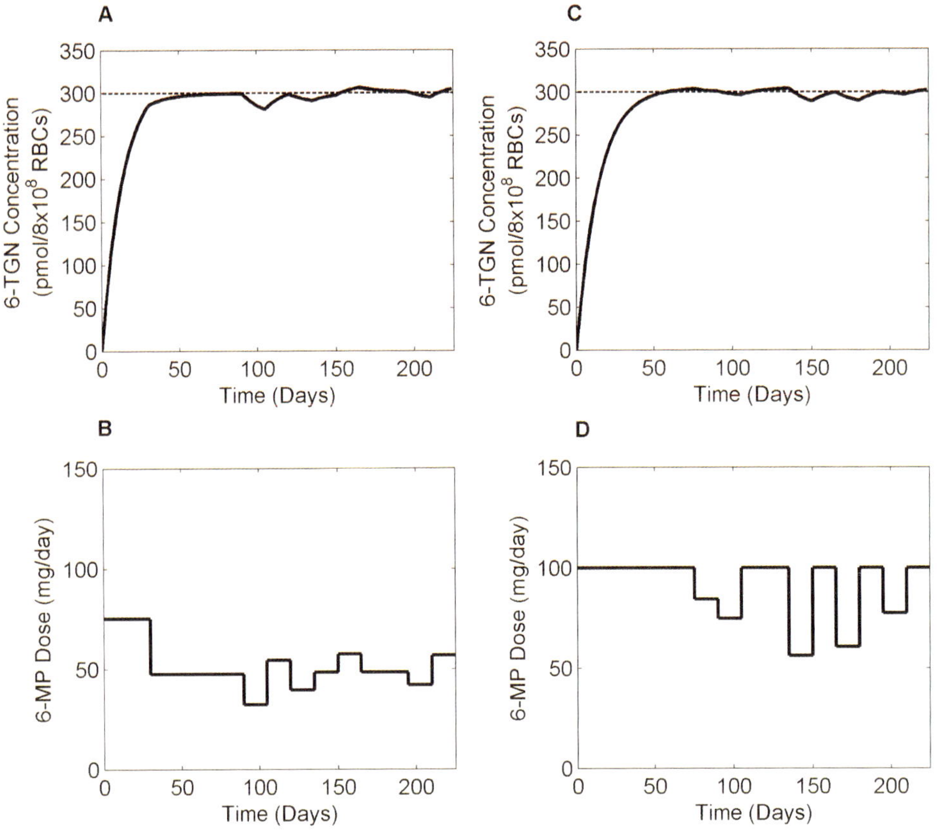

Figure 12. Optimal dosing based on 6-TGN concentration as therapeutic target. A & B. Optimal 6-TGN concentration and optimal 6-MP regimen respectively, for a patient with low TPMT enzyme activity. C & D. Optimal profiles for a patient with high TPMT enzyme activity. Patient with low TPMT activity required significantly lower dose compared to the standard treatment and vice versa. Dashed line shows the therapeutic target level.

desired level whereas in others, the feedback is weak which is a common phenomenon in leukopoiesis [42].

Individual MCV measurements from pediatric ALL patients were obtained from Riley Hospital for Children in Indianapolis. The data was de-identified and collected according to approved IRB protocol (0505002519). Patients were undergoing MT with 6-MP and MTX. Patients were given a standard initial 6-MP dose of 75 mg/m^2 and subsequent doses were adjusted in accordance with observed leukocyte count. Hence, the dosing pattern and dosage varied substantially among and within patients. 6-TGN levels were not measured in these patients, so average parameters were used in 6-MP model. The model fitting to individual patient data are shown in Fig. 9 and the estimated parameters are listed in Table 5.

3.3.1. Predicting Response through Virtual Patient Simulation. In order to appraise the variations in response to the treatment, we have created virtual patients by assuming a correspondence across the parameter sets of the three models, i.e. all possibilities of parameter set combinations across three models. This has produced 56 virtual patients for leukocyte response and 70 virtual patients for MCV response. Figures 10A & 10B show three representative patient responses for leukocytes and RBCs, respectively. It is apparent from these figures that, for the same pattern of drug dosing, individual patients varied widely in their response. The comparison between the published results and model predicted values for the three models are summarized in Table 6. The results are statistically significant using t-test (for mean comparison) and F-test (for variance comparison) and thus show that the model prediction and clinical results are the same. The model predicted standard deviation (SD) for ΔMCV is significantly higher than the literature values as there were many dose adjustments in our study; whereas Decaux et al. study was conducted at stable dose.

Fig. 11 shows the profiles of standard deviation in leukocyte and MCV responses. The variations predicted by the models are physiologically anticipated. For leukocytes, the variation spikes at the start of the therapy as there are huge variation in response to the therapy. As the treatment progresses, the feedback mechanism gets underway and brings the leukocyte population back to the base line which is relatively constant for all the patients. This helps to subside the variation at the later stages of the treatment. In contrast, for ΔMCV, the variation at the onset of the treatment is small compared to that of the later stage. This is expected since the treatment response is based on the MCV change after four months of continuous therapy.

In order to validate the model's ability to predict future response, we estimated parameters for individual patients with $(N-3)$ original data points. With these parameters, the remaining data points were predicted and the SSEs are calculated for full and $(N-3)$ data points. For all patients, the differences in SSEs are less than 2% for 6-MP model, and less than 5% for leukocyte and MCV models.

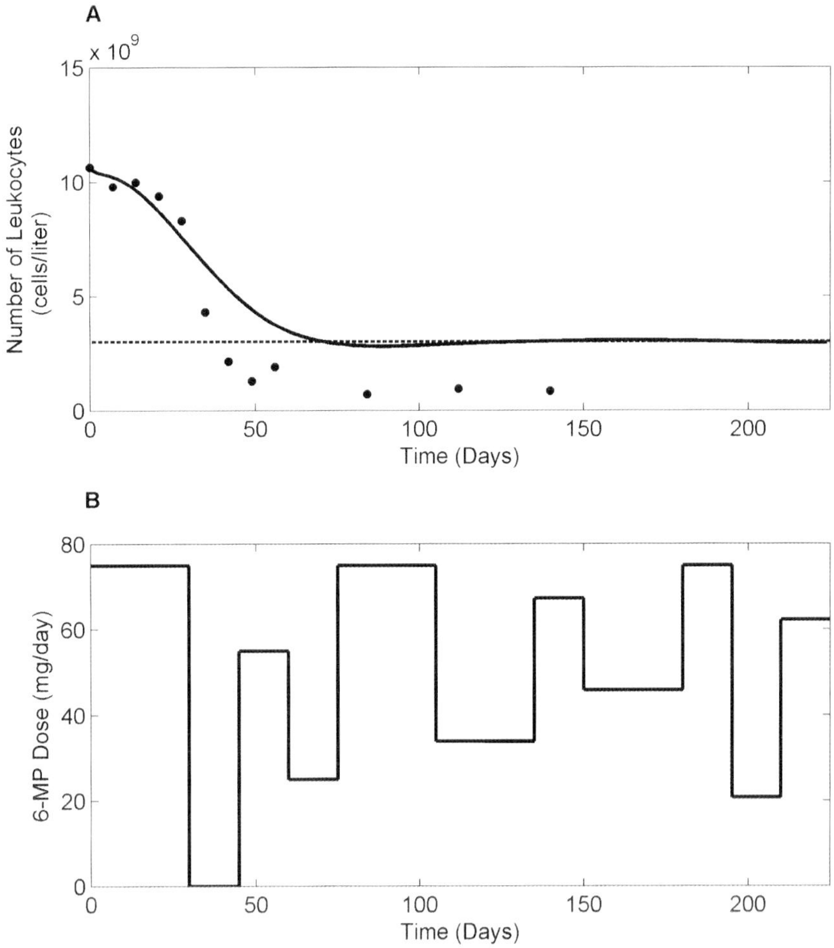

Figure 13. Optimal dosing based on leukocyte count as target. A. Evolution of leukocyte count in response to optimum 6-MP dosing. Dashed line represents critical leukocyte level and solid dots represent clinical data for an average patient. B. Optimum 6-MP dosing profile predicted by NMPC. The standard daily 6-MP dosing is 75 mg/day.

3.4. Dose Optimization

NMPC control strategy was applied to clinical scenarios using three different therapeutic targets: i) 6-TGN, ii) leukocyte count, iii) both leukocyte count and ΔMCV. All dosing calculations are based on 15 days sampling horizon with 75 days treatment window. Clinical studies propose a therapeutic window of 235–400 pmol/8×10^8 RBCs for 6-TGN concentration for effective management of both efficacy and toxicity [20,58]. Hence, we optimized 6-MP input with a target 6-TGN concentration of 300 pmol/8×10^8 RBCs. Fig. 12 shows the optimal 6-MP input together with resultant 6-TGN concentration for low and high TPMT activity patients. Dose inputs for different patients suggest that dosage varies mainly as a function of the 6-TGN conversion ratek_{pt}. From the figure, low TPMT patient required 31.82% less dose compared to the standard dose whereas, high TPMT patient needed 20.25% higher. Although 6-TGN concentration is not an ideal target, as there are further variability in pharmacodynamics, it proves useful in certain clinical conditions where efficacy measures are categorical and highly subjective. Fig. 13 shows the optimal dosage for current clinical practice where the dosing decisions are primarily driven by leukocyte count. Currently, patients are 'titrated' to a target leukocyte level of 3×10^9 cells/liter using a trial-and-error approach. However, with the help of NMPC, the oncoming leukopenia is predicted and dosing adjustments are made in a timely manner so that the leukocyte count remained close to the critical level for fighting infection. Fig. 14 shows the optimal 6-MP profile with simultaneous optimization of both therapeutic targets, i.e. maximizing efficacy without causing severe toxicity. The significance of these dose optimization should be viewed from the maximization of therapeutic benefits rather than the reduction of drug input as the cost of drug is only a fraction of the overall healthcare spending. Interestingly, cumulative optimal dosage for some of the patients are equivalent to their actual cumulative clinical dosage, but timely reduction or suspension of treatment predicted by NMPC has proven vital for forestalling life-threatening toxicity or compromising efficacy.

Discussion

We have presented here a modeling and individualized dosing approach to predict the treatment outcome and optimize the dosage during chemotherapy of childhood ALL. It should become transparent from this paper and other similar efforts [59,60] that mathematical models could in fact be an eminent substitute for empirical treatment adjustments. Mathematical models were developed and validated for 6-MP metabolism, MCV dynamics (a surrogate marker for treatment efficacy) and leukopenia (a dose-

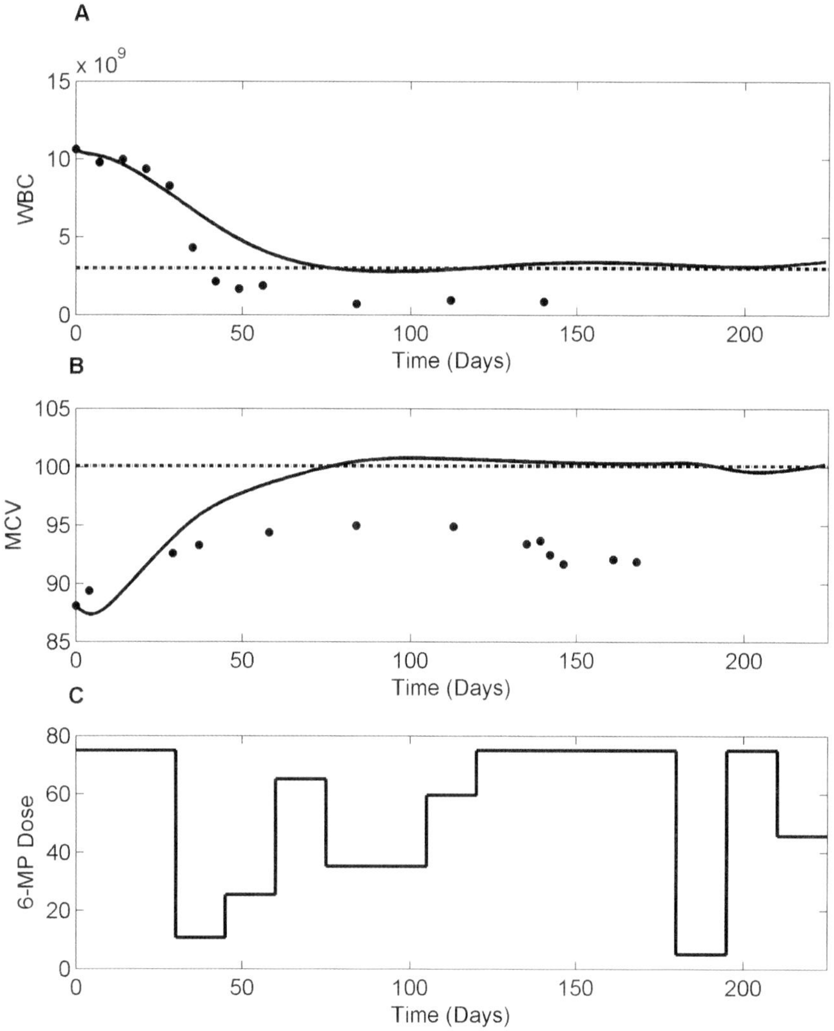

Figure 14. Optimal dosing based on leukocyte count and MCV as target. A. Evolution of leukocyte count in response to optimum 6-MP dosing. B. Evolution of ΔMCV response with optimum 6-MP dose. Dashed lines represent critical leukocyte and target MCV levels and solid dots represent clinical data for an average patient. C. Optimum 6-MP dosing profile predicted by NMPC. The standard daily 6-MP dosing is 75 mg/day.

limiting side-effect during treatment). The models were fitted to real patient data obtained from clinical settings. It is evident from the figures 8–10 that the models fit the data well with reduced parameter space. It is important to note that the data needed for this study did not come from the same source so we had to assume that the 6-TGN concentration was that of an average patient in leukopoiesis and MCV models. Some of the variations observed in the patient-specific parameters of leukopoiesis and MCV models may have arisen from the fact that the patients have performed significantly different from the average patient's 6-TGN concentration.

The implementation of the proposed approach in clinical practice can be envisioned as follows: When the new patient completes the induction treatment and is ready to start the 6-MP based consolidation and maintenance therapy, TPMT enzyme activity has to be measured. This actual TPMT enzyme activity will replace the estimate e in the 6-MP model and dictate the initial 6-MP dosing based on therapeutic window based NMPC. As the metabolite measurements and CBC become available, parameters can be progressively estimated from the most sensitive to the least sensitive in the reduced parameter group and the models are adapted to the new patient. Once a patient-specific model is obtained, future course of action can be predicted and optimized using NMPC.

It is a known fact that the global sensitivity indices for various parameters are not identical at different time points. Given the fact that only a few sensitive parameters are estimated to individualize the model, future experiments for new patients have to be designed carefully to estimate these parameters with precision. In this line, dynamic model-based design of experiment strategies can be exploited to estimate the optimum measurement points and other design variables. Efforts are in progress to determine the optimal experimental points for each of these models and compare the parameter precision and prediction capabilities of the models with a reduced data set.

It has been the aim of this work to address issues concerning the survival and well-being of children afflicted by ALL. The methodology, however, has import for treatment of other cancers or diseases as well where treatment involves the same or similar drugs. For instance, 6-MP is the major drug in treating autoimmune diseases and inflammatory bowel disease (IBD) whose incidence rate far exceeds that of ALL. Similar issues to that of ALL have been reported in IBD treatment with 6-MP. Hence the proposed techniques have the potential to be extended to a broader class of diseases and medical conditions. Admittedly, besides the technical solutions described here, there are other challenges to individualized treatment such as physiological, logistical, economical and societal in nature. When addressed together, it has the potential to reduce healthcare cost as well as improve the quality-of-life among patients by effectively tuning the therapy for each patient based upon their own response instead of the statistics of prior trials.

Acknowledgements

The authors would like to thank Dr.Hyun-Seob Song and Dr. Eric Sherer for their valuable suggestions and discussions.

Author Contributions

Conceived and designed the experiments: DJ AR DR. Performed the experiments: DJ AR DR. Analyzed the data: DJ AR RH. Contributed reagents/materials/analysis tools: TV. Wrote the paper: DJ AR RH TV DR. Clinical Consultation: TV RH.

References

1. Jemal A, Siegel R, Xu J, Ward E (2010) Cancer statistics, 2010. CA: a cancer journal for clinicians: caac. 20073v20071.
2. Pui CH, Evans WE (2006) Treatment of acute lymphoblastic leukemia. New England Journal of Medicine 354: 166–178.
3. Mody R, Li S, Dover DC, Sallan S, Leisenring W, et al. (2008) Twenty-five-year follow-up among survivors of childhood acute lymphoblastic leukemia: a report from the Childhood Cancer Survivor Study. Blood 111: 5515.
4. Harila MJ, Salo J, Lanning M, Vilkkumaa I, Harila Saari AH (2010) High health related quality of life among long term survivors of childhood acute lymphoblastic leukemia. Pediatric blood & cancer 55: 331–336.
5. Haupt R, Fears TR, Robison LL, Mills JL, Nicholson HS, et al. (1994) Educational attainment in long-term survivors of childhood acute lymphoblastic leukemia. JAMA: The Journal of the American Medical Association 272: 1427.
6. Tucker M, Meadows A, Boice Jr J, Stovall M, Oberlin O, et al. (1987) Leukemia after therapy with alkylating agents for childhood cancer. Journal of the National Cancer Institute 78: 459.
7. Dickerman JD (2007) The late effects of childhood cancer therapy. Pediatrics 119: 554.
8. Armstrong GT, Liu Q, Yasui Y, Neglia JP, Leisenring W, et al. (2009) Late mortality among 5-year survivors of childhood cancer: a summary from the Childhood Cancer Survivor Study. Journal of Clinical Oncology 27: 2328.
9. Sklar CA, Mertens AC, Mitby P, Occhiogrosso G, Qin J, et al. (2002) Risk of disease recurrence and second neoplasms in survivors of childhood cancer treated with growth hormone: a report from the Childhood Cancer Survivor Study. Journal of Clinical Endocrinology & Metabolism 87: 3136.
10. Cavé H, van der Werff ten Bosch J, Suciu S, Guidal C, Waterkeyn C, et al. (1998) Clinical significance of minimal residual disease in childhood acute lymphoblastic leukemia. New England Journal of Medicine 339: 591–598.
11. Childhood A (1996) Collaborative Group. Duration and intensity of maintenance chemotherapy in acute lymphoblastic leukaemia: overview of 42 trials involving 12,000 randomised children. Lancet 347: 1783–1788.
12. Tolar J, Bostrom B, Lee M, Sather H (2000) Oral 6-mercaptopurine protects against fatal relapses in childhood acute lymphoblastic leukemia: a report from the Children's Cancer Group study CCG 1922. Journal of Pediatric Hematology/Oncology 22: 378.
13. Schmiegelow K, Al-Modhwahi I, Andersen MK, Behrendtz M, Forestier E, et al. (2009) Methotrexate/6-mercaptopurine maintenance therapy influences the risk of a second malignant neoplasm after childhood acute lymphoblastic leukemia: results from the NOPHO ALL-92 study. Blood 113: 6077.
14. Schmiegelow K, Forestier E, Kristinsson J, Söderhäll S, Vettenranta K, et al. (2008) Thiopurine methyltransferase activity is related to the risk of relapse of childhood acute lymphoblastic leukemia: results from the NOPHO ALL-92 study. Leukemia 23: 557–564.
15. Aricó M, Baruchel A, Bertrand Y, Biondi A, Conter V, et al. (2005) The seventh international childhood acute lymphoblastic leukemia workshop report: Palermo, Italy, January 29–30, 2005. Leukemia 19: 1145–1152.
16. Chessells J, Harrison G, Lilleyman J, Bailey C, Richards S (1997) Continuing (maintenance) therapy in lymphoblastic leukaemia: lessons from MRC UKALL X. British journal of haematology 98: 945–951.
17. Evans WE, Relling MV, Rodman JH, Crom WR, Boyett JM, et al. (1998) Conventional compared with individualized chemotherapy for childhood acute lymphoblastic leukemia. New England Journal of Medicine 338: 499–505.
18. Lennard L (1992) The clinical pharmacology of 6-mercaptopurine. European journal of clinical pharmacology 43: 329–339.
19. Lilleyman J, Lennard L (1994) Mercaptopurine metabolism and risk of relapse in childhood lymphoblastic leukaemia. The Lancet 343: 1188–1190.
20. Gearry R, Barclay M, Roberts R, Harraway J, Zhang M, et al. (2005) Thiopurine methyltransferase and 6-thioguanine nucleotide measurement: early experience of use in clinical practice. Internal medicine journal 35: 580–585.
21. Lennard L, Lilleyman J, Van Loon J, Weinshilboum R (1990) Genetic variation in response to 6-mercaptopurine for childhood acute lymphoblastic leukaemia. The Lancet 336: 225–229.
22. Koren G, Ferrazini G, Sulh H, Langevin AM, Kapelushnik J, et al. (1990) Systemic exposure to mercaptopurine as a prognostic factor in acute lymphocytic leukemia in children. New England Journal of Medicine 323: 17–21.
23. Decaux G, Prospert F, Horsmans Y, Desager J (2000) Relationship between red cell mean corpuscular volume and 6-thioguanine nucleotides in patients treated with azathioprine* 1. Journal of Laboratory and Clinical Medicine 135: 256–262.
24. Thomas Jr CW, Lowry PW, Franklin CL, Weaver AL, Myhre GM, et al. (2003) Erythrocyte mean corpuscular volume as a surrogate marker for 6-thioguanine nucleotide concentration monitoring in patients with inflammatory bowel disease treated with azathioprine or 6-mercaptopurine. Inflammatory Bowel Diseases 9: 237–245.
25. Noble SL, Sherer E, Hannemann RE, Ramkrishna D, Vik T, et al. (2010) Using adaptive model predictive control to customize maintenance therapy chemotherapeutic dosing for childhood acute lymphoblastic leukemia. J Theor Biol 264: 990–1002.
26. Rombout F, Aarons L, Karlsson M, Man A, Mentre F, et al. (2004) Modelling and simulation in the development and use of anti-cancer agents: An underused tool? Journal of Pharmacokinetics and Pharmacodynamics 31: 419–440.
27. Nowak M, May RM (2000) Virus Dynamics: Mathematical Principles of Immunology and Virology: Mathematical Principles of Immunology and Virology: Oxford university press.
28. Doyle III F (2011) Dynamics and Control for the Artificial Pancreas. The Impact of Control Technology.
29. Deisboeck TS, Wang Z, Macklin P, Cristini V (2011) Multiscale cancer modeling. Annual review of biomedical engineering 13.
30. Stefanini MO, Qutub AA, Mac Gabhann F, Popel AS (2012) Computational models of VEGF-associated angiogenic processes in cancer. Mathematical Medicine and Biology 29: 85–94.
31. Kiran KL, Jayachandran D, Lakshminarayanan S (2009) Mathematical modelling of avascular tumour growth based on diffusion of nutrients and its validation. The Canadian Journal of Chemical Engineering 87: 732–740.
32. Bell B, Brockway G, Shuster J, Erdmann G, Sterikoff S, et al. (2004) A comparison of red blood cell thiopurine metabolites in children with acute lymphoblastic leukemia who received oral mercaptopurine twice daily or once daily: A Pediatric Oncology Group study (now The Children's Oncology Group). Pediatric blood & cancer 43: 105–109.
33. Brandalise SR, Pinheiro VR, Aguiar SS, Matsuda EI, Otubo R, et al. (2010) Benefits of the Intermittent Use of 6-Mercaptopurine and Methotrexate in Maintenance Treatment for Low-Risk Acute Lymphoblastic Leukemia in Children: Randomized Trial From the Brazilian Childhood Cooperative Group—Protocol ALL-99. Journal of Clinical Oncology 28: 1911.
34. Hawwa AF, Collier PS, Millership JS, McCarthy A, Dempsey S, et al. (2008) Population pharmacokinetic and pharmacogenetic analysis of 6-mercaptopurine in paediatric patients with acute lymphoblastic leukaemia. British journal of clinical pharmacology 66: 826–837.
35. Hawwa AF, Millership JS, Collier PS, Vandenbroeck K, McCarthy A, et al. (2008) Pharmacogenomic studies of the anticancer and immunosuppressive thiopurines mercaptopurine and azathioprine. British journal of clinical pharmacology 66: 517–528.
36. Lennard L, Hale J, Lilleyman J (1993) Red blood cell hypoxanthine phosphoribosyltransferase activity measured using 6-mercaptopurine as a substrate: a population study in children with acute lymphoblastic leukaemia. British journal of clinical pharmacology 36: 277.
37. Foley C, Mackey M (2009) Dynamic hematological disease: a review. Journal of mathematical biology 58: 285–322.
38. Testart-Paillet D, Girard P, You B, Freyer G, Pobel C, et al. (2007) Contribution of modelling chemotherapy-induced hematological toxicity for clinical practice. Critical reviews in oncology/hematology 63: 1–11.
39. Friberg LE, Henningsson A, Maas H, Nguyen L, Karlsson MO (2002) Model of chemotherapy-induced myelosuppression with parameter consistency across drugs. Journal of clinical oncology 20: 4713.
40. Hillman RS, Finch CA (1996) Red cell manual: FA Davis.
41. Terashi K, Oka M, Ohdo S, Furukubo T, Ikeda C, et al. (1999) Close association between clearance of recombinant human granulocyte colony-stimulating factor (G-CSF) and G-CSF receptor on neutrophils in cancer patients. Antimicrobial agents and chemotherapy 43: 21–24.
42. Bernard S, Belair J, Mackey MC (2003) Oscillations in cyclical neutropenia: New evidence based on mathematical modeling. Journal of theoretical biology 223: 283–298.

43. Mackey MC (1978) Unified hypothesis for the origin of aplastic anemia and periodic hematopoiesis. Blood 51: 941.
44. Adimy M, Crauste F, Ruan S (2005) A mathematical study of the hematopoiesis process with applications to chronic myelogenous leukemia. SIAM Journal on Applied Mathematics 65: 1328–1352.
45. Matlab U (1760) The MathWorks. Inc, Natick, MA 1992.
46. Saltelli A, Chan K, Scott EM (2000) Sensitivity analysis: Wiley New York.
47. Sobol IM (2001) Global sensitivity indices for nonlinear mathematical models and their Monte Carlo estimates. Mathematics and Computers in Simulation 55: 271–280.
48. Morari M (1999) Model predictive control: past, present and future* 1. Computers & Chemical Engineering 23: 667–682.
49. Campo PJ, Morari M (1987) Robust model predictive control. IEEE: pp. 1021–1026.
50. Hindorf U, Lindqvist M, Peterson C, Söderkvist P, Ström M, et al. (2006) Pharmacogenetics during standardised initiation of thiopurine treatment in inflammatory bowel disease. Gut 55: 1423.
51. Balis FM, Holcenberg JS, Poplack DG, Ge J, Sather HN, et al. (1998) Pharmacokinetics and pharmacodynamics of oral methotrexate and mercaptopurine in children with lower risk acute lymphoblastic leukemia: a joint children's cancer group and pediatric oncology branch study. Blood 92: 3569.
52. Krynetski EY, Krynetskaia NF, Yanishevski Y, Evans WE (1995) Methylation of mercaptopurine, thioguanine, and their nucleotide metabolites by heterologously expressed human thiopurine S-methyltransferase. Molecular pharmacology 47: 1141.
53. Innocenti F, Danesi R, Bocci G, Fogli S, Di Paolo A, et al. (1999) Metabolism of 6-mercaptopurine in the erythrocytes, liver, and kidney of rats during multiple-dose regimens. Cancer chemotherapy and pharmacology 43: 133–140.
54. Hindorf U, Peterson C, Almer S (2004) Assessment of thiopurine methyltransferase and metabolite formation during thiopurine therapy: results from a large Swedish patient population. Therapeutic drug monitoring 26: 673.
55. Fransson M (2007) Towards Individualized Drug Dosage-General Methods and Case Studies. Statistics 2009: 04–27.
56. Lohrmann HP, Schreml W (1982) Cytotoxic drugs and the granulopoietic system. Recent results in cancer research Fortschritte der Krebsforschung Progrès dans les recherches sur le cancer 81: 1.
57. Haurie C, Dale DC, Mackey MC (1998) Cyclical neutropenia and other periodic hematological disorders: a review of mechanisms and mathematical models. Blood 92: 2629–2640.
58. Armstrong L, Sharif JA, Galloway P, McGrogan P, Bishop J, et al. (2011) Evaluating the use of metabolite measurement in children receiving treatment with a thiopurine. Alimentary pharmacology & therapeutics 34: 1106–1114.
59. Kiran KL, Jayachandran D (2009) Multi-objective optimization of cancer immuno-chemotherapy. Springer: pp. 1337–1340.
60. Laínez JM, Blau G, Mockus L, Orçun S, Reklaitis GV (2011) Pharmacokinetic based design of individualized dosage regimens using a Bayesian approach. Industrial & Engineering Chemistry Research.

Gene Expression Profiling Identifies IRF4-Associated Molecular Signatures in Hematological Malignancies

Ling Wang[1], Zhi Q. Yao[1,2], Jonathan P. Moorman[1,2], Yanji Xu[3], Shunbin Ning[1]*

1 Center for Inflammation, Infectious Diseases and Immunity, Quillen College of Medicine, East Tennessee State University, Johnson City, Tennessee, United States of America, **2** HIV/HCV Program, James H. Quillen VA Medical Center, Johnson City, Tennessee, United States of America, **3** Shaun and Lilly International, LLC, Collierville, Tennessee, United States of America

Abstract

The lymphocyte-specific transcription factor Interferon (IFN) Regulatory Factor 4 (IRF4) is implicated in certain types of lymphoid and myeloid malignancies. However, the molecular mechanisms underlying its interactions with these malignancies are largely unknown. In this study, we have first profiled molecular signatures associated with IRF4 expression in associated cancers, by analyzing existing gene expression profiling datasets. Our results show that IRF4 is overexpressed in melanoma, in addition to previously reported contexts including leukemia, myeloma, and lymphoma, and that IRF4 is associated with a unique gene expression pattern in each context. A pool of important genes involved in B-cell development, oncogenesis, cell cycle regulation, and cell death including BATF, LIMD1, CFLAR, PIM2, and CCND2 are common signatures associated with IRF4 in non-Hodgkin B cell lymphomas. We confirmed the correlation of IRF4 with LIMD1 and CFLAR in a panel of cell lines derived from lymphomas. Moreover, we profiled the IRF4 transcriptome in the context of EBV latent infection, and confirmed several genes including IFI27, IFI44, GBP1, and ARHGAP18, as well as CFLAR as novel targets for IRF4. These results provide valuable information for understanding the IRF4 regulatory network, and improve our knowledge of the unique roles of IRF4 in different hematological malignancies.

Editor: Luwen Zhang, University of Nebraska - Lincoln, United States of America

Funding: This work is supported by the American Society of Hematology Scholar Award to SN (http://www.hematology.org/Awards/Career-Training/463.aspx). The funders had no role in study design, data collection and analysis, decision to publish, or preparation of the manuscript.

Competing Interests: YX is employed by a commercial company (Shaun and Lilly International, LLC, Collierville, TN 38017).

* Email: nings1@etsu.edu

Introduction

IRF4 is a lymphocyte-specific transcription factor, and its expression is confined to immune cells including B cells, macrophages, and CD11b+ DCs. IRF4 can be induced by various mitogenic stimuli which commonly activate NFκB for the activation of the IRF4 gene promoter [1]. As a transcription factor, IRF4 exerts its functions through regulation of its transcriptional targets involved in cell development, immune response, and oncogenesis. IRF4 is a quintessential 'context-dependent' transcription factor, and regulates distinct groups of targets in different contexts. Its DNA-binding specificity depends on lineage-specific transcriptional co-regulators. Many of these co-regulators have been identified, including two Ets family members PU.1 and SPIB, BATF, DEF6, STAT3, NFAT, FKBP52 and PGC-1α [2–12]. Ets and BATF are dominant co-regulators for IRF4 in B and T lymphocytes, respectively [6,9,11,13]. When interacting with one of the Ets family members, IRF4, like its closest family member IRF8, binds to a composite Ets/ISRE-consensus element (EICE) with the consensus sequence 5′-GGAANNGAAA-3′, that fuses the Ets-binding motif (5′-GGAA-3′) with the IRF-binding motif (5′-AANNGAAA-3′), or to the Ets/IRF-responsive element (EIRE) with the consensus sequence 5′-GGAAANNGAAA-3′, or to the IRF/Ets-consensus sequence (IECS) 5′-GAAANN(N)GGAA-3′. When IRF4 interacts with BATF that belongs to the AP1/ATF superfamily of transcription factors, the complex IRF4-BATF binds to a composite DNA element called AICE (TGANTCA/GAAA) [14,15].

Increasing evidence has implicated IRF4 in hematological malignancies. IRF4 overexpression is a hallmark of the activated B-cell-like (ABC) type of diffuse large B-cell lymphoma (DLBCL) and multiple myeloma (MM) [3,13], and is also overexpressed in almost 100% cases of classical Hodgkin lymphoma (cHL), plasma cell myeloma and primary effusion lymphoma (PEL) [16]. Interestingly, high levels of IRF4 protein exist in Epstein-Barr virus (EBV)-transformed cells and associated B-cell lymphomas with Type 3 latency [17–20], as well as in Human T-cell Leukemia Virus-1 (HTLV1)-infected cell lines and associated Adult T-cell Leukemia (ATL) [21–25]. Chromosomal translocation and genetic mutation of IRF4 have been identified in MM, peripheral T-cell lymphomas [26], and Chronic Lymphocytic Leukemia (CLL) [27]. In clinical practice, IRF4 serves as an important prognostic and diagnostic marker for certain types of hematological malignancies [28–30]. These lines of evidence highlight the importance of IRF4 in hematological malignancies. However, only very limited transcriptional targets have been identified for IRF4 in these malignancies, and the role of IRF4 in tumorigenesis remains to be elucidated.

In this study, we aim to profile IRF4-associated unique molecular signatures in different types of hematological malignancies, by analyzing existing gene expression profile databases obtained from clinical samples. Results show that IRF4 is overexpressed in melanoma, in addition to previously reported myeoloma, lymphoma, and leukemia, and that IRF4 is associated with a unique gene expression pattern in each of these settings. Some of these genes are known IRF4 transcriptional targets, whereas some others may represent a new group of IRF4 targets. We have verified LIMD1 and CFLAR as two novel genes whose expression is correlated with IRF4 in non-Hodgkin lymphomas, and shown that CFLAR is likely an IRF4 target. Moreover, we have profiled the IRF4 transcriptome in EBV latency by using Microarray analysis and further confirmed a panel of genes including IFI27, IFI44, GBP1, and ARHGAP18 as novel IRF4 targets.

Materials and Methods

Datasets and Oncomine Bioinformatics

All datasets selected for this study are available on Oncomine website (www.oncomine.org). These datasets were log-transformed, median centered per array, and standard deviation normalized to one per array. Bioinformatic analysis was performed at Oncomine website, with the default parameters on the site for IRF4 co-expression analysis (threshold by p value: 10^{-4}, fold change: 2, and gene rank: top 10%).

GEO Bioinformatics

Raw data from existing Gene Expression Omnibus (GEO) datasets were downloaded. The intensity values were extracted using GeneSpring GX 12.5 software from Agilent and scaled and Quantile normalized. Values were then log transformed (base 2) to the median of all samples on the R/Bioconductor package. Two probes assigned to IRF4 gene, 204562_at and 216986_s_at, were used to divide the samples into IRF4+ and IRF4− groups. Probe 216987_at was not used as it has small variance and low expression value (mean value: 5.527 and variance 0.042). Differentially expressed genes between the two groups (IRF4+ and IRF4−) were identified using limma R package from Bioconductor with a simple two group design matrix (cut-off $p \leq 0.05$ and fold change ≥ 1.5). Limma is a popular library for analysis of gene expression microarray data, it uses linear model to accommodate complicated experimental design and Empirical Bayesian to provide stable results for small datasets. Benjamin-Hochberg was used for multiple testing correction.

Cell Lines

These cell lines used in this study are well established B cell lines and have been worldwide used for EBV research for many years [31–34]. Akata, Sav I, Sav III, JiJoye, and P3HR1 are Burkitt's lymphoma cell lines which were derived from patients. DG75 is an EBV-negative B cell line. IB4 and LCL.Jul are lymphoblastic cell lines *in vitro* transformed with EBV. All B cell lines are cultured in RPMI1640 medium plus 10% FBS and antibiotics.

Plasmids, Reagents and Antibodies

The shIRF4 and retrovirus-mediated transfection and selection of stable transfectants were described in our previous publication [35]. Anti-LIMD1 clone H-4 (Santa Cruz), anti-FLIPs clone G-11 (Santa Cruz), anti-LMP1 CS1–4 (Dako), anti-IRF4 H140 (Santa Cruz), and anti-GAPDH (Sigma) were used for Western blotting.

RNA Isolation, Microarray Analysis and Real-time PCR

Total RNAs from JiJoye and IB4 cell lines stably expressing shIRF4 or control were isolated using RNeasy mini kit (Qiagen) according to the manufacturer's protocols. The eluted RNA was subjected to reverse transcriptase reactions, which were performed with the use of GoScript RT kit (Promega) following the manufacturer's instructions. cDNAs were subjected to MOgene company (Saint Louis, MO) for Microarray analysis, with Agilent HD 4×44 k format (G4845F 026652) chips. A cross-labeling duplicate, i.e. Cy5-labeled cDNA chip for shCtl/Cy3-labeled cDNA chip for shIRF4 and Cy3-labeled chip for shCtl/Cy5-labeled chip for shIRF4, were performed for each cell line. Genes were selected with 2-fold changes as threshold.

Selected genes were confirmed by real-time PCR, as described in our previous publication [35], with specific primers. IFI27 forward: 5′-TGGCCAGGATTGCTACAGTTG-3′, and reverse: 5′-TATGGAGGACGAGGCGATTC-3′, GBP1 forward: 5′-TGGAACGTGTGAAAGCTGAG-3′, and reverse: 5′-TGACAGGAAGGCTCTGGTCT-3′, IFI44 forward: 5′- TACCAGTTTAATCCCATGGAATCA-3′, and reverse: 5′- CAAATACAAATGCCACACAATGAA-3′, and ARHGAP18 forward: 5′-AAGAGTACAAATGATGCTGACG-3′ and reverse: 5′-CCTGGCAAGTACATCACTGG-3′.

Results

IRF4 Expression Levels in Different Cancers

We initially checked the expression levels of IRF4 in different cancer cell lines. To this end, the gene expression data, obtained from 917 cell lines in a previous study [36], was analyzed at Oncomine (http://www.oncomine.org). As shown in Fig. 1A, in 18 selected cancer types, the expression level of IRF4 was the highest in myeloma, followed by lymphoma, melanoma and leukemia. Overexpression of IRF4 has been well documented in all these cancers but only a few publications have reported the association between IRF4 genetic variants or abnormal expression and skin cancer [29,37–40]. Our results have confirmed the overexpression of IRF4 in melanoma and supported the claim that IRF4 may play an important role in the development of this cancer.

Next, we analyzed the gene expression profiles for IRF4 expression in different types of B cell lymphomas with a total of 336 samples which include 36 cancer cell lines (10.7%), 125 experimentally manipulated B cell lines (37.2%), and 25 normal B cell samples (7.4%) [41]. As shown in Fig. 1B, amongst the analyzed lymphoma types, PEL has the highest level of IRF4. PEL, also known as AIDS-associated body cavity-based lymphoma (BCBL), is a malignant B cell lymphoma (non-Hodgkin lymphoma). PELs are 100% positive for Kaposi sarcoma herpesvirus (KSHV), and often contain EBV as well. Among 3 types of DLBCL (Activated, Germinal center, and Type 3), analysis results from 414 samples reveal that activated DLBCL has the highest expression level of IRF4 (Fig. 1, C) [42].

In regard to myeloma, analysis results from 304 multiple myeloma patient samples reveal that there is no significant difference of IRF4 expression levels among different stages, including smoldering (Fig. 1, D) [43].

Together, these results indicate that IRF4 is overexpressed in specific hematological malignancies including myeloma, lymphoma, and leukemia, and also in melanoma.

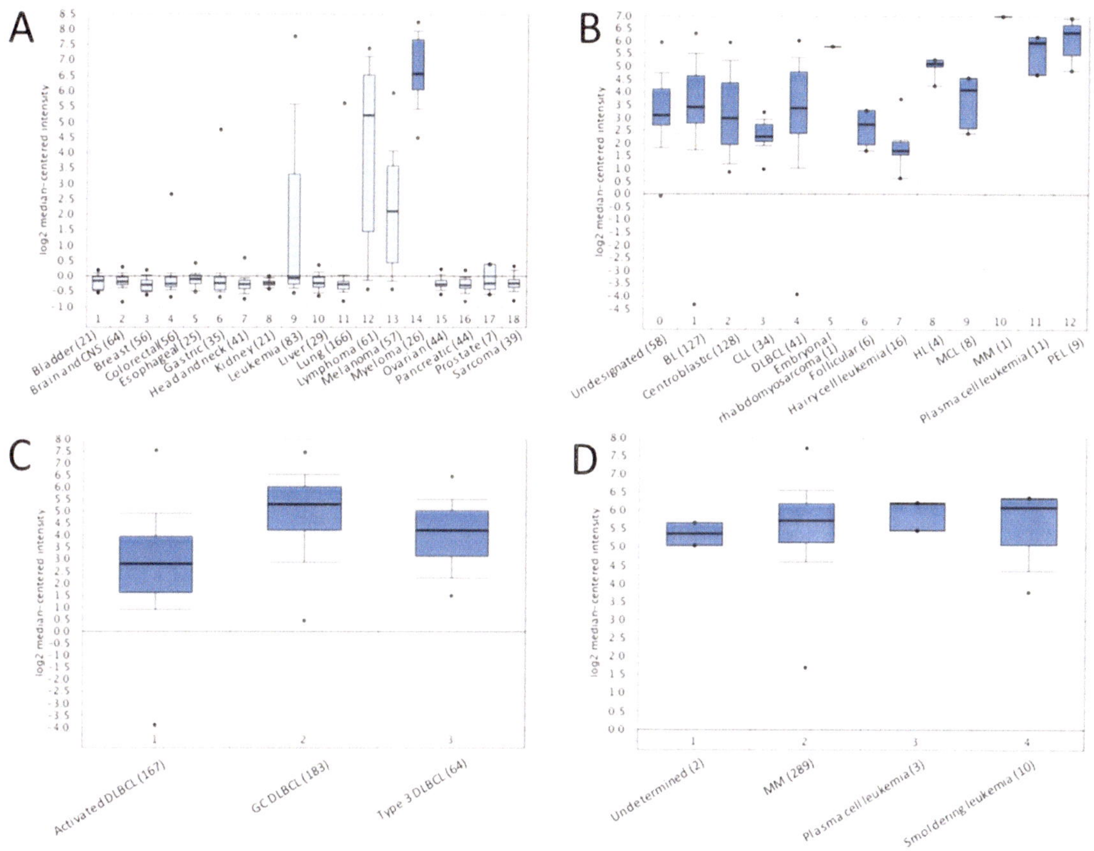

Figure 1. Differential expression of IRF4 in different cancer contexts. A. IRF4 is differentially expressed in a panel of cancer cell lines [36]. 1. Bladder cancer (21 samples); 2. Brain and CNS cancers (64 samples); 3. Breast cancer (56 samples); 4. Colorectal cancer (56 samples); 5. Esophageal cancer (25 samples); 6. Gastric cancer (35 samples); 7. Head and neck cancer (41 samples); 8. Kidney cancer (21 samples); 9. Leukemia (83 samples); 10. Liver cancer (29 samples); 11. Lung cancer (166 samples); 12. Lymphoma (61 samples); 13. Melanoma (57 samples); 14. Myeloma (26 samples); 15. Ovarian cancer (44 samples); 16. Pancreatic cancer (44 samples); 17. Prostate cancer (7 samples). 18. Sarcoma (39 samples). **B.** Differential expression of IRF4 in lymphomas [41]. 0. Undesignated (58 samples); 1. Burkitt's lymphoma (127 samples); 2. Centroblastic lymphoma (28 samples); 3. Chronic lymphocytic leukemia (34 samples); 4. DLBCL (41 samples); 5. Embryonal rhabdomyosarcoma (1 sample); 6. Follicular lymphoma (6 samples); 7. Hairy cell leukemia (16 samples); 8. Hodgkin lymphoma (4 samples); 9. Mantle cell lymphoma (8 samples); 10. Multiple myeloma (1 sample); 11. Plasma cell leukemia (11 samples); 12. Primary effusion lymphoma (9 samples). **C.** Differential expression of IRF4 in different DLBCLs [42]. 1. Activated B cell-like DLBCL (167 samples); 2. Germinal center B cell-like DLBCL (183 samples); 3. Type 3 DLBCL (64 samples). **D.** Differential expression of IRF4 in myeloma [43]. 1. Monoclonal gammopathy of undetermined significance (2 samples). 2. Multiple myeloma (289 samples); 3. Plasma cell leukemia (3 samples); 4. Smoldering leukemia (10 samples).

Molecular Signatures Associated with IRF4 in Different Cancers

Since IRF4 is a "context-dependent" factor, it is necessary to analyze the patterns of gene expression associated with IRF4 in individual cancer types.

First, a pool of gene expression profile datasets obtained from different types of hematological malignancies were analyzed for genes whose expression is correlated with IRF4 using the Oncomine website. As to multiple myeloma, the dataset including 124 clinical samples and 7 cell lines (5.3%) was selected for analysis [44], with default parameters (p value: 10^{-4}, fold change: 2, and gene rank: top 10%). Top 20 genes/probes correlating with IRF4 including ATXN1, HEXB, PSEN2, CASP10, are shown in Fig. 2A, and top 60 genes are shown in Table S1.

For leukemia, we analyzed the dataset which includes 288 B- and T-cell acute lymphoblastic leukemia samples [45]. As shown in Fig. 2B, IRF4 is frequently expressed in B-cell ALL, but not in T-cell ALL. Top 20 genes/probes correlating with IRF4 include QRSL1, FAM3C, KIAA0802, WASF1, BLK, ELL3, etc. Top 60 genes are shown in Table S1.

For melanoma, we analyzed the dataset which includes 28 cutaneous melanoma patient samples [46]. Top 20 genes/probes correlated with IRF4 are shown in Fig. 2C, and top 60 genes/probes are shown in Table S1. Among these genes, the transcription factor MITF, the pigmentation enzyme TYR, and MLANA and GPR143 that are involved in melanosome biogenesis, are important players in melanoma. MITF is known to cooperate with IRF4 in regulation of the expression of TYR in melanocytes [38]. Similar results were obtained from another dataset (data not shown) [47].

To analyze the molecular signature for IRF4 in cHL, the dataset including 64 Hodgkin's lymphoma, 3 T-cell/histiocyte-rich B-cell lymphoma, 3 Hodgkin's lymphoma cell lines, and 3 lymphadenitis samples (60 cHL samples in total), was selected for analysis [48]. As shown in Fig. 2D, overexpression of IRF4 in cHL is not dependent on EBV infection. Top 20 genes/probes include SLC26A3, ZNF674, TOX3, FUT9, etc. Top 60 genes/probes are shown in Table S1.

As to non-Hodgkin's lymphoma DLBCL, we analyzed a dataset comprising 414 DLBCL samples [42]. Results indicate that IRF4

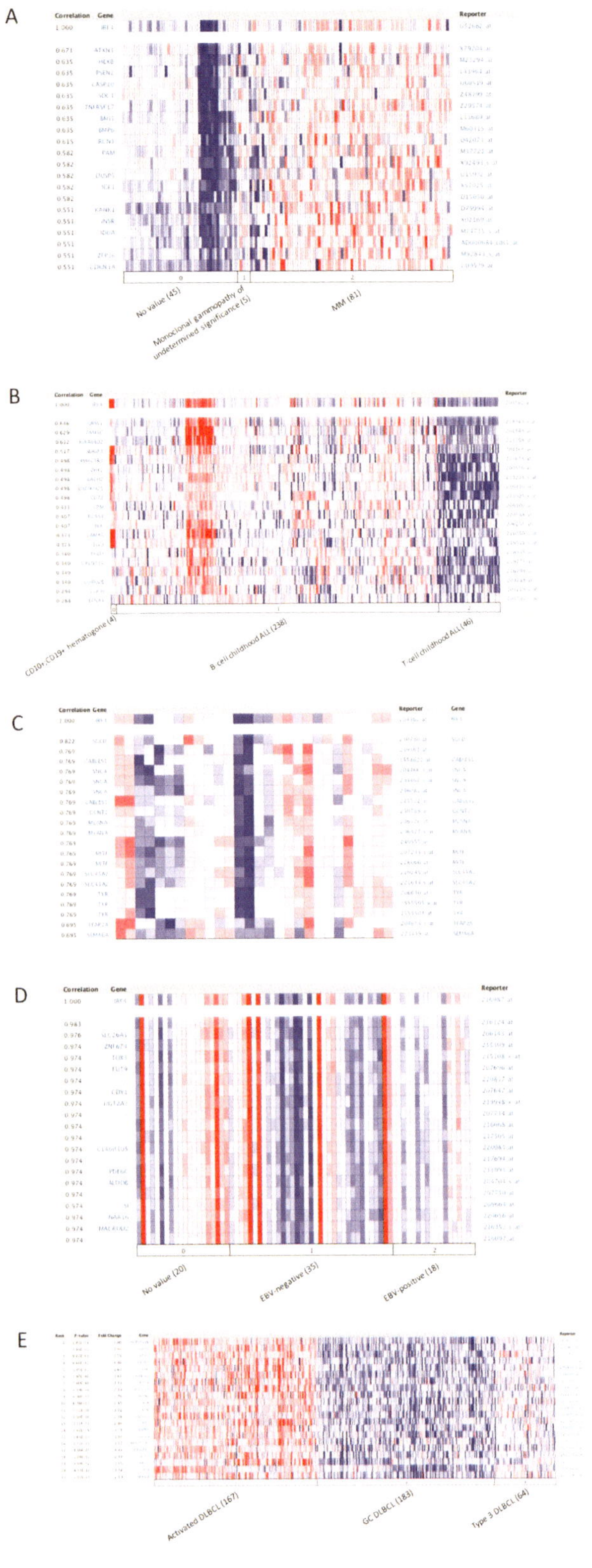

Figure 2. Molecular signature associated with IRF4 in hematological malignancies. A. IRF4-associated gene expression pattern in myeloma. The dataset includes 131 samples [44]. Analysis was performed with default parameters (p value: 10^{-4}, fold change: 2, and gene rank: top 10%). 0. No value (45 samples); 1. Monoclonal gammopathy of undetermined significance (5 samples); 2. Multiple myeloma (81 samples including 74 clinical samples and 7 cell lines). **B.** IRF4-associated gene expression pattern in leukemia. The dataset includes 288 B- and T-cell acute lymphoblastic leukemia samples [45]. 0. CD10+;CD19+ hematogone (4 samples); 1. B-Cell childhood acute lymphoblastic leukemia (238 samples); 2. T-cell childhood acute lymphoblastic leukemia (46 samples). **C**. IRF4-associated gene expression pattern in melanoma. The dataset includes 28 cutaneous melanoma patient samples [46]. **D**. IRF4-associated gene expression pattern in classic Hodgkin lymphoma. The dataset includes 64 Hodgkin's lymphoma, 3 T-cell/histiocyte-rich B-cell lymphoma, 3 Hodgkin's lymphoma cell lines, and 3 lymphadenitis samples (60 cHL samples in total) [48]. 0. No value (20 samples); 1. EBV negative (35 samples); 2. EBV positive (18 samples). **E**. The gene expression pattern correlated with IRF4 in non-Hodgkin lymphoma DLBCL. The dataset comprises 414 DLBCL samples [42]. 1. Activated B cell-like DLBCL (167 samples); 2. Germinal center B cell-like DLBCL (183 samples); 3. Type 3 DLBCL (64 samples).

is expressed at a high level in activated DLBCL, along with a panel of other genes including BATF, LIMD1, CFLAR, PIM2, CCND2, IL16, miR-155, etc (Fig. 2, E and Table S1). BATF is an AP1-like transcription factor known to cooperate with IRF4 in gene transcription in B, T, and dendritic cells [6,8,9,11]. Interestingly, we have previously identified the miR-155-encoding gene BIC as a target for IRF4 in viral cancer cells [35]. However, IRF4 is expressed at a lower level in Type 3 DLBCL, and at the least level in germinal center DLBCL (Fig. 2, E). Similar results were obtained with another dataset which comprises 271 DLBCL samples (data not shown) [49].

We also chose the GEO dataset GSE4475 which includes 220 BL and DLBCL samples [50], and performed differential expression and gene set enrichment analyses, using Limma R package and MSigDB. Our results show that, similar to other datasets from Oncomine analysis, BATF, PIM2, LIMD1, CFLAR, and CCND2, along with a panel of other genes such as STAT3, CD44, and IL16, are correlated with IRF4. Expression of some genes such as SSBP2 and MYBL1 is inversely correlated with IRF4 (Fig. 3). Results with cut-off p value<0.01 and fold change ≥ 2 are shown in Fig. 3 and Table S2. CD44 is known to be targeted by IRF4 in ABC DLBCL but not in MM [51]. Similar results were obtained from the GEO datasets GSE4732 which includes 303 Burkitt's and B-cell lymphoma samples [52], and GSE38885 which includes 65 PTLD samples (data not shown).

Taken together, we concluded that IRF4 is associated with unique molecular signatures in myeloma, leukemia, myeloma, Hodgkin's and non-Hodgkin's lymphomas, and that common molecular signatures associated with IRF4 in different types of non-Hodgkin's lymphomas include BATF, LIMD1, CFLAR, PIM2, and CCND2, amongst others.

Verification of the Correlation of IRF4 with LIMD1 and CFLAR in EBV-associated B-cell Lymphoma

The LIMD1 (LIM domain-containing protein 1) gene is located in a chromosomal region which undergoes frequent loss of heterozygosity in many solid tumors [53]. Expression of LIMD1 is absent or decreased in many cancers including breast cancer, lung carcinoma and blood cancers [53–55]. LIMD1 is an adapter protein that is involved in the assembly of numerous protein complexes such as Rb [56] and TRAF6, and participates in several cellular processes such as repression of gene transcription, cell-cell adhesion, cell differentiation, proliferation and migration. LIMD1 also positively regulates microRNA (miRNA)-mediated gene silencing by binding to the core proteins of the microRNA induced silencing complex (miRISC) such as Ago1/2 [57].

To verify the correlation between IRF4 and LIMD1, a panel of EBV-negative and -positive B cell lines derived from B lymphomas or transformed with EBV *in vitro* were subjected to immunoblotting analysis with IRF4- and LIMD1-specific antibodies. As shown

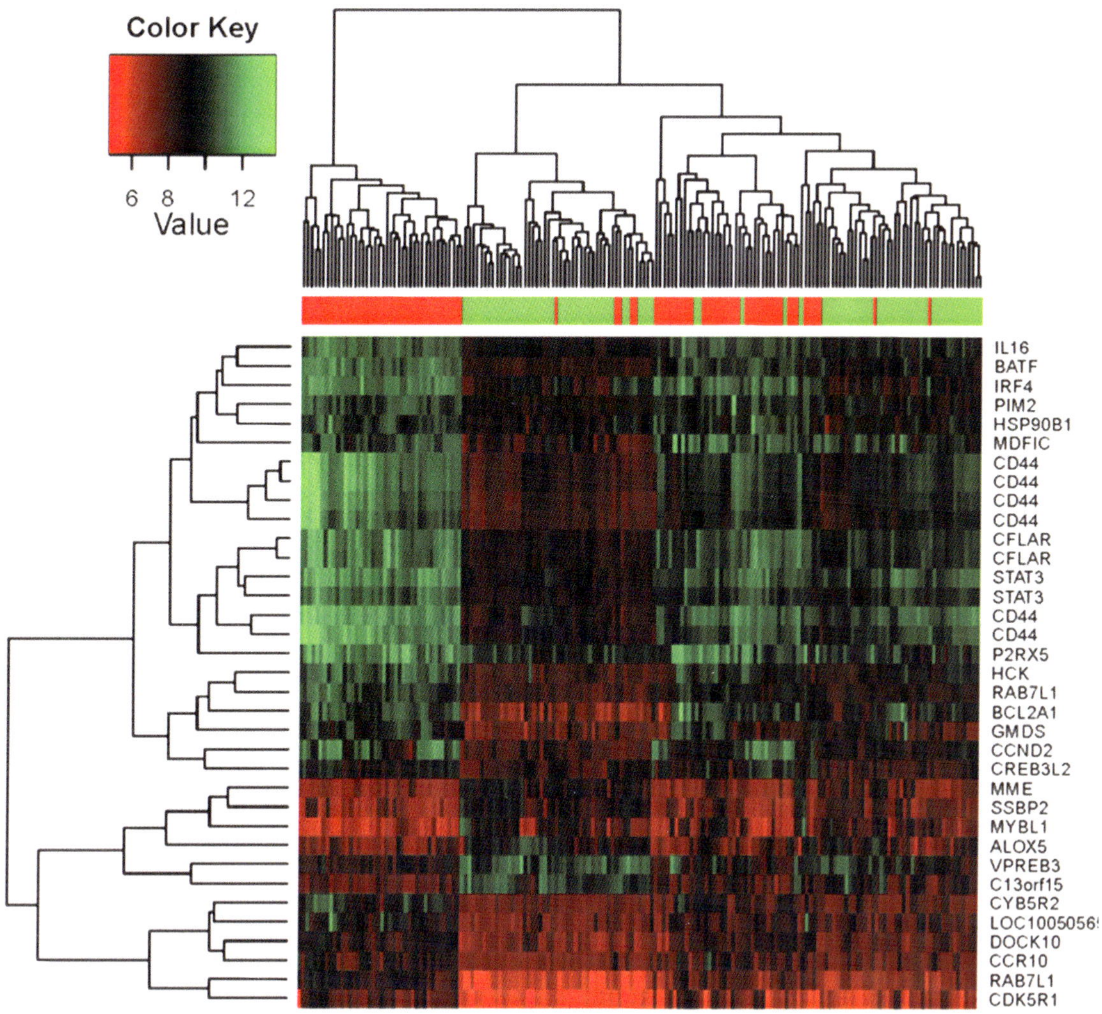

Figure 3. IRF4-associated gene expression pattern in lymphomas. The GEO dataset GSE4475 which includes 220 BL and DLBCL samples [50], was subjected to bioinformatic analysis for differential gene expression pattern correlated with IRF4 and gene set enrichment, as detailed in Materials and Methods. The heat map shows results from analysis with cut-off p value<0.01 and fold change≥2.

in Fig. 4A, LIMD1 is expressed at high levels in EBV latency 3, in which both IRF4 and LMP1 are also expressed at high levels. However, in EBV-negative and type I latency, LIMD1 is not detectable.

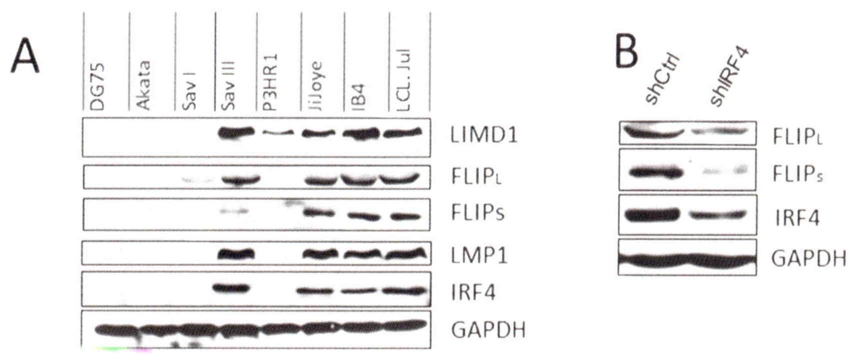

Figure 4. Verification of the correlation of IRF4 with LIMD1 and CFLAR. A. A panel of EBV negative and -positive B cell lines were subjected for immunoblotting analysis for IRF4, LIMD1, CFLAR (c-Flip), and LMP1 expression, with specific antibodies. DG75: EBV-negative. Akata and SavI: EBV-positive with Type I latency. SavIII, P3HR1, and JiJoye were derived from EBV+ Burkitt's lymphomas. IB4 and LCL.Jul are LCLs established in vitro by EBV transformation. **B**. Knockdown of IRF4 in JiJoye cells downregulates the c-Flip protein level in JiJoye cells.

CFLAR encodes c-FLIP, a master inhibitor of Fas/TRAIL/TNFα-induced apoptosis [58]. Resistance to Fas/TRAIL-mediated apoptosis is a common mechanism used by tumors to evade the immune system [59]. Similar to LIMD1, CFLAR expression is high in type 3 latency, but was not detected in EBV-negative B cells and EBV type I latency (Fig. 4, A). Furthermore, depletion of IRF4 in JiJoye cells decreases endogenous CFLAR protein level (Fig. 4, B). However, depletion of IRF4 did not affect the protein level of LIMD1 (data not shown), suggesting that LIMD1 and IRF4 are both upregulated by a common transcription factor rather than LIMD1 is a direct target for IRF4.

These results confirm that IRF4 is correlated with LIMD1 and CFLAR in B lymphomas, and strongly suggest that CFLAR is a transcriptional target for IRF4.

IRF4 Transcriptome in EBV Latency

IRF4 is overexpressed in EBV type 3 latency [17–20]. To our knowledge, BIC/miR-155 and IRF5 are the only two IRF4 targets identified in the context of EBV infection [35,60]. To better understand the role of IRF4 in EBV latency and oncogenesis, we performed microarray analysis to profile the IRF4 transcriptome in EBV latency. Endogenous IRF4 expression in JiJoye and IB4 cells was depleted with shIRF4 as described in our previous work [35]. Knockdown efficiency of IRF4 is shown in Fig. 5, A. Total RNAs were subjected to microarray analysis. Results show that 434 genes were upregulated (>2.0 fold) and 428 were downregulated (<2.0 fold) in JiJoye cells stably expressing shIRF4 compared to cells expressing scramble control shRNA, and 324 were upregulated (>2.0 fold) and 198 were downregulated (<2.0 fold) in IB4 cells after IRF4 depletion (Fig. 5, B and Table S3).

Because these two cell lines have different genetic background (JiJoye is a BL cell line established from a BL patient and IB4 is a LCL cell line by in vitro transformation of umbilical cord B-lymphocytes with EBV), only a small portion (about 10%) of overlapping genes were identified between these two cell lines, with 54 in the upregulated gene group and 14 in the downregulated gene group (Fig. 5, B). This observation is consistent with the fact that IRF4 is a quintessential "context-dependent" factor which regulates distinct groups of targets in different contexts [5,16].

Among the overlapping target genes between JiJoye and IB4, we confirmed the regulation of IFI27, IFI44, IFIT1, GBP1, CD88, CXCL10, and ARHGAP18 by IRF4 using real-time PCR with specific primers. IFI27, IFI44, IFIT1, CXCL10 and GBP1 are known IFN-stimulated genes (ISGs). As shown in Fig. 5C, real-time PCR results confirmed that IFI27, IFI44 and GBP1 expression levels are significantly elevated after IRF4 depletion, and ARHGAP18 level is significantly decreased (data for IFIT1, CD88 and CXCL10 are not shown). IFI27 is a mitochondrial protein involved in IFN-induced apoptosis [61,62]. IFI44 has anti-proliferative activity and is known to be associated with HCV infection [63]. GBP1 acts as a tumor suppressor in colorectal cancer cells [64], and also plays a role in chronic active EBV infection and interacts with HCV NS5B [65]. ARHGAP18 a Rho GTPase-activating protein for RhoA and modulates cell shape, spreading, and motility [66].

Of note, CFLAR is also downregulated by shIRF4 in JiJoye cells (1.32 fold) in the microarray results, consistent with the results from GEO bioinformatics that IRF4 correlates with CFLAR in non-Hodgkin's lymphomas and depletion of IRF4 downregulated CFLAR protein level in EBV+ lymphoma cells (Fig. 4). These data indicate that CFLAR is also a transcriptional target for IRF4. In fact, CFLAR is a known target for IRF8 [67], the closest member to IRF4 in the IRF family.

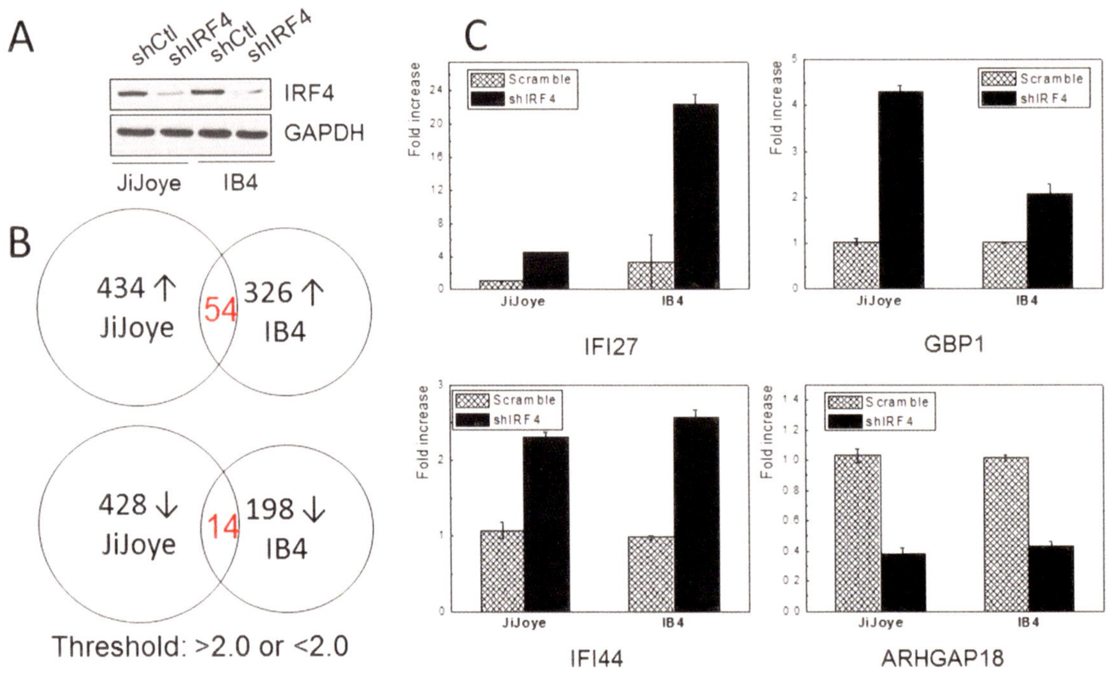

Figure 5. IRF4 transcriptome in EBV latency. A. Expression of endogenous IRF4 in JiJoye (EBV+ Burkitt's lymphoma cell line) and IB4 (EBV+ LCL) cell lines were depleted by retrovirus-mediated transfection of shIRF4 (or control)-expressing retrovirus. Stable transfectants were selected with hygromycin and shIRF4 (or control) was induced by 1 μg/ml doxycycline. **B**. Total RNAs were extracted and subjected for Microarray analysis. Genes with >2.0 and <2.0 fold changes were selected. **C**. Real-time PCR confirmation of IRF4 transcriptional targets IFI27, GBP1, IFI44, and ARHGAP18.

Discussion

In this study, we have systematically profiled the molecular signatures associated with IRF4 expression in a subset of hematological malignancies including melanoma in which IRF4 is overexpressed. In addition, we have identified a panel of novel transcriptional targets including IFI27, IFI44, GBP1, CFLAR and ARHGAP18 for IRF4 in lymphomas.

Gene expression profiling datasets are available online and are convenient for identification of differential expression of a given gene and for related high throughput comparison among different cancers or under different conditions of treatments. Since a large portion of these datasets were derived from clinical patient samples, they provide an important resource which complements *in vitro* studies. In our analyses, the IRF4-associated molecular signatures include a subset of IRF4 transcriptional targets such as CFLAR verified in this study. Other signature genes should be co-regulated with IRF4 by upstream transcription factors such as NFκB. In future pursuits, we will combine with other strategies including cell culture systems to identify IRF4-regulated networks in individual cancer contexts.

We and others have shown that IRF4 promotes proliferation of EBV-transformed cells and IRF4 deficiency results in death of cells derived from different hematological malignancies [17,28,35], indicating that IRF4 plays a non-redundant role in tumorigenesis of hematological malignancies. Expression of IRF4 is associated with resistance to treatment of viral cancers with IFN/AZT, and AZT specifically induces apoptosis as well as initiates the viral lytic program in Type I EBV+ Burkitt's lymphomas [21]. However, the mechanism of action of IRF4 accounting for this important clinical observation is unclear. Further study on the interaction between IRF4 and the IFN-inducible genes including IFI27 and IFI44 may disclose the mechanism through which IRF4 confers resistance to IFN treatment of vial cancers by regulating their expression.

Consistent with our finding that CFLAR is a transcriptional target for IRF4, CFLAR has been shown to be targeted by IRF8, the closest family member of IRF4 [67]. Correspondingly, we have identified a potential IRF4/8-binding site EICE in the CFLAR gene promoter (not shown). We will verify if this EICE is functional and responsible for IRF4/8 regulation. Targeting CFLAR by IRF4 may implicate a role for IRF4 in Fas/TRAIL/TNFα-induced apoptosis in non-Hodgkin lymphomas.

The implication of IRF4 in hematological malignancies is increasingly recognized. However, most evidence has emerged from clinical observations. Recent efforts have focused on the identification of "context-dependent" co-factors for IRF4 [2–11]. To date, only limited targets including miR-155 [35], IRF5 [60], Blimp1, CCNB1, BCL6, CDK6, Myc, and several others have been identified as IRF4 targets in cancers [7,25,28,68]. Clearly, identification of IRF4-specific gene regulation networks will improve our understanding of its functional roles in distinct cancer contexts. Our following work will aim to disclose the roles of the novel IRF4 targets identified in our study in EBV oncogenesis.

In addition to the downstream gene regulatory networks, our recent observation that IRF4 is activated through Src-mediated tyrosine phosphorylation in EBV-associated lymphomas [69], represents another important topic and a novel challenge for studying the interaction of IRF4 with hematological malignancies. We are encouraged to identify lymphocyte-specific signaling pathways leading to IRF4 activation, which potentially opens new avenues for targeting IRF4 networks for future clinical treatments.

Supporting Information

Table S1 IRF4-associated molecular signatures in different hematological malignancies.

Table S2 Bioinformatic analysis of GEO dataset GSE4475 for IRF4-assoicated molecular signatures in B cell lymphoma.

Table S3 Microarray analysis for IRF4 transcriptome in EBV latently infected B lymphocytes.

Acknowledgments

This publication is the result of work supported with resources and the use of facilities at the James H. Quillen Veterans Affairs Medical Center. The contents in this publication do not represent the views of the Department of Veterans Affairs or the United States Government.

Author Contributions

Conceived and designed the experiments: LW SN. Performed the experiments: LW YX SN. Analyzed the data: SN. Contributed reagents/materials/analysis tools: YX SN. Contributed to the writing of the manuscript: ZY JM SN.

References

1. Gualco G, Weiss LM, Bacchi CE (2010) MUM1/IRF4: A review. Appl Immunohistochem Mol Morphol 18: 301–310.
2. Eisenbeis CF, Singh H, Storb U (1995) Pip, a novel IRF family member, is a lymphoid-specific, PU.1-dependent transcriptional activator. Genes Dev 9: 1377–1387.
3. Shaffer AL, Emre NC, Romesser PB, Staudt LM (2009) IRF4: immunity. malignancy! therapy? Clin Cancer Res 15: 2954–2961.
4. Mamane Y, Sharma S, Petropoulos L, Lin R, Hiscott J (2000) Posttranslational regulation of IRF-4 activity by the immunophilin FKBP52. Immunity 12: 129–140.
5. Biswas PS, Bhagat G, Pernis AB (2010) IRF4 and its regulators: evolving insights into the pathogenesis of inflammatory arthritis? Immunol Rev 233: 79–96.
6. Glasmacher E, Agrawal S, Chang AB, Murphy TL, Zeng W, et al. (2012) A genomic regulatory element that directs assembly and function of immune-specific AP-1-IRF complexes. Science 16: 975–980.
7. Kwon H, Thierry-Mieg D, Thierry-Mieg J, Kim HP, Oh J, et al. (2009) Analysis of Interleukin-21-induced Prdm1 gene regulation reveals functional cooperation of STAT3 and IRF4 transcription factors. Immunity 31: 941–952.
8. Tussiwand R, Lee WL, Murphy TL, Mashayekhi M, KC W, et al. (2012) Compensatory dendritic cell development mediated by BATF-IRF interactions. Nature 490: 502–507.
9. Li P, Spolski R, Liao W, Wang L, Murphy TL, et al. (2012) BATF-JUN is critical for IRF4-mediated transcription in T cells. Nature 490: 543–546.
10. Farrow MA, Kim EY, Wolinsky SM, Sheehy AM (2011) NFAT and IRF proteins regulate transcription of the anti-HIV protein, APOBEC3G. J Biol Chem 286: 2567–2577.
11. Murphy TL, Tussiwand R, Murphy KM (2013) Specificity through cooperation: BATF-IRF interactions control immune-regulatory networks. Nat Rev Immunol 13: 499–509.
12. Kong X, Banks A, Liu T, Kazak L, Rao RR, et al. (2014) IRF4 is a key thermogenic transcriptional partner of PGC-1a. Cell 158: 69–83.
13. Rui L, Schmitz R, Ceribelli M, Staudt LM (2011) Malignant pirates of the immune system. Nat Immunol 12: 933–940.
14. Tamura T, Yanai H, Savitsky D, Taniguchi T (2008) The IRF family transcription factors in immunity and oncogenesis. Annu Rev Immunol 26: 535–584.
15. Lu R (2008) Interferon regulatory factor 4 and 8 in B-cell development. Trends Immunol 29: 487–492.
16. Ning S (2013) IRF4 as an oncogenic biomarker for hematological malignancies. Journal of Oncobiomarkers 1: 6.
17. Xu D, Zhao L, Del Valle L, Miklossy J, Zhang L (2008) Interferon regulatory factors 4 is involved in Epstein-Barr virus-mediated transformation of human B lymphocytes. J Virol 82: 6251–6258.

18. Martin HJ, Lee JM, Walls D, Hayward SD (2007) Manipulation of the Toll-Like Receptor 7 signaling pathway by Epstein-Barr Virus. J Virol 81: 9748–9758.
19. Spender LC, Lucchesi W, Bodelon G, Bilancio A, Karstegl CE, et al. (2006) Cell target genes of Epstein-Barr virus transcription factor EBNA-2: induction of the p55α regulatory subunit of PI3-kinase and its role in survival of EREB2.5 cells. J Gen Virol 87: 2859–2867.
20. Cahir-McFarland ED, Carter K, Rosenwald A, Giltnane JM, Henrickson SE, et al. (2004) Role of NF-κB in cell survival and transcription of latent membrane protein 1-expressing or Epstein-Barr Virus latency III-infected cells. J Virol 78: 4108–4119.
21. Ramos JC, Ruiz P, Jr., Ratner L, Reis IM, Brites C, et al. (2007) IRF4 and c-Rel expression in antiviral-resistant adult T-cell leukemia/lymphoma. Blood 109: 3060–3068.
22. Sharma S, Grandvaux N, Mamane Y, Genin P, Azimi N, et al. (2002) Regulation of IFN regulatory factor 4 expression in human T cell leukemia virus-I-transformed T cells. J Immunol 169: 3120–3130.
23. Sharma S, Mamane Y, Grandvaux N, Bartlett J, Petropoulos L, et al. (2000) Activation and regulation of interferon regulatory factor 4 in HTLV type 1-infected T lymphocytes. AIDS Res Hum Retrov 16: 1613–1622.
24. Mamane Y, Sharma S, Grandvaux N, Hernandez E, Hiscott J (2002) IRF-4 activities in HTLV-I-induced T cell leukemogenesis. J Interferon Cytokine Res 22: 135–143.
25. Mamane Y, Grandvaux N, Hernandez E, Sharma S, Innocente SA, et al. (2002) Repression of IRF-4 target genes in human T cell leukemia virus-1 infection. Oncogene 21: 6751–6765.
26. Feldman AL, Law M, Remstein ED, Macon WR, Erickson LA, et al. (2009) Recurrent translocations involving the IRF4 oncogene locus in peripheral T-cell lymphomas. Leukemia 23: 574–580.
27. Iida S, Rao PH, Butler M, Corradini P, Boccadoro M, et al. (1997) Deregulation of MUM1/IRF4 by chromosomal translocation in multiple myeloma. Nat Genet 17: 226–230.
28. Shaffer AL, Emre NCT, Lamy L, Ngo VN, Wright G, et al. (2008) IRF4 addiction in multiple myeloma. Nature 454: 226–231.
29. Sundram U, Harvell JD, Rouse RV, Natkunam Y (2003) Expression of the B-cell proliferation marker MUM1 by melanocytic lesions and comparison with S100, gp100 (HMB45), and MelanA. Mod Pathol 16: 802–810.
30. Chang CC, Lorek J, Sabath DE, Li Y, Chitambar CR, et al. (2002) Expression of MUM1/IRF4 correlates with clinical outcome in patients with B-cell chronic lymphocytic leukemia. Blood 100: 4671–4675.
31. Hurley EA, Klaman LD, Agger S, Lawrence JB, Thorley-Lawson DA (1991) The prototypical Epstein-Barr virus-transformed lymphoblastoid cell line IB4 is an unusual variant containing integrated but no episomal viral DNA. J Virol 65: 3958–3963.
32. Takada K, Horinouchi K, Ono Y, Aya T, Osato T, et al. (1991) An Epstein-Barr virus-producer line Akata: Establishment of the cell line and analysis of viral DNA. Virus Genes 5: 147–156.
33. Nonkwelo C, Skinner J, Bell A, Rickinson A, Sample J (1996) Transcription start sites downstream of the Epstein-Barr virus (EBV) Fp promoter in early-passage Burkitt lymphoma cells define a fourth promoter for expression of the EBV EBNA-1 protein. J Virol 70: 623–627.
34. Contreras-Brodin BA, Anvret M, Imreh S, Altiok E, Klein G, et al. (1991) B cell phenotype-dependent expression of the Epstein-Barr virus nuclear antigens EBNA-2 to EBNA-6: studies with somatic cell hybrids. J Gen Virol 72: 3025–3033.
35. Wang L, Toomey NL, Diaz LA, Walker G, Ramos JC, et al. (2011) Oncogenic IRFs provide a survival advantage for EBV- or HTLV1-transformed cells through induction of BIC expression. J Virol 85: 8328–8337.
36. Barretina J, Caponigro G, Stransky N, Venkatesan K, Margolin AA, et al. (2012) The Cancer Cell Line Encyclopedia enables predictive modelling of anticancer drug sensitivity. Nature 483: 603–307.
37. Duffy DL, Iles MM, Glass D, Zhu G, Barrett JH, et al. (2010) IRF4 variants have age-specific effects on nevus count and predispose to melanoma. The American Journal of Human Genetics 87: 6–16.
38. Praetorius C, Grill C, Stacey SN, Metcalf AM, Gorkin DU, et al. (2013) A polymorphism in IRF4 affects human pigmentation through a tyrosinase-dependent MITF/TFAP2A pathway. Cell 155: 1022–1033. S0092-8674(13)01298-1 [pii];10.1016/j.cell.2013.10.022 [doi].
39. Pena-Chilet M, Blanquer-Maceiras M, Ibarrola-Villava M, Martinez-Cadenas C, Martin-Gonzalez M, et al. (2013) Genetic variants in PARP1 (rs3219090) and IRF4 (rs12203592) genes associated with melanoma susceptibility in a Spanish population. BMC Cancer 13: 160.
40. Alonso SR, Ortiz P, PollÃ¡n M, PÃ©rez-GÃ3mez B, SÃ¡nchez L, et al. (2004) Progression in cutaneous malignant melanoma is associated with distinct expression profiles: A tissue microarray-based study. The American Journal of Pathology 164: 193–203.
41. Basso K, Margolin AA, Stolovitzky G, Klein U, Dalla-Favera R, et al. (2005) Reverse engineering of regulatory networks in human B cells. Nat Genet 37: 382–390. ng1532 [pii];10.1038/ng1532 [doi].
42. Lenz G, Wright G, Dave SS, Xiao W, Powell J, et al. (2008) Stromal gene signatures in large-B-cell lymphomas. N Engl J Med 359: 2313–2323.
43. Chapman MA, Lawrence MS, Keats JJ, Cibulskis K, Sougnez C, et al. (2011) Initial genome sequencing and analysis of multiple myeloma. Nature 471: 467–472.
44. Zhan F, Hardin J, Kordsmeier B, Bumm K, Zheng M, et al. (2002) Global gene expression profiling of multiple myeloma, monoclonal gammopathy of undetermined significance, and normal bone marrow plasma cells. Blood 99: 1745–1757.
45. Coustan-Smith E, Song G, Clark C, Key L, Liu P, et al. (2011) New markers for minimal residual disease detection in acute lymphoblastic leukemia. Blood 117: 6267–6276.
46. Beasley GM, Riboh JC, Augustine CK, Zager JS, Hochwald SN, et al. (2011) Prospective multicenter phase II trial of systemic ADH-1 in combination with melphalan via isolated limb infusion in patients with advanced extremity melanoma. Journal of Clinical Oncology 29: 1210–1215.
47. Hoek KS, Schlegel NC, Brafford P, Sucker A, Ugurel S, et al. (2006) Metastatic potential of melanomas defined by specific gene expression profiles with no BRAF signature. Pigment Cell Research 19: 290–302.
48. Chetaille B, Bertucci Fo, Finetti P, Esterni B, Stamatoullas A, et al. (2008) Molecular profiling of classical Hodgkin lymphoma tissues uncovers variations in the tumor microenvironment and correlations with EBV infection and outcome. Blood 113: 2765–3775.
49. Salaverria I, Philipp C, Oschlies I, Kohler CW, Kreuz M, et al. (2011) Translocations activating IRF4 identify a subtype of germinal center-derived B-cell lymphoma affecting predominantly children and young adults. Blood 118: 139–147.
50. Hummel M, Bentink S, Berger H, Klapper W, Wessendorf S, et al. (2006) A biologic definition of Burkitt's lymphoma from transcriptional and genomic profiling. N Engl J Med 354: 2419–2430.
51. Yang Y, Shaffer III AL, Emre NC, Ceribelli M, Zhang M, et al. (2012) Exploiting synthetic lethality for the therapy of ABC Diffuse Large B Cell Lymphoma. Cancer Cell 21: 723–737.
52. Dave SS, Fu K, Wright GW, Lam LT, Kluin P, et al. (2006) Molecular diagnosis of Burkitt's lymphoma. N Engl J Med 354: 2431–2442.
53. Tsuzuki S, Karnan S, Horibe K, Matsumoto K, Kato K, et al. (2007) Genetic abnormalities involved in t(12; 21) TEL-AML1 acute lymphoblastic leukemia: Analysis by means of array-based comparative genomic hybridization. Cancer Sci 98: 698–706.
54. Huggins CJ, Andrulis IL (2008) Cell cycle regulated phosphorylation of LIMD1 in cell lines and expression in human breast cancers. Cancer Letters 267: 55–66.
55. Sharp TV, Al-Attar A, Foxler DE, Ding L, de A, V, et al. (2008) The chromosome 3p21.3-encoded gene, LIMD1, is a critical tumor suppressor involved in human lung cancer development. Proc Natl Acad Sci USA 105: 19932–19937.
56. Sharp TV, Munoz F, Bourboulia D, Presneau N, Darai E, et al. (2004) LIM domains-containing protein 1 (LIMD1), a tumor suppressor encoded at chromosome 3p21.3, binds pRB and represses E2F-driven transcription. Proc Natl Acad Sci USA 101: 16531–16536.
57. James V, Zhang Y, Foxler DE, de Moor CH, Kong YW, et al. (2010) LIM-domain proteins, LIMD1, Ajuba, and WTIP are required for microRNA-mediated gene silencing. Proc Natl Acad Sci USA 107: 12499–12504.
58. Safa AR (2012) c-FLIP, a master anti-apoptotic regulator. Exp Oncol 34: 176–184. 3429 [pii].
59. Johnstone RW, Frew AJ, Smyth MJ (2008) The TRAIL apoptotic pathway in cancer onset, progression and therapy. Nat Rev Cancer 8: 782–798.
60. Xu D, Meyer F, Ehlers E, Blasnitz L, Zhang L (2011) Interferon regulatory factor 4 (IRF-4) targets IRF-5 to regulate Epstein-Barr virus transformation. J Biol Chem 286: 18261–18267.
61. Cheriyath V, Leaman DW, Borden EC (2011) Emerging roles of FAM14 family members (G1P3/ISG 6-16 and ISG12/IFI27) in innate immunity and cancer. J Interferon Cytokine Res 31: 173–181. 10.1089/jir.2010.0105 [doi].
62. Rosebeck S, Leaman D (2008) Mitochondrial localization and pro-apoptotic effects of the interferon-inducible protein ISG12a. Apoptosis 13: 562–572.
63. Hallen LC, Burki Y, Ebeling M, Broger C, Siegrist F, et al. (2007) Antiproliferative activity of the human IFN-alpha-inducible protein IFI44. J Interferon Cytokine Res 27: 675–680. 10.1089/jir.2007.0021 [doi].
64. Britzen-Laurent N, Lipnik K, Ocker M, Naschberger E, Schellerer VS, et al. (2013) GBP-1 acts as a tumor suppressor in colorectal cancer cells. Carcinogenesis 34: 153–162.
65. Itsui Y, Sakamoto N, Kakinuma S, Nakagawa M, Sekine-Osajima Y, et al. (2009) Antiviral effects of the interferon-induced protein guanylate binding protein 1 and its interaction with the hepatitis C virus NS5B protein. Hepatology 50: 1727–1737.
66. Maeda M, Hasegawa H, Hyodo T, Ito S, Asano E, et al. (2011) ARHGAP18, a GTPase-activating protein for RhoA, controls cell shape, spreading, and motility. Mol Biol Cell 22: 3840–3852.
67. Yang D, Wang S, Brooks C, Dong Z, Schoenlein PV, et al. (2009) IFN Regulatory Factor 8 sensitizes soft tissue sarcoma cells to death receptor-initiated apoptosis via repression of FLICE-like Protein expression. Cancer Res 69: 1080–1088.
68. Saito M, Gao J, Basso K, Kitagawa Y, Smith PM, et al. (2007) A signaling pathway mediating downregulation of BCL6 in germinal center B cells is blocked by BCL6 gene alterations in B cell lymphoma. Cancer Cell 12: 280–292.
69. Wang L, Ning S (2013) IRF4 is activated through c-Src-mediated tyrosine phosphorylation in virus-transformed cells. J Virol 87: 9672–9679.

Pharmacologic Blockade of JAK1/JAK2 Reduces GvHD and Preserves the Graft-Versus-Leukemia Effect

Jaebok Choi[1]*, Matthew L. Cooper[1], Bader Alahmari[1], Julie Ritchey[1], Lynne Collins[2], Matthew Holt[1], John F. DiPersio[1]

1 Division of Oncology, Department of Medicine, Washington University School of Medicine, St. Louis, Missouri, United States of America, **2** BRIGHT Institute, and Molecular Imaging Center, Mallinckrodt Institute of Radiology, and Department of Cell Biology & Physiology, Washington University School of Medicine, St. Louis, Missouri, United States of America

Abstract

We have recently reported that interferon gamma receptor deficient (IFNγR−/−) allogeneic donor T cells result in significantly less graft-versus-host disease (GvHD) than wild-type (WT) T cells, while maintaining an anti-leukemia or graft-versus-leukemia (GvL) effect after allogeneic hematopoietic stem cell transplantation (allo-HSCT). We demonstrated that IFNγR signaling regulates alloreactive T cell trafficking to GvHD target organs through expression of the chemokine receptor CXCR3 in alloreactive T cells. Since IFNγR signaling is mediated via JAK1/JAK2, we tested the effect of JAK1/JAK2 inhibition on GvHD. While we demonstrated that pharmacologic blockade of JAK1/JAK2 in WT T cells using the JAK1/JAK2 inhibitor, INCB018424 (Ruxolitinib), resulted in a similar effect to IFNγR−/− T cells both *in vitro* (reduction of CXCR3 expression in T cells) and *in vivo* (mitigation of GvHD after allo-HSCT), it remains to be determined if *in vivo* administration of INCB018424 will result in preservation of GvL while reducing GvHD. Here, we report that INCB018424 reduces GvHD and preserves the beneficial GvL effect in two different murine MHC-mismatched allo-HSCT models and using two different murine leukemia models (lymphoid leukemia and myeloid leukemia). In addition, prolonged administration of INCB018424 further improves survival after allo-HSCT and is superior to other JAK1/JAK2 inhibitors, such as TG101348 or AZD1480. These data suggest that pharmacologic inhibition of JAK1/JAK2 might be a promising therapeutic approach to achieve the beneficial anti-leukemia effect and overcome HLA-barriers in allo-HSCT. It might also be exploited in other diseases besides GvHD, such as organ transplant rejection, chronic inflammatory diseases and autoimmune diseases.

Editor: Vassiliki A. Boussiotis, Beth Israel Deaconess Medical Center, Harvard Medical School, United States of America

Funding: J.C. is supported by the Siteman Cancer Center Research Development Awards and SPORE-CDP (P50 CA171063-01). J.F.D. is supported by the National Cancer Institute (P50 CA94056-09 and P50 CA171063-01) and the Bryan Thomas Campbell Foundation. The funders had no role in study design, data collection and analysis, decision to publish, or preparation of the manuscript.

Competing Interests: The authors have declared that no competing interests exist.

* Email: jchoi@dom.wustl.edu

Introduction

Allo-HSCT is often the most effective and curative treatment for patients with hematologic malignancies such as relapsed or refractory leukemia and marrow failure states such as myelodysplastic syndromes (MDS), myelofibrosis, and aplastic anemia [1]. The therapeutic benefits of allo-HSCT are primarily derived from an anti-leukemia effect (graft-versus-leukemia effect or GvL) that is mediated by mature donor T cells present in the donor graft. Unfortunately, these donor T cells also induce GvHD, the major life-threatening complication of allo-HSCT [2]. Thus, the clinical goal is to minimize GvHD without abrogating the beneficial GvL effect.

The current treatment of GvHD involves the reduction of T cell numbers or function resulting in loss of donor engraftment, alloreactivity (GvHD), and an anti-leukemia effect (GvL), thereby potentially undermining of the beneficial effects of allo-HSCT leading to enhanced leukemia relapse. Managing the threat of GvHD while maximizing the beneficial GvL effect would broaden the scope and usefulness of allo-HSCT procedures and mitigate the major cause of morbidity and mortality in patients with hematologic malignancies undergoing allo-HSCT. The development of simple and innovative pharmacologic approaches to modulate alloreactive donor T cell trafficking to GvHD target organs without affecting T cell trafficking to leukemia cells *in vivo* represents a significant advance in allo-HSCT prophylaxis.

Recently, we reported that IFNγR is upregulated in activated T cells and that IFNγR−/− allogeneic donor T cells result in significantly less GvHD than WT T cells, while preserving GvL with normal allo-reactivity. In addition, we demonstrated that IFNγR signaling is essential for a chemokine receptor, CXCR3, expression and T cell trafficking to GvHD target organs [3]. IFNγR signaling is mediated via JAK1 and JAK2. INCB018424 is a commercially available potent JAK1/JAK2-specific inhibitor [4,5], that is FDA-approved for advanced myelofibrosis and currently being tested in clinical trials for the treatment of other myeloproliferative disorders [4,5]. We found that this small molecule inhibitor dramatically reduces the expression of CXCR3 in both human and murine activated T cells [3]. Most importantly, INCB018424 significantly reduced GvHD and improved survival after allo-HSCT by modulating allogeneic donor T cell trafficking to GvHD target organs as seen in IFNγR−/− T cells [3]. Based on these data, we hypothesize that

INCB018424 will preserve the beneficial GvL effect while mitigating GvHD after allo-HSCT.

Materials and Methods

Ethics statement

This study was carried out in strict accordance with current National Institutes of Health guidelines. The animal care, use, and euthanasia protocols were approved by the Washington University School of Medicine Animal Studies Committee (Approval Number: 20120058).

Mice

All mice were obtained from Jackson Laboratory (Bar Harbor, ME).

Cell culture

Mouse pan T cells (CD4+ and CD8+ T cells) were isolated from mouse spleens using Miltenyi pan T cell isolation kit and an AutoMACS (Miltenyi Biotech, Auburn, CA) [6]. The isolated pan T cells were activated for three days in the presence of anti-CD3/CD28 antibody-coated beads (bead:cell = 1:1) (Invitrogen, Carlsbad, CA) in Xcyte media with IL-2 (10 IU/ml) [7].

Flow cytometric analysis

The antibodies used for flow cytometric analyses are as follows. CD4, CD8, H-$2K^b$, CD3, B220, CD45.2, STAT1 (clone: 1/Stat1), STAT1 (pY701) (clone: 4a) (BD Pharmingen) and CD183 (clone: CXCR3-173) (eBioscience). All data were collected on a FACScan cytometer (BD Biosciences, Mountain View, CA) and analyzed using FlowJo (Tree Star Inc, Ashland, OR).

Allo-HSCT

Allo-HSCT was performed as previously described [6,7]. In brief, 5×10^6 T cell-depleted bone marrow cells (TCD BM) (CD45.1+ B6 (H-2^b)) and 5×10^5 pan T cells (CD45.2+ B6 (H-2^b)) were injected into lethally irradiated (900–925cGy) Balb/c recipient mice (H-2^d, CD45.2+). The Balb/c-derived B cell lymphoma cell line, A20, was used in both systemic leukemia and solid tumor models. The primary acute promyelocytic leukemia (APL) cells, which were harvested from the human PML-RARα knock-in mice [8], were used in myeloid leukemia model.

In vivo bioluminescence imaging (BLI)

GvL effect assessment and BLI of animals were done as previously described [6,9]. BLI was performed once every week starting on day 1 until day 43 post allo-HSCT. Mice were injected intraperitoneally with 150 mg/g D-luciferin (Biosynth, Naperville, IL) in PBS, anesthetized with 2.5% isoflurane, and imaged with a charge-coupled device (CCD) camera-based BLI system (IVIS 100; Caliper, Hopkinton, MA; exposure time 1–60 seconds, binning 16, field of view 12, f/stop 1, open filter. Signal was displayed as photons/sec/cm^2/sr [9].

JAK1/JAK2 inhibitors

INCB018424, TG101348, and AZD1480 were purchased from Selleck Chemicals (Houston, TX) and prepared for injection as described in the manufacturer's instructions.

Statistical analysis

The significance of differences in survival between treatment groups was analyzed using the log-rank test. For all other analyses, the unpaired *t*-test was used.

Results

In vivo administration of INCB018424 preserves a strong anti-leukemia effect

Since the clinical goal of allo-HSCT is to prevent GvHD without abrogating GvL, we examined if the *in vivo* administration of INCB018424 preserves the beneficial anti-leukemia effect by performing BLI in two different mouse models of tumor growth; one a systemic leukemia model (**Fig. 1**) and the other a solid tumor lymphoma model (**Fig. 1**) [3,7]. Using murine T-cell depleted allo-HSCT model, B6 (H-2^b) → Balb/c (H-2^d) (925 cGy TBI), with infusion of pan T cells (5×10^5) (i.v.) and CBRluc-expressing A20 leukemia cells (Balb/c-derived) either i.v. (systemic leukemia) or s.c. (solid tumor) at day 0, followed by administration of INCB018424, we examined the effect of this small molecule inhibitor on GvL. BLI was performed once every week starting day 1 until day 43 (**Fig. 1A, B**).

We found that INCB018424 treatment preserves the potent anti-leukemia effect in both tumor models (**Fig. 1A, B**). These data suggest that pharmacologic modulation of JAK1/JAK2 using INCB018424 would be a promising therapeutic approach to overcome HLA-barriers in allo-HSCT.

Prolonged administration of INCB018424 prevents GvHD and is superior to other JAK inhibitors

As we previously reported, INCB018424 treatment improves survival by mitigating GvHD after allo-HSCT. Although the survival after INCB018424 treatment was statistically significant in that study, the overall survival rate after INCB018424 (40% at day 35 post allo-HSCT) was not as effective as that seen in IFNγR−/− T cells (80% at day 35 post allo-HSCT) [3]. Likewise, in the current study, we observed a statistically significant improvement of survival after allo-HSCT along with infusion of leukemia cells. However, the overall survivals at day 30 in the systemic leukemia and solid tumor models were 50% (5% survival in the control group) and 26.7% (0% survival in the control group), respectively (**Fig. 1C**). The critical difference between the previous genetic study and the current pharmacologic approach is the duration of JAK1/JAK2 activation. While IFNγR-mediated JAK1/JAK2 signaling in IFNγR−/− T cells is presumably inactive (although JAK1 and JAK2 activation mediated by other signaling pathways might not be affected), the pharmacologic blockade of JAK1/JAK2 in WT T cells by INCB018424 was maintained for only three weeks after allo-HSCT. Thus, we hypothesized that a prolonged administration of INCB018424 (greater than three weeks *in vivo*) would result in improvement in overall survival. As demonstrated in **Fig. 2A**, we found that the prolonged administration of INCB018424 (for one month) significantly improved overall survival (75% at day 30 and 50% at day 60) in this fully MHC-mismatched mouse allo-HSCT model. In addition, this improved survival was similarly observed in A20 bearing mice when these mice were treated for one month with INCB018424 (**Fig. 2B–C**). Furthermore, we observed a similar immunomodulatory effect of INCB018242 in a different mouse model (Balb/c to B6) in terms of overall survival (80% - DMSO vs. 100% - INCB), clinical GvHD score (**Fig. 2D**), and weight change (**Fig. 2E**). Westervelt et al generated an APL mouse model (B6; H-2^b, CD45.2+) in which the human PML-RARα gene is inserted into the 5′ UTR of the murine cathepsin G

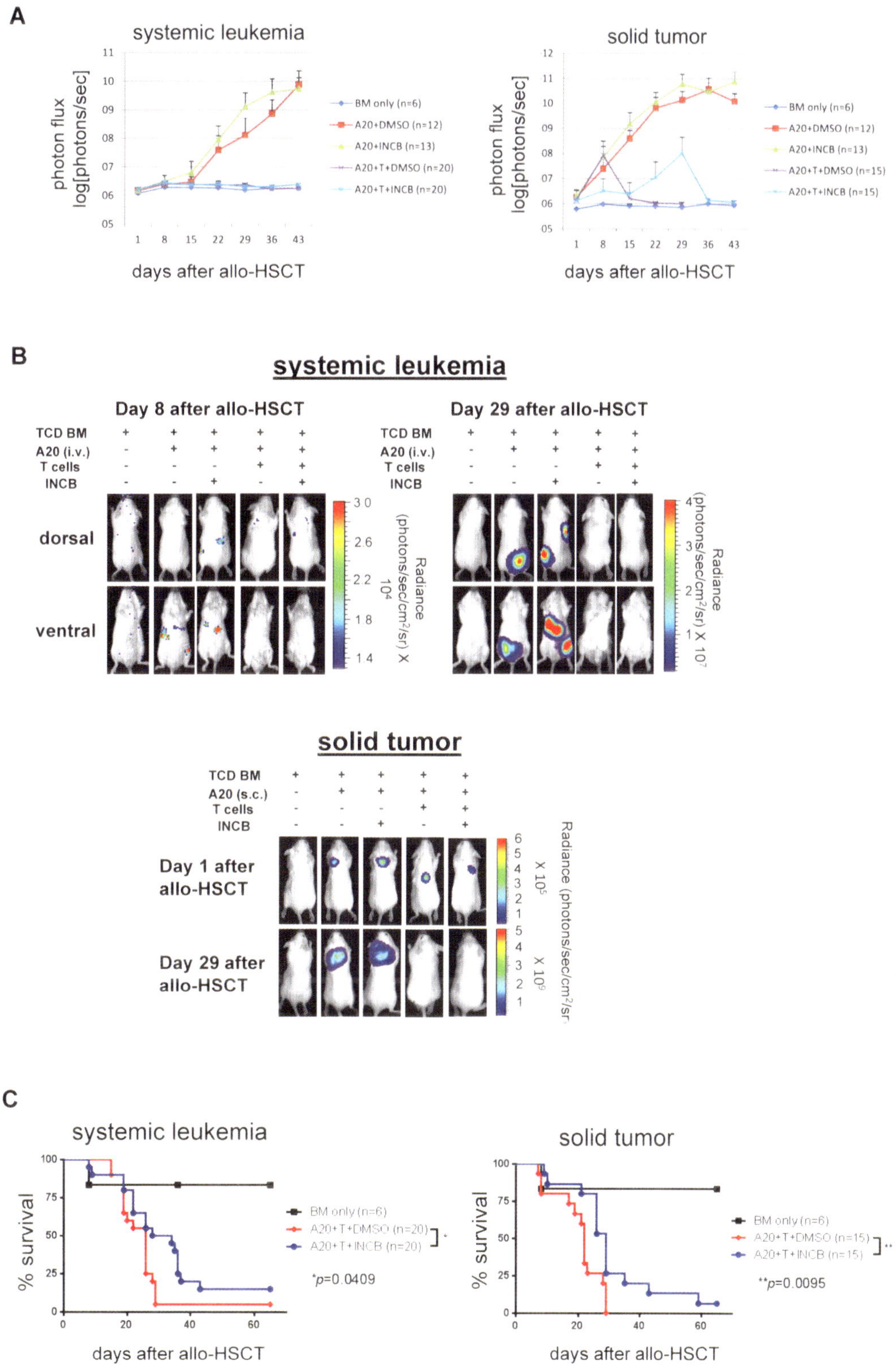

Figure 1. ***In vivo*** **administration of INCB018424 maintains a beneficial GvL effect and improves survival after allo-HSCT.** Allo-HSCT was performed as described in the Materials and Method. CBRluc-expressing A20 B cell lymphoma cells were injected either i.v. (1×10^4 cells) or s.c. (1×10^5 cells in 100 ul PBS). *In vivo* BLI imaging technique was used to measure tumor burden once every week starting day 1 to day 43 after allo-HSCT. INCB018424 was injected for three weeks (days 3–23) twice a day (100 µg/injection, i.p.). (**A**) Systemic leukemia (left panel) and solid tumor (right panel) models. Photon flux was measured with a region of interest drawn over the entire body of each mouse. (**B**) Actual images of 1 representative mouse from each group are shown. Data represents the pool of three independent experiments. Systemic A20 lymphoid leukemia model is shown in upper panels and solid tumor A20 lymphoid leukemia model shown in bottom panel. (**C**) Survival of mice shown in Kaplan-Meier plots of both a systemic (left panel) and a solid tumor model (right panel).

gene [8]. These mice develop a fatal myeloid leukemia with 90–100% penetrance [8]. The leukemia is characterized by marked peripheral leukocytosis [8]. Banked primary APL cells (5×10^5 cells) obtained from these mice were injected (i.v.) into the lethally irradiated B6 recipient mice along with TCD BM (5×10^6 cells) and splenic pan T cells (5×10^6 cells) isolated from Balb/c donor mice at day 0. Starting at day 16 post transplantation, we determined leukemic burden of these mice by measuring percent APL cells in the PB once every week. We found that administration of INCB018424 preserves GvL activity in this myeloid leukemia model (**Fig. 2F**) while significantly reducing GvHD (**Fig. 2G**). These data and our previous report [3], in which altered T cell trafficking was found in another allo-HSCT model (FVB to Balb/c) after INCB018424 treatment, suggest that the effect of *in vivo* blockade of JAK1/JAK2 on GvHD and GvL might not be model-specific. We also found that INCB018424 is superior to other JAK inhibitors, such as TG101348 and AZD1480 (**Fig. 2A**). Since IFNγR-mediated activation of JAK1 and JAK2 results in phosphorylation of STAT1, we examined if there are any differences in the ability of these three JAK inhibitors to inhibit STAT1 phosphorylation. We observed that INCB018424 is the most effective at blocking STAT1 phosphorylation (**Fig. 2H**). These data suggest that INCB018424 is superior in inhibiting IFNγR-mediated JAK1/JAK2 signaling and phosphorylation of STAT1 *in vitro* and *in vivo* than the other JAK1/JAK2 inhibitors tested and may potentially be an ideal drug to test in the context of GvHD prophylaxis in human allo-HSCT in the future.

Although we demonstrated that IFNγR signaling can be modulated by targeting JAK1/JAK2, we cannot exclude the possibility that JAK1/JAK2 inhibitors have off-target effects, considering JAK1 and JAK2 function as signal transducers of multiple cytokine receptors and activation pathways. Thus, we examined if INCB018424 could further reduce GVHD in the recipients of IFNγR−/− T cells. Interestingly, INCB018424 administration resulted in 100% survival (**Fig. 2I**) and negligible evidence of clinical GvHD in 90% of the recipients; 1/10 mouse had grade 2 denuded skin based on the Cooke et al. GvHD scoring system [10]. These data suggest that INCB018424 may modulate signaling pathways other than, and in addition to, JAK1/JAK2. Alternatively, JAK1/JAK2 inhibitors perhaps reduce IFNγR signaling in recipients or donor BM-derived antigen presenting cells (APCs), which may also contribute to reduction of MHC I and II expression in recipient APCs [11,12].

Discussion

In our previous report, we demonstrated that either genetic deficiency of IFNγR signaling or pharmacologic inhibition of its downstream targets JAK1 and JAK2 using INCB018424 results in less GvHD after allo-HSCT by reducing alloreactive T cell trafficking to GvHD target organs [3]. In the current study, we further demonstrate and confirm that the pharmacologic inhibition of JAK1/JAK2 preserves the beneficial anti-leukemia effect previously reported by our group in IFNγR−/− T cells [3] in two different leukemia models (A20 lymphoid leukemia and APL myeloid leukemia).

We also show that extending the duration of INCB018424 administration by 10 days (from 21 days in our previous study to 31 days in our current study) [3] significantly reduces GvHD and improves the overall survival of major MHC-mismatched allo-HSCT recipients. Spoerl et al. recently reported similar results [13]. While the overall survivals are comparable between the two studies (relative survival rates comparing to the BM only groups: 65% - Spoerl et al. vs 58.3% - current study), there are several differences in the experimental designs of our study and that of Spoerl et al. First, Spoerl et al used a dose of INCB018424 three times higher than that used in our current study (Spoerl et al.: 30 mg/kg/day; current study: equivalent to 10 mg/kg/day with an average body weight of recipient mice, approximately 20 g/mouse). It is possible that this high dose of INCB018424 resulted in the reduction of T cell expansion in their BLI study [13] while our previous study demonstrated that the lower dose of INCB018424 altered T cell trafficking but did not affect T cell expansion [3]. Second, Spoerl et al. used only 60% of the T cell dose used in our study (0.3×10^6 T cells vs. 0.5×10^6 T cells). It is possible that this modest difference may also contribute to the observed marginal improved survival reported by Spoerl et al. Third, the duration of INCB018424 administration was from day -1 to day +20 by oral gavage in the Spoerl study, while in our study it was started on day +1 and continued to day +31 by s.c. injection.

There are several possible reasons why INCB018424 might be more effective at reducing GvHD than TG101348 and AZD1480 in spite of them all being potent JAK inhibitors. Since others have shown that plasma concentrations of both TG101348 and AZD1480 are well maintained when administered twice a day and these drugs are effective in reducing tumor burden *in vivo* [14–16], we speculate that the drug efficacy and stability *in vivo* is likely not the issue. First, it is conceivable that the preferential inhibition of JAK2 over JAK1 by TG101348 (35 fold) and AZD1480 (5 fold), compared to 1.18 fold with INCB018424, may possibly lead to reduced inhibition of IFNγR signaling (via STAT1) [16–18]. Therefore TG101348 and AZD1480 may preferentially inhibit other signaling pathways involving only JAK2, such as IL-12 (via STAT4), leptin (via STAT3), and IL-3, IL-5 or GM-CSF (via STAT5) [19]. Indeed, Dey *et al* demonstrated that IL-12 is protective against GvHD by inhibiting activation of alloreactive CD4+ T cells [20]. In addition, it has been reported that STAT3 signaling is essential for myeloid-derived suppressor cells [21], which may have an important role in the suppressing the proliferation of alloreactive T cells [22]. Furthermore, the Blazar group reported that constitutive activation of STAT5b reduces GvHD [23], suggesting that inhibition of STAT5 by these compounds could aggravate GvHD. Second, it has been shown that AZD1480 and TG101348 can reduce the expression of PD-L1 and PD-L2 [24,25], which are ligands of programed cell death 1 (PD1). Thus, it is possible that reduction of PD-L1 and PD-L2 on target tissues by AZD1480 might lead to an increase of alloreactive T cells in GvHD target organs [26,27], offsetting the reduced T cell trafficking to the GvHD target organs. Lastly, there might be off-target effects by these drugs which may be proinflammatory rather than anti-inflammatory.

It has been recently reported that aberrant function of JAK kinases is found often in AML [28,29], suggesting that JAK1/JAK2 inhibitors may also induce direct negative regulatory effects on AML survival and proliferation. If successful in humans, this strategy (the use of JAK1/JAK2 inhibitors as GvHD prophylaxis for allo-HSCT) may limit the need for expensive and labor intensive *ex vivo* cellular manipulations, such as T cell depletion to reduce GvHD while maintaining GvL. In addition, this approach may also result in the reduced use of post-transplant immunosuppressive agents which, may themselves, contribute to both morbidity and mortality after allo-HSCT. Consistent with our study, Spoerl et al. recently demonstrated that INCB018424 was able to reduce established GVHD of 6/6 patients treated [13], suggesting that blockade of JAK1/JAK2 would be an effective therapeutic strategy for established GvHD as well as a rational approach as GvHD prophylaxis. Furthermore, pharmacologic

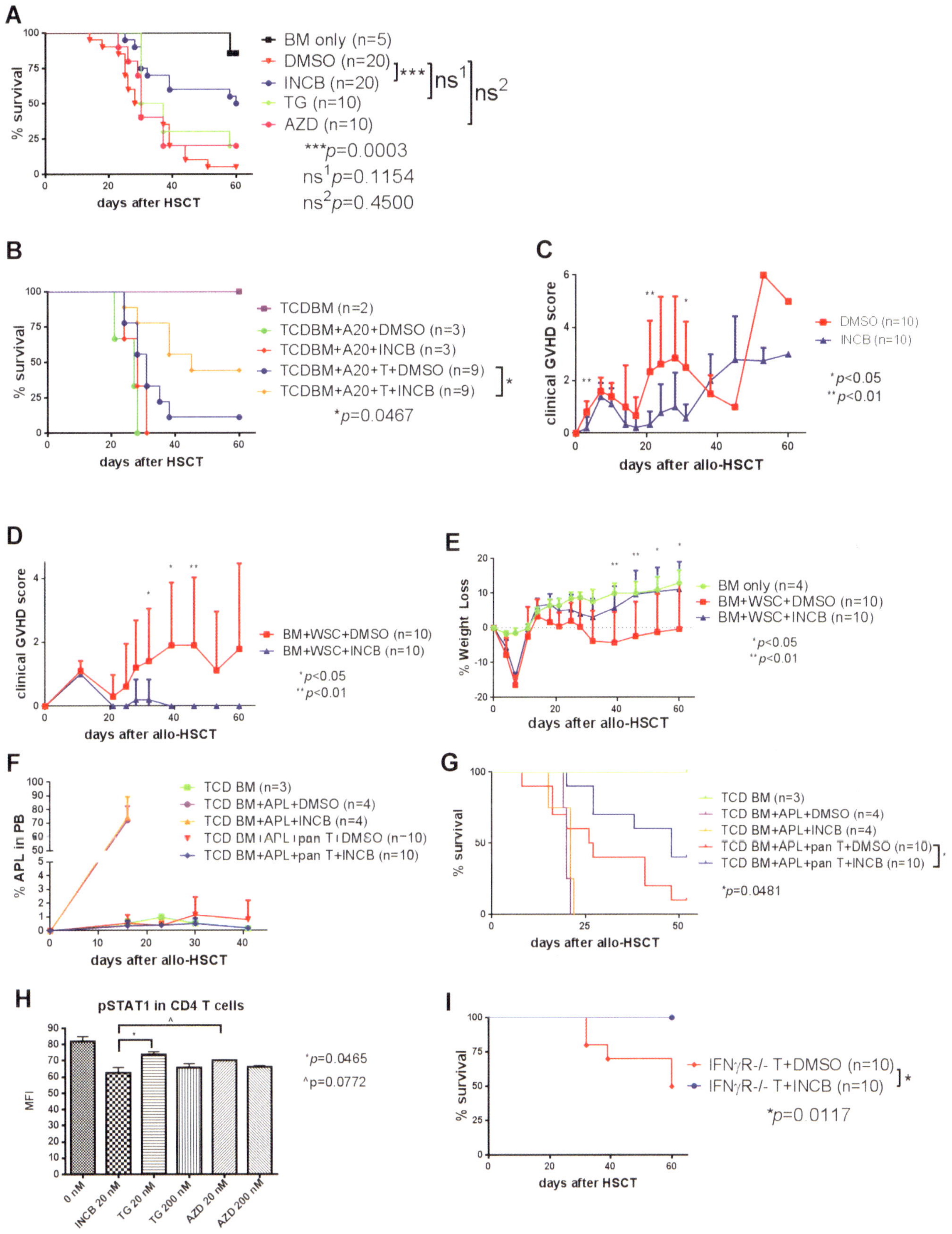

Figure 2. Prolonged administration of INCB018424 further improves survival after allo-HSCT. (**A**) Administration of INCB018424 for one month (days +1–+31) twice a day (100 μg/injection, s.c.) significantly improves survival after allo-HSCT ($p = 0.0003$). (**B–C**) Prolonged administration of INCB018424 improves survival while preserving GvL (**B**). 1×10^5 A20 cells (i.v) were transplanted along with allogeneic TCD BM and pan T cells at day

0. Clinical GvHD scores according to Cooke et al [10] (**C**). (**D–E**) B6 mice were lethally irradiated (1,200 cGy) at day -1 and injected (i.p.) with 50 μg of anti-NK1.1 mAb (PK136). BM cells (5×10^6) and whole splenocytes (20×10^6) harvested from Balb/c were transplanted into lethally irradiated B6 at day 0, followed by INCB018424 for 31 days (days +1–+31). Clinical GvHD scores according to Cooke et al [10] (**D**) and weight change (**E**). (**F–G**) B6 mice were lethally irradiated (1,200 cGy) at day -1 and injected (i.p.) with 50 μg of anti-NK1.1 mAb (PK136). TCD BM (5×10^6) and pan T cells (5×10^6) isolated from Balb/c were transplanted into the lethally irradiated B6 at day 0. Banked primary APL cells (5×10^5) were injected (i.v.) along with TCD BM and pan T cells at day 0. INCB018424 was administered s.c. twice a day for 31 days (days +1–+31). (**F**) Percentage of APL cells in the PB was measured by flow cytometry after staining PB cells starting at day +16 once every week until day +41. Anti-H-2Kb and anti-CD45.2 antibodies were used to identify the APL cells. H-2^b+ CD45.1+ B6 recipients and H-2^d+ CD45.2+ Balb/c donors were used to discriminate APL from all other cells. (**G**) Shown is a Kaplan-Meier survival curve. (**H**) INCB018424 is superior to other JAK inhibitors, such as TG101348 and AZD1480, in blocking IFNγR signaling. As an indicator of IFNγR signaling, we assessed STAT1 phosphorylation by intracellular pSTAT1 staining and FACS. MFI: geometric mean fluorescence intensity. (**I**) Lethally irradiated (900 cGy) Balb/c mice were transplanted with TCD BM (5×10^6) obtained from B6 WT mice and pan T cells (5×10^5) isolated from B6 WT or IFNγR−/− mice at day 0. INCB018424 was administered s.c. twice a day for 31 days (days +1–+31). INCB018424 treatment for 31 days results in free of GvHD in 90% of recipients and 100% survival when mice are transplanted with IFNγR−/− T cells.

JAK1/JAK2 blockade, either alone or in conjunction with other methods of GvHD prophylaxis may permit for those patients who lack a human leukocyte antigen (HLA)-matched sibling or matched unrelated donor (approximately 50% of patients) to proceed to transplant with limited GvHD and a well preserved GvL effect. Taken together, our data suggests that JAK1/JAK2 is a promising therapeutic target to prevent GvHD while maintaining GvL.

Acknowledgments

We thank Mike Rettig and Ezhilarasi Chendamarai for help with the APL model.

Author Contributions

Conceived and designed the experiments: JC JFD. Performed the experiments: JC MLC BA JR LC MH. Analyzed the data: JC MLC JR LC JFD. Wrote the paper: JC MLC JFD.

References

1. Miller JS, Warren EH, van den Brink MR, Ritz J, Shlomchik WD, et al. (2010) NCI First International Workshop on The Biology, Prevention, and Treatment of Relapse After Allogeneic Hematopoietic Stem Cell Transplantation: Report from the Committee on the Biology Underlying Recurrence of Malignant Disease following Allogeneic HSCT: Graft-versus-Tumor/Leukemia Reaction. Biol Blood Marrow Transplant 16: 565–586.
2. Paczesny S, Hanauer D, Sun Y, Reddy P (2010) New perspectives on the biology of acute GVHD. Bone Marrow Transplant 45: 1–11.
3. Choi J, Ziga ED, Ritchey J, Collins L, Prior JL, et al. (2012) IFNgammaR signaling mediates alloreactive T-cell trafficking and GVHD. Blood 120: 4093–4103.
4. Tyner JW, Bumm TG, Deininger J, Wood L, Aichberger KJ, et al. (2010) CYT387, a novel JAK2 inhibitor, induces hematologic responses and normalizes inflammatory cytokines in murine myeloproliferative neoplasms. Blood 115: 5232–5240.
5. Wilson LJ (2010) Recent patents in the discovery of small molecule inhibitors of JAK3. Expert Opin Ther Pat 20: 609–623.
6. Rettig MP, Ritchey JK, Prior JL, Haug JS, Piwnica-Worms D, et al. (2004) Kinetics of in vivo elimination of suicide gene-expressing T cells affects engraftment, graft-versus-host disease, and graft-versus-leukemia after allogeneic bone marrow transplantation. J Immunol 173: 3620–3630.
7. Choi J, Ritchey J, Prior JL, Holt M, Shannon WD, et al. (2010) In vivo administration of hypomethylating agents mitigate graft-versus-host disease without sacrificing graft-versus-leukemia. Blood 116: 129–139.
8. Westervelt P, Lane AA, Pollock JL, Oldfather K, Holt MS, et al. (2003) High-penetrance mouse model of acute promyelocytic leukemia with very low levels of PML-RARalpha expression. Blood 102: 1857–1865.
9. Gross S, Piwnica-Worms D (2005) Real-time imaging of ligand-induced IKK activation in intact cells and in living mice. Nat Methods 2: 607–614.
10. Cooke KR, Kobzik L, Martin TR, Brewer J, Delmonte J, Jr., et al. (1996) An experimental model of idiopathic pneumonia syndrome after bone marrow transplantation: I. The roles of minor H antigens and endotoxin. Blood 88: 3230–3239.
11. van den Elsen PJ, Gobin SJ, van Eggermond MC, Peijnenburg A (1998) Regulation of MHC class I and II gene transcription: differences and similarities. Immunogenetics 48: 208–221.
12. Schroder K, Hertzog PJ, Ravasi T, Hume DA (2004) Interferon-gamma: an overview of signals, mechanisms and functions. J Leukoc Biol 75: 163–189.
13. Spoerl S, Mathew NR, Bscheider M, Schmitt-Graeff A, Chen S, et al. (2014) Activity of therapeutic JAK 1/2 blockade in graft-versus-host disease. Blood.
14. Sonbol MB, Firwana B, Zarzour A, Morad M, Rana V, et al. (2013) Comprehensive review of JAK inhibitors in myeloproliferative neoplasms. Ther Adv Hematol 4: 15–35.
15. Plimack ER, Lorusso PM, McCoon P, Tang W, Krebs AD, et al. (2013) AZD1480: a phase I study of a novel JAK2 inhibitor in solid tumors. Oncologist 18: 819–820.
16. Wernig G, Kharas MG, Okabe R, Moore SA, Leeman DS, et al. (2008) Efficacy of TG101348, a selective JAK2 inhibitor, in treatment of a murine model of JAK2V617F-induced polycythemia vera. Cancer Cell 13: 311–320.
17. Quintas-Cardama A, Vaddi K, Liu P, Manshouri T, Li J, et al. (2010) Preclinical characterization of the selective JAK1/2 inhibitor INCB018424: therapeutic implications for the treatment of myeloproliferative neoplasms. Blood 115: 3109–3117.
18. Hedvat M, Huszar D, Herrmann A, Gozgit JM, Schroeder A, et al. (2009) The JAK2 inhibitor AZD1480 potently blocks Stat3 signaling and oncogenesis in solid tumors. Cancer Cell 16: 487–497.
19. Rawlings JS, Rosler KM, Harrison DA (2004) The JAK/STAT signaling pathway. J Cell Sci 117: 1281–1283.
20. Dey BR, Yang YG, Szot GL, Pearson DA, Sykes M (1998) Interleukin-12 inhibits graft-versus-host disease through an Fas-mediated mechanism associated with alterations in donor T-cell activation and expansion. Blood 91: 3315–3322.
21. Markowitz J, Wesolowski R, Papenfuss T, Brooks TR, Carson WE, 3rd (2013) Myeloid-derived suppressor cells in breast cancer. Breast Cancer Res Treat 140: 13–21.
22. Highfill SL, Rodriguez PC, Zhou Q, Goetz CA, Koehn BH, et al. (2010) Bone marrow myeloid-derived suppressor cells (MDSCs) inhibit graft-versus-host disease (GVHD) via an arginase-1-dependent mechanism that is up-regulated by interleukin-13. Blood 116: 5738–5747.
23. Vogtenhuber C, Bucher C, Highfill SL, Koch LK, Goren E, et al. (2010) Constitutively active Stat5b in CD4+ T cells inhibits graft-versus-host disease lethality associated with increased regulatory T-cell potency and decreased T effector cell responses. Blood 116: 466–474.
24. Derenzini E, Lemoine M, Buglio D, Katayama H, Ji Y, et al. (2011) The JAK inhibitor AZD1480 regulates proliferation and immunity in Hodgkin lymphoma. Blood Cancer J 1: e46.
25. Hao Y, Chapuy B, Monti S, Sun HH, Rodig SJ, et al. (2014) Selective JAK2 inhibition specifically decreases Hodgkin lymphoma and mediastinal large B-cell lymphoma growth in vitro and in vivo. Clin Cancer Res 20: 2674–2683.
26. Blazar BR, Carreno BM, Panoskaltsis-Mortari A, Carter L, Iwai Y, et al. (2003) Blockade of programmed death-1 engagement accelerates graft-versus-host disease lethality by an IFN-gamma-dependent mechanism. J Immunol 171: 1272–1277.
27. Yi T, Chen Y, Wang L, Du G, Huang D, et al. (2009) Reciprocal differentiation and tissue-specific pathogenesis of Th1, Th2, and Th17 cells in graft-versus-host disease. Blood 114: 3101–3112.
28. Wartman LD, Larson DE, Xiang Z, Ding L, Chen K, et al. (2011) Sequencing a mouse acute promyelocytic leukemia genome reveals genetic events relevant for disease progression. J Clin Invest 121: 1445–1455.
29. Lee HJ, Daver N, Kantarjian HM, Verstovsek S, Ravandi F (2013) The role of JAK pathway dysregulation in the pathogenesis and treatment of acute myeloid leukemia. Clin Cancer Res 19: 327–335.

Association of ITPA Genotype with Event-Free Survival and Relapse Rates in Children with Acute Lymphoblastic Leukemia Undergoing Maintenance Therapy

Alenka Smid[1], Natasa Karas-Kuzelicki[1], Miha Milek[1¤], Janez Jazbec[2], Irena Mlinaric-Rascan[1*]

1 Faculty of Pharmacy, University of Ljubljana, Ljubljana, Slovenia, 2 University Children's Hospital, University Medical Centre Ljubljana, Ljubljana, Slovenia

Abstract

Although the treatment of acute lymphoblastic leukemia (ALL) has improved significantly over recent decades, failure due to treatment-related toxicities and relapse of the disease still occur in about 20% of patients. This retrospective study included 308 pediatric ALL patients undergoing maintenance therapy and investigated the effects of genetic variants of enzymes involved in the 6-mercaptopurine (6-MP) metabolism and folate pathway on survival and relapse rates. The presence of at least one of the non-functional *ITPA* alleles (94C>A and/or IVS2+21A>C variant) was associated with longer event-free survival compared to patients with the wild-type *ITPA* genotype ($p = 0.033$). Furthermore, patients carrying at least one non-functional *ITPA* allele were shown to be at a lower risk of suffering early ($p = 0.003$) and/or bone marrow relapse ($p = 0.017$). In conclusion, the *ITPA* genotype may serve as a genetic marker for the improvement of risk stratification and therapy individualization for patients with ALL.

Editor: David R. Booth, University of Sydney, Australia

Funding: This work was supported by Slovenian Research Agency grant No. J3-3615. The funder had no role in study design, data collection and analysis, decision to publish, or preparation of the manuscript.

Competing Interests: The authors have declared that no competing interests exist.

* Email: irena.mlinaric@ffa.uni-lj.si

¤ Current address: Max-Delbrück-Center for Molecular Medicine, Berlin Institute for Medical Systems Biology, Berlin, Germany

Introduction

Treatment of pediatric acute lymphoblastic leukemia (ALL) has improved drastically over the last forty years, with the long term-survival rate for children diagnosed with ALL now such that approximately 85% survive for 5 years or more after diagnosis [1]. This great improvement can be attributed both to risk-adjusted treatment based on the identification of several biological and clinical prognostic factors which facilitated the definition of patient subgroups with different relapse risks, and the implementation of rationally designed phases in the treatment backbone of ALL [2]. Despite this remarkable progress, treatment failure due to treatment-related toxicities, which can be life threatening, and drug resistance, which leads to relapse, still occur in about 20% of patients [3], for whom there is a very low likelihood of long-term survival [1,4,5,6].

Genetic polymorphisms in thiopurine-S-methyltransferase (*TPMT*) influence the toxicity of 6-mercaptopurine (6-MP), used as the backbone of the maintenance therapy of ALL, and thus represent one of the best examples of clinically important pharmacogenetic markers [7,8]. Patients on 6-MP therapy exhibiting decreased TPMT activity have been shown to be at greater risk of developing toxic effects, due to undesirably high thioguanine nucleotides (TGN) accumulation in cells [9]. On the other hand, ultra-high enzyme activity can lead to superior 6-MP tolerability but also an increased risk of relapse [10]. Despite the very well characterized influences of genetic polymorphisms on TPMT activity, it is known that there are other genetic and non-genetic factors influencing it. Our previous study in ALL patients revealed that the presence of low-activity methylenetetrahydrofolate reductase (*MTHFR*) alleles contributes to 6-MP toxicity, presumably by limiting S-adenosylmethionine (SAM) synthesis [11]. Further molecular and functional studies carried out *in vitro* on several cancer cell lines have demonstrated that SAM is responsible for direct post-translational TPMT stabilization, resulting in increased TPMT activity [12]. Since folate and methionine pathways are crucial for SAM synthesis, other polymorphisms in enzyme-coding genes (such as 5-methyltetrahydrofolate-homocysteine methyltransferase reductase (*MTRR*), methylenetetrahydrofolate dehydrogenase 1 (*MTHFD1*), betaine homocysteine S-methyltransferase (*BHMT*), and glycine N-methyltransferase (*GNMT*)) could influence TPMT activity and thus affect the safety and efficacy of 6-MP therapy. A recent study in ALL patients conducted by Stocco et al. [13] has shown that genetic variation in *PACSIN2* also influences TPMT activity and is significantly associated with the incidence of 6-MP-related gastrointestinal toxicity [13].

Inosine triphosphate pyrophosphatase (ITPA) is an enzyme involved in 6-MP metabolism whose activity is determined by polymorphisms in the *ITPA* gene and is currently being extensively studied in relation to 6-MP treatment outcome. ITPA catalyses the pyrophosphohydrolysis of inosine triphosphate (ITP) into inosine monophosphate (Figure 1), and prevents the accumulation of potentially toxic compounds, such as ITP and deoxy-ITP or xanthosine triphosphate (XTP), that may be incorporated into RNA and DNA; in this way, it rescues the cell from apoptosis [14]. Although *ITPA* has been linked to 6-MP toxicity, different studies on patients with inflammatory bowel disease, liver transplant recipients and ALL patients showed inconsistent results [7,15,16,17,18,19,20,21,22,23,24]. Two SNPs in the *ITPA* gene, namely a non-synonymous C94A transition and the intronic IVS2+21A>C variant, with a frequency of approximately 6% and 13%, respectively, in Caucasians [25], have been correlated with defective enzyme activity [14,26] leading to a higher risk of myelotoxicity and hepatotoxicity in pediatric ALL patients [7,22,27]. Furthermore, a recent Korean study suggested the *ITPA* 94C>A polymorphism might be associated with survival rate in pediatric ALL patients [21].

Despite intense efforts devoted to precise risk classification, patient characteristics at relapse reveal that more than half of relapsed patients were originally classified as non-high risk [28]. This highlights the need for the identification of additional prognostic markers.

In the present retrospective study we aimed to investigate the association of selected polymorphisms in genes involved in the folate and methionine pathway (*MTHFR* 677C>A, *MTHFR* 1298A>C, *MTRR* 66A>G, *MTHFD1* 1958G>A, *BHMT* 742G>A, *GNMT* 1298C>T), as well as polymorphisms of *PACSIN2* (rs2413739) and *ITPA* (94C>A and IVS2+21A>C), and long-term outcome and relapse rates in pediatric ALL patients undergoing maintenance therapy with 6-MP.

Patients and Methods

Study subjects

ALL patients diagnosed and treated at University Children's Hospital, University Medical Centre, Ljubljana, Slovenia from 1970 to 2006 were identified through the National Cancer Registry. Of 408 registered patients with childhood ALL, adequate documentation and intact genetic material was obtained from 308, which represented the final study group. Ethical approval for this study was obtained from the National Medical Ethics Committee of Slovenia (59/07/10) which waived the need for written informed consent, since the data was collected retrospectively and was analyzed anonymously.

The following therapy protocols were applied: from 1970 to 1983 the USA Pediatric Oncology Group (POG) protocols were used; from 1983 the therapy was changed to the German Berlin-Frankfurt-Muenster (BFM) protocols (BFM-83, -86, -90, -95 and IC2002). Maintenance therapy was included in all protocols and lasted from 1 to 3 years. The maintenance phase consisted of 6-MP taken daily per os (50 mg/m^2) and weekly oral low-dose methotrexate (MTX) (20 mg/m^2).

Patients' characteristics, such as gender, age at diagnosis, therapy protocol and risk group allocation, were obtained from their medical records. Patients were grouped according to age at diagnosis in 4 groups: (a) <1 year, (b) 1–6 years, (c) 6–12 years, and (d)>12 years, and according to treatment protocols to 3 groups: (a) POG protocol, (b) BFM83 or BFM86 protocol, and (c) BFM90, BFM95 or IC BFM2002 protocol.

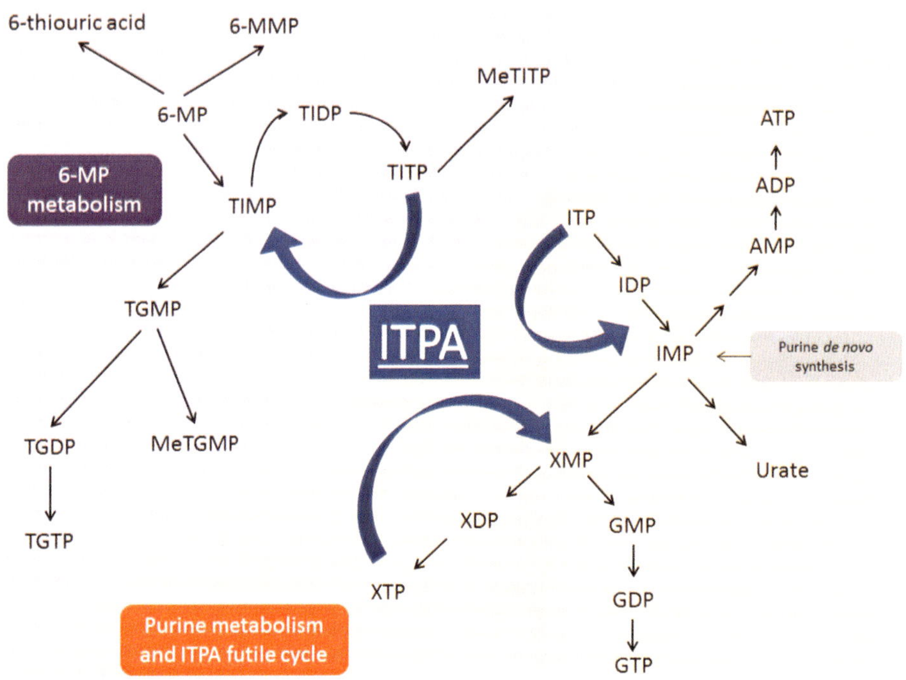

Figure 1. Schematic representation of the *ITPA* involvement in 6-MP metabolism and endogenous purine metabolism. 6-MP, 6-mercaptopurine; 6-MMP, 6-methylmercaptopurine; TIMP, thioinosine monophosphate; TIDP, thioinosine diphosphate; TITP, thioinosine triphosphate; MeTITP, methylthioinosine triphosphate; TGMP, thioguanosine monophosphate; TGDP, thioguanosine diphosphate; TGTP, thioguanosine triphosphate; MeTGMP, methylthioguanosine monophosphate; ITPA, inosine triphosphate pyrophosphatase; IMP, inosine monophosphate; XMP, xanthosine monophosphate; XDP, xanthosine diphosphate; XTP, xanthosine triphosphate; GMP, guanosine monophosphate; GDP, guanosine diphosphate; GTP, guanosine triphosphate; ITP, inosine triphosphate; IDP, inosine diphosphate; AMP, adenosine monophosphate; ADP, adenosine diphosphate; ATP, adenosine triphosphate.

Event and risk group definition

The event in the calculation of event-free survival (EFS) probability was defined as any relapse, death, or secondary malignant neoplasm.

Patients were stratified into risk groups according to criteria described previously [29,30,31,32]. The standard risk group included the low-risk group of POG, SR-L and SR-H groups of BFM-83 and SR groups of protocols BFM-86, -90 and -95. Intermediate or high-risk groups included the high-risk group of POG, R-group of BFM-86, MR groups of BFM-83, -90, -95 and HR groups of BFM-83, -90, -95 protocols.

DNA extraction and genotyping

DNA extraction was performed as previously described [11,33]. All the analyzed polymorphisms were determined by means of TaqMan chemistry using either the ABI Prism 7000 Sequence Detection system or the Roche LightCycler 480 system, in accordance with the manufacturers' instructions. The amount of DNA used in each individual assay was 10 ng. The TaqMan SNP Genotyping Assay part numbers are available in Table S1.

Statistical analysis

The distributions of genotypes and possible deviations from the Hardy-Weinberg equilibrium were assessed by Fisher's exact test. Odds ratios, 95% confidence intervals (95% CI) and P values, showing the association of occurrence of relapse with studied genotypes, were calculated using logistic regression analysis. Covariates considered to be potential confounders, such as gender, age at diagnosis, ALL therapy protocol and risk group, were also placed in the model.

Kaplan-Meier event-free survival curves (EFS) for ALL patients were created, and the survival differences according to different genetic polymorphisms and prognostic variables were analyzed by log-rank test. The starting point for the observation time was date of diagnosis. Multivariate analysis was conducted using the Cox proportional-hazards regression model to analyze predictive factors. Cumulative incidence curves of the different types of relapses were estimated, adjusting for competing risks of the other events, and compared with the Gray's test. In both analyses, the observation time was censored at the last follow-up date if no event was observed.

To explore the independent and synergistic effects of the studied SNPs on the occurrence of relapse we performed a multifactor dimensionality reduction (MDR) analysis [34].

Statistical analyses were performed using R, IBM SPSS for Windows, version 21.0 and MDR software. For all tests, a 2-sided $p<0.05$ was considered statistically significant.

Results

Patients and genotyping

In total, 308 patients with childhood ALL were included in this study. Their clinical characteristics are presented in Table 1.

Genotyping was performed once the clinical data were extracted from patients' medical files and analyzed by researchers who were blinded to patients' medical data. All genotype distributions were in Hardy-Weinberg equilibrium ($p>0.05$). The variant allele frequencies of the analyzed polymorphisms are presented in Table 2 and summary of genotype data provided in Table S2.

Analysis of patient survival and characteristics of relapsed patients

All the included patients were followed up for at least 5 years after diagnosis. The most significant improvement in overall, as well as event-free, survival rate was observed when patients were treated in accordance with later protocols, increasing from 58% (5-year OS) and 43% (5-year EFS) in patients treated by POG protocol to 91% (5-year OS) and 83% (5-year EFS) in patients treated by protocols BFM90/95/2002, as described in Table 3. Overall and event-free survival rates were not different in patients stratified to different risk groups (Table 3).

A total of 102 (33.1%) patients relapsed during the median follow-up time of 155 months, 5 patients (1.6%) died because of therapy-related complications and 6 patients (1.9%) developed secondary malignancy.

Of all relapsed patients, 36 (35.3%) were stratified to a standard risk group and only 21 (20.6%) to an intermediate or high risk group; 45 relapsed patients treated using POG protocols were not allocated to any risk group since stratification according to risk factors was not well established then. Clinical characteristics of relapsed patients are shown in Table 4.

Association of selected genotypes with relapse rate, overall and event-free survival

In search of novel biomarkers for the prediction of long-term outcomes and the occurrence of relapse, we addressed the involvement of selected polymorphisms in genes involved in 6-MP metabolism and folate and methionine pathways.

Multiple logistic regression analysis revealed that among all genes tested, only *ITPA* had a statistically significant effect on the occurrence of relapse, when the model was adjusted to treatment protocol group, age group and gender; namely, that *ITPA* wild-type patients were at higher risk of relapse than patients carrying at least one variant *ITPA* allele (odds ratio (OR) = 1.9; 95% CI = 1.1–3.4; $p = 0.026$).

In the univariate analysis using the Kaplan-Meier curve, the event-free survival (EFS) was affected by treatment protocol group, gender and *ITPA* genotype. EFS was lower in earlier protocols (43% in POG, 63% in BFM83/86 and 83% in BFM90/96/2002, $p<0.001$), in male patients as compared to female patients (60% and 72%, respectively; $p = 0.022$) and in the wild-type *ITPA* patients as compared to variant *ITPA* patients (62% and 74%, respectively; $p = 0.030$) (Figure 2A).

Multivariate analysis conducted with the Cox proportional-hazards regression model adjusted for treatment protocol group, gender and age group confirmed that among the genotypes tested, the *ITPA* 94CC/IVS2+21AA genotype was the only risk factor for lower EFS (HR 1.6, 95% CI 1.0–2.4; $p = 0.033$) (Table 5).

Influence of *ITPA* genotype on the site of relapse

Next, we aimed to explore whether the *ITPA* genotype has different effects in accordance with the relapse site. Patients experiencing relapse were divided into subgroups based on the site of the first relapse; namely, into those experiencing isolated bone marrow relapse (50 patients), combined bone marrow and extramedullary relapse (21 patients) and isolated extramedullary relapse (31 patients). The results of the multinomial logistic regression analysis adjusted to protocol treatment group, age group and gender revealed that wild-type *ITPA* patients were at higher risk of suffering medullary relapse (HR 2.5, 95% CI 1.2–5.2; $p = 0.017$) compared to variant *ITPA* patients, whereas the risk of experiencing a combined or isolated extramedullary relapse was not significantly different in patients with different *ITPA*

Table 1. Clinical characteristics of patients with childhood ALL (N = 308).

Characteristic	No	%
Gender		
Female	143	46.4
Male	165	53.6
Mean age at diagnosis ± standard deviation		5.9±4.3 years
<1 year	10	3.2
1<6 years	192	62.3
6<12 years	68	22.1
>12 years	38	12.3
ALL therapy protocol, n (%)		
POG	92	29.9
BFM 83/BFM 86	89	28.9
BFM 90/BFM 95/IC-BFM 2002	127	41.2
Risk group, n (%)		
Standard risk	134	43.5
Intermediate or high risk	94	30.5
undetermined	80	26

Abbreviations: POG, Pediatric Oncology Group; BFM, Berlin-Frankfurt-Muenster.

genotypes. Furthermore, in competing risk regression analysis the risk of suffering a bone marrow relapse was two times higher for wild-type *ITPA* patients compared to variant *ITPA* patients ($p = 0.040$). The model was adjusted for age, gender and treatment protocol group. The cumulative incidence of bone marrow relapse in wild-type *ITPA* patients was 19.6%, while it was 10.7% in variant *ITPA* patients (Figure 2B).

Influence of the *ITPA* genotypes on the time to relapse

Patients suffering relapse were divided into 3 subgroups in accordance with time to relapse criteria: very early (less than18 months from diagnosis), early (more than 18 months after diagnosis and less than 6 months after the end of treatment) and late relapse (more than 6 months after the end of treatment).

The frequency of *ITPA* wild-type patients was significantly higher in the group of patients suffering early relapse (84%) compared to the group having no relapse (60%), very early relapse (59%) or late relapse (67%) (Fisher's exact test, $p = 0.020$). After adjustment to treatment protocol group, age and gender, the multinomial regression model confirmed that the effect of *ITPA* genotype was significant only for the occurrence of early relapse, such that *ITPA* wild-type patients are at higher risk of experiencing an early relapse than *ITPA* variant patients (HR 3.9, 95% CI 1.6–9.6; $p = 0.003$) (Figure 3).

Table 2. Frequency of the analyzed polymorphisms in patients with childhood ALL.

Gene	Variant	Wild type (N)	Heterozygous (N)	Homozygous variant (N)	Variant allele frequency (%)
TPMT	rs1142345 and rs1800460 (*3A)	290	18	0	3
TPMT	rs1800460 (*3B)	308	0	0	0
TPMT	rs1142345 (*3C)	305	3	0	0
MTHFR	rs1801133 (677C>A)	134	134	40	35
MTHFR	rs1801131 (1298 A>C)	143	131	34	33
MTRR	rs1801394 (66A>G)	59	140	109	58
MTHFD1	rs2236225 (1958G>A)	94	149	65	45
BHMT	rs3733890 (742G>A)	144	122	42	33
GNMT	rs10948059 (1289C>T)	89	139	80	49
PACSIN2	rs2413739[†]	111	139	55	41
ITPA	rs1127354 (94C>A)	268	40	0	6
ITPA	rs7270101 (IVS2+21A>C)	235	68	5	13

[†]PACSIN2 rs2413739 could not be determined in 3 patients.
Abbreviations: TPMT, Thiopurine S-methyltransferase; MTHFR, methylenetetrahydrofolate reductase; MTRR, 5-methyltetrahydrofolate-homocysteine methyltransferase reductase; MTHFD1, methylenetetrahydrofolate dehydrogenase 1; BHMT, betaine—homocysteine S-methyltransferase; GNMT, glycine N-methyltransferase; PACSIN2, protein kinase C and casein kinase substrate in neurons protein; ITPA, Inosine triphosphate pyrophosphatase.

Table 3. Overall and event-free survival rates in patients with childhood ALL, according to treatment protocol and risk group stratification.

	5-year OS/EFS	Log-rank p	10-year OS/EFS	Log-rank p
Overall survival rate ± SE %				
Treatment protocol (n)				
POG (92)	60±5	<0.001	51±5	<0.001
BFM 83/86 (89)	74±5		71±5	
BFM 90/95/2002 (127)	91±2		91±3	
Risk group (n)[1]				
Standard (94)	83±3	0.983	81±3	0.983
Intermediate or high (134)	84±4		80±4	
Event-free survival rate ± SE %				
Treatment protocol (n)				
POG (92)	43±5	<0.001	40±5	<0.001
BFM 83/86 (89)	64±5		61±5	
BFM 90/95/2002 (127)	83±3		82±3	
Risk group (n)[1]				
Standard (94)	72±4	0.645	70±4	0.645
Intermediate or high (134)	76±4		74±5	

[1]Risk group was not determined for 80 patients (those who were treated under POG protocol).
Abbreviations: POG, Pediatric Oncology Group; BFM, Berlin-Frankfurt-Muenster.

Gene-gene interactions

Gene-gene interactions between the variants and event-free survival or relapse were analysed using multifactor dimensionality reduction. There was no statistically significant multi-gene interaction model for event or relapse (data not shown).

Discussion

The remarkable improvements in risk-directed treatments of childhood ALL observed over recent decades have resulted in an impressive increase in long term survival rates, currently approaching 85% in the developed world [35]. In contrast to the steadily improving outcome for patients with newly diagnosed ALL, little progress has been made in the treatment of relapsed ALL patients whose long-term survival rates range only from about 35% to 40% [1,36,37]. Relapse of the disease, therefore, remains a major concern in the treatment of ALL.

Due to the well-known importance of maintenance therapy for event-free and overall survival, this retrospective study, including all patients treated in Slovenia from 1970 to 2006 receiving at least one cycle of maintenance therapy, was conducted. We selected 8 candidate genes and identified 12 polymorphisms that could influence the metabolism of 6-MP, either by being directly involved in the metabolism or indirectly by altering TPMT activity, and evaluated their effects on survival and relapse rates.

We found that the inheritance of at least one of the non-functional *ITPA* alleles (94C>A and/or IVS2+21A>C) is associated with improved event-free survival and lower relapse rates in patients undergoing maintenance treatment for ALL.

ITPA is a human ITPase, a 'house-cleaning' enzyme, which protects cells from endogenous non-canonical nucleotides and, in the case of thiopurine therapy, from exogenous nucleotides, such as thio-ITP and methyl-thio-ITP, derived from thiopurines [38]. One possible explanation for the protective role of non-functional *ITPA* polymorphisms in relation to the relapse of ALL could be that the absence of functional ITPA activity can lead to the accumulation of non-canonical nucleotides that may cause DNA damage; such has also been demonstrated in an *in vitro* study on human HeLa cells with a knockdown *ITPA* gene [39]. Leukaemic blasts of the relapsed disease are more drug-resistant than blasts at initial diagnosis, which is probably the result of drug-resistant subclones being present at diagnosis or developing during therapy through the acquisition of additional genomic lesions [35]. It is possible that the action of 6-MP during the maintenance is partially reversed by the fully functional ITPA activity; this may then lead to the increased survival of leukemic blasts, which can, in turn, progress to relapse of the disease.

A more in-depth analysis of the impact of the *ITPA* genotype on relapse revealed that wild-type *ITPA* patients were at higher risk of suffering early relapse (HR 3.9, 95% CI 1.6–9.6; $p=0.003$), whereas its effect on very early or late relapse was not statistically significant.

A study by Henderson et al. investigating the mechanism of relapse in ALL demonstrated that a shorter time interval to first relapse correlated with a higher quantity of the relapsing clone at diagnosis [40]. It is, therefore, possible that in the event of very early relapse occurring less than 18 months after the diagnosis, the amount of therapy-resistant sub-clones of leukemic blasts is too high for maintenance therapy to be effective in eradicating them. However, since the number of leukemic blasts in early relapse occurring more than 18 months after the diagnosis and less than 6 months after the end of treatment is lower, the influence of the *ITPA* genotype emerges by counteracting the 6-MP action. In the case of the wild-type *ITPA* genotype, the leukemic blasts are better protected against the therapy and are able to survive longer, resulting in a later expansion and onset of the relapse. On the other hand, the influence of the *ITPA* genotype diminishes again in late relapse occurring more than 6 months after the end of treatment. A possible explanation for this could lie in observed differences in gene expression between early and late relapse.

Table 4. Clinical characteristics of relapsed patients (N = 102).

Characteristic	No	%
Gender		
Female	39	38.2
Male	63	61.8
Time to relapse		
Median time (range) 24 (4–163) months		
Very early relapse[1]	32	31.4
Early relapse[2]	43	42.1
Late relapse[3]	27	26.5
Site of first relapse		
Bone marrow	50	49.0
Combined[4]	21	20.6
Isolated EMD[5]	31	30.4
Site of any relapse		
Bone marrow (with or without EMD)	89	87.3
Only isolated EMD[5]	13	12.7
Treatment protocol		
POG	53	52.0
BFM 83/86	30	29.4
BFM 90/95/2002	19	18.6
Initially assigned risk group		
Standard risk	36	35.3
Intermediate or high risk	21	20.6
Undetermined	45	44.1

Abbreviations: POG, Pediatric Oncology Group; BFM, Berlin-Frankfurt-Muenster; EMD, extramedullary disease.
[1]less than18 months from diagnosis.
[2]more than 18 months after diagnosis and less than 6 months after the end of treatment.
[3]more than 6 months after the end of treatment.
[4]Bone marrow with or without extramedullary disease.
[5]CNS/testes/Other (spinal channel, liver, iris, mesenterium, lymph nodes neck, labia major).

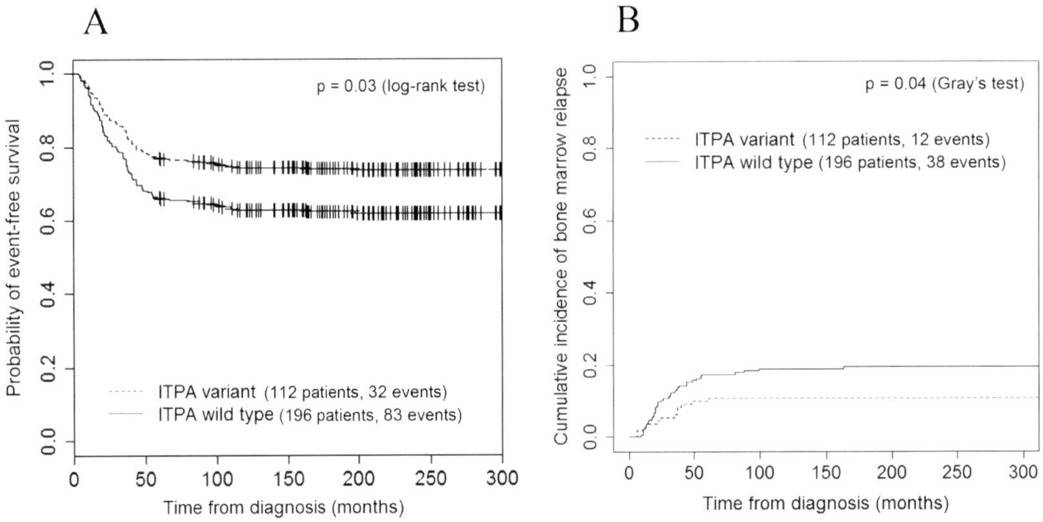

Figure 2. Event-free survival and cumulative incidence of bone marrow relapse by *ITPA* genotype (N = 308). A) *ITPA* wild-type genotype was shown to be an independent risk factor for lower event-free survival rate. 5-year EFS rates were 62% in wild-type patients and 74% in patients with at least 1 variant allele (log-rank test, p = 0.03). **B**) Cumulative incidences of bone marrow relapse in patients with wild-type *ITPA* and patients with at least one variant *ITPA* allele were 19.6% and 10.7%, respectively (Gray's test, p = 0.04).

Table 5. Results of analysis of genotypes' influence on survival rates.

		Univariate		*Multivariate*	
		(Log rank)		**(Cox regression)**	
Genotype (No. of patients)	**No. of events (% patients)**	**5-year EFS (%)**	**p**	**Hazard ratio (95% CI)**	**p**
Overall survival					
ITPA **genotype (94C>A/IVS2+21A>C)**					
CC/AA (196)	59 (30%)	71%	0.164		
at least 1 variant allele[1] (112)	25 (22%)	77%			
Event-free survival					
ITPA **genotype (94C>A/IVS2+21A>C)**					
CC/AA (196)	83 (42%)	62%	**0.030***	1.6 (1.04–2.37)	**0.033***
at least 1 variant allele[1] (112)	32 (29%)	74%			
TPMT **genotype**					
1*/1* (287)	107 (37%)	79%	0.919		
1*/3*[2] (21)	8 (38%)	69%			
MTHFR **genotype (677C>A/1298 A>C)**					
CC/AA (31)	15 (48%)	58%	0.298		
at least 1 variant allele[3] (277)	100 (36%)	67%			
MTRR **66A>G**					
AA (59)	21 (36%)	66%	0.757		
AG/GG (249)	94 (38%)	66%			
MTHFD **1958G>A**					
GG (94)	34 (36%)	68%	0.865		
GA/AA (214)	81 (38%)	65%			
BHMT **742G>A**					
GG (144)	55 (38%)	67%	0.843		
GA/AA (164)	60 (37%)	67%			
GNMT **1298C>T**					
CC (89)	32 (36%)	67%	0.841		
CT/TT (219)	83 (38%)	66%			
PACSIN2 **rs2413739**					
CC (111)	40 (36%)	68%	0.727		
CT/TT (194)	73 (38%)	64%			

*denotes statistically significant difference.
[1]*ITPA* genotype combinations with at least one variant allele (94CA/IVS2+21AA, 94CA/IVS2+21AC, 94CA/IVS2+21CC, 94CC/IVS2+21AC, 94CC/IVS2+21CC).
[2]either a *1/*3A or *1/*3C *TPMT* genotype.
[3]*MTHFR* genotype combinations with at least variant allele (677CC/1298AC, 677CT/1298AA, 677CC/1298CC, 677TT/1298AA, 677CT/1298AC, 677TT/1298AC).
Abbreviations: *TPMT*, Thiopurine S-methyltransferase; *MTHFR*, methylenetetrahydrofolate reductase; *MTRR*, 5-methyltetrahydrofolate-homocysteine methyltransferase reductase; *MTHFD1*, methylenetetrahydrofolate dehydrogenase 1; *BHMT*, betaine–homocysteine S-methyltransferase; *GNMT*, glycine N-methyltransferase; *PACSIN2*, protein kinase C and casein kinase substrate in neurons protein; *ITPA*, Inosine triphosphate pyrophosphatase.

Hogan et al. found that a set of genes involved in nucleotide biosynthesis and folate metabolism were specifically up-regulated in late relapse [41]. Another previous study by Zaza et al. has shown that the down-regulation of genes involved in purine metabolism correlates with the decreased *de novo* purine synthesis in EVT6/RUNX1 ALL and it has been postulated that this accounts for the chemosensitivity of this genetic subtype [42]. Overexpression in the blasts of patients who experience a late relapse offers an explanation for the resistance to antimetabolites and the lack of influence of the *ITPA* genotype in these patients.

The observation that *ITPA* genotype was associated only with bone marrow relapse could be explained by the role of the blood-brain and blood-testes barriers; these protect the leukemic blasts hidden in the CNS or testes (the so-called sanctuary sites) from the action of chemotherapeutics [43] and so the genes involved in the metabolism of anticancer drugs do not play such an important role in extramedullary relapse cases.

Several studies have previously been conducted studying the effects of *ITPA* polymorphisms on treatment outcome in ALL patients [7,21,22,24,25]; however, most of them focused on evaluating the effect of *ITPA* genotype on treatment-related toxicities and only a few on long-term survival. Stocco *et al.* reported that on maintenance therapy dosages, once the adjustment for *TPMT* had been made, the additional influence of *ITPA* genotype on 6-MP toxicity emerged [7]. No effect on long-term survival was seen therein. The effects of the combined *TPMT* and *ITPA* genotype on the mercaptopurine pharmacokinetics were also shown in a study by de Beaumais *et al.* [25]

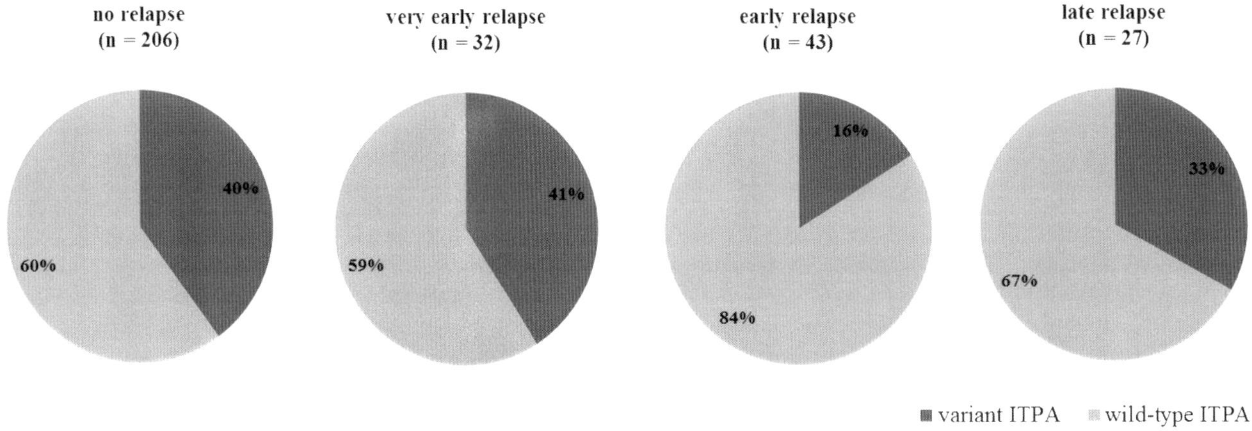

Figure 3. Influence of *ITPA* genotype on the incidence of relapses grouped according to time to relapse. Pie chart slices represent the percent of patients with different *ITPA* genotypes; wild-type *ITPA*: 94CC/IVS2+21AA ITPA genotype combination, variant *ITPA*: 94CA/IVS2+21AA, 94CA/IVS2+21AC, 94CA/IVS2+21CC, 94CC/IVS2+21AC, 94CC/IVS2+21CC ITPA genotype combinations. Very early relapse, <18 months after diagnosis; early relapse,>18 months after diagnosis and <6 months after the end of treatment; late relapse,>6 months after discontinuation of therapy (multinomial regression model adjusted to treatment protocol group, age group at diagnosis and gender; reference category = no relapse; p = 0.003).

Furthermore, a study conducted in Indian ALL patients showed an independent role for both *TPMT* and *ITPA* in terms of association with the incidence of hematological toxicity [24]. The only study that associated *ITPA* genotype with survival rate was that conducted by Kim *et al.* in 100 Korean patients with pediatric ALL. They evaluated 18 loci in 16 candidate genes of pharmacogenetic interest, finding that the *ITPA* genotype, though not *TPMT*, had a significant effect on the event-free survival rate, which was lower in *ITPA* variants [21]. Like Kim *et al.*, we have not seen any effect of the *TPMT* genotype on event-free survival in pediatric ALL patients. However, and in contrast to their study, we found a different effect of the *ITPA* genotype on the event-free survival rate, such that it was lower in wild-type *ITPA* patients. A significant effect was observed most particularly on the occurrence of relapse, with patients carrying at least one *ITPA* variant allele being at lower risk of suffering early and/or bone marrow relapse. One possible explanation for the observed differences may be the fact that the study by Kim *et al.* was evaluating only one of the two non-functional polymorphisms of the *ITPA* gene, which is probably due to ethnic differences in *ITPA* genotype frequencies between Asian and Caucasian populations. Although the *ITPA* 94C>A polymorphism has been more frequently associated with 6-MP related toxicities, we believe that genotyping for *ITPA* IVS2+21A>C is also important due to its higher frequency in Caucasian populations. Indeed, when the two polymorphisms were evaluated independently, no significant correlation with event-free survival and/or relapse rate could be shown in our study. However, since both of these variants lower ITPA activity, we considered it rational to evaluate them together, thus producing only two variables: (a) wild-type *ITPA* and (b) variant *ITPA*. This could also explain why other studies, such as that by Stocco *et al.* evaluating only the *ITPA* 94C>A polymorphism, did not detect a significant effect of the *ITPA* genotype on survival or relapse rate [7]. Furthermore, since no association between *ITPA* genotype and treatment-related toxicity (especially febrile neutropenia) could be observed in the Korean study, they postulated that the lower survival rate in the variant group might not be influenced by accumulated toxic metabolites but by different factors, such as other genetic polymorphisms that were linked with *ITPA* 94C>A [21]. In contrast, our results support the hypothesis that variant *ITPA* alleles potentiate the effects of maintenance therapy by increasing the levels of toxic metabolites such that leukemic blasts are not protected and, therefore, unable to survive the attack of 6-MP. The effect is more pronounced in leukemic blasts in bone marrow and less so in blasts hidden in the sanctuary sites. Unfortunately, this hypothesis cannot be supported by measurements of toxic metabolites levels, since this was a retrospective study.

Our study evaluated a limited number of patients and, although we have taken into account - and adjusted our statistical models to - other factors influencing survival rates (the most important being treatment protocol), the effect of *ITPA* genotype should be evaluated in a larger cohort of patients treated according to the recent treatment protocols. In addition, we would like to point out that our conclusions are drawn from the analysis of DNA samples isolated from archival bone marrow smears prepared at the time of diagnosis of ALL. Since they contained a mixture of cells with different ratios of leukemic blasts and non-leukemic cells, the presence of hyperdiploid blasts and the potentially confounding effect of the acquisition of additional copies of chromosomes containing polymorphic genes on the concordance between the genotype and inherited phenotype could not be taken into account. Furthermore, additional molecular studies should be performed to elucidate the possible role of ITPA in relation to 6-MP therapy for the survival and expansion of leukemic blasts.

In summary, this study of pediatric ALL patients undergoing maintenance therapy shows that the *ITPA* genotype might be associated with event-free survival, with patients carrying at least one non-functional *ITPA* allele having higher event-free survival rates and a lower risk of suffering early and/or bone marrow relapse than wild-type *ITPA* patients.

Supporting Information

Table S1 List of TaqMan assays used for genotyping. Footnotes: Abbreviations: TPMT, Thiopurine S-methyltransferase; MTHFR, methylenetetrahydrofolate reductase; MTRR, 5-methyltetrahydrofolate-homocysteine methyltransferase reductase; MTHFD1, methylenetetrahydrofolate dehydrogenase 1; BHMT, betaine–homocysteine S-methyltransferase; GNMT, glycine N-methyltransferase; PACSIN2, protein kinase C and casein kinase substrate in neurons protein; ITPA, Inosine triphosphate pyrophosphatase.

Table S2 Summary of genotype data of ALL patients analysed in the study. Footnotes: [1] less than 18 months from diagnosis. [2] more than 18 months after diagnosis and less than 6 months after the end of treatment. [3] more than 6 months after the end of treatment. [4] percentage of patients within genotype group. Abbreviations: TPMT, Thiopurine S-methyltransferase; MTHFR, methylenetetrahydrofolate reductase; MTRR, 5-methyltetrahydrofolate-homocysteine methyltransferase reductase; MTHFD1, methylenetetrahydrofolate dehydrogenase 1; BHMT, betaine homocysteine S-methyltransferase; GNMT, glycine N-methyltransferase; PACSIN2, protein kinase C and casein kinase substrate in neurons protein; ITPA, Inosine triphosphate pyrophosphatase.

Acknowledgments

We thank Ms. Klavdija Stare for her dedicated work and Mr. Benedict Dries-Jenkins for proofreading the manuscript.

Author Contributions

Conceived and designed the experiments: IMR AS. Performed the experiments: AS MM. Analyzed the data: AS NKK MM JJ. Contributed reagents/materials/analysis tools: IMR JJ. Wrote the paper: AS IMR.

References

1. Freyer DR, Devidas M, La M, Carroll WL, Gaynon PS, et al. (2011) Postrelapse survival in childhood acute lymphoblastic leukemia is independent of initial treatment intensity: a report from the Children's Oncology Group. Blood 117: 3010–3015.
2. van der Veer A, Waanders E, Pieters R, Willemse ME, Van Reijmersdal SV, et al. (2013) Independent prognostic value of BCR-ABL1-like signature and IKZF1 deletion, but not high CRLF2 expression, in children with B-cell precursor ALL. Blood.
3. Pui CH, Robison LL, Look AT (2008) Acute lymphoblastic leukaemia. Lancet 371: 1030–1043.
4. Malempati S, Gaynon PS, Sather H, La MK, Stork LC (2007) Outcome after relapse among children with standard-risk acute lymphoblastic leukemia: Children's Oncology Group study CCG-1952. J Clin Oncol 25: 5800–5807.
5. Reismuller B, Attarbaschi A, Peters C, Dworzak MN, Potschger U, et al. (2009) Long-term outcome of initially homogenously treated and relapsed childhood acute lymphoblastic leukaemia in Austria a population-based report of the Austrian Berlin-Frankfurt-Munster (BFM) Study Group. Br J Haematol 144: 559–570.
6. Nguyen K, Devidas M, Cheng SC, La M, Raetz EA, et al. (2008) Factors influencing survival after relapse from acute lymphoblastic leukemia: a Children's Oncology Group study. Leukemia 22: 2142–2150.
7. Stocco G, Cheok MH, Crews KR, Dervieux T, French D, et al. (2009) Genetic polymorphism of inosine triphosphate pyrophosphatase is a determinant of mercaptopurine metabolism and toxicity during treatment for acute lymphoblastic leukemia. Clin Pharmacol Ther 85: 164–172.
8. Krynetski EY, Evans WE (1998) Pharmacogenetics of cancer therapy: getting personal. Am J Hum Genet 63: 11–16.
9. Karas-Kuzelicki N, Mlinaric-Rascan I (2009) Individualization of thiopurine therapy: thiopurine S-methyltransferase and beyond. Pharmacogenomics 10: 1309–1322.
10. Schmiegelow K, Forestier E, Kristinsson J, Soderhall S, Vettenranta K, et al. (2009) Thiopurine methyltransferase activity is related to the risk of relapse of childhood acute lymphoblastic leukemia: results from the NOPHO ALL-92 study. Leukemia 23: 557–564.
11. Karas-Kuzelicki N, Jazbec J, Milek M, Mlinaric-Rascan I (2009) Heterozygosity at the TPMT gene locus, augmented by mutated MTHFR gene, predisposes to 6-MP related toxicities in childhood ALL patients. Leukemia 23: 971–974.
12. Milek M, Smid A, Tamm R, Kuzelicki NK, Metspalu A, et al. (2012) Post-translational stabilization of thiopurine S-methyltransferase by S-adenosyl-L-methionine reveals regulation of TPMT*1 and *3C allozymes. Biochem Pharmacol 83: 969–976.
13. Stocco G, Yang W, Crews KR, Thierfelder WE, Decorti G, et al. (2012) PACSIN2 polymorphism influences TPMT activity and mercaptopurine-related gastrointestinal toxicity. Hum Mol Genet 21: 4793–4804.
14. Sumi S, Marinaki AM, Arenas M, Fairbanks L, Shobowale-Bakre M, et al. (2002) Genetic basis of inosine triphosphate pyrophosphohydrolase deficiency. Hum Genet 111: 360–367.
15. Zabala-Fernandez W, Barreiro-de Acosta M, Echarri A, Carpio D, Lorenzo A, et al. (2011) A pharmacogenetics study of TPMT and ITPA genes detects a relationship with side effects and clinical response in patients with inflammatory bowel disease receiving Azathioprine. J Gastrointestin Liver Dis 20: 247–253.
16. Shipkova M, Franz J, Abe M, Klett C, Wieland E, et al. (2011) Association between adverse effects under azathioprine therapy and inosine triphosphate pyrophosphatase activity in patients with chronic inflammatory bowel disease. Ther Drug Monit 33: 321–328.
17. Kim JH, Cheon JH, Hong SS, Eun CS, Byeon JS, et al. (2010) Influences of thiopurine methyltransferase genotype and activity on thiopurine-induced leukopenia in Korean patients with inflammatory bowel disease: a retrospective cohort study. J Clin Gastroenterol 44: e242–248.
18. Jung YS, Cheon JH, Park JJ, Moon CM, Kim ES, et al. (2010) Correlation of genotypes for thiopurine methyltransferase and inosine triphosphate pyrophosphatase with long-term clinical outcomes in Korean patients with inflammatory bowel diseases during treatment with thiopurine drugs. J Hum Genet 55: 121–123.
19. Uchiyama K, Nakamura M, Kubota T, Yamane T, Fujise K, et al. (2009) Thiopurine S-methyltransferase and inosine triphosphate pyrophosphohydrolase genes in Japanese patients with inflammatory bowel disease in whom adverse drug reactions were induced by azathioprine/6-mercaptopurine treatment. J Gastroenterol 44: 197–203.
20. Breen DP, Marinaki AM, Arenas M, Hayes PC (2005) Pharmacogenetic association with adverse drug reactions to azathioprine immunosuppressive therapy following liver transplantation. Liver Transpl 11: 826–833.
21. Kim H, Kang HJ, Kim HJ, Jang MK, Kim NH, et al. (2012) Pharmacogenetic analysis of pediatric patients with acute lymphoblastic leukemia: a possible association between survival rate and ITPA polymorphism. PLoS One 7: e45558.
22. Wan Rosalina WR, Teh LK, Mohamad N, Nasir A, Yusoff R, et al. (2012) Polymorphism of ITPA 94C>A and risk of adverse effects among patients with acute lymphoblastic leukaemia treated with 6-mercaptopurine. J Clin Pharm Ther 37: 237–241.
23. Adam de Beaumais T, Fakhoury M, Medard Y, Azougagh S, Zhang D, et al. (2011) Determinants of mercaptopurine toxicity in paediatric acute lymphoblastic leukemia maintenance therapy. Br J Clin Pharmacol 71: 575–584.
24. Dorababu P, Nagesh N, Linga VG, Gundeti S, Kutala VK, et al. (2012) Epistatic interactions between thiopurine methyltransferase (TPMT) and inosine triphosphate pyrophosphatase (ITPA) variations determine 6-mercaptopurine toxicity in Indian children with acute lymphoblastic leukemia. Eur J Clin Pharmacol 68: 379–387.
25. Adam de Beaumais T, Jacqz-Aigrain E (2012) Pharmacogenetic determinants of mercaptopurine disposition in children with acute lymphoblastic leukemia. Eur J Clin Pharmacol 68: 1233–1242.
26. Heller T, Oellerich M, Armstrong VW, von Ahsen N (2004) Rapid detection of ITPA 94C>A and IVS2 + 21A>C gene mutations by real time fluorescence PCR and in vitro demonstration of effect of ITPA IVS2 + 21A>C polymorphism on splicing efficiency. Clin Chem 50: 2182–2184.
27. Hawwa AF, Millership JS, Collier PS, Vandenbroeck K, McCarthy A, et al. (2008) Pharmacogenomic studies of the anticancer and immunosuppressive thiopurines mercaptopurine and azathioprine. Br J Clin Pharmacol 66: 517–528.
28. Moricke A, Zimmermann M, Reiter A, Henze G, Schrauder A, et al. (2010) Long-term results of five consecutive trials in childhood acute lymphoblastic leukemia performed by the ALL-BFM study group from 1981 to 2000. Leukemia 24: 265–284.
29. Reiter A, Schrappe M, Ludwig WD, Hiddemann W, Sauter S, et al. (1994) Chemotherapy in 998 unselected childhood acute lymphoblastic leukemia patients. Results and conclusions of the multicenter trial ALL-BFM 86. Blood 84: 3122–3133.
30. Schrappe M, Reiter A, Ludwig WD, Harbott J, Zimmermann M, et al. (2000) Improved outcome in childhood acute lymphoblastic leukemia despite reduced use of anthracyclines and cranial radiotherapy: results of trial ALL-BFM 90. German-Austrian-Swiss ALL-BFM Study Group. Blood 95: 3310–3322.
31. Laks D, Longhi F, Wagner MB, Garcia PC (2003) [Survival evaluation of children with acute lymphoblastic leukemia treated with Berlin-Frankfurt-Munich trial]. J Pediatr (Rio J) 79: 149–158.
32. Riehm H, Reiter A, Schrappe M, Berthold F, Dopfer R, et al. (1987) [Corticosteroid-dependent reduction of leukocyte count in blood as a prognostic factor in acute lymphoblastic leukemia in childhood (therapy study ALL-BFM 83)]. Klin Padiatr 199: 151–160.
33. Karas Kuzelicki N, Milek M, Jazbec J, Mlinaric-Rascan I (2009) 5,10-Methylenetetrahydrofolate reductase (MTHFR) low activity genotypes reduce the risk of relapse-related acute lymphoblastic leukemia (ALL). Leuk Res 33: 1344–1348.

34. Hahn LW, Ritchie MD, Moore JH (2003) Multifactor dimensionality reduction software for detecting gene-gene and gene-environment interactions. Bioinformatics 19: 376–382.
35. Bhojwani D, Pui CH (2013) Relapsed childhood acute lymphoblastic leukaemia. Lancet Oncol 14: e205–217.
36. Tallen G, Ratei R, Mann G, Kaspers G, Niggli F, et al. (2010) Long-term outcome in children with relapsed acute lymphoblastic leukemia after time-point and site-of-relapse stratification and intensified short-course multidrug chemotherapy: results of trial ALL-REZ BFM 90. J Clin Oncol 28: 2339–2347.
37. Raetz EA, Bhatla T (2012) Where do we stand in the treatment of relapsed acute lymphoblastic leukemia? Hematology Am Soc Hematol Educ Program 2012: 129–136.
38. Marinaki AM, Ansari A, Duley JA, Arenas M, Sumi S, et al. (2004) Adverse drug reactions to azathioprine therapy are associated with polymorphism in the gene encoding inosine triphosphate pyrophosphatase (ITPase). Pharmacogenetics 14: 181–187.
39. Menezes MR, Waisertreiger IS, Lopez-Bertoni H, Luo X, Pavlov YI (2012) Pivotal role of inosine triphosphate pyrophosphatase in maintaining genome stability and the prevention of apoptosis in human cells. PLoS One 7: e32313.
40. Henderson MJ, Choi S, Beesley AH, Sutton R, Venn NC, et al. (2008) Mechanism of relapse in pediatric acute lymphoblastic leukemia. Cell Cycle 7: 1315–1320. Epub 2008 Feb 1329.
41. Hogan LE, Meyer JA, Yang J, Wang J, Wong N, et al. (2011) Integrated genomic analysis of relapsed childhood acute lymphoblastic leukemia reveals therapeutic strategies. Blood 118: 5218–5226.
42. Zaza G, Yang W, Kager L, Cheok M, Downing J, et al. (2004) Acute lymphoblastic leukemia with TEL-AML1 fusion has lower expression of genes involved in purine metabolism and lower de novo purine synthesis. Blood 104: 1435–1441.
43. Buhrer C, Hartmann R, Fengler R, Dopfer R, Gadner H, et al. (1993) Superior prognosis in combined compared to isolated bone marrow relapses in salvage therapy of childhood acute lymphoblastic leukemia. Med Pediatr Oncol 21: 470–476.

NIAM-Deficient Mice Are Predisposed to the Development of Proliferative Lesions including B-Cell Lymphomas

Sara M. Reed[1,2], Jussara Hagen[1], Viviane P. Muniz[1,3], Timothy R. Rosean[4], Nick Borcherding[5], Sebastian Sciegienka[1], J. Adam Goeken[5], Paul W. Naumann[5], Weizhou Zhang[4,5], Van S. Tompkins[5], Siegfried Janz[4,5], David K. Meyerholz[5], Dawn E. Quelle[1,2,3,5]*

1 Department of Pharmacology, University of Iowa, Iowa City, Iowa, United States of America, **2** Medical Scientist Training Program, University of Iowa, Iowa City, Iowa, United States of America, **3** Molecular and Cellular Biology Program, University of Iowa, Iowa City, Iowa, United States of America, **4** Interdisciplinary Program in Immunology, University of Iowa, Iowa City, Iowa, United States of America, **5** Department of Pathology, University of Iowa, Iowa City, Iowa, United States of America

Abstract

Nuclear Interactor of ARF and Mdm2 (NIAM, gene designation *Tbrg1*) is a largely unstudied inhibitor of cell proliferation that helps maintain chromosomal stability. It is a novel activator of the ARF-Mdm2-Tip60-p53 tumor suppressor pathway as well as other undefined pathways important for genome maintenance. To examine its predicted role as a tumor suppressor, we generated *NIAM* mutant (*NIAM*$^{m/m}$) mice homozygous for a β-galactosidase expressing gene-trap cassette in the endogenous gene. The mutant mice expressed significantly lower levels of NIAM protein in tissues compared to wild-type animals. Fifty percent of aged *NIAM* deficient mice (14 to 21 months) developed proliferative lesions, including a uterine hemangioma, pulmonary papillary adenoma, and a Harderian gland adenoma. No age-matched wild-type or *NIAM*$^{+/m}$ heterozygous animals developed lesions. In the spleen, *NIAM*$^{m/m}$ mice had prominent white pulp expansion which correlated with enhanced increased reactive lymphoid hyperplasia and evidence of systemic inflammation. Notably, 17% of *NIAM* mutant mice had splenic white pulp features indicating early B-cell lymphoma. This correlated with selective expansion of marginal zone B cells in the spleens of younger, tumor-free *NIAM*-deficient mice. Unexpectedly, basal p53 expression and activity was largely unaffected by NIAM loss in isolated splenic B cells. In sum, *NIAM* down-regulation *in vivo* results in a significant predisposition to developing benign tumors or early stage cancers. These mice represent an outstanding platform for dissecting NIAM's role in tumorigenesis and various anti-cancer pathways, including p53 signaling.

Editor: Sumitra Deb, Virginia Commonwealth University, United States of America

Funding: This work was supported by the NIH through a pre-doctoral fellowship 5F30CA165736 (S.M.R.), pre-doctoral training grant 5T32AI007485 (T.R.R.), NCI Core Grant P30CA086862 in support of the University of Iowa Holden Comprehensive Cancer Center, and R01CA151354 (S.J.), as well as an Oberley Award through the Holden Comprehensive Cancer Center (S.J. and D.E.Q). The funders had no role in study design, data collection and analysis, decision to publish or preparation of the manuscript.

Competing Interests: The authors have declared that no competing interests exist.

* Email: dawn-quelle@uiowa.edu

Introduction

The p53 tumor suppressor forms the core of an extensive signaling network that protects cells against genomic instability and neoplastic transformation in response to genotoxic insults [1–3]. Once activated, p53 transactivates or represses a wide array of genes that cause cell cycle arrest, promote DNA repair, restrict metabolism or kill irreparably damaged cells, among other anti-cancer activities [4]. Loss of p53 function occurs in the vast majority of human cancers, if not all, due to *TP53* gene mutation or alteration of its many regulators and targets [2,5]. Mouse models that lack p53 or express naturally occurring p53 mutants are highly tumor prone and develop the broad range of malignancies found in humans with impaired p53 signaling [6–8]. Understanding how p53 activity is controlled, and the importance of its regulators in tumor biology, has been a top priority in cancer research for more than two decades [1–3,9].

NIAM (Nuclear Interactor of ARF and Mdm2, also called *Tbrg1*) is a new p53 regulator and anti-proliferative factor whose role in cancer is not yet defined [10–13]. Mechanistically, it engages the p53 pathway at multiple levels. First, NIAM promotes the relocalization of ARF (Alternative Reading Frame protein), a major activator of p53 [14], from nucleoli into the nucleoplasm where it is more effective at activating p53 [10,15,16]. Second, NIAM binds to Mdm2, the primary antagonist of p53 [17], and reduces the formation of p53-Mdm2 complexes [10,12]. As such, NIAM impairs Mdm2-mediated polyubiquitylation and proteasomal degradation of p53, thereby stabilizing and activating p53 signaling [12]. Third, NIAM is a chromatin-bound protein that associates with the histone acetyltransferase, Tip60 (Tat-interacting protein of 60 kDa) [12], which is essential for p53-dependent cell cycle arrest and death [18–20]. Tip60 knockdown studies demonstrated that it contributes to NIAM-mediated p53

Table 1. Reduced *NIAM* mRNA levels in cancer tissues.

Tumor Type	No. of Studies*	References
Brain	9	[63–67]
B-cell Lymphoma	7	[33–37]
Lung	2	[68]
Breast	10	[69–71]
Prostate	2	[72]

*Microarray analyses identified through ONCOMINE showing a statistically significant decrease in *NIAM* mRNA in tumors. ($p<0.05$).

activation, revealing that NIAM induces p53 activity through multiple mechanisms involving Tip60 association as well as Mdm2 inhibition [12]. Notably, like p53 and Tip60, NIAM is normally kept at low expression levels in cells by Mdm2-dependent ubiquitylation [10].

The interplay of NIAM with p53 and its established partners (ARF, Mdm2 and Tip60), all of which are frequently disrupted in human cancers [3,14,17,21,22], suggests NIAM may have tumor suppressive activity. That idea is supported by *in silico* evidence from microarray databases suggesting significant down-regulation of NIAM mRNA levels in many advanced human cancers [23,24]. Interestingly, NIAM can act independently of ARF-Mdm2-p53 signaling. It can inhibit proliferation in cells lacking ARF, Mdm2 and/or p53, and its depletion in *ARF/Mdm2/p53*-null mouse embryo fibroblasts results in chromosomal instability [10]. These findings imply that NIAM plays an important role in other anti-cancer pathways outside of the ARF-Mdm2-p53 tumor suppressor pathway.

Here, we describe the generation and initial characterization of the first *NIAM* mutant mouse model. These animals have hypomorphic *NIAM* alleles that result in greatly impaired expression of NIAM protein in tissues, similar to what may occur in human malignancies in which its mRNA expression is down-regulated. Spontaneous tumor formation was assessed and NIAM down-regulation found to increase tumor susceptibility in aged animals. B-cell lymphoma was among the tumors identified and this correlated with a marked expansion of splenic marginal zone B cells in young, tumor-free *NIAM*-deficient mice. Interestingly, p53 inactivation in B cells promotes splenic marginal zone B cell expansion and B-cell lymphoma [25,26], implicating impaired p53 function in the *NIAM* knockout phenotype. At least under non-stressed conditions, however, splenic B cells from young *NIAM*-deficient mice showed no significant effect on basal p53 activity. We suggest that the *NIAM* mutant mice described in this study represent a unique model of B-cell lymphoma that should help resolve NIAM's biological role in p53 signaling and other cancer pathways.

Results

Decreased NIAM mRNA expression in human tumors

It is well established that ARF-Mdm2-Tip60-p53 signaling plays a dominant role in carcinogenesis [1–3,17,21,27]. Since NIAM has important roles in regulating this pathway, we probed various online databases for the most recent information on *NIAM* alterations in human cancers. A previous analysis of the ONCOMINE microarray database in 2007 suggested that *NIAM* mRNA expression is down-regulated in multiple advanced human cancers [10]. The addition of large amounts of microarray results to ONCOMINE since that time only strengthens that conclusion, once again suggesting significant reduction of *NIAM* mRNA levels in many cancers including lung, breast, brain, prostate, and B-cell lymphoma (**Table 1**). Recent RNA sequencing data from The Cancer Genome Atlas (TCGA) project is now available for certain cancers and verifies that there is a marked decrease in *NIAM* (gene name *Tbrg1*) mRNA levels in human lung, liver, bladder, and breast cancers as compared to paired, normal tissues (**Fig. 1**). These data demonstrate that *NIAM* expression is reduced in many different types of human malignancies, consistent with the prediction that it plays an important role in inhibiting tumorigenesis.

Generation of NIAM-deficient mice

A *NIAM* gene targeting construct was inserted between exon 1 (which contains the ATG start site) and exon 2 in C57BL/6N embryonic stem cells by the Knockout Mouse Project (KOMP) (**Fig. 2A**). The cassette contains a poly (A) adenylation site, a neomycin resistance gene (Neo), and β-galactosidase trap for tracking normal *NIAM* expression patterns in tissues. It also contains FRT sites for removal of neomycin and β-galactosidase cassettes by flippase, which would restore normal gene function of *NIAM*. Two intronic LoxP sites enable conditional deletion of exon 2 using Cre-expressing mice should the cassette not lead to sufficient loss of the *NIAM* gene. This construct is predicted to interfere with splicing or, at minimum, generate a severely

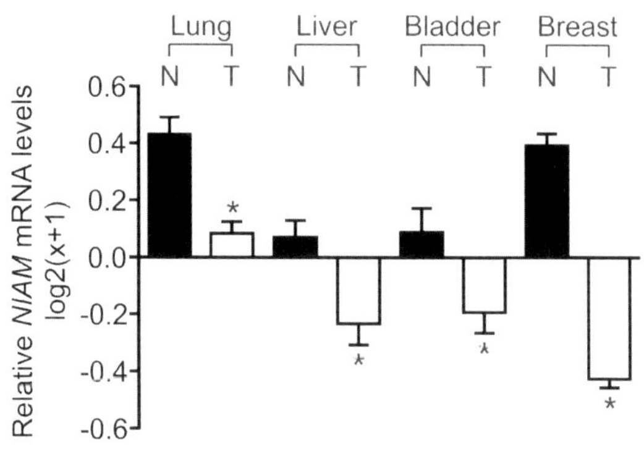

Figure 1. *NIAM* mRNA expression is downregulated in multiple human cancers. *NIAM* mRNA levels are significantly reduced in primary tumor (T) samples relative to normal (N) tissue, according to RNA-seq data obtained from the TCGA project database. The number of samples analyzed for each tissue was as follows: lung (N = 58, T = 488), liver (N = 50, T = 147), bladder (N = 19, T = 211), and breast (N = 108, T = 992). Error bars represent a 95% CI as calculated using the standard error, and an unpaired Welch's T-test was used to calculate statistical significance (*, $p<0.0001$).

truncated chimeric protein containing only 48 N-terminal residues of NIAM.

We obtained chimeric mice expressing the mutant (m) *NIAM* allele from KOMP and generated NIAM heterozygous (+/m) mice by crossing them to C57BL/6N breeders. After obtaining germline transmission, we interbred heterozygous mice to obtain homozygous offspring (m/m) (**Fig. 2B**). Heterozygous mouse matings (n = 31) produced litter sizes between 1 to 9 pups (avg = 5.58). The genotype (+/+, +/m, m/m) was determined for 173 mice and the expected Mendelian ratios of 1:2:1 were not met ($p = 0.0035$, using the χ^2-test) (**Fig. 2C**). The number of heterozygous $NIAM^{+/m}$ and homozygous $NIAM^{m/m}$ mice was higher than expected, possibly suggesting that *NIAM* loss may provide a selective advantage during embryogenesis. The $NIAM^{m/m}$ mice also successfully mated and produced offspring demonstrating no crucial effects of NIAM on fertility and viability.

To determine if the gene-trap cassette effectively interfered with *NIAM* expression, mouse tissues from each genotype were obtained and assessed for levels of NIAM protein. NIAM expression was greatly diminished although some level of expression remained in all $NIAM^{m/m}$ mouse tissues examined, demonstrating that these animals have hypomorphic *NIAM* alleles (**Fig. 3**). Effective down-regulation of NIAM expression was observed in the bladder, lung, pancreas and spleen of homozygous m/m mice. By comparison, protein extracts from the brain (**Fig 3**) and testes (not shown) of the $NIAM^{m/m}$ mice showed decreased yet substantial remaining expression of NIAM as compared to wild-type mice. Interestingly, many bands for NIAM protein were detected in some tissues, such as brain, consistent with database predictions for the existence of numerous alternative transcripts of *NIAM*. Tissues were also examined for expression of p53, Mdm2 and p21. NIAM would be predicted to reduce their levels; however, we did not expect to detect significant changes in their expression since p53 signaling is generally kept off in normal tissues under non-stressed conditions. Indeed, basal expression of all three factors was low, and in some cases undetectable, in whole tissue lysates with no consistent differences observed between $NIAM^{m/m}$ and wild-type mice (data not shown). Immunohistochemical analyses of tissues to identify cell-specific changes in naïve versus stressed mice exposed to p53 activating stimuli (e.g., irradiation) should more effectively reveal effects of NIAM down-regulation on the p53 pathway *in vivo*. Overall, a significant decrease in NIAM expression was observed in $NIAM^{+/m}$ and $NIAM^{m/m}$ mice relative to wild-type controls, indicating these animals are a useful model for examining the biological effects of reduced NIAM expression *in vivo*.

Loss of NIAM *in vivo* promotes spontaneous tumor formation

$NIAM^{m/m}$ mice grow to adulthood and normal size, are fertile, and are externally indistinguishable from wild-type mice. Moreover, full pathological examination of young *NIAM* mutant animals at approximately 8 weeks of age showed no apparent tissue abnormalities, suggesting that tissue development is unaffected by *NIAM* deficiency. However, NIAM carries out a variety of anti-cancer activities in cultured cells [10,12] and our database analyses (**Table 1** and **Fig. 1**) indicate its expression is down-regulated in many human cancers, suggesting it may normally prevent tumor development. Thus, we assessed aged mice of all three *NIAM* genotypes for spontaneous tumorigenesis. As shown in **Table 2**, 50% of $NIAM^{m/m}$ mice developed a neoplastic lesion whereas no wild-type and heterozygous mice of similar age showed obvious signs of tumorigenesis ($p = 0.0025$, Fisher's exact test). The $NIAM^{m/m}$ mice developed different types of benign tumors including a uterine hemangioma (**Fig. 4A**), an early lung papillary adenoma (**Fig. 4B**), and a Harderian gland adenoma (**Fig. 4C**). In addition, a focus of cellular alteration (FCA) was seen in the liver of one $NIAM^{m/m}$ mouse (**Fig. 4D**), a precancerous lesion seen in other mouse models [28]. These histopathological findings suggest that NIAM normally suppresses neoplasia.

Inflammation and early B-cell lymphoma develop in $NIAM^{m/m}$ mice

A prominent finding within the cohort was the pathological changes in the spleens of older *NIAM* mutant mice, which were significantly increased in size compared to wild-type and heterozygous mouse spleens ($p < 0.05$) (**Fig. 5A**). Hematoxylin and Eosin (H&E) staining showed that NIAM deficiency led to a significant expansion of the splenic white pulp compared to control age matched cohorts (**Fig. 5B, C**). These white pulp changes in $NIAM^{m/m}$ mice were often due to reactive hyperplasia. This, along with perivascular lymphoid aggregates in various visceral organ, was consistent with systemic inflammation in mice [29]. In addition, one $NIAM^{m/m}$ mouse had severe diffuse eosinophilic crystalline pneumonia (ECP) whereas only one control had minor localized ECP disease (**Fig. 5D**). ECP may be seen in certain strains of mice including those with immunodeficiency and Th2 prone inflammatory environments [30,31]. Altogether, these data suggest that NIAM mutant mice have a

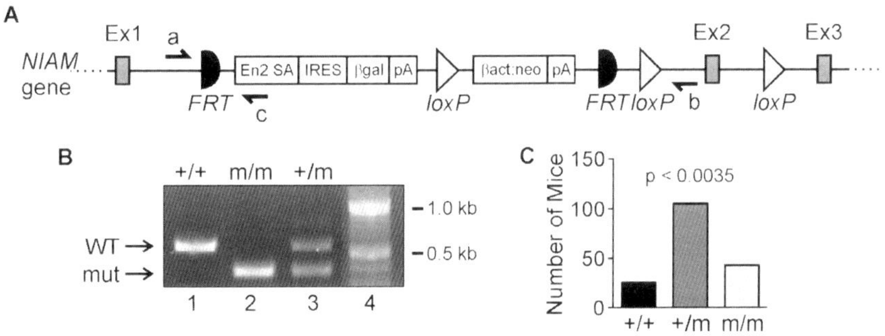

Figure 2. Generating and verifying *NIAM* gene disruption in mice. A. The targeted *NIAM* gene locus for the conditional-ready mouse knockout model. Cre-recombinase LoxP sites and Flippase targeted FRT sites are shown, as are locations for the PCR primers to detect the endogenous *NIAM* allele (a+b) or the mutant allele (a+c). Ex, exon. **B.** PCR amplification of the mutant (mut) allele results in a 380 bp product whereas the 548 bp product reflects the wild-type (WT) *NIAM* allele. DNA standards are shown in lane 4. **C.** Number of mice with each genotype (+/+, +/m, m/m) from heterozygous mouse crossings. Chi-square analysis shows a statistically significant difference from the Mendelian distribution of 1:2:1.

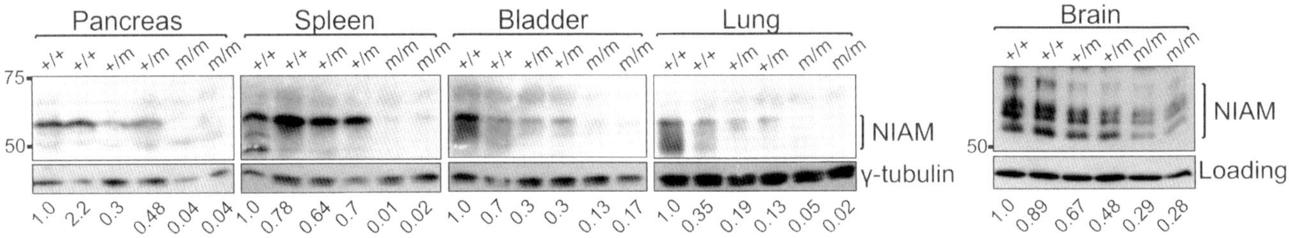

Figure 3. NIAM protein expression in tissues of *NIAM* mutant mice. NIAM protein levels were assessed in mouse tissues from two mice of each genotype (+/+, +/m, m/m). Equivalent amounts of protein lysates from spleen, bladder, lung, brain, and pancreas were analyzed by immunoblotting with antibodies to NIAM and γ-tubulin. The relative expression of NIAM in each sample, as compared to the first wild-type (+/+) sample in each tissue set, is denoted below the lanes. Relative NIAM levels were determined by Image J analysis of band intensities followed by normalization of those values to quantified intensities of the loading control (γ-tubulin or the non-specific band in brain lysates) in each sample.

proinflammatory phenotype. Additionally, two of the twelve (17%) $NIAM^{m/m}$ mice developed early B-cell lymphoma. Their spleens had multifocal loss of the white pulp architecture (e.g. small lymphocytes, germinal centers and tingible body macrophages) with replacement by highly mitotic centrocytic and centroblastic cells (**Fig. 5E**) [32]. When considered with the development of various benign neoplasms in other $NIAM^{m/m}$ animals, these results indicate that NIAM expression is required to prevent spontaneous tumorigenesis.

Marginal zone B cells are increased in $NIAM^{m/m}$ mice

Since aged $NIAM^{m/m}$ mice have enlarged spleens and some develop B-cell lymphoma, we evaluated B cell development in younger, tumor-free mice (6 months of age, 3 of each *NIAM* genotype) to identify potential pre-malignant changes that could give rise to B-cell tumors. Analysis of B cell development in the bone marrow of $NIAM^{m/m}$ mice revealed no alterations compared to wild-type control animals (**Fig. S1**). Specifically, there were no significant differences in the frequency of pro/pre (B220+IgM-, $p = 0.4783$), immature (B220+IgM+, $p = 0.7693$) or mature ($B220^{hi}IgM+$, $p = 0.8048$) B cells. Analysis of B cells from the spleen likewise showed no difference in the frequency of transitional ($CD21^{lo}$/CD23-) or follicular (CD21+/CD23+) B cells (**Fig. 6A, B**; p values of 0.5068 and 0.9325, respectively). In contrast, splenic marginal zone B cells ($CD21^{hi}$/CD23-) were significantly increased in frequency ($p = 0.0281$) and number ($p = 0.0144$) in $NIAM^{m/m}$ mice compared to wild-type controls (**Fig. 6**). These results uncover a specific sensitivity of splenic marginal zone B cells to NIAM loss, which may suggest that NIAM normally restricts their proliferation.

Selective expansion of splenic marginal zone B cells also occurs in mice with conditional inactivation of p53 in B cells and it is associated with their development of B-cell lymphomas [25,26]. Since NIAM is a positive regulator of p53 expression and transcriptional activation [12], and some NIAM mice developed B-cell lymphoma, we wondered if the B cell phenotype in $NIAM^{m/m}$ mice could be associated with reduced p53 signaling. Therefore, we examined p53 status in LPS-stimulated splenic B cells isolated from five wild-type $NIAM^{+/+}$ and five mutant $NIAM^{m/m}$ mice. Western analyses showed complete NIAM loss in $NIAM^{m/m}$ cells compared to wild-type B cells (**Fig. 7**). We expected NIAM loss would reduce p53 levels and activity, but surprisingly it had no effect on basal expression of p53 or its targets, Mdm2 and p21, in the B cells of most $NIAM^{m/m}$ mice (4 of 5) relative to NIAM-positive B cells (**Fig. 7**, set A). These results were seen in B cells isolated from both 8 week and 6 month old mice, suggesting the marginal zone B cell expansion in 6 month old *NIAM* mutant mice is likely independent of p53. Notably, one *NIAM* mutant mouse had decreased B cell expression of p53 although this did not correlate with reduced expression of Mdm2 or p21, at least under these stress-free conditions (**Fig. 7**, set B). These analyses show that NIAM is not required for basal p53 activity in splenic B cells but may, depending on the context, predispose to p53 down-regulation. Additional studies examining p53 stimulation and checkpoint activation following DNA damage or other genotoxic insults in *NIAM*-deficient B cells are warranted.

Discussion

This study is the first investigation of NIAM function *in vivo* using newly generated *NIAM*-deficient mice. A tumor suppressor role for NIAM was anticipated given its ability to activate p53 and other currently undefined anti-cancer pathways involved in growth inhibition and genome maintenance [10,12]. Consistent with that prediction, reduced NIAM expression in mice yielded a tumor phenotype characterized by the development of both benign and cancerous lesions, including early B-cell lymphoma. No neoplasms developed in similarly aged heterozygote or wild-type controls, strongly suggesting that tumor formation was due to

Table 2. Neoplastic lesions in *NIAM*-deficient mice.

Genotype	Avg. Age at Necropsy (weeks)	# of mice with Neoplasms*	Types of neoplasms
$NIAM^{+/+}$	68.2	0/8	-
$NIAM^{+/m}$	68.5	0/8	-
$NIAM^{m/m}$	66	6/12	Early B-cell lymphoma (2) Uterine hemangioma (1) Preputial gland cyst (1) Harderian gland adenoma (1) Lung adenoma (1)

*, $p < 0.0025$ by Fisher's Exact Test between control ($NIAM^{+/+}$ and $NIAM^{+/m}$) mice and $NIAM^{m/m}$ mice.

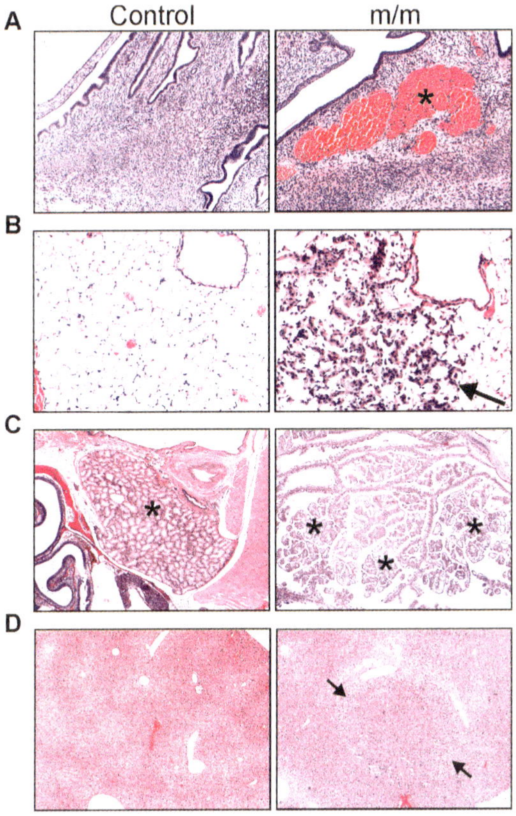

Figure 4. *NIAM*$^{m/m}$ mice are predisposed to proliferative lesions. Histopathologic analyses of multiple mouse tissues. **A**. A hemangioma (asterisk, right panel) found in the uterus of a *NIAM*$^{m/m}$ mouse compared to normal uterine tissue (left panel). (H&E, 100x) **B**. Pulmonary papillary adenoma in a homozygous *NIAM*$^{m/m}$ mouse (arrow, right panel). A depiction of normal lung tissue from a control mouse is shown (left panel). (H&E, 20x) **C**. Harderian gland adenoma of a *NIAM*$^{m/m}$ mouse (asterisks, right panel). A representative image of a normal Harderian gland (asterisk) from a control mouse is depicted (left panel). (H&E, 40x) **D**. A representative image of a normal liver from a control mouse (left panel) versus a focus of cellular alteration (arrows) in a *NIAM*$^{m/m}$ mouse (right panel). (H&E, 40x) Controls represent tissues from similarly aged wild-type (panels B and C) and *NIAM*$^{+/m}$ heterozygous (panels A and D) mice, which were found to be indistinguishable in our analyses.

NIAM loss. It is noteworthy that systemic inflammation was seen in multiple mice as that often precedes tumorigenesis. Although mice from each genotype (+/+, +/m, m/m) in our cohort showed signs of heightened inflammation, only the *NIAM*$^{m/m}$ animals develop lesions. Thus, it is possible that reduced NIAM expression may accelerate or exacerbate the tumor promoting effects of a chronic inflammatory response.

The development of B-cell lymphoma in *NIAM*$^{m/m}$ mice is consistent with several observations. First, microarray analyses suggest that *NIAM* mRNA levels are significantly reduced in human B-cell lymphomas [33–37]. Second, NIAM's functional partners, ARF, Mdm2, and p53 each play a critical role in that disease. ARF and p53 are commonly inactivated whereas Mdm2 is overexpressed in a majority of B-cell lymphomas in patients [38–40], and genetically engineered mice that mimic those alterations effectively model the disease [41–43]. Finally, NIAM is a growth inhibitor whose activation of p53 in cultured cells results in induction of *p21* (*CDKN1A/Waf1/Cip1*) [10,12], a key transcriptional target of p53 [44,45]. Others previously showed that a significant fraction (14%) of tumors that develop in *p21* knockout mice are B-cell lymphomas [46], which is similar in incidence (17%) to the B-cell lymphomas arising in *NIAM*$^{m/m}$ mice.

Our data show that NIAM contributes to tumor suppression but to a lesser extent than p53 or ARF. Half of *NIAM*$^{m/m}$ mice developed benign and early cancerous lesions at an average age of 16.5 months (66 weeks). By comparison, mice lacking p53 in all tissues develop a range of malignancies (mainly T-cell lymphomas and sarcomas) with full penetrance at approximately 5 months of age [6,7]. Less pronounced *in vivo* effects are observed for disruption of p53 regulators and targets relative to loss of p53 itself [2]. For example, animals lacking ARF, a major positive regulator of p53, develop tumors at a slower rate (~10 months average age) than *p53*-null mice [47,48]. Among p53 targets, loss of *PUMA* causes no increased susceptibility to tumorigenesis [49] while deletion of *p21* yields a moderate tumor phenotype [46]. Specifically, *p21*-null animals develop tumors at an average age of 16 months and with reduced incidence (27% in females, 55% in males) compared to mice lacking *p53*. Thus, a milder tumor phenotype for *NIAM*$^{m/m}$ mice is not surprising since it represents just one of many p53 regulators [1,3].

We currently know very little about the normal physiological or pathological signals that control NIAM expression and where its function is required. The expression of β-galactosidase in these mutant mice will provide an excellent surrogate for tracking normal patterns of NIAM expression during development, in particular tissue and cell types, and in response to different stimuli. The interplay between NIAM, p53, and ARF, as well as NIAM's regulation of p21 expression, may be instructive. For instance, loss of each factor (p53, ARF, or p21) is associated with impaired stem cell maintenance and renewal for a variety of cellular lineages, including hematopoietic and neuronal cells, suggesting a possible contribution by NIAM to those processes and cell types [50–52]. Similarly, one of the most significant cellular stresses that stimulate p53 activity is DNA damage [1]. We recently found that treatment of MCF10A mammary epithelial cells causes NIAM protein upregulation (**Fig. S2**), implying a role for NIAM in the DNA damage response. The importance of NIAM to p53 activation and maintenance of DNA integrity in different tissues in response to DNA damage or other diverse stimuli may now be evaluated in an *in vivo* context.

A link between *NIAM* and *p53* in B cell development and lymphoma was strongly suggested by findings that mice lacking those genes each display splenic marginal zone B cell expansion and B-cell lymphoma ([25,26] and this study). Yet NIAM loss had minimal effects on basal p53 expression and activity in B cells from young animals, with just one of five *NIAM*$^{m/m}$ mice displaying lower p53 levels. That unexpected result suggests the splenic marginal zone B cell enrichment in young *NIAM*$^{m/m}$ mice is independent of p53. However, it remains to be determined if p53 function in response to DNA damage or other cellular stresses is diminished in *NIAM*$^{m/m}$ cells and contributes to tumor development in older animals. Indeed, it is conceivable that lower basal p53 expression in splenic B cells observed in some *NIAM*$^{m/m}$ mice impairs stress-induced p53 signaling and checkpoint activation, ultimately fostering B-cell lymphomagenesis in aging mice. Future studies will assess that possibility.

Crosses between *NIAM* mutant mice with other genetic models of cancer will be instrumental in determining NIAM's contribution to p53 signaling as well as other cancer pathways. In that regard, *in vivo* studies should help resolve the biological relevance of NIAM's association with the ARF tumor suppressor [10–12]. Initial studies showed NIAM is capable of mobilizing ARF into the nucleoplasm [10], where ARF is known to more effectively bind

Mdm2 and activate p53 [15,16], yet NIAM and ARF can nonetheless act independent of each other to transiently activate p53 [10,12]. It is possible that NIAM's inhibition of Mdm2 and association with Tip60 may help sustain ARF-p53 signaling and promote senescence in cells following DNA damage or oncogene activation. If so, this would represent an important anti-cancer function since p53-mediated cellular senescence (induced by ARF or other mechanisms) is thought to play a pivotal role in tumor suppression [53–56].

Earlier work on NIAM and much of this Discussion has revolved around the idea that NIAM would prevent tumorigenesis, at least in part, through its effects on p53. However, it is likely that NIAM has significant anti-cancer functions *in vivo* that are independent of p53. One reason is that NIAM can inhibit proliferation and promote chromosomal stability independent of ARF, Mdm2, and p53, indicating it acts in other important pathways relevant to maintaining genomic stability [10]. Moreover, in this study basal p53 expression in splenic B cells was unchanged by NIAM loss in most animals. One factor besides p53 that could contribute to the tumor phenotype in $NIAM^{m/m}$ mice is transforming growth factor beta 1 (TGF-β1). *NIAM* was originally identified as a TGF-β1 responsive gene [13] and we previously found it is induced in TGF-β1-arrested cells [10]. TGF-β1 is a potent inhibitor of proliferation in many cell types (epithelial, endothelial, hematopoietic, etc), but alterations of its signaling components in neoplastic cells ultimately causes it to drive proliferation and cancer progression [57,58]. If NIAM is an effector of TGF-β signaling, its down-regulation in $NIAM^{m/m}$ mice may diminish the anti-proliferative activities of the pathway and consequently enhance its tumor-promoting effects.

Another factor of interest is the nuclear transcription factor, NF-kappa B. NF-κB was originally identified in B cells, contributes to marginal zone B cell formation, and is often constitutively activated in numerous inflammatory conditions and human cancers, including B cell lymphomas [59,60]. NF-κB is activated by a multitude of stimuli and cross-talks with many essential molecules (e.g., p53 and STAT3) and complex signaling pathways (including TGF-β) that control inflammation, cell survival and cell proliferation, among other key biological processes. The enrichment of marginal zone B cells as well as progressive expansion of splenic white pulp and development of B-cell lymphomas in *NIAM* mutant mice supports the prediction that NF-κB signaling may be hyper-activated when NIAM is down-regulated.

Overall, our data show that *NIAM* deficiency is associated with a proinflammatory phenotype and facilitates spontaneous tumorigenesis. Based on the literature, we speculate that the marginal

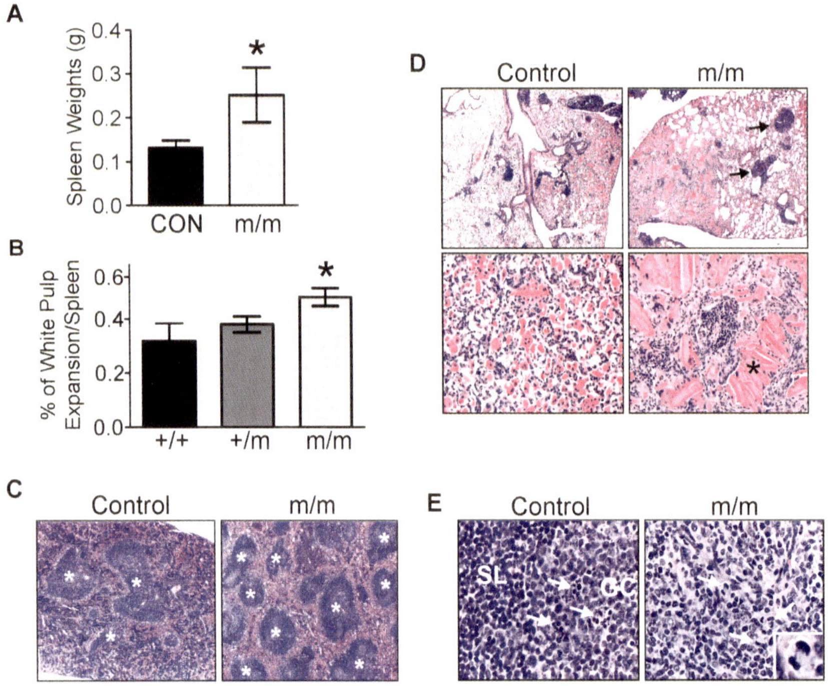

Figure 5. Loss of NIAM promotes reactive lymphoid hyperplasia and B-cell lymphoma in the spleen. A. Weights of spleens from +/+ and +/m mice (CON, n = 15) compared to $NIAM^{m/m}$ mice (m/m, n = 12). Note: one WT (+/+) mouse with an incidental case of severe chronic pyometra was excluded from the analysis. Statistical significance was shown by a Mann-Whitney test (*, $p<0.05$) **B**. The percentage of splenic white pulp per total splenic area was calculated for each genotype. $NIAM^{m/m}$ mice (n = 8) are statistically different from both wild-type (+/+, n = 5) and heterozygous (+/m, n = 6) mice as calculated by an unpaired two-tailed T-test. (*, $p<0.05$) Note: one WT (+/+) and one mutant (m/m) mouse were excluded from the analysis because extensive extramedullary hematopoiesis prevented accurate visualization of the white pulp **C**. Representative images of spleens from control wild-type (+/+) and homozygous m/m mice (H&E, 40x). Splenic white pulp (asterisks) was increased in $NIAM^{m/m}$ mice. Note: these samples show a range of variation in the extent of red pulp extramedullary hematopoiesis that was seen for both groups. **D**. Eosinophilic crystalline pneumonia in the lungs of control $NIAM^{+/m}$ heterozygous and $NIAM^{m/m}$ mice. Loss of NIAM resulted in more severe disease with extensive pulmonary lymphoid inflammation (arrows) and large extracellular crystals (asterisks) in the affected $NIAM^{m/m}$ mouse. (H&E, 40× top and 100× bottom panels) **E**. White pulp from control $NIAM^{+/m}$ heterozygous and $NIAM^{m/m}$ homozygous mice (H&E, 600x). A spleen from a heterozygous mouse with chronic ulcerative dermatitis and reactive hyperplasia of white pulp characterized by a germinal center (GC) and tingible body macrophages full of cellular debris (arrows) on a background of small lymphocytes (SL) (left panel). In two homozygous m/m mice, typical white pulp architecture was multifocally depleted and effaced by centroblasts and centrocytes with multiple mitotic figures (inset and arrows) (right panel). Note that $NIAM^{+/m}$ heterozygous and $NIAM^{+/+}$ wild-type mice appeared identical in our analyses and were therefore used interchangeably as controls.

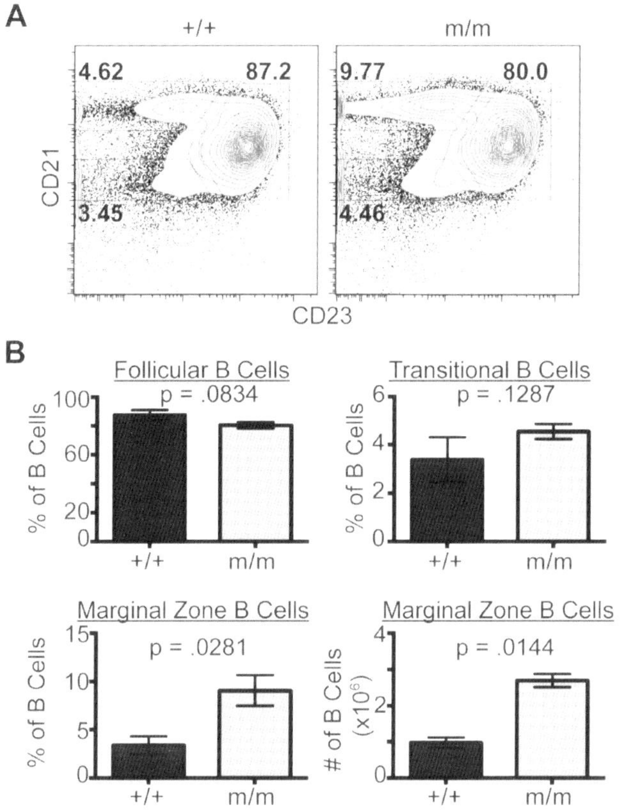

Figure 6. Marginal zone B cells are increased in *NIAM*$^{m/m}$ mice. Flow cytometric analyses of splenic B cell development. Splenic B cells were isolated from young, 6 month old tumor-free wild-type (+/+) and *NIAM* mutant (m/m) mice (three of each genotype). **A**. Representative flow cytometry plots of *NIAM* wild-type versus m/m IgM positive splenocytes. Transitional (CD21^{lo}/CD23-), follicular (CD21+/CD23+) and marginal zone (CD21^{hi}/CD23-) B cells are identified. **B**. Average frequency of follicular (top left), transitional (top right), and marginal zone (bottom left) B cells from mice of the indicated genotypes. Average marginal zone B cell numbers are also shown (bottom right). All p values were calculated using unpaired, two-tailed Student's T tests.

zone B cell expansion in *NIAM* mutant mice is intimately related to their development of systemic inflammation [61] and B cell lymphomagenesis [25,26]. We also predict that NIAM, as a regulator of ARF-Mdm2-Tip60-p53 signaling and other undefined pathways affecting maintenance of chromosomal stability, normally cooperates with multiple anti-cancer pathways to suppress tumor development. The *NIAM*$^{m/m}$ mice described here are an outstanding model to explore those concepts.

Materials and Methods

Animal Husbandry and Ethics Statement

Mice were housed in the University of Iowa Animal Care barrier facility. Mice were kept in rooms with a 12 hour light-dark cycle and free access to water and food. All mouse experiments were conducted according to protocols approved by the University of Iowa Institutional Animal Care and Use Committee (protocol#1204079). All efforts were made to minimize suffering. Mice were euthanized using carbon dioxide inhalation.

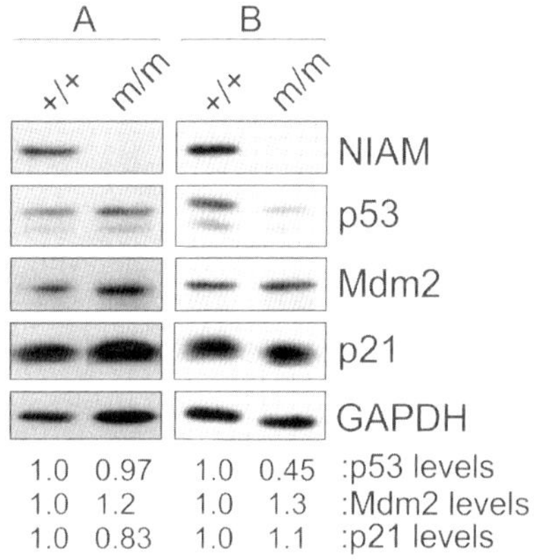

Figure 7. NIAM is not required for basal p53 activity in splenic B cells. Splenic B cells from young, tumor-free wild-type *NIAM*$^{+/+}$ or *NIAM*$^{m/m}$ homozygous mutant mice were isolated and expression of endogenous NIAM, p53, Mdm2 and p21 proteins was assessed by western blotting. Relative levels of p53, Mdm2 and p21 (normalized to GAPDH loading and compared to the untreated, wild-type control sample) were determined following quantification of bands using Image J. Representative results from 4 of 5 pairs of mice (both 8 week and 6 months of age) are shown in Set A, while Set B shows data for one pair of 6 month old mice. Set A and B samples were analyzed on separate gels, and lanes within each set were spliced together from the same autoradiogram for image clarity.

Generation of NIAM Mutant Mice

The Knockout Mouse Project (KOMP) generated male chimeras by injecting embryonic stem cells containing a *NIAM (TBRG1)* allele with a β-galactosidase cassette and LoxP sites around Exon2 into C57BL/6 blastocysts (www.komp.org, Project ID: CSD41510). Chimeric mice were then bred with C57BL/6N females to obtain germline transmission of the mutant *TBRG1* allele. To confirm mouse genotypes, the REDExtract-N-Amp Tissue PCR Kit (Sigma Aldrich, XNAT-100RXN) was used to isolate DNA from mouse tails and to perform PCR. PCR genotyping primers were: Primer a: 5′- GGTCAAAGCTG-TAAGCATAGAGAGTC -3′; Primer b: 5′- CTTGAGG-CTCCTTTCTGGTG -3′; Primer c: 5′- CCAACTGACCT-TGGGCAAGAACAT -3′. PCR reactions consisted of 2 μL DNA added to 5 μl RedExtract PCR Master Mix (Sigma Aldrich), 0.8 μl of each primer and 0.6 μL PCR grade water to a total reaction volume of 10 μL. PCR was performed as follows: 95°C for 5 min, 35 cycles of 95°C for 1 min, annealing of primers at 54°C for 1 min, and extension at 72°C for 1.5 min on a PCR Sprint thermal cycler (Thermo Scientific Hybaid).

Database Analyses

The Cancer Genome Atlas Pan-Cancer analysis project's individual RNAseq datasets were downloaded from the UCSC Cancer Genome Browser (https://genome-cancer.ucsc.edu/). The UCSC Cancer Browser Team utilized level 3 TCGA RNAseq datasets (available at https://tcga-data.nci.nih.gov/tcga/), log2(x+1) transformed, and renormalized to the expression of all available TCGA cancer cohorts. PanCan normalized, log2(x+1) expression for available paired normal and primary tumor samples were compared for each TCGA cancer cohort utilizing an unpaired Welch's T-test.

Protein Analyses in Mouse Tissues

Mouse tissues were isolated, flash frozen in liquid nitrogen, and crushed into a powder by mortar and pestle. Tissues were lysed with RIPA buffer (50 mM Tris, pH 8.0, 150 mM NaCl, 1% Triton X-100, 0.1% SDS, 0.5% Sodium deoxycholate) supplemented with 1 mM NaF, protease inhibitor cocktail (Sigma, P8340), phosphatase inhibitor cocktail (Sigma, P0044), and 30 µM phenylmethylsulfonyl fluoride for 1 hour on ice. After brief sonication (2×5s pulses), protein lysates were centrifuged at 14,000 rpm for 15 min at 4°C. The concentration of protein for each tissue was assessed by BCA assay (Pierce, Rockford, IL). Equivalent amounts of total cellular protein was loaded and separated by SDS-PAGE, transferred to polyvinylidene difluoride (PVDF) membranes (Millipore), and analyzed by immunoblotting. Proteins were detected on membranes by ECL (Amersham Biosciences) with antibodies against NIAM (rabbit polyclonal antibody at 1.5 µg/ml [10] and mouse monoclonal antibody [clone 11E12] at 1:5 dilution [62]) and γ-tubulin (Sigma, T6557, mouse monoclonal antibody, 1:10,000).

Primary B Cell Analyses

Bone marrow and spleens were harvested from wild-type and NIAM mutant mice (three 6 month old littermate males per genotype) and minced between frosted glass slides to liberate cells. ACK lysis (Lonza, Radnor, PA) was used to lyse red blood cells. For flow cytometric analyses of B cells, one million lymphocytes were washed and resuspended in staining buffer that consisted of balanced salt solution, 5% bovine calf serum and 0.1% sodium azide. Non-specific binding of antibody was blocked using 10 µl rat serum (Jackson Immunoresearch, West Grove, PA) and 10 µg 2.4G2 (BioXCell, West Lebanon, NH). Cells were then incubated on wet ice in the dark with antibodies to B220-PE-Cy7 (6B2, eBioscience, San Diego, CA), CD23-PE (B3B4, eBioscience), CD21-APC (7G6, BD Biosciences, San Jose, CA), and IgM-FITC (RMM-1, Biolegend, San Diego, CA). Samples were run on a BD FACSCANTO II instrument (Becton Dickinson, San Jose, CA) and data were analyzed using FlowJo (Tree Star, Ashland, OR).

For analyses of p53, B cells were isolated from spleens of 6 month and 8 week old wild-type and NIAM mutant mice using B220 micro beads (Miltenvi Biotec, San Diego, CA) according to manufacturer's specifications. Cells were plated at 5×10^5 c/ml in B-cell media (RPMI, 10% fetal calf serum, 2 mM Glutamine, 1 mM Sodium Pyruvate, 0.055 mM β-mercaptoethanol and 100 units/ml of penicillin with 100 µg/ml streptomycin) supplemented with LPS (Sigma) at 20 µg/ml to maintain viability. After overnight incubation at 37°C, 5% CO_2, cells were harvested and lysed directly in 1× SDS-PAGE sample buffer. Samples (1×10^6 cell equivalents) were subjected to SDS-PAGE and protein expression examined by western blotting as described above using antibodies to p53 (Santa Cruz, Sc-6243 [FL-393] rabbit polyclonal, 1:200), Mdm2 (2A10 mouse monoclonal, 1:10), p21 (Calbiochem, PC55 [Ab-5], rabbit polyclonal, 2 µg/ml), and GAPDH (Abcam, Ab8245, mouse monoclonal, 1:20,000).

Mouse Necropsy and Histopathological Analyses

Individual organs were harvested from mice euthanized by CO_2 asphyxiation. A total of 28 mice (8 $NIAM^{+/+}$, 8 $NIAM^{+/m}$ and 12 $NIAM^{m/m}$) between the ages of 14 to 21 months were subjected to pathological examination. Organs assessed by macroscopic and histopathological analyses included pancreas, liver, spleen, gastrointestinal tract, reproductive tract for males and females, kidney, urinary bladder, lung, heart, head sections (e.g., eyes, nasal cavity, etc), and sagittal section of the brain (cerebellum, cerebrum and brain stem). Organ weights (e.g., spleen and liver) were collected and then tissues were formalin fixed and paraffin embedded. Tissue sections (~4 µm) were made from paraffin blocks and stained with hematoxylin and eosin (H&E). Mouse tissues were analyzed and reviewed for abnormal findings by a pathologist. Quantification of the white pulp of individual mouse spleens stained with H&E was measured by Image J software. The splenic white pulp was evaluated as a percentage of the total splenic area in tissue sections.

Supporting Information

Figure S1 Early B cell development is not altered in NIAM-deficient mice. Flow cytometric analysis of early B cell development. **A.** Representative flow cytometry plots of bone marrow lymphocytes from *NIAM* wild-type (+/+) or mutant (m/m) mice. Early (B220+/IgM-), immature (B220+/IgM+) and mature (B220high/IgM+) B cells are identified. **B.** Average frequency of immature (left), mature (middle) and early (right) B cells in *NIAM* +/+ versus m/m mice. No significant differences were observed. For these studies, bone marrow was isolated and analyzed from six mice total (the same analyzed in Figure 6), three of each genotype.

Figure S2 Sustained DNA damage induces NIAM expression. Western analyses show that endogenous NIAM protein is induced by DNA damage caused by exposure to doxorubicin (Dxn, 66 ng/mL) for the indicated times (hrs) in human MCF10A mammary epithelial cells. GAPDH levels serve as control for equivalent loading.

Acknowledgments

The authors thank Jennifer Stivers for technical assistance and personnel in the animal care facility for their mouse expertise and guidance. We also thank Drs. Adam Dupuy and Fred Quelle for helpful discussions.

Author Contributions

Conceived and designed the experiments: SMR TRR VST DKM DEQ. Performed the experiments: SMR JH VPM TRR NB SS JAG PN VST DKM DEQ. Analyzed the data: SMR DEQ WZ NB DKM JAG PN TRR VST SJ. Contributed reagents/materials/analysis tools: WZ SJ DKM DEQ. Wrote the paper: SMR TRR DKM DEQ.

References

1. Vousden KH, Prives C (2009) Blinded by the Light: The Growing Complexity of p53. Cell 137: 413–431.
2. Vogelstein B, Lane D, Levine AJ (2000) Surfing the p53 network. Nature 408: 307–310.
3. Levine AJ, Oren M (2009) The first 30 years of p53: growing ever more complex. Nature Reviews Cancer 9: 749–758.
4. Riley T, Sontag E, Chen P, Levine A (2008) Transcriptional control of human p53-regulated genes. Nat Rev Mol Cell Biol 9: 402–412.
5. Muller PAJ, Vousden KH (2013) p53 mutations in cancer. Nat Cell Biol 15: 2–8.
6. Donehower LA, Harvey M, Slagle BL, McArthur MJ, Montgomery CA Jr, et al. (1992) Mice deficient for p53 are developmentally normal but susceptible to spontaneous tumours. Nature 356: 215–221.
7. Jacks T, Remington L, Williams BO, Schmitt EM, Halachmi S, et al. (1994) Tumor spectrum analysis in p53-mutant mice. Current Biology 4: 1–7.
8. Garcia PB, Attardi LD (2014) Illuminating p53 function in cancer with genetically engineered mouse models. Seminars in Cell & Developmental Biology.
9. Lane DP (1992) p53, guardian of the genome. Nature 358: 15–16.
10. Tompkins VS, Hagen J, Frazier AA, Lushnikova T, Fitzgerald MP, et al. (2007) A Novel Nuclear Interactor of ARF and MDM2 (NIAM) That Maintains Chromosomal Stability. Journal of Biological Chemistry 282: 1322–1333.
11. Tompkins V, Hagen J, Zediak VP, Quelle DE (2006) Identification of novel ARF binding proteins by two-hybrid screening. Cell Cycle 5: 641–646.

12. Reed SM, Hagen J, Tompkins V, Thies K, Quelle FW, et al. (2014) Nuclear Interactor of ARF and Mdm2 regulates multiple pathways to activate p53. Cell Cycle 13: 1288–1298.
13. Babalola GO, Schultz RM (1995) modulation of gene-expression in the preimplantation mouse embryo by TGF-alpha and TGF-beta. Molecular Reproduction and Development 41: 133–139.
14. Sherr CJ (2006) Divorcing ARF and p53: an unsettled case. Nature Reviews Cancer 6: 663–673.
15. Llanos S, Clark PA, Rowe J, Peters G (2001) Stabilisation of p53 by p14ARF without relocalization of Mdm2 to the nucleolus. Nature Cell Biology 3: 445–452.
16. Korgaonkar C, Hagen J, Tompkins V, Frazier AA, Allamargot C, et al. (2005) Nucleophosmin (B23) Targets ARF to Nucleoli and Inhibits Its Function. Molecular and Cellular Biology 25: 1258–1271.
17. Momand J, Wu HH, Dasgupta G (2000) MDM2 - master regulator of the p53 tumor suppressor protein. Gene 242: 15–29.
18. Legube G, Linares LK, Tyteca S, Caron C, Scheffner M, et al. (2004) Role of the Histone Acetyl Transferase Tip60 in the p53 Pathway. Journal of Biological Chemistry 279: 44825–44833.
19. Sykes SM, Mellert HS, Holbert MA, Li K, Marmorstein R, et al. (2006) Acetylation of the p53 DNA-Binding Domain Regulates Apoptosis Induction. Molecular Cell 24: 841–851.
20. Tang Y, Luo J, Zhang W, Gu W (2006) Tip60-dependent acetylation of p53 modulates the decision between cell-cycle arrest and apoptosis. Molecular Cell 24: 827–839.
21. Sapountzi V, Logan IR, Robson CN (2006) Cellular functions of TIP60. International Journal of Biochemistry & Cell Biology 38: 1496–1509.
22. Senturk E, Manfredi JJ (2012) Mdm2 and Tumorigenesis: Evolving Theories and Unsolved Mysteries. Genes & Cancer 3: 192–198.
23. Rhodes DR, Yu JJ, Shanker K, Deshpande N, Varambally R, et al. (2004) ONCOMINE: A cancer microarray database and integrated data-mining platform. Neoplasia 6: 1–6.
24. Rhodes DR, Kalyana-Sundaram S, Mahavisno V, Varambally R, Yu J, et al. (2007) Oncomine 3.0: Genes, pathways, and networks in a collection of 18,000 cancer gene expression profiles. Neoplasia 9: 166–180.
25. Gostissa M, Bianco JM, Malkin DJ, Kutok JL, Rodig SJ, et al. (2013) Conditional inactivation of p53 in mature B cells promotes generation of nongerminal center-derived B-cell lymphomas. Proceedings of the National Academy of Sciences of the United States of America 110: 2934–2939.
26. Chiang YJ, Difilippantonio MJ, Tessarollo L, Morse HC, Hodes RJ (2012) Exon 1 Disruption Alters Tissue-Specific Expression of Mouse p53 and Results in Selective Development of B Cell Lymphomas. Plos One 7: e49305.
27. Lowe SW, Sherr CJ (2003) Tumor suppression by Ink4a-Arf: progress and puzzles. Current Opinion in Genetics & Development 13: 77–83.
28. Carter JH, Carter HW, Deddens JA, Hurst BM, George MH, et al. (2003) A 2-year dose-response study of lesion sequences during hepatocellular carcinogenesis in the male B6C3F(1) mouse given the drinking water chemical dichloroacetic acid. Environmental Health Perspectives 111: 53–64.
29. Percy DH, Barthold SW (2007) Pathology of laboratory rodents and rabbits 2nd Edition: 90.
30. Liu Q, Cheng LI, Yi L, Zhu N, Wood A, et al. (2009) p47(phox) Deficiency Induces Macrophage Dysfunction Resulting in Progressive Crystalline Macrophage Pneumonia. American Journal of Pathology 174: 153–163.
31. Hoenerhoff MJ, Starost MF, Ward JM (2006) Eosinophilic crystalline pneumonia as a major cause of death in 129S4/SvJae mice. Veterinary Pathology 43: 682–688.
32. Ward JM, Rehg JE, Morse HC III (2012) Differentiation of Rodent Immune and Hematopoietic System Reactive Lesions from Neoplasias. Toxicologic Pathology 40: 425–434.
33. Alizadeh AA, Eisen MB, Davis RE, Ma C, Lossos IS, et al. (2000) Distinct types of diffuse large B-cell lymphoma identified by gene expression profiling. Nature 403: 503–511.
34. Rosenwald A, Wright G, Chan WC, Connors JM, Campo E, et al. (2002) The use of molecular profiling to predict survival after chemotherapy for diffuse large-B-cell lymphoma. New England Journal of Medicine 346: 1937–1947.
35. Brune V, Tiacci E, Pfeil I, Doering C, Eckerle S, et al. (2008) Origin and pathogenesis of nodular lymphocyte-predominant Hodgkin lymphoma as revealed by global gene expression analysis. Journal of Experimental Medicine 205: 2251–2268.
36. Eckerle S, Brune V, Doering C, Tiacci E, Bohle V, et al. (2009) Gene expression profiling of isolated tumour cells from anaplastic large cell lymphomas: insights into its cellular origin, pathogenesis and relation to Hodgkin lymphoma. Leukemia 23: 2129–2138.
37. Storz MN, van de Rijn M, Kim YH, Mraz-Gernhard S, Hoppe RT, et al. (2003) Gene expression profiles of cutaneous B cell lymphoma. Journal of Investigative Dermatology 120: 865–870.
38. Ghobrial IM, McCormick DJ, Kaufmann SH, Leontovich AA, Loegering DA, et al. (2005) Proteomic analysis of mantle-cell lymphoma by protein microarray. Blood 105: 3722–3730.
39. Watanabe T, Ichikawa A, Saito H, Hotta T (1996) Overexpression of the MDM2 oncogene in leukemia and lymphoma. Leukemia & Lymphoma 21: 391–397.
40. Wilda M, Bruch J, Harder L, Rawer D, Reiter A, et al. (2004) Inactivation of the ARF-MDM-2-p53 pathway in sporadic Burkitt's lymphoma in children. Leukemia 18: 584–588.
41. Eischen CM, Weber JD, Roussel MF, Sherr CJ, Cleveland JL (1999) Disruption of the ARF-Mdm2-p53 tumor suppressor pathway in Myc- induced lymphomagenesis. Genes & Development 13: 2658–2669.
42. Alt JR, Greiner TC, Cleveland JL, Eischen CM (2003) Mdm2 haplo-insufficiency profoundly inhibits Myc-induced lymphomagenesis. EMBO Journal 22: 1442–1450.
43. Wang P, Greiner TC, Lushnikova T, Eischen CM (2006) Decreased Mdm2 expression inhibits tumor development induced by loss of ARF. Oncogene 25: 3708–3718.
44. el-Deiry WS, Tokino T, Velculescu VE, Levy DB, Parsons R, et al. (1993) WAF1, a potential mediator of p53 tumor suppression. Cell 75: 817–825.
45. el-Deiry WS, Harper JW, O'Connor PM, Velculescu VE, Canman CE, et al. (1994) WAF1/CIP1 is induced in p53-mediated G1 arrest and apoptosis. Cancer Research 54: 1169–1174.
46. Martin-Caballero J, Flores JM, Garcia-Palencia P, Serrano M (2001) Tumor Susceptibility of p21Waf1/Cip1-deficient Mice. Cancer Research 61: 6234–6238.
47. Kamijo T, Zindy F, Roussel MF, Quelle DE, Downing JR, et al. (1997) Tumor suppression at the mouse INK4a locus mediated by the alternative reading frame product p19(ARF). Cell 91: 649–659.
48. Kamijo T, Bodner S, van de Kamp E, Randle DH, Sherr CJ (1999) Tumor spectrum in ARF-deficient mice. Cancer Research 59: 2217–2222.
49. Jeffers JR, Parganas E, Lee Y, Yang CY, Wang JL, et al. (2003) Puma is an essential mediator of p53-dependent and -independent apoptotic pathways. Cancer Cell 4: 321–328.
50. Kippin TE, Martens DJ, van der Kooy D (2005) P21 loss compromises the relative quiescence of forebrain stem cell proliferation leading to exhaustion of their proliferation capacity. Genes & Development 19: 756–767.
51. Cheng T, Rodrigues N, Shen HM, Yang YG, Dombkowski D, et al. (2000) Hematopoietic stem cell quiescence maintained by p21(cip1/waf1). Science 287: 1804–1808.
52. Yu H, Yuan YZ, Shen HM, Cheng T (2006) Hematopoietic stem cell exhaustion impacted by p18(INK4C) and p21(Cip1/Waf1) in opposite manners. Blood 107: 1200–1206.
53. Jiang D, Attardi LD (2013) Engaging the p53 metabolic brake drives senescence. Cell Res 23: 739–740.
54. Christophorou MA, Ringshausen I, Finch AJ, Swigart LB, Evan GI (2006) The pathological response to DNA damage does not contribute to p53-mediated tumour suppression. Nature 443: 214–217.
55. Ventura A, Kirsch DG, McLaughlin ME, Tuveson DA, Grimm J, et al. (2007) Restoration of p53 function leads to tumour regression in vivo. Nature 445: 661–665.
56. Xue W, Zender L, Miething C, Dickins RA, Hernando E, et al. (2007) Senescence and tumour clearance is triggered by p53 restoration in murine liver carcinomas. Nature 445: 656–660.
57. Massague J, Blain SW, Lo RS (2000) TGF beta signaling in growth control, cancer, and heritable disorders. Cell 103: 295–309.
58. Derynck R, Akhurst RJ, Balmain A (2001) TGF-beta signaling in tumor suppression and cancer progression. Nature Genetics 29: 117–129.
59. Hoesel B, Schmid JA (2013) The complexity of NF-kappa B signaling in inflammation and cancer. Molecular Cancer 12: 86.
60. Gerondakis S, Siebenlist U (2010) Roles of the NF-kappa B Pathway in Lymphocyte Development and Function. Cold Spring Harbor Perspectives in Biology 2: a000182.
61. Cerutti A, Cols M, Puga I (2013) Marginal zone B cells: virtues of innate-like antibody-producing lymphocytes. Nature Reviews Immunology 13: 118–132.
62. Hagen J, Tompkins V, Dudakovic A, Weydert JA, Quelle DE (2008) Generation and characterization of monoclonal antibodies to NIAM: A nuclear interactor of ARF and Mdm2. Hybridoma 27: 159–166.
63. Bredel M, Bredel C, Juric D, Harsh GR, Vogel H, et al. (2005) Functional network analysis reveals extended gliomagenesis pathway maps and three novel MYC-interacting genes in human gliomas. Cancer Research 65: 8679–8689.
64. Sun LX, Hui AM, Su Q, Vortmeyer A, Kotliarov Y, et al. (2006) Neuronal and glioma-derived stem cell factor induces angiogenesis within the brain. Cancer Cell 9: 287–300.
65. Liang Y, Diehn M, Watson N, Bollen AW, Aldape KD, et al. (2005) Gene expression profiling reveals molecularly and clinically distinct subtypes of glioblastoma multiforme. Proceedings of the National Academy of Sciences of the United States of America 102: 5814–5819.
66. French PJ, Swagemakers SMA, Nagel JHA, Kouwenhoven MCM, Brouwer E, et al. (2005) Gene expression profiles associated with treatment response in oligodendrogliomas. Cancer Research 65: 11335–11344.
67. Murat A, Migliavacca E, Gorlia T, Lambiv WL, Shay T, et al. (2008) Stem cell-related "Self-Renewal" signature and high epidermal growth factor receptor expression associated with resistance to concomitant chemoradiotherapy in glioblastoma. Journal of Clinical Oncology 26: 3015–3024.
68. Hou J, Aerts J, den Hamer B, van Ijcken W, den Bakker M, et al. (2010) Gene Expression-Based Classification of Non-Small Cell Lung Carcinomas and Survival Prediction. Plos One 5: e10312.

69. Zhao HJ, Langerod A, Ji Y, Nowels KW, Nesland JM, et al. (2004) Different gene expression patterns in invasive lobular and ductal carcinomas of the breast. Molecular Biology of the Cell 15: 2523–2536.
70. Blum JL, Kohles J, McKenna E, Scotto N, Hu S, et al. (2011) Association of age and overall survival in capecitabine-treated patients with metastatic breast cancer in clinical trials. Breast Cancer Research and Treatment 125: 431–439.
71. Richardson AL, Wang ZGC, De Nicolo A, Lu X, Brown M, et al. (2006) X chromosomal abnormalities in basal-like human breast cancer. Cancer Cell 9: 121–132.
72. Tomlins SA, Mehra R, Rhodes DR, Cao X, Wang L, et al. (2007) Integrative molecular concept modeling of prostate cancer progression. Nature Genetics 39: 41–51.

Major Molecular Response Achievement in CML Patients Can Be Predicted by *BCR-ABL1/ABL1* or *BCR-ABL1/GUS* Ratio at an Earlier Time Point of Follow-Up than Currently Recommended

Sarah Huet[1,2]*, Pascale Cony-Makhoul[3], Maël Heiblig[4], Isabelle Tigaud[1], Sophie Gazzo[1], Amine Belhabri[5], Denis Souche[1], Mauricette Michallet[4], Jean-Pierre Magaud[1,2], Sandrine Hayette[1,2], Franck Nicolini[4]

1 Laboratoire d'hématologie, Centre de Biologie Sud, Centre Hospitalier Lyon Sud, Pierre-Benite, France, **2** Unité Mixte de Recherche 5239 Centre National de la Recherche Scientifique, Faculté de médecine Lyon Sud, Oullins, France, **3** Service clinique d'hématologie, Centre Hospitalier d'Annecy, Pringy, France, **4** Service clinique d'hématologie 1G, Centre Hospitalier Lyon Sud, Pierre-Benite, France, **5** Service clinique d'hématologie, Centre Régional de Lutte Contre le Cancer Léon Bérard, Lyon, France

Abstract

Recent studies demonstrate that early molecular response to tyrosine-kinase inhibitors is strongly predictive of outcome in chronic myeloid leukemia patients and that early response landmarks may identify patients at higher risk for transformation who would benefit from an early switch to second-line therapy. In this study, we evaluated the ability of the control gene *GUS* to identify relevant thresholds for known therapeutic decision levels (*BCR-ABL1/ABL1^{IS}* = 10% and 0.1%). We then defined the most relevant cut-offs for early molecular response markers (transcript level at 3 months, halving time and log reduction between diagnosis and 3 months of treatment) using *GUS* or *ABL1*. We demonstrated that, although both control genes could be used (in an equivalent way) to accurately assess early molecular response, the *BCR-ABL1/GUS* level at diagnosis is impacted by the higher *GUS* copy number over-expressed in CML cells, thus negatively impacting its ability to completely replace *ABL1* at diagnosis. Furthermore, we pointed out, for the first time, that it would be helpful to monitor *BCR-ABL1* levels at an earlier time point than that currently performed, in order to assess response to first-line tyrosine-kinase inhibitors and consider a potential switch of therapy as early as possible. We evaluated this optimal time point as being 19 days after the start of treatment in our cohort.

Editor: Zhuang Zuo, UT MD Anderson Cancer Center, United States of America

Funding: The authors have no support or funding to report.

Competing Interests: The authors have read the journal's policy and the authors of this manuscript have the following competing interests: Cony-Makhoul P: BMS: Honoraria. Michallet M: MSD: consultancy, Honoraria, Research Funding; Astellas: Consultancy, Honoraria, Research Funding; Novartis: Consultancy, Honoraria, Research Funding; Pfizer: Consultancy, Honoraria, Research Funding; Bristol-Myers Squibb: Consultancy, Honoraria, Research Funding; Genzyme: consultancy, Honoraria, Research Funding. Nicolini FE: Ariad, Teva, BMS and Pfizer: Honoraria. Novartis: Honoraria and grants. Huet S, Heiblig M, Tigaud I, Gazzo S, Belhabri A, Souche D, Magaud JP, and Hayette S have declared that no competing interests exist.

* Email: sarah.huet@chu-lyon.fr

Introduction

The European Leukemia Network (ELN) recommendations for the management of chronic myeloid leukemia (CML) patients define optimal response, warning or failure according to cytogenetic and/or molecular criteria obtained at 3, 6 and 12 months on tyrosine-kinase inhibitors (TKI) therapy [1] and optimal response is associated with best long-term outcome. Indeed, several studies have highlighted that the achievement of early molecular and cytogenetic responses on TKI was predictive of long term event-free survival (EFS), treatment-free survival (TFS) and overall survival (OS) and that this ability to predict outcome is observed for all TKI although with different kinetics [2–11]. Marin et al. reported that *BCR-ABL1^{IS}* levels at 3 and 6 months on Imatinib were significantly correlated with 8-year progression-free survival (PFS) and OS [12], and Hanfstein et al. proposed *BCR-ABL1^{IS}* levels of 10% at 3 months and 1% at 6 months as clinically important thresholds correlated with 5-year PFS and OS [3]. Therefore, early molecular response (EMR) to TKI is currently identified as being one of the most important prognostic factors, and early response landmarks may identify patients at higher risk for transformation and poor outcome, who may benefit from alternative treatments in order to improve response and thereby minimize exposure to risk over time.

Is was also demonstrated that EMR at 3 and 6 months correlates with future major molecular response (MMR) and deep molecular response (ie, molecular response ≥4.5-log reduction [MR$^{4.5}$] and beyond) [5,9,10,13]. Although the prognostic significance of achieving MMR at 12 or 18 months has been controversial in the past [14,15], Hughes et al. showed that patients who achieved MMR by 12 and 18 months while on Imatinib therapy had significantly improved 7-year EFS and PFS rates [4], thus demonstrating a strong association between MMR achievement and long-term clinical outcome. Moreover, reaching the 12-month MMR still represents an ELN criterion of optimal response and should be a main goal in the management of the patient.

This growing interest in the assessment of EMR led to reconsider the use of *ABL1* as control gene (CG) when quantifying the *BCR-ABL1* transcript. This CG was selected by a Europe Against Cancer (EAC) study group [16,17] but has the disadvantage of inducing a quantification bias in determining *BCR-ABL1* transcript levels. Indeed the location of *ABL1* primers leads to the simultaneous amplification of the non-translocated allele of *ABL1* and the fusion gene *BCR-ABL1*, then quantifying total-*ABL1* (figure 1). This may lead to underestimation of *BCR-ABL1*/*ABL1*% when *BCR-ABL1* expression is high. Although *BCR-ABL1* level at diagnosis has not been clearly identified as being of prognostic significance by itself and has been cause for controversy [18,19], it allows (at least) the assessment of early transcript kinetics (for example between diagnosis and 3–6 months of treatment), which recently arose as an important parameter of the EMR [1,19,20]. Thus, the fact that *BCR-ABL1* transcript level at diagnosis should be measured as accurately as possible encouraged efforts to find another CG. Accordingly, the *GUS* gene, encoding for beta-glucuronidase, previously identified as a suitable CG in CML [16], attracted interest for quantifying *BCR-ABL1* and assessing EMR to TKI [18,19].

Our study intended (i) to assess the ability of *GUS* to normalize the *BCR-ABL1* level without technical bias at diagnosis and validate its potential predictive value at this time (ii) to evaluate its ability to accurately define the relevant thresholds for known therapeutic decision levels (10% and major molecular response MMR: 0.1%) and (iii) to compare different markers of EMR (IS cut off, halving time and fold reduction of transcript ratios) using *GUS* and *ABL1* to predict the achievement of MMR after 12 months of TKI in a series of front line therapy patients. We describe the optimal cut-offs for the different markers to predict the 12-month MMR achievement with confirmation in a validation cohort. We highlight that it could be appropriate to add a new, earlier time point to patient monitoring earlier than those currently recommended in clinical practice in order to identify patients likely to benefit from an early switch of TKI.

Subjects and Methods

1. Patients and samples

CML patients included in this retrospective analysis were diagnosed and monitored on TKI in our institutions since August 2000 and the blood samples were collected between August 2000 and January 2013. Patients gave written informed consent for their data to be used in this analysis and the procedures followed were in accordance to the Helsinki declaration as revised in 2008. Samples were stored in the Biological Resource Center Bank according to the French "Comité de Protection des Personnes" specifications. The review board protocol of the Hospices Civils de Lyon approved this study. To address the main questions of the study, samples were collected as follows:

- First, we focused on the transcript values obtained by using *GUS* as a CG. Therefore, we studied 3 groups of samples according to their transcript values: the first group comprised diagnostic samples (n = 124), the second group comprised follow-up samples with a *BCR-ABL1/ABL1*^{IS} ratio between 6 and 14% (n = 18) and the third group consisted of samples at the MMR IS threshold of 0.1% (n = 42). We were particularly interested in these transcript values since (i) diagnosis is highly impacted by the quantification bias but is crucial to assess the EMR (for example between diagnosis and 3–6 months of treatment) and (ii) they represent the relevant thresholds for known therapeutic decision levels (10% and major molecular response MMR: 0.1%).
- We then went on to evaluate the prognostic value (probability of obtaining MMR one year after diagnosis) of different parameters described in the literature for assessing the early molecular response (EMR) value. We then selected patients with available samples at diagnosis and after 3 months of TKI therapy. Of the 124 patients obtained at diagnosis, patients with the following criteria were included: (1) TKI therapy started less than 60 days after diagnosis (median, 29 days; range, 0–58 days), (2) the patient should have received TKI between 60 and 120 days before the follow-up so-called "3-month" sample (median, 90 days; range, 62–117 days; 4 of them received between 60 and 75 days of TKI) and (3) molecular follow-up assessed for at least 1 year after diagnosis in order to evaluate the achievement of MMR (median follow-up 3.9 years; range 1.1–9.7 years). One patient who simultaneously presented another haematological malignancy and died before 1 year of treatment was excluded. Patient characteristics at diagnosis are listed in table 1. Of the 84 patients who met the inclusion criteria, 55 were treated with Imatinib and 29 received second-generation TKI (Nilotinib, n = 12 or Dasatinib, n = 17). Treatment interruption and/or switching was documented for 7 patients on Imatinib (temporary interruption, n = 4 and switch to Nilotinib, n = 3)

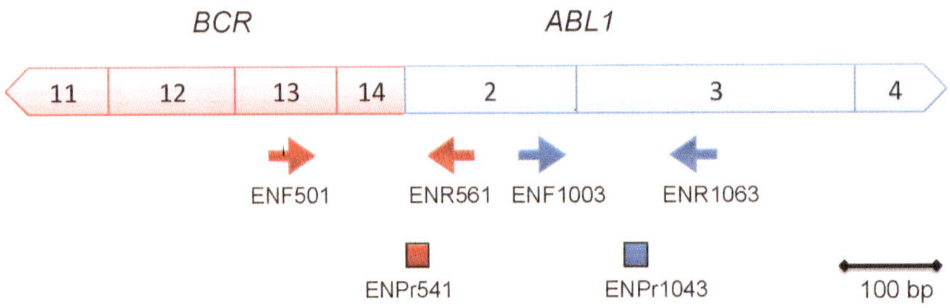

Figure 1. Quantification bias in the assessment of *BCR-ABL1* transcript levels by using *ABL1* as control gene. Localization of primers (arrows) and probes (rectangles) used for the relative quantification of the *M-BCR-ABL1* transcript according to the EAC protocol [16,17] are represented. Boxes represented the exon number. Red signs indicate primers and probe relative to the fusion transcript, blue signs to the control gene *ABL1*. The *ABL1* primers localization explains both amplification of *ABL1* and *BCR-ABL1* during the Q-RT-PCR reaction. ENF = forward primer, ENPr = TaqMan reverse probe, ENR = reverse primer.

and 2 patients on Nilotinib (1 temporary interruption and 1 switch to Imatinib then Dasatinib because of blast crisis).

- We validated our results in a supplemental cohort of patients (n = 58) selected according to the same criteria. Forty patients were on Imatinib as first-line treatment, 9 on Dasatinib and 9 on Nilotinib. Treatment interruption and/or switching was documented for 6 patients on Imatinib (switch to Nilotinib, n = 3; switch to Dasatinib, n = 3).

2. Molecular analysis

RNA was extracted from peripheral blood sample and reverse transcription (RT) and Quantitative Real-time-PCR (RQ-PCR) to amplify *BCR-ABL1* fusion transcript *ABL1* and *GUS* were performed according to standardised EAC protocols previously described [16,17]. Only patients expressing typical *BCR-ABL1* transcripts (b2a2 or b3a2) were considered. The final results are expressed as *BCR-ABL1/ABL1* ratios in percent according to the international scale IS (i.e. the conversion factor was applied for raw ratios ≤10%, and not for raw values >10%) as it was previously recommended [21,22] or as *BCR-ABL1/GUS*, without transformation of the original values since no conversion factor was defined for this CG. Samples with copy numbers that were too low (CN< 10,000) for either *ABL1* or *GUS* were presumably degraded samples (according to the GBMHM [Groupe des Biologistes Moléculaires de Hémopathies Malignes] recommendation guidelines: https://sites.google.com/site/gbmhmassociation/) and were excluded.

3. Statistical and result analysis

The alignment between both methods using (*BCR-ABL1/ABL1*)^{IS} and *BCR-ABL1/GUS* values was performed by setting a new conversion factor (CF), following the procedure that has been used previously to set the international conversion factor IS [21]. To determine this new CF, each measurement generated by using *ABL1* as CG was compared with that generated with *GUS* for the same sample. The bias between both measurements reflects the tendency of a method using one given CG to exceed the method using another CG. It was calculated as the difference between both measurements: bias = log(*BCR-ABL1/ABL1*^{IS}) − log(*BCR-ABL1/GUS*) for each sample. The CF is calculated as the antilog of the mean bias between measurements with both methods.

Three markers of EMR were used: halving time, transcript level at 3 months and log reduction between diagnosis and 3 months on TKI. The halving time defines the number of days over which the *BCR-ABL1* transcript value shows a 2-fold decrease [20,23]. According to Branford et al, the following formula was used: halving time = ln2*d/[ln(a)-ln(b)] where (a) is the transcript value at diagnosis, (b) the transcript value of the 3-month follow-up and (d) the number of days between both measurements. The log reduction in transcript level is another measurement of early molecular response [19]. This was defined as log(Transcript level at diagnosis/Transcript level at 3 months). All the analyses were performed on an intention-to-treat basis. Groups were compared using the ANOVA or the Kruskal-Wallis test adjusted for multiple comparisons when relevant. The Fisher Exact test and χ^2 test were used to compare frequencies. Correlations between different variables were investigated using the Pearson test.

Table 1. Patient Characteristics (N = 84)

Characteristics	No.	%
Age, years		
Median	58	
Range	20–89	
Sex		
Male	58	69
Female	26	31
Sokal risk group*		
Low	19	24
Intermediate	34	43
High	23	29
Accelerated phase at diagnosis	3	4
Chromosomal abnormalities in addition to the Philadelphia chromosome**	8	10

*We could not calculate Sokal score in 5 patients because of missing data.
**Information relative to chromosomal abnormalities was not available for 2 patients.

Results and Discussion

1. The use of *GUS* as CG requires the application of a conversion factor

In the first group of patients, the *BCR-ABL1/ABL1* median ratio at diagnosis was 69.3% (range: 25.0–121.0%) whereas the *BCR-ABL1/GUS* median ratio was 15.1% (range: 8.3–51.1%).

In the second group (patients chosen for their transcript *BCR-ABL1*^{IS} values comprised between 6% and 14%), the median ratios of these transcripts were 11.1% for *BCR-ABL1/ABL1* (range: 6.7–13.8%) and 3.1% (range: 2.2–5.8%) for *BCR-ABL1/GUS*.

In the third group (patients with transcript levels at 0.1%), the median ratios were 0.089% for *BCR-ABL1/ABL1* (range: 0.047–0.183%) and 0.035% (range: 0.016–0.072%) for *BCR-ABL1/GUS*. As samples were chosen according to their transcript value of 0.1% when analysed in laboratory routine practice, and that all measurement were performed again simultaneously for this study, ratios vary slightly in this range of values. Therefore, we will refer to this group of samples as "MMR-related samples" later in this study.

As expected, *BCR-ABL1/ABL1*^{IS} and *BCR-ABL1/GUS* values showed a direct correlation ($\rho = 0.762$; $p<0.001$).

These results indicate that the conversion from *BCR-ABL1/ABL1* to *BCR-ABL1/GUS* values would require the introduction of a further conversion factor in order to adapt them to the decision thresholds currently used for MRD monitoring. This conversion is exemplified in figure 2 for the MMR threshold, for which the transcript ratio of 0.1% using *ABL1* corresponds to a ratio of 0.036% using *GUS*.

The bias between measurements using *ABL1* or *GUS* was calculated for each sample. In diagnostic samples, the mean bias was 0.65 (standard deviation SD: 0.12) whereas it valued at 0.45 (SD: 0.16) in samples with a 6–14% *BCR-ABL1/ABL1* ratio and was somewhat similar, 0.42 (SD: 0.12) in the third group. The CF was then calculated as the antilog of the mean bias and valued at 4.45, 2.84, and 2.65 in the three groups of samples, respectively (table 2). A CF of 2.14 was reported by Hanfstein et al [19]. Nevertheless, we observed that the mean bias (and therefore the CF) differed within the different groups of samples (table 2 and figure 3). In particular, it was significantly different in the group of diagnostic samples ($p<0.001$, adjusted for multiple comparison test) whereas it did not differ significantly between the two other groups. Therefore, the conversion factor from *BCR-ABL1/ABL1* to *BCR-ABL1/GUS* is not constant within the different disease times and contrary to what was expected, is more pronounced at diagnosis implying that *GUS* is not a better GC than *ABL1* at diagnosis.

2. *GUS* is overexpressed at diagnosis

This difference in CF values during the course of the disease was due to the overexpression of *GUS* at diagnosis, with *GUS* mean copy number of 290 800, 117 200 and 110 900 in the 3 groups, respectively ($p<0.001$). Thus the higher copy number of *GUS* at diagnosis is responsible for the higher CF. Although *ABL1* is also overestimated at diagnosis due to the quantification test bias ($p<0.001$), *GUS* expression varies at least in the same range of values as *ABL1* (mean copy number: 66 500, 37 900 and 33 700, respectively) (Figure 4). The values of transcripts, gene copy number and conversion factor for the 3 groups are summarized in table 2.

This higher copy number of *GUS* at diagnosis is not due to the higher number of cells at this point in the disease, since the reverse-transcription protocol is designed to ensure that the same amounts of RNA are used whatever the sample is (MRD or diagnosis) [16,17].

It was previously reported that *GUS* was overexpressed at CML diagnosis compared to healthy donors [16]. We thus hypothesized that *GUS* may be overexpressed in leukemic cells compared to normal cells and that *GUS* quantification may be correlated to the *BCR-ABL1* transcript level. Indeed, a significant correlation was found between *GUS* and *BCR-ABL1* copy number ($R^2 = 0.704$; $p<0.001$, figure 5).

This overexpression of *GUS*, impacts the *BCR-ABL1/GUS* ratio at diagnosis and warrants the use of a unique conversion factor for all disease levels. Nevertheless, the number of copies of *GUS* did not differ significantly between the 6–14% samples and MMR-related samples, nor did the *ABL1* copy number. Therefore, the quantification bias observed for diagnostic samples does not seem to impact the values under 14%.

3. The transcript level at diagnosis does not impact on the achievement of MMR

In order to determine whether the transcript level at diagnosis could be used as a prognostic indicator for disease evolution, we compared patients who achieved the MMR threshold 1 year after TKI introduction (n = 70) and those who did not (n = 54). The *BCR-ABL1/GUS* median ratio at diagnosis was 13.78% in the first group and 15.96% in the second, and it did not differ significantly between both groups; neither did the *BCR-ABL1/ABL1* median ratio (69.3% in both groups). The sub-group analysis for patients receiving TKI 1st or 2nd generation did not

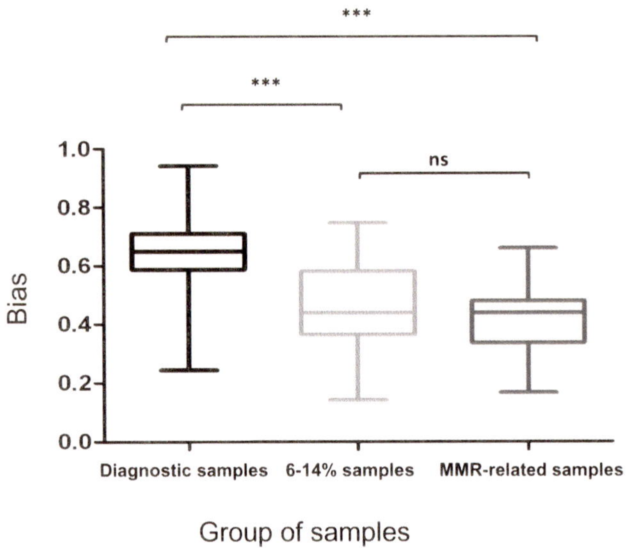

Figure 3. Box plot of the bias between *(BCR-ABL1/ABL1)^{IS}* and *BCR-ABL1/GUS* measurement in the 3 groups of samples. The bias (leading to conversion factor calculation) was compared between 3 groups of samples: diagnostic samples, samples with 6–14% and 0.1% transcript levels. It is significantly higher in the group of diagnostic samples (*** represents p-value<0.001; ns, non-significant).

show any other difference for the *BCR-ABL1/GUS* or *BCR-ABL1/ABL1* ratios. Besides, no prognostic cut-off could be identified for either *BCR-ABL1/GUS* or *BCR-ABL1/ABL1* at diagnosis. Therefore, the transcript level at this time, whatever CG is used, does not predict the achievement of MMR after one year of treatment. Another group reported that elevated *BCR-ABL1/GUS* at diagnosis correlated with inferior probabilities of optimal response [18]. We could not confirm these findings since we did not identify any prognostic cut-off, which is in accordance with a recent report assessing the absence of prognostic significance of transcript level at diagnosis on OS and PFS [19].

4. The transcript kinetics between diagnosis and 3 months of treatment predicts reaching the MMR levels at 12 months

The median *BCR-ABL1^{IS}* level in this 84-patient cohort was 69.6% (range, 25.0–95.7%) at diagnosis and 0.98% (range, 0.01–

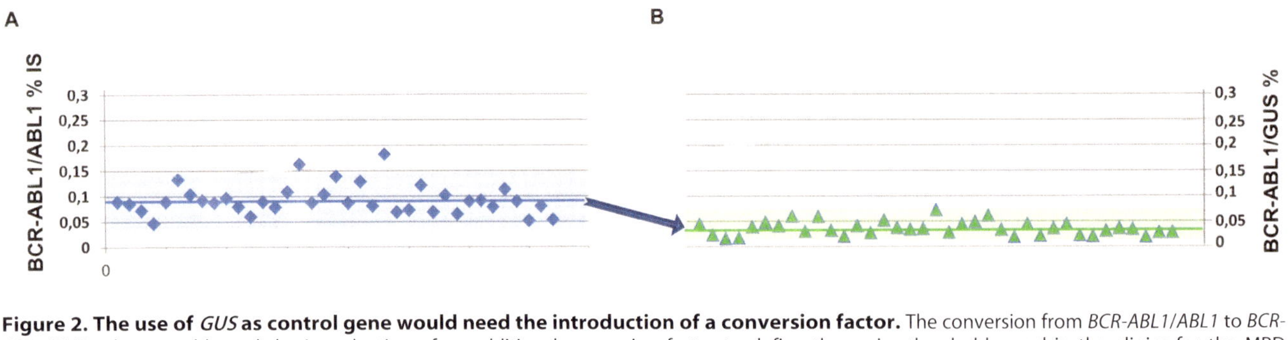

Figure 2. The use of *GUS* as control gene would need the introduction of a conversion factor. The conversion from *BCR-ABL1/ABL1* to *BCR-ABL1/GUS* values would need the introduction of an additional conversion factor to define the major thresholds used in the clinics for the MRD monitoring, as exemplified for the MMR threshold. (**a**) Graph A plots the *(BCR-ABL1/ABL1)^{IS}* % value of each patient close to the MMR threshold. The mean of 42 samples was 0.092%, 2 s.d. range 0.038–0.147%. (**b**) Graph B plots the *BCR-ABL1/GUS* % value of the same samples. The mean was 0.036% and 2 s.d. range 0.010–0.062%.

Table 2. Summary of the results obtained in the 3 groups of samples.

	Diagnosis samples	6–14% samples	0,1% samples	p
n	**124**	**18**	**42**	**/**
***BCR-ABL1/ABL1^{IS}* ratio (%)**				
median	69.3	11.1	0.089	/
range	25.0–121.0	6.7–13.8	0.047–0.183	
***BCR-ABL1/GUS* ratio (%)**				
median	15.1	3.1	0.035	/
range	8.3–51.1	2.2–5.8	0.016–0.072	
Bias				
mean	0.65	0.45	0.42	<0.001
standard deviation	0.12	0.16	0.12	
antilog of bias = Conversion Factor	4.45	2.84	2.65	
***GUS* copy number**				
mean	290,800	117,200	110,900	<0.001
standard deviation	164,400	46,700	28,900	
***ABL1* copy number**				
mean	66,500	37,900	33,700	<0.001
standard deviation	49,300	16,700	9,200	

36.9%) at 3 months. We used a receiver operating characteristic (ROC) curve to identify the optimal cut-off for the different variables tested that would allow us to classify the patients as presumably achieving or not the MMR at 12 months with maximal sensitivity and specificity (table 3).

Transcript level at 3 months. It was recently demonstrated that the persistence of *BCR-ABL1^{IS}* transcript levels above 10% at 3 months identified a group of high-risk patients that would benefit from treatment optimization [3,12]. Similarly, Marin et al. found that patients with a transcript value ≤2.81% had a significantly higher rate of MMR achievement during an 8-year follow-up [12]. Branford et al. reported a cut-off level for MMR achievement of 1.4% [20]. We tested, in our cohort, whether another cut-off point could predict long-term achievement of MMR at 12 months. Patients with *BCR-ABL1^{IS}* transcript levels >0.99% at 3 months had less chance of attaining the 1-year MMR threshold (18% vs. 84%, p<0.001). These results were concordant with recent reports regarding the 3-month landmark analysis predictive of 1-year MMR [3], including for separate analysis of patients on TKI 1st and 2nd generation [5]. The use of *BCR-ABL1/GUS* levels with a cut-off at 0.36% (corresponding to the 0.99% *BCR-ABL1^{IS}* corrected by the conversion factor of 2.65 defined for this MRD

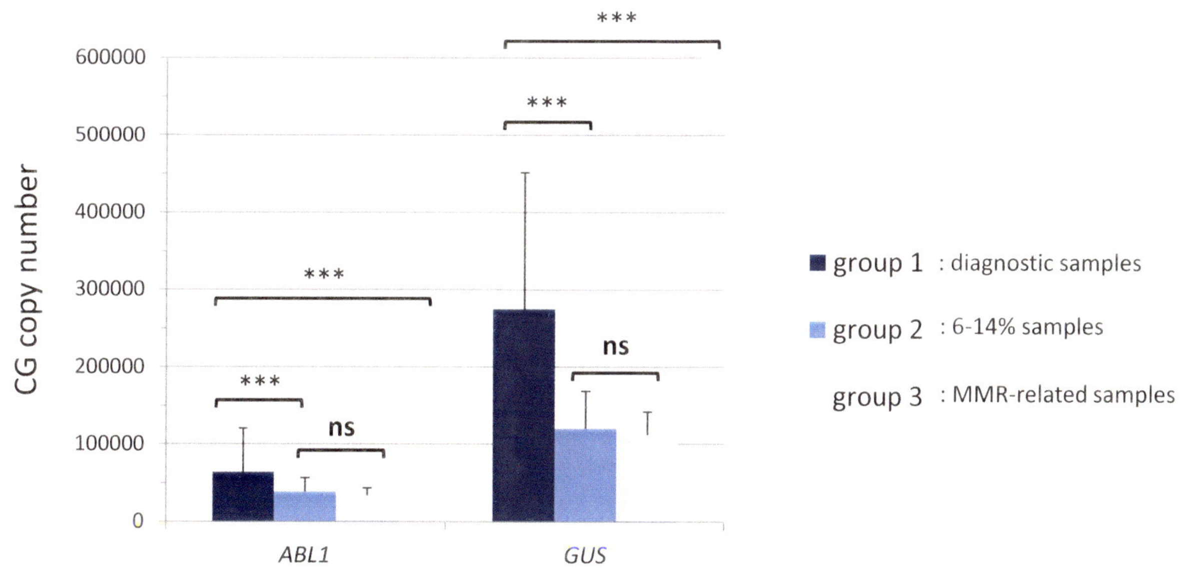

Figure 4. Mean copy number of both control genes for the 3 groups of samples. *GUS* and *ABL1* copy number is significantly higher at diagnosis (*** represents p-value<0.001; ns, non-significant).

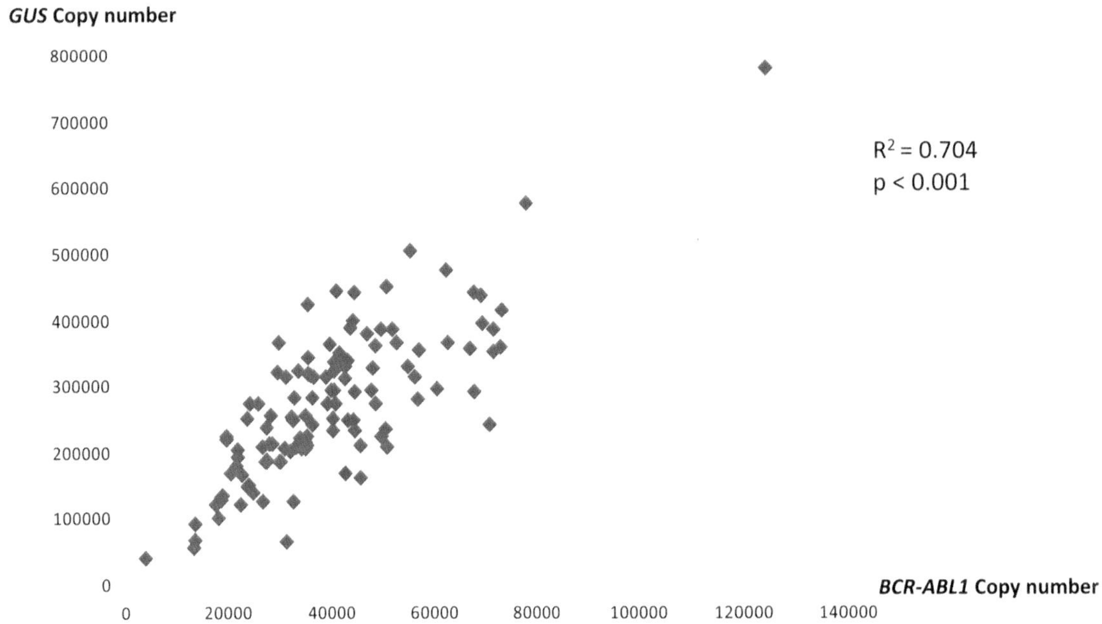

Figure 5. The copy number of *GUS* and *BCR-ABL1* are highly correlated. This supports the hypothesis that *GUS* may be overexpressed in leukemic cells compared to normal cells.

level) led to the same conclusions ($p<0.001$), for both generation of TKI.

Halving time. The halving time defines the number of days over which the *BCR-ABL1* transcript value shows a 2-fold decrease [20,23]. The median halving time was 18 days (range, 9–202 days) and was similar between Imatinib (18 days) and 2nd generation TKI (19 days). Using *(BCR-ABL1/ABL1)* ^{IS}, we found that patients with a halving time ≤19 days (n = 46) had a superior rate of MMR achievement at 12 months than patients with halving time >19 days (n = 38) (85% vs. 18%, $p<0.001$). Similarly to the predictive cut-off for transcript level at 3 months which varies according to the end-point of the study, our halving time cut-off value for 1-year MMR is lower than the 90-day cut-off used by Branford et al. to predict survival [20], but confirms that the transcript kinetics also represents an important information to predict the MMR achievement. Using *BCR-ABL1/GUS*, we found that the cut-off of 21 days separated both groups with the maximal accuracy (22.5% vs. 84%, $p<0.001$). The same results were obtained by TKI sub-group analysis.

Log reduction between diagnosis and 3 months. Similarly, the reduction of the transcript *BCR-ABL1/GUS* ratio between diagnosis and 3 months of treatment was reported as a predictor of survival [3,19]. The median reduction in our cohort was a 43-time decrease, corresponding to a 1.63 log reduction, and we identified the value of 1.45 log reduction at 3 months as the best predictive cut-off for MMR achievement. Eighty-one % of patients who obtained a log reduction >1.45 achieved the MMR threshold at 12 months, vs. 19% of patients with a log reduction ≤1.45 ($p<0.001$). By using the *(BCR-ABL1/ABL1)* ^{IS} ratio, the median log reduction was 1.86 and a cut-off of 1.70 log reduction allowed the best discrimination for MMR achievement (83% vs. 19%, $p<0.001$). The same results were obtained by TKI sub-group analysis. Of note, all the patients with a *BCR-ABL1* ^{IS} transcript level ≤0.99% at 3 months also obtained a log reduction >1.70.

Therefore, the use of halving time, log reduction or transcript level at 3 months seem to have similar capacity to predict the molecular evolution of a patient, whatever CG is used. The comparison of EMR obtained according to the 3 markers using *ABL1* as CG is shown figure 6. Nevertheless, 7 patients still did not achieve MMR at 12 months although they obtained all the cut-offs listed here (*BCR-ABL1* ^{IS} ratio ≤0.99% at 3 and 6 months, a halving time ≤19 days and a log reduction <1.70) (7 patients out of 43: 16%). No treatment interruption or transformation was reported for these patients and all of them achieved the 0.1% threshold 15 to 22 months after treatment initiation without changing therapy (3 patients on Imatinib, 3 Dasatinib, 1 Nilotinib), suggesting that some patients may respond more slowly to TKI therapy. Conversely, 6 patients obtained MMR at 12 months although they were classified as high-risk patients according to each of these early molecular markers (*BCR-ABL1* ^{IS} ratio >0.99% at 3 months, a halving time >19 days and a log reduction <1.70) (6 patients out of 35: 17%). Interestingly, of these 6 patients, 5 had a *BCR-ABL1* ^{IS} ratio ≤1% at 6 months (3 on Imatinib, 1 Dasatinib, 1 Nilotinib) and 4 obtained a deep molecular response level of at least MR^4 at a later stage. It is noteworthy that the cohort of discordant patients is too small to identify the best EMR marker (if one of them would be superior to others). Although all the markers seem to be relevant, the halving time cut-off identified allows the earliest detection of EMR failure.

5. Validation of the early 19 days monitoring time point

The observation that a halving time cut-off of 19 days may distinguish patients more likely to achieve MMR 1 year after diagnosis is a new finding that could change the current practices of molecular follow-up. In other words, a patient whose transcript level has not decreased by half after 19 days of treatment would benefit from an early switch of TKI. In order to confirm this finding, we evaluated this cut-off in a validation cohort of 58 patients. Only the *BCR-ABL1/ABL1* ratios were determined in this cohort, since we demonstrated the equivalence of both CG for the determination of EMR markers. The median halving time was 11 days (range, 3–171 days). MMR achievement rate was 70% in patients with a halving time ≤19 days (n = 43) and 7% in patients with a halving time >19 days (n = 15) ($p<0.001$), thus confirming

Table 3. Prediction of MMR achievement at 12 months with the use of different EMR markers.

EMR marker	Analysis with *(BCR-ABL1/ABL1)*^{IS}					Analysis with *BCR-ABL1/GUS*				
	Cut-off	**No. of patients**	**OR**	**95% CI**	**p**	**Cut-off**	**No. of patients**	**RR**	**95% CI**	**p**
Transcript level at 3 months (%)										
TKI1										
Low risk	≤0.99	28	23.81	5.45–104.1	<0.001	≤0.36	27	20.00	4.67–85.60	<0.001
High risk	>0.99	27				>0.36	28			
TKI2										
Low risk	≤0.99	16	16.50	2.51–108.6	0.003	≤0.36	14	6.88	1.35–35.07	0.027
High risk	>0.99	13				>0.36	15			
All TKI										
Low risk	≤0.99	44	18.21	6.08–54.54	<0.001	≤0.36	41	12.55	4.38–35.92	<0.001
High risk	>0.99	40				>0.36	43			
Halving time (days)										
TKI1										
Low risk	≤19	31	33.25	7.39–149.6	<0.001	≤21	30	36.00	7.69–168.6	<0.001
High risk	>19	24				>21	25			
TKI2										
Low risk	≤19	15	10.08	1.82–56.02	0.009	≤21	14	6.88	1.35–35.07	0.027
High risk	>19	14				>21	15			
All TKI										
Low risk	≤19	46	20.89	6.81–64.08	<0.001	≤21	44	18.21	6.08–54.54	<0.001
High risk	>19	38				>21	40			
Log reduction										
TKI1										
Low risk	≤1.70	31	25.65	6.08–108.3	<0.001	≤1,45	32	19.44	4.91–76.96	<0.001
High risk	>1.70	24				>1,45	23			
TKI2										
Low risk	≤1.70	15	16.50	2.51–108.6	0.003	≤1,45	16	16.50	2.51–108.6	0.003
High risk	>1.70	13				>1,45	13			
All TKI										
Low risk	≤1.70	47	20.89	6.81–64.08	<0.001	≤1,45	48	17.95	5.98–53.86	<0.001
High risk	>1.70	37				>1,45	36			

We compared the ability 3 early molecular response (EMR) markers recently described (transcript level at 3 months, Halving time and transcript log reduction) to accurately predict the achievement of major molecular response (MMR) after 12 months of treatment, either with the use of *ABL1* or *GUS* as control gene. Optimal cut-off for each marker was identified by using receiver operating characteristic (ROC) curve. Relative risks are expressed as odds ratios (OR) with 95% confidence interval (95% CI).

the reliability of this cut-off. Similarly, cut-offs of 1.70 for log reduction and 0.99% for the 3-month ratio also showed a good distinction between patients achieving MMR and those who did not (log reduction: 89% vs 20%, $p<0.001$; 3–month ratio: 88% vs 27%, $p<0.001$).

6. Conclusions

Does *GUS* represent a better CG than *ABL1*? Although *GUS* may be used as CG to quantify the *BCR-ABL1* transcript, our study highlights that the use of *BCR-ABL1/GUS* instead of *BCR-ABL1/ABL1* would have several consequences.

Firstly, *GUS* and *ABL1* are not expressed in the same range of values, which impacts the ratio *BCR-ABL1*/[CG] and requires a conversion factor to assess the connection between both measurements. This signifies that the use of *GUS* as CG would (i) imply a new standardization of the international scale and (ii) change in particular the MRD thresholds defined in the international recommendations to assess patient's response to therapy as the MMR threshold [1].

Secondly, we highlighted that *GUS* transcript levels at diagnosis show a direct correlation with *BCR-ABL1* levels, thus raising the hypothesis that *GUS* expression may depend on *BCR-ABL1* transcript level. Therefore, although *GUS* measurement is not affected by a technical quantification bias as observed with *ABL1*, this overexpression (directly linked to *BCR-ABL1* expression or not) does not allow more precise quantification of *BCR-ABL1* at diagnosis. Furthermore, *GUS* expression varies in a greater range of values than *ABL1* between the different disease times, which may preclude its use to assess the *BCR-ABL1* transcript kinetics of the EMR. Given the limitations described, we therefore do not consider that the replacement of *ABL1* by *GUS* represents an ideal option to assess EMR in CML patients.

Evaluation of molecular response with time-dependent variables. In the second part of our study, we investigated different ways recently described to assess the EMR and evaluated the ability of *BCR-ABL1/GUS* and *BCR-ABL1/ABL1* kinetics to predict the achievement of MMR 12 months after the TKI introduction. Using stringent inclusion criteria to ensure the reliability of our findings, we confirmed the strong predictive value of several early molecular markers in CML patients treated with 1st or 2nd generation TKI: the transcript level at 3 months of treatment, the halving time and the log-reduction of transcript levels between diagnosis and 3 months. We described the optimal cut-offs for the different markers for predicting 12-month MMR achievement in our cohort. In accordance with previous studies [3,10,12], we found that these molecular markers may predict patient molecular evolution with accuracy since the rate of molecular response was lower in patients with EMR failure than in patients who achieved EMR. Thus, in a near future the evaluation of the molecular response of each patient to TKI therapy will not only use the raw transcript levels but also different time-dependent variables assessing the transcript kinetics which are predictive of future molecular response and survival. Of note, there is currently no evidence that the use of *GUS* enables the prediction of patient evolution with more accuracy than *ABL1*. We identified a time point of 19 days after TKI introduction to assess whether halving time has been reached and these results were confirmed in an additional validation cohort. Patients whose transcript level has not decreased by half after 19 days of treatment are less likely to achieve MMR 1 year after diagnosis. It would therefore be appropriate to add this time point to patient monitoring in order to identify those patients likely to benefit from an early switch of TKI. Although these results remain to be validated on larger cohorts of patients, they suggest that it would be helpful to monitor *BCR-ABL1* levels at an earlier time point (close to 19 days) than

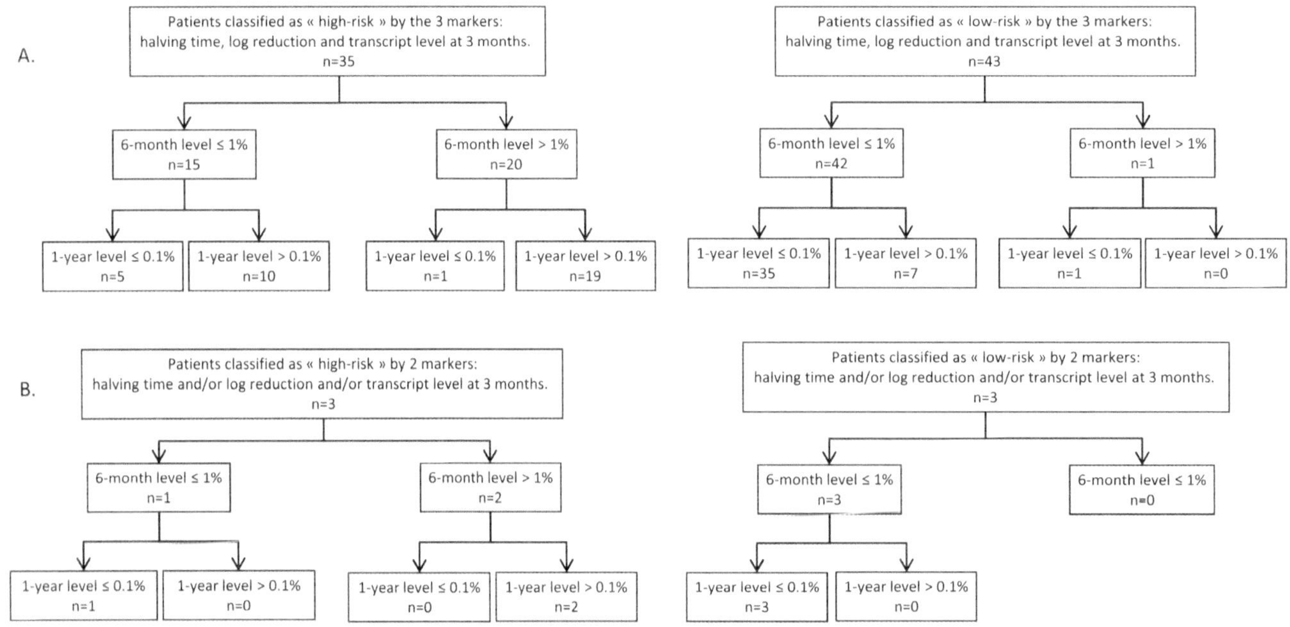

Figure 6. *BCR-ABL1/ABL1*^{IS} transcript evolution of patients according to their classification with the 3 EMR markers. Three markers were used to assess early molecular response (EMR) with the use of *BCR-ABL1/ABL1*^{IS} ratio: transcript level at 3 months, halving time and log reduction. Patients are classified as "high-risk" or "low-risk" according to the cut-offs described for each marker (see table 3) and their transcript level evolution at 6 and 12 months is reported. A: In most cases, all three markers were consistent to classify these patients as high risk (left part) or low risk (right part). B: In some discordant cases one of the markers showed a predictive value that differed from the other two. In this latter case, we took into account both concordant markers to classify the patients.

realized in the current practice, in order to accurately assess response to TKI.

Acknowledgments

We thank Mrs Barbara White-Meunier, MBA, for her kind reading of our manuscript.

Author Contributions

Conceived and designed the experiments: S. Hayette FN MM JPM. Performed the experiments: DS. Analyzed the data: S. Huet IT SG MH AB S. Hayette. Contributed to the writing of the manuscript: S. Huet PCM S. Hayette FN.

References

1. Baccarani M, Deininger MW, Rosti G, Hochhaus A, Soverini S, et al. (2013) European LeukemiaNet recommendations for the management of chronic myeloid leukemia: 2013. Blood 122: 872–884.
2. Marin D, Hedgley C, Clark RE, Apperley J, Foroni L, et al. (2012) Predictive value of early molecular response in patients with chronic myeloid leukemia treated with first-line dasatinib. Blood 120: 291–294.
3. Hanfstein B, Müller MC, Hehlmann R, Erben P, Lauseker M, et al. (2012) Early molecular and cytogenetic response is predictive for long-term progression-free and overall survival in chronic myeloid leukemia (CML). Leukemia 26: 2096–2102.
4. Hughes TP, Hochhaus A, Branford S, Müller MC, Kaeda JS, et al. (2010) Long-term prognostic significance of early molecular response to imatinib in newly diagnosed chronic myeloid leukemia: an analysis from the International Randomized Study of Interferon and STI571 (IRIS). Blood 116: 3758–3765.
5. Hughes TP, Saglio G, Kantarjian HM, Guilhot F, Niederwieser D, et al. (2013) Early molecular response predicts outcomes in patients with chronic myeloid leukemia in chronic phase treated with frontline nilotinib or imatinib. Blood 123: 1353–1360.
6. Jabbour E, Kantarjian HM, Saglio G, Steegmann JL, Shah NP, et al. (2014) Early response with dasatinib or imatinib in chronic myeloid leukemia: 3-year follow-up from a randomized phase 3 trial (DASISION). Blood 123: 494–500.
7. Rousselot P, Guilhot J, Preudhomme C, Mahon F-X, Rea D, et al. (2012) Relationship Between Molecular Responses and Disease Progression in Patients (Pts) Treated First Line with Imatinib (Im) Based Regimens: Impact of Treatment Arm within the French Spirit Trial From the French CML Group (FI LMC). ASH Annu Meet Abstr 120: 168.
8. Jain P, Kantarjian H, Nazha A, O'Brien S, Jabbour E, et al. (2013) Early responses predict better outcomes in patients with newly diagnosed chronic myeloid leukemia: results with four tyrosine kinase inhibitor modalities. Blood 121: 4867–4874.
9. Brummendorf TH, Kantarjian HM, Gambacorti-Passerini C, Guilhot F, Akard L, et al. (2012) Assessment of Early Molecular Response As a Predictor of Long-Term Clinical Outcomes in the Phase 3 BELA Study. ASH Annu Meet Abstr 120: 69.
10. Branford S, Kim D-W, Soverini S, Haque A, Shou Y, et al. (2012) Initial Molecular Response at 3 Months May Predict Both Response and Event-Free Survival at 24 Months in Imatinib-Resistant or -Intolerant Patients With Philadelphia Chromosome Positive Chronic Myeloid Leukemia in Chronic Phase Treated With Nilotinib. J Clin Oncol 30: 4323–4329.
11. Neelakantan P, Gerrard G, Lucas C, Milojkovic D, May P, et al. (2013) Combining BCR-ABL1 transcript levels at 3 and 6 months in chronic myeloid leukemia: implications for early intervention strategies. Blood 121: 2739–2742.
12. Marin D, Ibrahim AR, Lucas C, Gerrard G, Wang L, et al. (2012) Assessment of BCR-ABL1 transcript levels at 3 months is the only requirement for predicting outcome for patients with chronic myeloid leukemia treated with tyrosine kinase inhibitors. J Clin Oncol Off J Am Soc Clin Oncol 3: 232–238.
13. Hehlmann R, Müller MC, Lauseker M, Hanfstein B, Fabarius A, et al. (2013) Deep Molecular Response Is Reached by the Majority of Patients Treated With Imatinib, Predicts Survival, and Is Achieved More Quickly by Optimized High-Dose Imatinib: Results From the Randomized CML-Study IV. J Clin Oncol Off J Am Soc Clin Oncol 32: 415–423.
14. Marin D, Milojkovic D, Olavarria E, Khorashad JS, Lavallade H de, et al. (2008) European LeukemiaNet criteria for failure or suboptimal response reliably identify patients with CML in early chronic phase treated with imatinib whose eventual outcome is poor. Blood 112: 4437–4444.
15. Druker BJ, Guilhot F, O'Brien SG, Gathmann I, Kantarjian H, et al. (2006) Five-Year Follow-up of Patients Receiving Imatinib for Chronic Myeloid Leukemia. N Engl J Med. 355: 2408–2417.
16. Beillard E, Pallisgaard N, van der Velden VHJ, Bi W, Dee R, et al. (2003) Evaluation of candidate control genes for diagnosis and residual disease detection in leukemic patients using "real-time" quantitative reverse-transcriptase polymerase chain reaction (RQ-PCR) - a Europe against cancer program. Leukemia 17: 2474–2486.
17. Gabert J, Beillard E, van der Velden VHJ, Bi W, Grimwade D, et al. (2003) Standardization and quality control studies of "real-time" quantitative reverse transcriptase polymerase chain reaction of fusion gene transcripts for residual disease detection in leukemia - a Europe Against Cancer program. Leukemia 17: 2318–2357.
18. Vigneri P, Stagno F, Stella S, Cupri A, Forte S, et al. (2013) High BCR-ABL/GUSIS Levels At Diagnosis Are Associated With Unfavorable Responses To Imatinib. Blood 122: 1495–1495.
19. Hanfstein B, Shlyakhto V, Lauseker M, Hehlmann R, Saussele S, et al. (2014) Velocity of early BCR-ABL transcript elimination as an optimized predictor of outcome in chronic myeloid leukemia (CML) patients in chronic phase on treatment with imatinib. Leukemia *In press*. doi:10.1038/leu.2014.153.
20. Branford S, Roberts N, Yeung DT, Altamura H, Parker WT, et al. (2013) Any BCR-ABL Reduction Below 10% At 6 Months Of Therapy Significantly Improves Outcome For CML Patients With a Poor Response At 3 Months. Blood 122: 254–254.
21. Branford S, Fletcher L, Cross NCP, Müller MC, Hochhaus A, et al. (2008) Desirable performance characteristics for BCR-ABL measurement on an international reporting scale to allow consistent interpretation of individual patient response and comparison of response rates between clinical trials. Blood 112: 3330–3338.
22. Hughes T, Deininger M, Hochhaus A, Branford S, Radich J, et al. (2006) Monitoring CML patients responding to treatment with tyrosine kinase inhibitors: review and recommendations for harmonizing current methodology for detecting BCR-ABL transcripts and kinase domain mutations and for expressing results. Blood 108: 28–37.
23. Branford S, Yeung DT, Prime JA, Choi S-Y, Bang J, et al. (2012) BCR-ABL1 doubling times more reliably assess the dynamics of CML relapse compared with the BCR-ABL1 fold rise: implications for monitoring and management. Blood 119: 4264–4271.

Induced Differentiation of Human Myeloid Leukemia Cells into M2 Macrophages by Combined Treatment with Retinoic Acid and 1α,25-Dihydroxyvitamin D_3

Hiromichi Takahashi[1,2], Yoshihiro Hatta[2], Noriyoshi Iriyama[2], Yuichiro Hasegawa[1], Hikaru Uchida[1], Masaru Nakagawa[1,2], Makoto Makishima[1]*, Jin Takeuchi[2¤], Masami Takei[2]

1 Division of Biochemistry, Department of Biomedical Sciences, Nihon University School of Medicine, Tokyo, Japan, **2** Division of Hematology and Rheumatology, Department of Medicine, Nihon University School of Medicine, Tokyo, Japan

Abstract

Retinoids and 1α,25-dihydroxyvitamin D_3 (1,25$(OH)_2D_3$) induce differentiation of myeloid leukemia cells into granulocyte and macrophage lineages, respectively. All-*trans* retinoic acid (ATRA), which is effective in the treatment of acute promyelocytic leukemia, can induce differentiation of other types of myeloid leukemia cells, and combined treatment with retinoid and 1,25$(OH)_2D_3$ effectively enhances the differentiation of leukemia cells into macrophage-like cells. Recent work has classified macrophages into M1 and M2 types. In this study, we investigated the effect of combined treatment with retinoid and 1,25$(OH)_2D_3$ on differentiation of myeloid leukemia THP-1 and HL60 cells. 9-*cis* Retinoic acid (9cRA) plus 1,25$(OH)_2D_3$ inhibited proliferation of THP-1 and HL60 cells and increased myeloid differentiation markers including nitroblue tetrazolium reducing activity and expression of CD14 and CD11b. ATRA and the synthetic retinoic acid receptor agonist Am80 exhibited similar effects in combination with 1,25$(OH)_2D_3$ but less effectively than 9cRA, while the retinoid X receptor agonist HX630 was not effective. 9cRA plus 1,25$(OH)_2D_3$ effectively increased expression of M2 macrophage marker genes, such as *CD163*, *ARG1* and *IL10*, increased surface CD163 expression, and induced interleukin-10 secretion in myeloid leukemia cells, while 9cRA alone had weaker effects on these phenotypes and 1,25$(OH)_2D_3$ was not effective. Taken together, our results demonstrate selective induction of M2 macrophage markers in human myeloid leukemia cells by combined treatment with 9cRA and 1,25$(OH)_2D_3$.

Editor: R. Keith Reeves, Beth Israel Deaconess Medical Center, Harvard Medical School, United States of America

Funding: This work was supported by "Strategic Research Base Development" Program for Private Universities subsidized by MEXT (2008–2012) and funds from Nihon University School of Medicine. The funders had no role in study design, data collection and analysis, decision to publish, or preparation of the manuscript.

* Email: makishima.makoto@nihon-u.ac.jp

¤ Current address: Department of Internal Medicine, International University of Health and Welfare Shioya Hospital, Yaita, Tochigi, Japan

Introduction

Retinoids play roles in numerous biological functions, such as cellular proliferation and differentiation, embryogenesis, immunity and metabolism [1]. An active natural retinoid, all-*trans* retinoic acid (ATRA), is effective in differentiation therapy for acute promyelocytic leukemia (APL) [2]. APL is a subtype of acute myeloid leukemia, which is characterized by a specific chromosomal abnormality t(15,17) associated with a genetic rearrangement between retinoic acid receptor α (RARα) (gene symbol, *RARA*) and the promyelocytic leukemia gene *PML* [2]. RARα plays a role in granulocytic differentiation of hematopoietic cells and the abnormal chimeric receptor PML-RARα has been implicated in APL pathogenesis by blocking the myeloid differentiation program and enhancing self-renewal of leukemic cells [3,4]. Pharmacological doses of ATRA induce differentiation of APL cells into granulocytes through degradation of PML-RARα and recovery of physiological RARα signaling [3,4].

Retinoids, including ATRA, 9-*cis* retinoic acid (9cRA) and synthetic RAR ligands, exhibit anti-tumor effects not only on APL but also on other malignancies, such as breast cancer, lung cancer, and head and neck cancer [5]. With regard to leukemia, ATRA was first reported to induce the differentiation of human myeloid leukemia HL60 cells towards the granulocytic lineage [6,7]. Importantly, HL60 cells are derived from non-APL leukemia without t(15,17) [8], and ATRA can also induce differentiation of leukemia cells from non-APL myeloid leukemia patients [9]. Retinoids in combination with other differentiation inducers, such as 1α,25-dihydroxyvitamin D_3 (1,25$(OH)_2D_3$) and dibutyryl cAMP, synergistically induce differentiation of leukemia cells [10–13]. However, the underlying mechanisms of retinoid-induced differentiation of leukemia cells remain poorly understood and retinoids have not been utilized in the treatment of myeloid leukemia other than APL.

The active form of vitamin D_3, 1,25$(OH)_2D_3$, regulates calcium and bone homeostasis, immunity, and cellular growth and differentiation through direct binding to the vitamin D receptor

(VDR), and has been demonstrated to inhibit the proliferation and to induce the differentiation of various types of malignant cells, including breast, prostate and colon cancers as well as myeloid leukemia cells [14,15]. The administration of 1,25(OH)$_2$D$_3$ and its analog has therapeutic effects in a mouse model of myeloid leukemia [16]. While ATRA induces granulocytic differentiation [6,7], 1,25(OH)$_2$D$_3$ induces the differentiation of HL60 cells and other myeloid leukemia cells towards the monocyte and macrophage lineage [17,18]. Interestingly, ATRA induces monocytic differentiation of monoblastic leukemia U937 and THP-1 cells [13,19]. Combined treatment with 1,25(OH)$_2$D$_3$ and retinoids induces the differentiation of HL60 cells and human monoblastic leukemia cells, such as THP-1 cells, to monocyte/macrophage-lineage cells more effectively than 1,25(OH)$_2$D$_3$ alone [10,12,20]. Although 1,25(OH)$_2$D$_3$ has been shown to exert its biological effects on cellular proliferation and differentiation by genomic and/or non-genomic pathways [21], the detailed mechanisms remain unclear. Macrophages have been classified into two cell types, classically activated M1 macrophages and alternatively activated M2 macrophages [22,23]. While M1 macrophages produce proinflammatory cytokines and enhance microbicidal and tumoricidal immunity, M2 macrophages are involved in wound healing and immune regulation. Although retinoids and 1,25(OH)$_2$D$_3$ play functional roles in monocytes and macrophages [4,24], the macrophage cell type resulting from 1,25(OH)$_2$D$_3$ and/or retinoid differentiation of myeloid leukemia cells has not been further characterized. In this study, we examined the effects of 1,25(OH)$_2$D$_3$ in combination with retinoids on differentiation of myeloid leukemia cells and found that 1,25(OH)$_2$D$_3$ in combination with 9cRA and ATRA induce the differentiation of myeloid leukemia cells to macrophages with M2-like phenotype.

Materials and Methods

Compounds

1,25(OH)$_2$D$_3$, ATRA and 9cRA were purchased from Wako Pure Chemical Industries (Osaka, Japan). Am80 (4-[(5,6,7,8-tetrahydro-5,5,8,8-tetramethyl-2-naphthalenyl)carbamoyl]benzoic acid) [25] and HX630 (4-[2,3-(2,5-dimethyl-2,5-hexano)dibenzo[*b,f*][1,4]-thiazepin-11-yl]benzoic acid) [26] were kindly provided by Dr. Koichi Shudo of Research Foundation ITSUU Laboratory (Tokyo, Japan).

Cell culture, cell growth, nitroblue tetrazolium (NBT) reduction, and interleukin-10 (IL-10) production

Human myeloid leukemia HL60 and THP-1 cells (RIKEN Cell Bank, Tsukuba, Japan) were maintained in RPMI1640 medium containing 10% fetal bovine serum, 100 unit/ml penicillin, and 100 μg/ml streptomycin in a humidified atmosphere containing 5% CO_2. Suspensions of cells (10^5 cells/ml) were cultured with or without test compounds at pharmacological concentrations (30–100 nM) according to our preliminary experiments and the previous reports [10–12,27]. Cell numbers were counted in a Z1S Coulter Counter (Beckman Coulter, Fullerton, CA). Cell morphology was examined in cell smears stained with May-Grünwald-Giemsa. NBT reduction was assayed colorimetrically and NBT-reducing activity data were normalized to the cell numbers [28]. IL-10 levels in culture media were determined with the Human IL-10 ELISA MAX Standard kit (BioLegend, San Diego, CA).

Flow cytometry

Expression of cell surface antigens, CD14, CD11b and CD163, were determined with immunofluorescence staining and flow cytometry [29]. FITC mouse anti-human CD14, PE mouse anti-human CD11b, PE mouse anti-human CD163, and isotype control antibodies were purchased from Becton, Dickinson and Company (Franklin Lakes, NJ). The stained cells were assayed with a flow cytometer (BD FACSCalibur; Becton, Dickinson and Company) and analyzed with the BD CellQuest software (Becton, Dickinson and Company).

Reverse transcription and real-time quantitative polymerase chain reaction

Total RNAs from samples were prepared by the acid guanidine thiocyanate-phenol/chloroform method [30]. cDNAs were synthesized using the ImProm-II Reverse Transcription system (Promega Corporation, Madison, WI). Intron-spanning primers were as follows: *CD163* (GenBank accession no. NM_004244), 5′-ACT GCA AGA ACT GGC AAT GG-3′ and 5′-CCA TGC TTC ACT TCA ACA CG-3′; *ARG1* (GenBank accession no. NM_000045), 5′-TCC AAG GTC TGT GGG AAA AG-3′ and 5′-ATT GCC AAA CTG TGG TCT CC-3′; *IL10* (GenBank accession no. NM_000572), 5′-CCA AGA CCC AGA CAT CAA GG-3′ and 5′-GGC CTT GCT CTT GTT TTC AC-3′; *IL12B* (GenBank accession no. NM_002187), 5′-ATT GAG GTC ATG GTG GAT GC-3′ and 5′-TTC TTG GGT GGG TCA GGT TT-3′; *TGFB1* (GenBank accession no. NM_000660), 5′-CAA CAA TTC CTG GCG ATA CCT C-3′ and 5′-AAA GCC CTC AAT TTC CCC TC-3′; *TNF* (GenBank accession no. NM_000594), 5′-TGC TTG TTC CTC AGC CTC TT-3′ and 5′-TGA GGT ACA GGC CCT CTG AT-3′; *IL6* (GenBank accession no. NM_000600), 5′-AAA GAG GCA CTG GCA GAA AA-3′ and 5′-AAA GCT GCG CAG AAT GAG AT-3′; *NOS2* (GenBank accession no. NM_000625), 5′-TAC CCC TCC AGA TGA GCT TC-3′ and 5′-TCT CCT TTG TTA CCG CTT CC-3′. Other primer sequences have been reported previously [28]. The mRNA values were normalized to the amount of β-actin mRNA.

Statistical analysis

All values are shown as mean ± S.D. We performed one-way ANOVA followed by Tukey's multiple comparisons or two-way ANOVA to assess significant differences using Prism 6 (Graphpad Software, La Jolla, CA).

Results

Induction of differentiation of human myeloid leukemia cells by retinoids plus 1,25(OH)$_2$D$_3$

We examined the effects of 9cRA and ATRA in the absence or presence of 1,25(OH)$_2$D$_3$ on NBT-reducing activity, a marker of myeloid differentiation, in monoblastic leukemia THP-1 cells and promyelocytic leukemia HL60 cells. 9cRA (100 nM) increased NBT-reducing activity in THP-1 and HL60 cells, while ATRA (100 nM) was not effective (Fig. 1A), consistent with the previous reports showing that 9cRA is more potent than ATRA in inducing differentiation of leukemia cells [20,31,32]. In combination with 1,25(OH)$_2$D$_3$, 9cRA and ATRA effectively increased NBT-reducing activity in these cells (Fig. 1A). Am80 (also called tamibarotene) is a potent synthetic RAR agonist that is used in the treatment of recurrent APL in Japan [33,34]. HX630 is an RXR selective agonist derived from LE135, an RAR antagonist [26]. HX630 does not exhibit RAR antagonistic activity but enhances the differentiation-inducing activity of Am80 in HL60 cells [33]. We also examined the effects of Am80 and HX630 in the absence or presence of 1,25(OH)$_2$D$_3$. Although Am80 and HX630 at 100 nM were not effective, the combination of

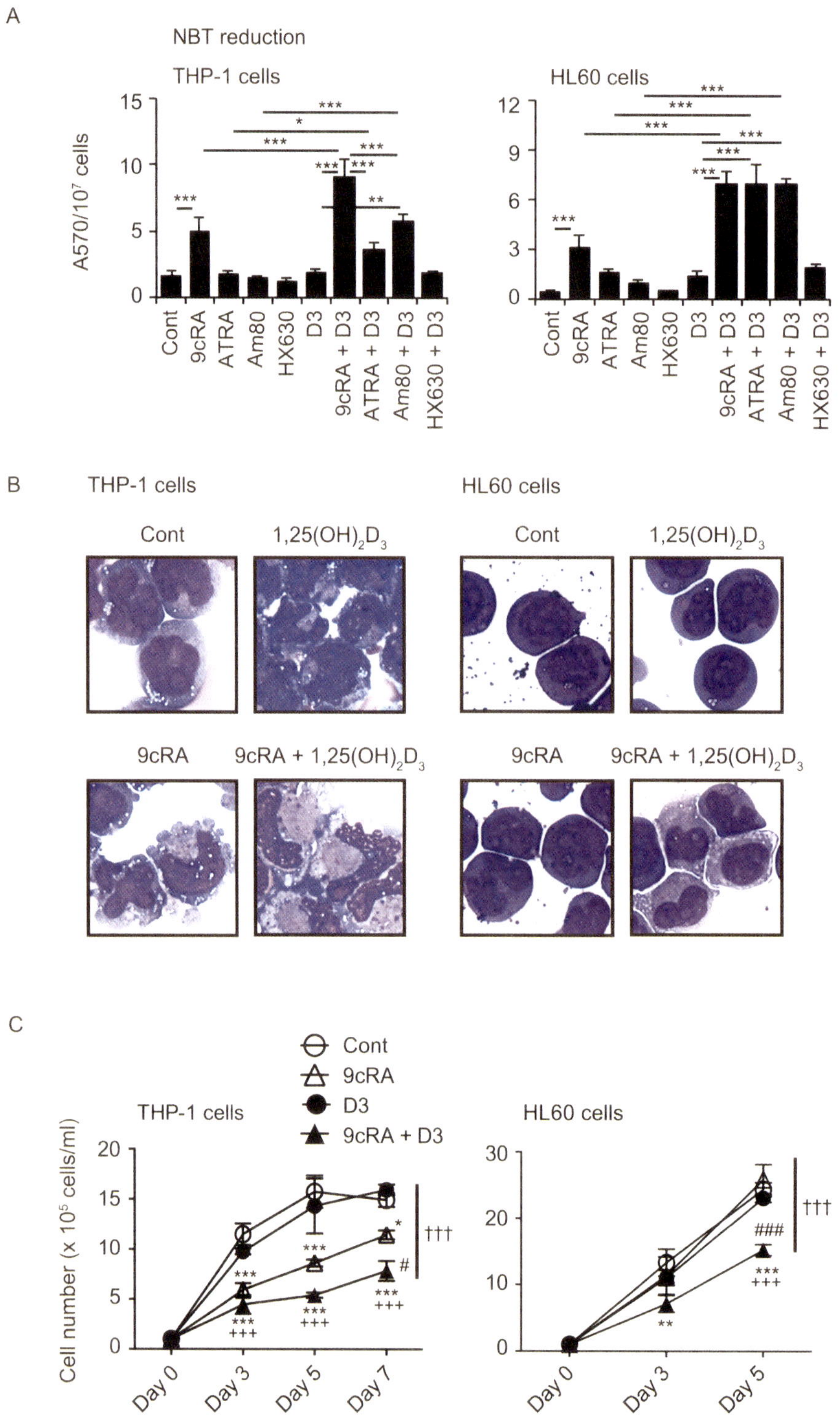

Figure 1. Induction of differentiation of THP-1 and HL60 cells by combined treatment with retinoid and $1,25(OH)_2D_3$. (A) NBT-reducing activities. Cells were treated with vehicle control (Cont), 100 nM 9cRA, ATRA, Am80 or HX630 in the absence or presence of 100 nM $1,25(OH)_2D_3$ (D3) for 5 days. *, $p<0.05$; **, $p<0.01$; ***, $p<0.001$ (one-way ANOVA followed by Tukey's multiple comparisons). (B) Morphological changes of THP-1 and HL60 cells treated with 9cRA and/or $1,25(OH)_2D_3$. Cells were treated with vehicle control (Cont), 100 nM 9cRA and/or 100 nM $1,25(OH)_2D_3$ for 5 days and the cell smears were stained with May-Grünwald-Giemsa. (C) Cell proliferations. Cells (1×10^5/ml) were cultured with vehicle control (Cont), 100 nM 9cRA and/or 100 nm $1,25(OH)_2D_3$ (D3), and cell numbers were counted at indicated days. *, $p<0.05$; **, $p<0.01$; ***, $p<0.001$ vs Cont; ###, $p<0.001$ vs 9cRA; +++, $p<0.001$ vs D3 (one-way ANOVA followed by Tukey's multiple comparisons). †††, $p<0.001$ (two-way ANOVA).

$1,25(OH)_2D_3$ with Am80 but not HX630 significantly increased NBT-reducing activity in THP-1 and HL60 cells (Fig. 1A).

THP-1 cells and HL60 cells were treated with $1,25(OH)_2D_3$ and/or 9cRA and the morphological features were examined. While untreated THP-1 cells had a basophilic cytoplasm and large nuclei with several nucleoli, cells treated with 9cRA (100 nM) had grayish, enlarged cytoplasm and slightly lobulated nuclei (Fig. 1B). Although $1,25(OH)_2D_3$ (100 nM) treatment did not induce an apparent morphological change, the combination of 9cRA and $1,25(OH)_2D_3$ enlarged the grayish cytoplasm area more effectively than 9cRA alone. Untreated HL60 cells have promyelocytic features, although they are not derived from APL having t(15;17) [8]. While HL60 treated with $1,25(OH)_2D_3$ (100 nM) had slightly less basophilic cytoplasm and decreased nuclear-cytoplasmic ratio, 9cRA (100 nM) induced differentiation of HL60 cells into myelocytic cells having slightly lobulated nuclei and a decreased nuclear-cytoplasmic ratio (Fig. 1B). Combined treatment with 9cRA and $1,25(OH)_2D_3$ enhanced the monocytic features of HL60 cells with enlarged grayish cytoplasm and a further decrease in the nuclear-cytoplasmic ratio. These findings are consistent with the previous reports showing monocytic differentiation of myeloid leukemia cells by $1,25(OH)_2D_3$ plus 9cRA or ATRA [32,35]. 9cRA (100 nM) suppressed the proliferation of THP-1 cells, and although $1,25(OH)_2D_3$ (100 nM) was not effective, combined treatment with $1,25(OH)_2D_3$ enhanced the anti-proliferative effect of 9cRA (Fig. 1C). While treatment with 9cRA (100 nM) or $1,25(OH)_2D_3$ (100 nM) alone was not effective, the combined treatment with 9cRA and $1,25(OH)_2D_3$ effectively suppressed HL60 proliferation (Fig. 1C).

We next examined the effects of combined treatment with retinoids and $1,25(OH)_2D_3$ on expression of surface antigens, CD14 and CD11b, additional markers of myelomonocytic differentiation. $1,25(OH)_2D_3$ at 100 nM slightly increased CD14 expression in THP-1 cells (Fig. 2A). 9cRA at 100 nM increased CD14 expression and the combination of 9cRA and $1,25(OH)_2D_3$ increased CD14 expression more strongly than single use of these compounds. Interestingly, although ATRA and Am80 were not effective, these retinoids enhanced CD14 expression in combination with $1,25(OH)_2D_3$. HX630 did not increase CD14 expression in the absence or presence of $1,25(OH)_2D_3$. $1,25(OH)_2D_3$ also slightly increased CD11b expression in THP-1 cells (Fig. 2B). 9cRA, ATRA and Am80 at 30 nM increased CD11b expression, and effectively enhanced CD11b expression induced by $1,25(OH)_2D_3$. HX630 did not increase CD11b expression in the absence or presence of $1,25(OH)_2D_3$. Transcriptional induction of *CD14*, a VDR target gene [36], is also associated with myeloid differentiation [28]. Retinoid treatment did not increase *CD14* mRNA levels in THP-1 and HL60 cells (Fig. 2C). Interestingly, while the effect of $1,25(OH)_2D_3$ (100 nM) alone was not significant, combinations of $1,25(OH)_2D_3$ with 9cRA, ATRA and Am80 effectively increased *CD14* mRNA expression in these cells. The combination of HX630 and $1,25(OH)_2D_3$ was not effective in *CD14* mRNA induction. Thus, when combined with $1,25(OH)_2D_3$, a RAR/RXR agonist (9cRA) and RAR agonists (ATRA and Am80), but not a RXR agonist (HX630), effectively induce differentiation of myeloid leukemia THP-1 and HL60 cells.

Induction of M2 macrophage markers in human myeloid leukemia cells by retinoids plus $1,25(OH)_2D_3$

As shown in Figure 1B and the previous reports [10,20,32], combined treatment with retinoid and $1,25(OH)_2D_3$ induces differentiation of myeloid leukemia cells into the monocytic lineage rather than the granulocytic lineage. We examined whether leukemia cells treated with retinoid plus $1,25(OH)_2D_3$ exhibit M1 or M2 macrophage phenotypes. Expression of the *CD163*, *ARG1*, *IL10* and *TGFB1* marker genes is associated with M2 macrophage activation, whereas *IL12B*, *TNF*, *IL6* and *NOS2* expression is increased in M1 macrophages [23]. Treatment of THP-1 cells with 9cRA, ATRA or $1,25(OH)_2D_3$ alone did not induce *CD163* mRNA expression, but the combination of 9cRA and $1,25(OH)_2D_3$ effectively increased *CD163* mRNA levels (Fig. 3A). ATRA plus $1,25(OH)_2D_3$ also increased *CD163* expression but less effectively than 9cRA plus $1,25(OH)_2D_3$. Although *CD163* mRNA expression was not detected in HL60 cells treated with 9cRA or ATRA alone, 9cRA plus $1,25(OH)_2D_3$ and ATRA plus $1,25(OH)_2D_3$ tended to increase *CD163* mRNA levels. 9cRA plus $1,25(OH)_2D_3$ also effectively increased *ARG1* mRNA expression in THP-1 cells, while ATRA plus $1,25(OH)_2D_3$ tended to increase its expression, an effect that did not reach statistical significance (Fig. 3B). Interestingly, combination of ATRA and $1,25(OH)_2D_3$ effectively increased *ARG1* mRNA levels in HL60 cells, while the combined effect of 9cRA and $1,25(OH)_2D_3$ did not reach statistical significance. *IL10* mRNA expression was also elevated in THP-1 cells treated with 9cRA plus $1,25(OH)_2D_3$ and, to a lesser extent, ATRA plus $1,25(OH)_2D_3$ (Fig. 3C). Although treatment of HL60 cells with $1,25(OH)_2D_3$ decreased *IL10* mRNA levels, the combination of $1,25(OH)_2D_3$ with 9cRA or ATRA increased them to control levels. Combination of $1,25(OH)_2D_3$ with 9cRA or ATRA did not increase *IL12B* mRNA levels in THP-1 and HL60 cells (Fig. 3D). *IL12B* mRNA levels in THP-1 cells treated with 9cRA were decreased by combined treatment with $1,25(OH)_2D_3$. Addition of 9cRA increased *TGFB1* mRNA levels in THP-1 cells treated with $1,25(OH)_2D_3$ (Fig. 3E). 9cRA increased *TNF* mRNA expression in THP-1 cells but combined treatment with $1,25(OH)_2D_3$ decreased its expression. *IL6* mRNA expression was increased by the combination of 9cRA and $1,25(OH)_2D_3$. 9cRA and/or $1,25(OH)_2D_3$ induced no significant change in *NOS2* mRNA expression. Thus, the combination of retinoid and $1,25(OH)_2D_3$ increases expression of genes associated with M2 macrophages.

We further examined expression of CD163 as a cell surface marker of M2 macrophages in THP-1 cells. Figure 4A shows representative flow cytometric analysis of THP-1 cells treated with or without 9cRA and $1,25(OH)_2D_3$ using anti-CD14 and anti-CD163 antibodies. 9cRA but not $1,25(OH)_2D_3$ increased CD163 mean fluorescence intensity in THP-1 cells, and the combination of 9cRA and $1,25(OH)_2D_3$ effectively enhanced the intensity values (Fig. 4B). 9cRA increased and $1,25(OH)_2D_3$ slightly decreased surface CD14 mean fluorescence intensity, but 9cRA plus $1,25(OH)_2D_3$ also strongly increased the CD14 intensity (Fig. 4B). 9cRA treatment increased the percentage of both CD163+/CD14+ cells and CD163−/CD14+ cells (Fig. 4B). Combination of $1,25(OH)_2D_3$ with 9CRA increased the percentage of CD163+/CD14+ cells but not of CD163−/CD14+ cells. These findings are consistent with induction of the M2 macrophage phenotype in THP-1 cells by 9cRA plus $1,25(OH)_2D_3$.

The combination of 9cRA and 1,25(OH)2D3 induces IL-10 protein secretion in THP-1 and HL60 cells

Finally, we examined IL-10 protein levels in conditioned media of THP-1 and HL60 cells treated with 9cRA and/or $1,25(OH)_2D_3$. IL-10 protein levels from THP-1 cells treated with 9cRA and $1,25(OH)_2D_3$ alone were below detection limits, but the combination of these compounds effectively induced IL-10 protein secretion from these cells (Fig. 5). While IL-10 protein was detected in the culture media of untreated HL60 cells, 9cRA increased and $1,25(OH)_2D_3$ decreased the protein level. 9cRA plus $1,25(OH)_2D_3$ effectively increased the IL-10 protein levels in

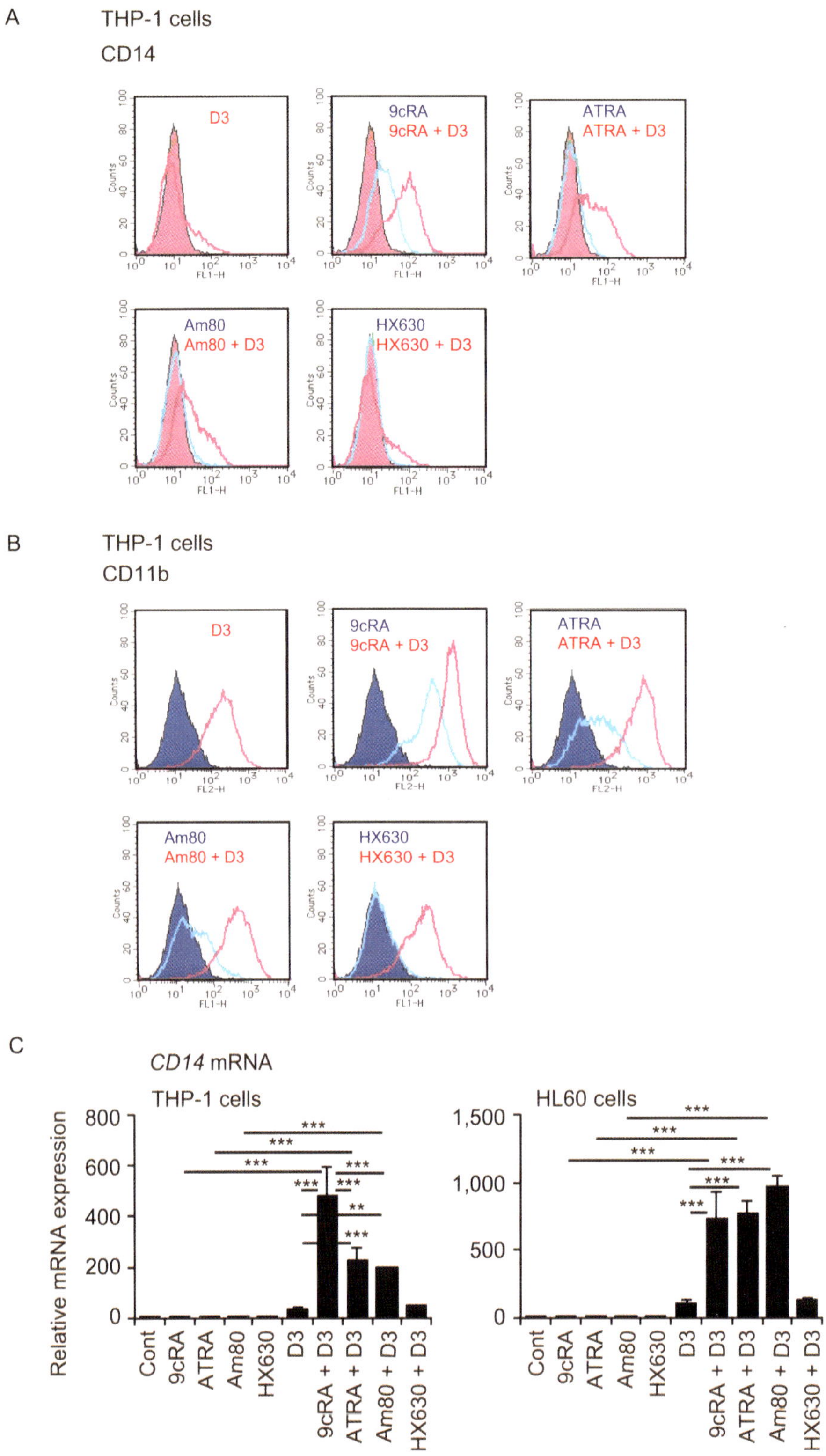

Figure 2. Effects of combined treatment with retinoid and $1,25(OH)_2D_3$ on cell surface CD14 and CD11b expression and *CD14* mRNA expression. Representative histograms of CD14 expression (A) and CD11b expression (B) in THP-1 cells. Cells were treated with vehicle control (Cont), 100 nM 9cRA, ATRA, Am80 or HX630 in the absence or presence of 100 nM $1,25(OH)_2D_3$ (D3) for 96 hours. Filled curves, vehicle control. Similar results were obtained from repeated experiments. (C) *CD14* mRNA levels in THP-1 and HL60 cells. Cells were treated with vehicle control (Cont), 30 nM 9cRA, ATRA, Am80 or HX630 in the absence or presence of 100 nM $1,25(OH)_2D_3$ (D3) for 72 hours. **, $p<0.01$; ***, $p<0.001$ (one-way ANOVA followed by Tukey's multiple comparisons).

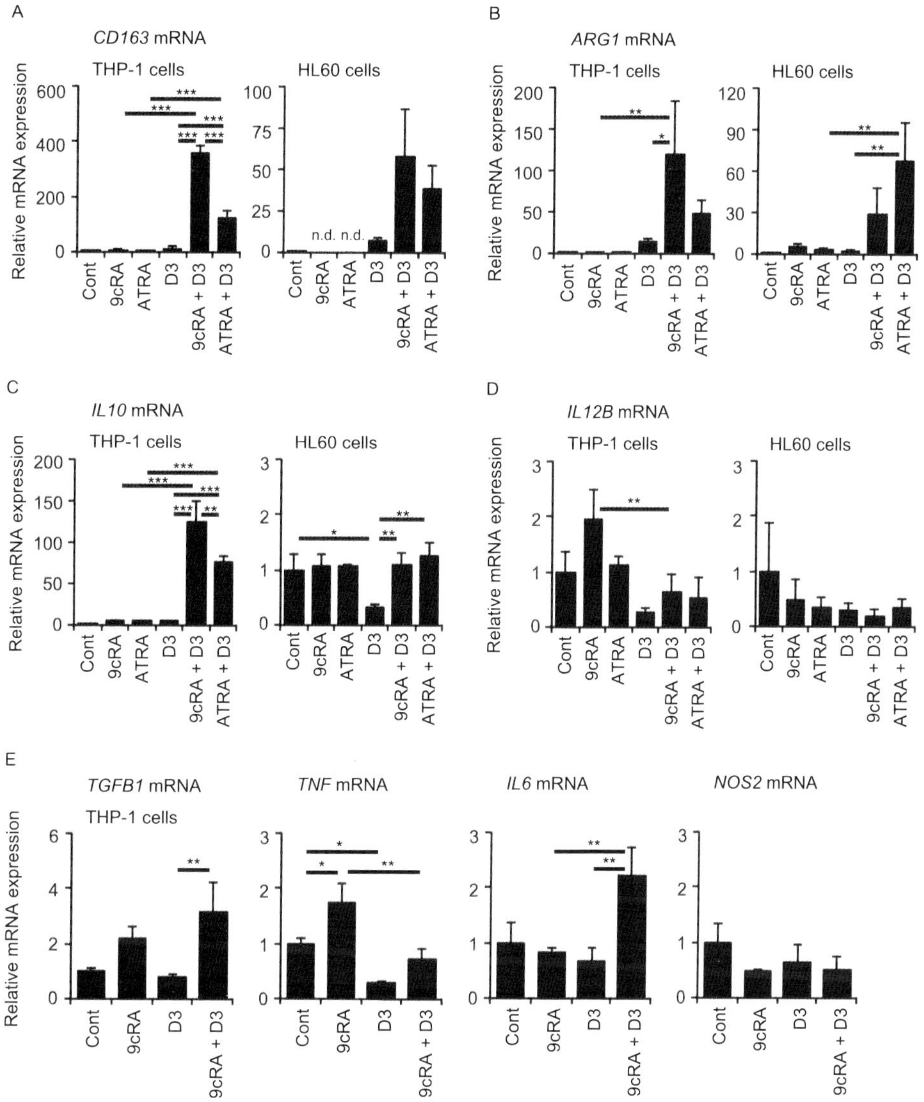

Figure 3. Expression of marker genes of M1 and M2 macrophages. mRNA levels of the M2 markers *CD163* (A), *ARG1* (B), *IL10* (C), and the M1 marker *IL12B* (D) in THP-1 and HL60 cells. (E) mRNA levels of the M2 marker *TGFB1*, the M1 markers *TNF*, *IL6*, and *NOS2* in THP-1 cells. Cells were treated with vehicle control (Cont), 30 nM 9cRA, or ATRA in the absence or presence of 100 nM 1,25(OH)$_2$D$_3$ (D3) for 72 hours. *, $p<0.05$; **, $p<0.01$; ***, $p<0.001$ (one-way ANOVA followed by Tukey's multiple comparisons). n.d., not detected.

media. Thus, combined treatment of leukemia cells with 9cRA and 1,25(OH)$_2$D$_3$ induces IL-10 protein secretion as well as increased expression of M2 macrophage markers.

Discussion

In this study, we found that combined treatment with retinoid and 1,25(OH)$_2$D$_3$ induces the differentiation of human myeloid leukemia THP-1 and HL60 cells into the monocytic lineage with a M2 macrophage phenotype. ATRA induces granulocytic differentiation of promyelocytic leukemia HL60 cells but monocytic differentiation of monoblastic U937 and THP-1 cells [6,7,13,19]. Combination of ATRA or 9cRA with 1,25(OH)$_2$D$_3$ effectively induces monocyte/macrophage phenotypes, such as phagocytic activity, monocyte-specific esterase, lysozyme secretion, and *CSF1R* expression, in HL60 and U937 cells [10,32,37]. We observed a monocytic morphology and increased CD14 expression in HL60 and THP-1 cells treated with 9cRA plus 1,25(OH)$_2$D$_3$ (Figs. 1 and 2). ATRA plus 1,25(OH)$_2$D$_3$ also induces differentiation of promyelocytic AML-193 cells into cells that display both a typical neutrophilic morphology and monocyte-specific properties, such as CD14 expression and monocyte-specific esterase, a hybrid granulomonocytic phenotype [35]. RAR signaling plays an important role in hematopoiesis and RARα is involved in neutrophil development [4]. RAR and RXR signaling pathways have been reported to regulate monocyte/macrophage function [4]. However, it remains to be determined how retinoid signaling enhances monocytic differentiation induced by 1,25(OH)$_2$D$_3$ in myeloid leukemia cells.

Among retinoids, 9cRA, ATRA and Am80, but not HX630, in combination with 1,25(OH)$_2$D$_3$ exhibit effective differentiation-inducing activity in these cells (Figs. 1 and 2). 1,25(OH)$_2$D$_3$ acts as a ligand for the nuclear receptor VDR, which forms a heterodimer with RXR [38], and the VDR−RXR heterodimer is not permissive to RXR ligand activation [39]. RAR selective ligands exhibit stronger synergistic effects with 1,25(OH)$_2$D$_3$ than RXR

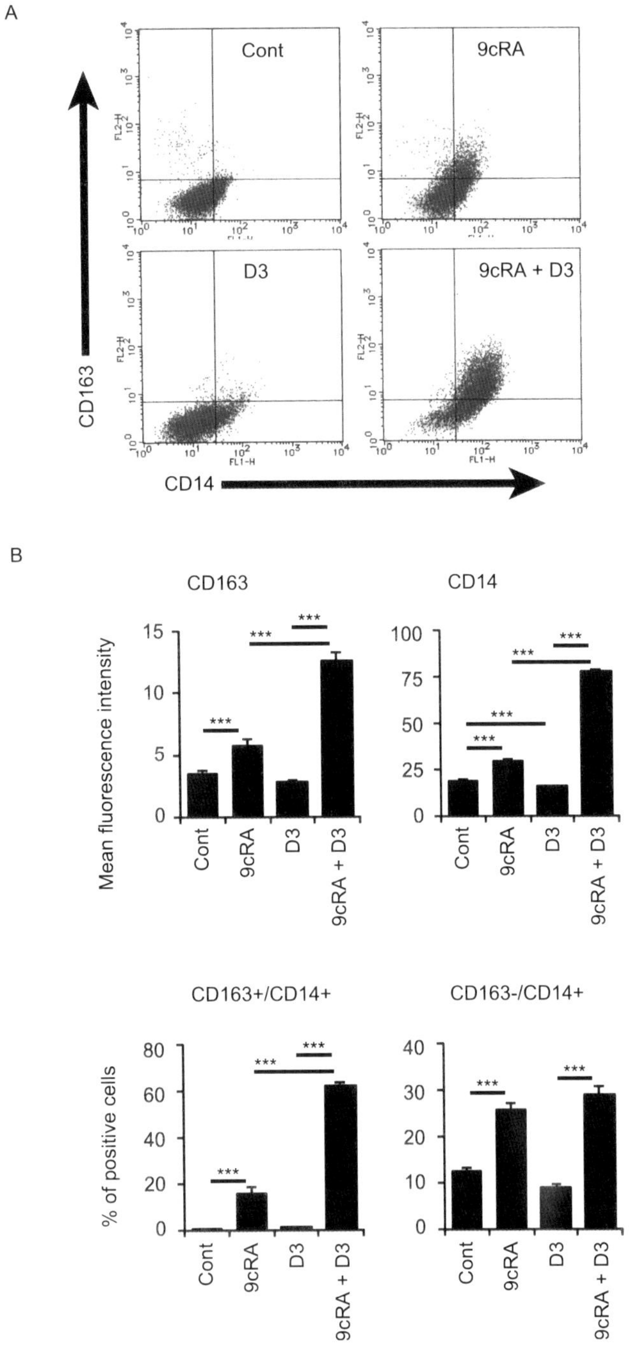

Figure 4. Cell surface expression of CD163 in THP-1 cells. (A) Representative histograms of CD14 and CD163 expression. (B) Quantification of mean fluorescence intensity of CD163 and CD14 expression. (C) Quantification of percentages of CD163+/CD14+ cells and CD163−/CD14+ cells. Cells were treated with vehicle control (Cont), 100 nM 9cRA and/or 100 nM $1,25(OH)_2D_3$ (D3) for 96 hours. **, $p<0.01$; ***, $p<0.001$ (one-way ANOVA followed by Tukey's multiple comparisons).

selective ligands in inhibiting proliferation and inducing differentiation of monoblastic U937 cells [27]. Combined effects of retinoid and $1,25(OH)_2D_3$ on differentiation of myelomonocytic leukemia cells are likely mediated by VDR and RAR activation. RXR also forms heterodimers with RAR and other nuclear receptors, including peroxisome proliferator-activated receptor (PPAR) and liver X receptor (LXR) [38]. The RAR−RXR heterodimer is activated by RXR ligand only in the presence of RAR ligand, a feature known as conditional permissivity [39]. 9cRA exhibits differentiation-inducing activity more effectively than ATRA in the absence or presence of $1,25(OH)_2D_3$ (Figs. 1 and 2), in agreement with previous reports [20,31,32]. Since 9cRA acts as a ligand for both RAR and RXR [40], synergistic activation may be due to binding to both RAR and RXR in the RAR−RXR heterodimer. In addition, RXR ligands can activate permissive heterodimers, such as PPAR−RXR and LXR−RXR [38]. PPARγ ligand and LXR ligand have been reported to induce differentiation of myeloid leukemia cells [41,42]. RXR ligand activation of these permissive heterodimers may also contribute to the effect of 9cRA. However, the pure RXR ligand HX630 alone and in combination with $1,25(OH)_2D_3$ was not effective in inducing differentiation of THP-1 and HL60 cells, while the combination of $1,25(OH)_2D_3$ with the RAR selective agonist Am80 induced the differentiation of these cells (Figs. 1 and 2). These findings suggest that cooperation between VDR signaling and RAR signaling, not RXR signaling, plays a role in the differentiation of myeloid leukemia cells. VDR activation changes expression of many genes, including those involved in cellular proliferation, differentiation and apoptosis [21]. $1,25(OH)_2D_3$ treatment can modulate intracellular kinase pathways via a non-genomic mechanism, and it remains unknown whether the non-genomic actions are mediated through VDR or other proteins [21]. Although both genomic and non-genomic effects of $1,25(OH)_2D_3$ have been shown to play roles in differentiation induction of leukemia cells, the detailed mechanisms remain to be elucidated. RAR signaling may modulate the vitamin D signaling pathway or regulate other differentiation mechanisms. Further studies are needed to elucidate molecular mechanisms involving VDR, RAR and RXR signaling pathways in the induced differentiation of leukemia cells.

Combined treatment with 9cRA and $1,25(OH)_2D_3$ increased mRNA expression of *CD163*, *ARG1*, *IL10*, and *TGFB1* genes (Fig. 3), surface expression of CD163 proteins (Fig. 4) and IL-10 secretion in THP-1 cells (Fig. 5). This combination also increased *CD163*, *ARG1* and *IL10* mRNA levels (Fig. 3) and IL-10 secretion in HL60 cells (Fig. 5). This phenotype has been characterized as M2 macrophages, although the classification of human macrophages remains controversial [23]. 9cRA plus $1,25(OH)_2D_3$ did not increase expression of the M1 macrophage gene *IL12B* in THP-1 and HL60 cells (Fig. 3). Although *TNF* mRNA levels were not increased, *IL6* mRNA expression was effectively induced by the combination of 9cRA and $1,25(OH)_2D_3$ in THP-1 cells. ATRA plus $1,25(OH)_2D_3$ has been reported to induce mRNA and protein levels of tumor necrosis factor (TNF) and IL-6 in U937 cells [43] and to increase expression of inducible nitric oxide synthase (encoded by *NOS2*) and nitric acid production in U937 cells [44], while we observed no significant change in *NOS2* mRNA expression in THP-1 and HL60 cells after treatment with ATRA or 9cRA in combination with $1,25(OH)_2D_3$ (Fig. 3, and data not shown). Tumor necrosis factor (TNF) and IL-6 are cytokines produced from M1 macrophages and *NOS2* expression is a M1 macrophage marker [22,23,45]. Macrophages with a mixed phenotype expressing both M1 and M2 markers have been identified [46]. Thus, differentiated leukemia cells by 9cRA plus $1,25(OH)_2D_3$ are macrophage-like cells expressing primarily M2 markers with some M1 markers. Further analysis is required to reveal their functional characteristics.

The RAR signaling pathways play an important role in hematopoiesis and granulocytic differentiation [4,47]. With regard

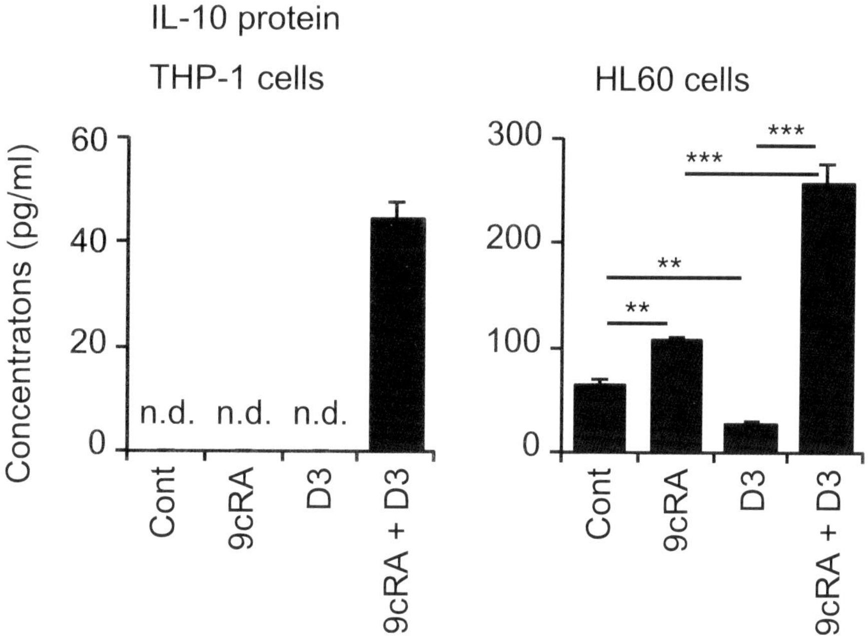

Figure 5. Secreted IL-10 production in THP-1 and HL60 cells. Cells were treated with vehicle control (Cont), 30 nM 9cRA and/or 100 nM 1,25(OH)$_2$D$_3$ (D3) for 72 hours and secreted IL-10 levels in media were measured. **, $p<0.01$; ***, $p<0.001$ (one-way ANOVA followed by Tukey's multiple comparisons). n.d., not detected.

to macrophages, ATRA inhibits TNF production in mouse peritoneal macrophages activated by lipopolysaccharide and interferon γ [48]. ATRA also reduces the synthesis of IL-12 and TNF and enhances IL-10 production in lipopolysaccharide-stimulated human macrophages [49]. Although VDR is dispensable for normal myelopoiesis [50], the vitamin D signaling pathway is involved in the regulation of macrophage/monocyte function [4]. 1,25(OH)$_2$D$_3$ suppresses activation of mouse macrophages by interferon γ [51], and enhances the immunoglobulin- and complement-dependent phagocytosis activity of human blood monocytes [52]. Thus, both ATRA and 1,25(OH)$_2$D$_3$ induce the macrophage/monocyte function common to M2 macrophages. Combined effects of retinoid and 1,25(OH)$_2$D$_3$ on physiological monocyte/macrophage function remain to be elucidated.

In contrast to 9cRA treatment, 1,25(OH)$_2$D$_3$ reduced *IL10* mRNA levels and IL-10 production in HL60 cells (Figs. 3 and 5). These findings agree with previous reports that show that 1,25(OH)$_2$D$_3$ suppresses *IL10* expression through VDR recruitment to the *IL10* promoter in monocytes [53,54]. Interestingly, 1,25(OH)$_2$D$_3$ enhances *IL10* expression of activated human B lymphocytes by recruiting VDR to the *IL10* promoter [55]. The combination of 9cRA with 1,25(OH)$_2$D$_3$ effectively induced IL-10 transcription and secretion in THP-1 and HL60 cells (Figs. 3 and 5). Thus, VDR activation induces or suppresses *IL10* expression in a manner dependent on cellular conditions. Treatment with 9cRA plus 1,25(OH)$_2$D$_3$ increased *CD163* mRNA levels and surface CD163 expression (Figs. 3 and 4). CD163 mediates IL-10 secretion in human monocytes [56]. IL-10 plays an important role in immune regulation by macrophages [46,57]. Our findings may provide an insight into mechanisms of IL-10 induction.

In conclusion, our results indicate that combined treatment with retinoid and 1,25(OH)$_2$D$_3$ induces differentiation of human myeloid leukemia THP-1 and HL60 cells into macrophage-like cells expressing M2 markers. Further study of human leukemia cell differentiation has the potential to extend differentiation-inducing therapy to the treatment of non-APL myeloid leukemia and to expand the understanding of human macrophage function.

Acknowledgments

The authors thank Dr. Shinya Suzu of Center for AIDS Research, Kumamoto University, Dr. Takayoshi Suganami and Dr. Yoshihiro Ogawa of Tokyo Medical and Dental University for helpful comments, members of the Makishima laboratory for technical assistance and helpful comments, and Dr. Andrew I. Shulman for editorial assistance.

Author Contributions

Conceived and designed the experiments: HT Y. Hatta MM. Performed the experiments: HT NI Y. Hatta HU MN. Analyzed the data: HT Y. Hatta Y. Hasegawa MM. Contributed reagents/materials/analysis tools: NI. Contributed to the writing of the manuscript: HT Y. Hatta MM JT MT.

References

1. Al Tanoury Z, Piskunov A, Rochette-Egly C (2013) Vitamin A and retinoid signaling: genomic and non-genomic effects. J Lipid Res 54: 1761–1775.
2. Wang ZY, Chen Z (2008) Acute promyelocytic leukemia: from highly fatal to highly curable. Blood 111: 2505–2515.
3. de Thé H, Chen Z (2010) Acute promyelocytic leukaemia: novel insights into the mechanisms of cure. Nat Rev Cancer 10: 775–783.
4. Nagy L, Szanto A, Szatmari I, Szeles L (2012) Nuclear hormone receptors enable macrophages and dendritic cells to sense their lipid environment and shape their immune response. Physiol Rev 92: 739–789.
5. Connolly RM, Nguyen NK, Sukumar S (2013) Molecular pathways: current role and future directions of the retinoic acid pathway in cancer prevention and treatment. Clin Cancer Res 19: 1651–1659.

6. Honma Y, Takenaga K, Kasukabe T, Hozumi M (1980) Induction of differentiation of cultured human promyelocytic leukemia cells by retinoids. Biochem Biophys Res Commun 95: 507–512.
7. Breitman TR, Selonick SE, Collins SJ (1980) Induction of differentiation of the human promyelocytic leukemia cell line (HL-60) by retinoic acid. Proc Natl Acad Sci USA 77: 2936–2940.
8. Dalton WJ, Ahearn M, McCredie K, Freireich E, Stass S, et al. (1988) HL-60 cell line was derived from a patient with FAB-M2 and not FAB-M3. Blood 71: 242–247.
9. Honma Y, Fujita Y, Kasukabe T, Hozumi M, Sampi K, et al. (1983) Induction of differentiation of human acute non-lymphocytic leukemia cells in primary culture by inducers of differentiation of human myeloid leukemia cell line HL-60. Eur J Cancer Clin Oncol 19: 251–261.
10. Brown G, Bunce CM, Rowlands DC, Williams GR (1994) All-*trans* retinoic acid and 1α,25-dihydroxyvitamin D_3 co-operate to promote differentiation of the human promyeloid leukemia cell line HL60 to monocytes. Leukemia 8: 806–815.
11. Taimi M, Chateau MT, Cabane S, Marti J (1991) Synergistic effect of retinoic acid and 1,25-dihydroxyvitamin D_3 on the differentiation of the human monocytic cell line U937. Leuk Res 15: 1145–1152.
12. Makishima M, Kanatani Y, Yamamoto-Yamaguchi Y, Honma Y (1996) Enhancement of activity of 1α,25-dihydroxyvitamin D_3 for growth inhibition and differentiation induction of human myelomonocytic leukemia cells by tretinoin tocoferil, an α-tocopherol ester of all-*trans* retinoic acid. Blood 87: 3384–3394.
13. Olsson IL, Breitman TR (1982) Induction of differentiation of the human histiocytic lymphoma cell line U-937 by retinoic acid and cyclic adenosine 3′:5′-monophosphate-inducing agents. Cancer Res 42: 3924–3927.
14. Nagpal S, Na S, Rathnachalam R (2005) Noncalcemic actions of vitamin D receptor ligands. Endocr Rev 26: 662–687.
15. Haussler MR, Whitfield GK, Kaneko I, Haussler CA, Hsieh D, et al. (2013) Molecular mechanisms of vitamin D action. Calcif Tissue Int 92: 77–98.
16. Honma Y, Hozumi M, Abe E, Konno K, Fukushima M, et al. (1983) 1α,25-Dihydroxyvitamin D_3 and 1α-hydroxyvitamin D_3 prolong survival time of mice inoculated with myeloid leukemia cells. Proc Natl Acad Sci USA 80: 201–204.
17. Abe E, Miyaura C, Sakagami H, Takeda M, Konno K, et al. (1981) Differentiation of mouse myeloid leukemia cells induced by 1α,25-dihydroxyvitamin D_3. Proc Natl Acad Sci USA 78: 4990–4994.
18. Mangelsdorf DJ, Koeffler HP, Donaldson CA, Pike JW, Haussler MR (1984) 1,25-Dihydroxyvitamin D_3-induced differentiation in a human promyelocytic leukemia cell line (HL-60): receptor-mediated maturation to macrophage-like cells. J Cell Biol 98: 391–398.
19. Mehta K, Lopez-Berestein G (1986) Expression of tissue transglutaminase in cultured monocytic leukemia (THP-1) cells during differentiation. Cancer Res 46: 1388–1394.
20. Defacque H, Sevilla C, Piquemal D, Rochette-Egly C, Marti J, et al. (1997) Potentiation of VD-induced monocytic leukemia cell differentiation by retinoids involves both RAR and RXR signaling pathways. Leukemia 11: 221–227.
21. Okamoto R, Koeffler HP (2011) Hematological malignancy. In: Feldman D, Pike JW, Adams JS, editors. Vitamin D. 3 ed. Waltham: Academic Press. 1731–1750.
22. Mosser DM, Edwards JP (2008) Exploring the full spectrum of macrophage activation. Nat Rev Immunol 8: 958–969.
23. Murray PJ, Allen JE, Biswas SK, Fisher EA, Gilroy DW, et al. (2014) Macrophage activation and polarization: nomenclature and experimental guidelines. Immunity 41: 14–20.
24. Hewison M (2012) Vitamin D and immune function: an overview. Proc Nutr Soc 71: 50–61.
25. Kagechika H, Kawachi E, Hashimoto Y, Himi T, Shudo K (1988) Retinobenzoic acids. 1. Structure-activity relationships of aromatic amides with retinoidal activity. J Med Chem 31: 2182–2192.
26. Umemiya H, Fukasawa H, Ebisawa M, Eyrolles L, Kawachi E, et al. (1997) Regulation of retinoidal actions by diazepinylbenzoic acids. Retinoid synergists which activate the RXR-RAR heterodimers. J Med Chem 40: 4222–4234.
27. Makishima M, Shudo K, Honma Y (1999) Greater synergism of retinoic acid receptor (RAR) agonists with vitamin D_3 than that of retinoid X receptor (RXR) agonists with regard to growth inhibition and differentiation induction in monoblastic leukemia cells. Biochem Pharmacol 57: 521–529.
28. Amano Y, Cho Y, Matsunawa M, Komiyama K, Makishima M (2009) Increased nuclear expression and transactivation of vitamin D receptor by the cardiotonic steroid bufalin in human myeloid leukemia cells. J Steroid Biochem Mol Biol 114: 144–151.
29. Iriyama N, Yuan B, Hatta Y, Horikoshi A, Yoshino Y, et al. (2012) Granulocyte colony-stimulating factor potentiates differentiation induction by all-*trans* retinoic acid and arsenic trioxide and enhances arsenic uptake in the acute promyelocytic leukemia cell line HT93A. Oncol Rep 28: 1875–1882.
30. Tavangar K, Hoffman AR, Kraemer FB (1990) A micromethod for the isolation of total RNA from adipose tissue. Anal Biochem 186: 60–63.
31. Sakashita A, Kizaki M, Pakkala S, Schiller G, Tsuruoka N, et al. (1993) 9-*cis*-retinoic acid: effects on normal and leukemic hematopoiesis *in vitro*. Blood 81: 1009–1016.
32. Nakajima H, Kizaki M, Ueno H, Muto A, Takayama N, et al. (1996) All-*trans* and 9-*cis* retinoic acid enhance 1,25-dihydroxyvitamin D_3-induced monocytic differentiation of U937 cells. Leuk Res 20: 665–676.
33. Kagechika H (2002) Novel synthetic retinoids and separation of the pleiotropic retinoidal activities. Curr Med Chem 9: 591–608.
34. Tobita T, Takeshita A, Kitamura K, Ohnishi K, Yanagi M, et al. (1997) Treatment with a new synthetic retinoid, Am80, of acute promyelocytic leukemia relapsed from complete remission induced by all-trans retinoic acid. Blood 90: 967–973.
35. Masciulli R, Testa U, Barberi T, Samoggia P, Tritarelli E, et al. (1995) Combined vitamin D_3/retinoic acid induction of human promyelocytic cell lines: enhanced phagocytic cell maturation and hybrid granulomonocytic phenotype. Cell Growth Differ 6: 493–503.
36. Carlberg C, Seuter S, de Mello VDF, Schwab U, Voutilainen S, et al. (2013) Primary vitamin D target genes allow a categorization of possible benefits of vitamin D_3 supplementation. PLoS ONE 8: e71042.
37. Bunce CM, Wallington LA, Harrison P, Williams GR, Brown G (1995) Treatment of HL60 cells with various combinations of retinoids and 1α,25 dihydroxyvitamin D_3 results in differentiation towards neutrophils or monocytes or a failure to differentiate and apoptosis. Leukemia 9: 410–418.
38. Evans RM, Mangelsdorf DJ (2014) Nuclear receptors, RXR, and the big bang. Cell 157: 255–266.
39. Shulman AI, Larson C, Mangelsdorf DJ, Ranganathan R (2004) Structural determinants of allosteric ligand activation in RXR heterodimers. Cell 116: 417–429.
40. Allenby G, Bocquel MT, Saunders M, Kazmer S, Speck J, et al. (1993) Retinoic acid receptors and retinoid X receptors: interactions with endogenous retinoic acids. Proc Natl Acad Sci USA 90: 30–34.
41. Tsao T, Kornblau S, Safe S, Watt JC, Ruvolo V, et al. (2010) Role of peroxisome proliferator-activated receptor-γ and its coactivator DRIP205 in cellular responses to CDDO (RTA-401) in acute myelogenous leukemia. Cancer Res 70: 4949–4960.
42. Sanchez PV, Glantz ST, Scotland S, Kasner MT, Carroll M (2014) Induced differentiation of acute myeloid leukemia cells by activation of retinoid X and liver X receptors. Leukemia 28: 749–760.
43. Taimi M, Defacque H, Commes T, Favero J, Caron E, et al. (1993) Effect of retinoic acid and vitamin D on the expression of interleukin-1β, tumour necrosis factor-α and interleukin-6 in the human monocytic cell line U937. Immunology 79: 229–235.
44. Dugas N, Mossalayi MD, Calenda A, Leotard A, Becherel P, et al. (1996) Role of nitric oxide in the anti-tumoral effect of retinoic acid and 1,25-dihydroxyvitamin D_3 on human promonocytic leukemic cells. Blood 88: 3528–3534.
45. Mantovani A, Sica A, Sozzani S, Allavena P, Vecchi A, et al. (2004) The chemokine system in diverse forms of macrophage activation and polarization. Trends Immunol 25: 677–686.
46. Noy R, Pollard JW (2014) Tumor-associated macrophages: from mechanisms to therapy. Immunity 41: 49–61.
47. Chanda B, Ditadi A, Iscove NN, Keller G (2013) Retinoic acid signaling is essential for embryonic hematopoietic stem cell development. Cell 155: 215–227.
48. Mehta K, McQueen T, Tucker S, Pandita R, Aggarwal BB (1994) Inhibition by all-*trans*-retinoic acid of tumor necrosis factor and nitric oxide production by peritoneal macrophages. J Leukoc Biol 55: 336–342.
49. Wang X, Allen C, Ballow M (2007) Retinoic acid enhances the production of IL-10 while reducing the synthesis of IL-12 and TNF-α from LPS-stimulated monocytes/macrophages. J Clin Immunol 27: 193–200.
50. O'Kelly J, Hisatake J, Hisatake Y, Bishop J, Norman A, et al. (2002) Normal myelopoiesis but abnormal T lymphocyte responses in vitamin D receptor knockout mice. J Clin Invest 109: 1091–1099.
51. Helming L, Bose J, Ehrchen J, Schiebe S, Frahm T, et al. (2005) 1α,25-Dihydroxyvitamin D_3 is a potent suppressor of interferon gamma-mediated macrophage activation. Blood 106: 4351–4358.
52. Xu H, Soruri A, Gieseler RK, Peters JH (1993) 1,25-Dihydroxyvitamin D3 exerts opposing effects to IL-4 on MHC class-II antigen expression, accessory activity, and phagocytosis of human monocytes. Scand J Immunol 38: 535–540.
53. Matilainen JM, Husso T, Toropainen S, Seuter S, Turunen MP, et al. (2010) Primary effect of 1α,25$(OH)_2D_3$ on IL-10 expression in monocytes is short-term down-regulation. Biochim Biophys Acta 1803: 1276–1286.
54. Matilainen JM, Rasanen A, Gynther P, Vaisanen S (2010) The genes encoding cytokines IL-2, IL-10 and IL-12B are primary 1α,25$(OH)_2D_3$ target genes. J Steroid Biochem Mol Biol 121: 142–145.
55. Heine G, Niesner U, Chang HD, Steinmeyer A, Zugel U, et al. (2008) 1,25-dihydroxyvitamin D_3 promotes IL-10 production in human B cells. Eur J Immunol 38: 2210–2218.
56. Philippidis P, Mason JC, Evans BJ, Nadra I, Taylor KM, et al. (2004) Hemoglobin scavenger receptor CD163 mediates interleukin-10 release and heme oxygenase-1 synthesis: antiinflammatory monocyte-macrophage responses *in vitro*, in resolving skin blisters *in vivo*, and after cardiopulmonary bypass surgery. Circ Res 94: 119–126.
57. Ng TH, Britton GJ, Hill EV, Verhagen J, Burton BR, et al. (2013) Regulation of adaptive immunity; the role of interleukin-10. Front Immunol 4: 129.

Permissions

All chapters in this book were first published in PLOS ONE, by The Public Library of Science; hereby published with permission under the Creative Commons Attribution License or equivalent. Every chapter published in this book has been scrutinized by our experts. Their significance has been extensively debated. The topics covered herein carry significant findings which will fuel the growth of the discipline. They may even be implemented as practical applications or may be referred to as a beginning point for another development.

The contributors of this book come from diverse backgrounds, making this book a truly international effort. This book will bring forth new frontiers with its revolutionizing research information and detailed analysis of the nascent developments around the world.

We would like to thank all the contributing authors for lending their expertise to make the book truly unique. They have played a crucial role in the development of this book. Without their invaluable contributions this book wouldn't have been possible. They have made vital efforts to compile up to date information on the varied aspects of this subject to make this book a valuable addition to the collection of many professionals and students.

This book was conceptualized with the vision of imparting up-to-date information and advanced data in this field. To ensure the same, a matchless editorial board was set up. Every individual on the board went through rigorous rounds of assessment to prove their worth. After which they invested a large part of their time researching and compiling the most relevant data for our readers.

The editorial board has been involved in producing this book since its inception. They have spent rigorous hours researching and exploring the diverse topics which have resulted in the successful publishing of this book. They have passed on their knowledge of decades through this book. To expedite this challenging task, the publisher supported the team at every step. A small team of assistant editors was also appointed to further simplify the editing procedure and attain best results for the readers.

Apart from the editorial board, the designing team has also invested a significant amount of their time in understanding the subject and creating the most relevant covers. They scrutinized every image to scout for the most suitable representation of the subject and create an appropriate cover for the book.

The publishing team has been an ardent support to the editorial, designing and production team. Their endless efforts to recruit the best for this project, has resulted in the accomplishment of this book. They are a veteran in the field of academics and their pool of knowledge is as vast as their experience in printing. Their expertise and guidance has proved useful at every step. Their uncompromising quality standards have made this book an exceptional effort. Their encouragement from time to time has been an inspiration for everyone.

The publisher and the editorial board hope that this book will prove to be a valuable piece of knowledge for researchers, students, practitioners and scholars across the globe.

List of Contributors

Hsin-Lien Huang and Hui-Yu Chen
Institute of Medicine, Chung Shan Medical University, Taichung, Taiwan

Shun-Fa Yang
Institute of Medicine, Chung Shan Medical University, Taichung, Taiwan
Department of Medical Research, Chung Shan Medical University Hospital, Taichung, Taiwan

Ming-Ju Hsieh
Institute of Medicine, Chung Shan Medical University, Taichung, Taiwan
Cancer Research Center, Changhua Christian Hospital, Changhua, Taiwan
School of Optometry, Chung Shan Medical University, Taichung, Taiwan

Ming-Hsien Chien
Graduate Institute of Clinical Medicine, College of Medicine, Taipei Medical University, Taipei, Taiwan
Wan Fang Hospital, Taipei Medical University, Taipei, Taiwan

Pei-Ching Hsiao
School of Medicine, Chung Shan Medical University, Taichung, Taiwan
Department of Internal Medicine, Chung Shan Medical University Hospital, Taichung, Taiwan

Shi-Jun Li, Hui-Ping Chen, Ying-Hua Chen, Li-hua Zhang, Yuan-Mao Tu and Zhi-hong Liu
National Clinical Research Center of Kidney Diseases, Jinling Hospital, Nanjing University of Medcine, Nanjing, China

Carmela Fimognari, Eleonora Turrini and Giorgio Cantelli-Forti
Department for Life Quality Studies, Alma Mater Studiorum-University of Bologna, Rimini, Italy

Piero Sestili and Cinzia Calcabrini
Department of Biomolecular Sciences, University of Urbino "Carlo Bo", Urbino, Italy

Giovanni Carulli, Giulia Fontanelli and Martina Rousseau
Division of Hematology, Department of Clinical and Experimental Medicine, University of Pisa, Pisa, Italy

Patrizia Hrelia
Department of Pharmacy and BioTechnology, Alma Mater Studiorum-University of Bologna, Bologna, Italy

Serena Ferraresso, Arianna Aricò, Maria Elena Gelain, Luca Bargelloni and Luca Aresu
Department of Comparative Biomedicine and Food Science, University of Padova, Padova, Italy

Silvia Bresolin and Geertruy te Kronnie
Department of Women's and Children's Health, University of Padova, Padova, Italy

Stefano Comazzi
Department of Animal Pathology Hygiene and Veterinary Public Health, University of Milano, Milano, Italy

Fulvio Riondato
Department Veterinary Science, University of Torino, Torino, Italy

Laura Marconato
Centro Oncologico Veterinario, Sasso Marconi, Italia

Ruihua Mi, Qian Wang, Xudong Wei, Qingsong Yin, Lin Chen, Xinghu Zhu and Yongping Song
Department of Hematology, Tumor Hospital of Zhengzhou University, Zhengzhou City, China

Haiping Yang
Department of Hematology, Tumor Hospital of Zhengzhou University, Zhengzhou City, China
Department of Hematology, First Affiliated Hospital of Henan University of Science and Technology, Zhengzhou City, China

Jingsong He, Li Yang, Xiaoyan Han, Gaofeng Zheng, Weiyan Zheng, Guoqing Wei, Wenjun Wu, Xiujin Ye, Jimin Shi, Wanzhuo Xie, Li Li, Jie Zhang, Weijia Huang, Yi Zhao, He Huang and Zhen Cai
The Bone Marrow Transplantation center and Multiple Myeloma Treatment Center, The First Affiliated Hospital of Medical College, Zhejiang University, Hangzhou, Zhejiang, P. R. China

Xuejin Zhang
Department of Hematology, Red Cross Hospital in Hangzhou, Zhejiang, P. R. China

Jiaping Fu
Department of Hematology, Shaoxing People's Hospital, Zhejiang, P. R. China

Chang Sook Hong
University of Pittsburgh Cancer Institute, Pittsburgh, Pennsylvania, United States of America

Laurent Muller
University of Pittsburgh Cancer Institute, Pittsburgh, Pennsylvania, United States of America
University Hospital, Department of Otolaryngology and Head and Neck Surgery, Basel, Switzerland

Michael Boyiadzis
University of Pittsburgh Cancer Institute, Pittsburgh, Pennsylvania, United States of America
University of Pittsburgh School of Medicine, Division of Hematology-Oncology, Pittsburgh, Pennsylvania, United States of America

Theresa L. Whiteside
University of Pittsburgh Cancer Institute, Pittsburgh, Pennsylvania, United States of America
University of Pittsburgh School of Medicine, Departments of Pathology, Immunology and Otolaryngology, Pittsburgh, Pennsylvania, United States of America

Yijiang Shi, Patrick Frost, Bao Hoang, Yonghui Yang, Carolyne Bardeleben, Joseph Gera and Alan Lichtenstein
Department of Medicine, Hematology-Oncology, Greater Los Angeles VA Healthcare Center, Los Angeles, California, United States of America
Department of Medicine, UCLA School of Medicine, Los Angeles, California, United States of America
Jonsson Comprehensive Cancer Center, Los Angeles, California, United States of America

Adam Cisterne, Rana Baraz, Naveed I. Khan, Robert Welschinger, Jordan Basnett, Carina Fung, Helen Rizos and Linda J. Bendall
Centre for Cancer Research, Westmead Millennium Institute, University of Sydney, Sydney, New South Wales, Australia

Kenneth F. Bradstock
Blood and Marrow Transplant Service, Department of Haematology, Westmead Hospital, Sydney, New South Wales, Australia

Minna Taskinen, Satu Koivula and Sirpa Leppä
Department of Oncology, Helsinki University Central Hospital, Helsinki, Finland
Genome Scale Biology Program, University of Helsinki, Helsinki, Finland

Riku Louhimo, Ping Chen, Ville Rantanen and Sampsa Hautaniemi
Genome Scale Biology Program, University of Helsinki, Helsinki, Finland

Harald Holte
Department of Oncology, Oslo University Hospital, Oslo, Norway

Jan Delabie
Department of Pathology, Oslo University Hospital, Oslo, Norway

Marja-Liisa Karjalainen-Lindsberg
Department of Pathology, Haartman Institute, University of Helsinki, Helsinki, Finland

Magnus Björkholm
Department of Medicine, Karolinska University Hospital, Stockholm, Sweden

Øystein Fluge
Department of Oncology and Medical Physics, Haukeland University Hospital, Bergen, Norway

Lars Møller Pedersen
Department of Hematology, Odense University Hospital, Odense, Denmark

Karin Fjordén, Mats Jerkeman and Mikael Eriksson
Department of Oncology, Lund University Hospital, Lund, Sweden

Brian M. Nolen
University of Pittsburgh Cancer Institute, University of Pittsburgh, Pittsburgh, Pennsylvania, United States of America

Frank J. Jenkins
University of Pittsburgh Cancer Institute, University of Pittsburgh, Pittsburgh, Pennsylvania, United States of America
Department of Pathology, School of Medicine, University of Pittsburgh, Pittsburgh, Pennsylvania, United States of America

Anna E. Lokshin
University of Pittsburgh Cancer Institute, University of Pittsburgh, Pittsburgh, Pennsylvania, United States of America
Department of Pathology, School of Medicine, University of Pittsburgh, Pittsburgh, Pennsylvania, United States of America
Department of Medicine, School of Medicine, University of Pittsburgh, Pittsburgh, Pennsylvania, United States of America
Department of Ob/Gyn, School of Medicine, University of Pittsburgh, Pittsburgh, Pennsylvania, United States of America

Elizabeth Crabb Breen
Department of Psychiatry and Biobehavioral Sciences, David Geffen School of Medicine at UCLA, University of California Los Angeles, Los Angeles, California, United States of America
UCLA AIDS Institute, University of California Los Angeles, Los Angeles, California, United States of America

Jay H. Bream
Department of Molecular Microbiology and Immunology, Johns Hopkins Bloomberg School of Public Health, Johns Hopkins University, Baltimore, Maryland, United States of America

Charles R. Rinaldo
Department of Pathology, School of Medicine, University of Pittsburgh, Pittsburgh, Pennsylvania, United States of America

Lawrence A. Kingsley
Department of Infectious Diseases and Microbiology, Graduate School of Public Health, University of Pittsburgh, Pittsburgh, Pennsylvania, United States of America

Helen Mahony, Athanasios Tsalatsanis and Ambuj Kumar
Department of Internal Medicine, Division of Evidence-Based Medicine and Health Outcomes Research, University of South Florida, Tampa, Florida, United States of America

Benjamin Djulbegovic
Department of Internal Medicine, Division of Evidence-Based Medicine and Health Outcomes Research, University of South Florida, Tampa, Florida, United States of America
H. Lee Moffitt Cancer Center and Research Institute, Department of Hematology and Health Outcomes and Behavior, Tampa, Florida, United States of America

Bei Xu
Department of Medical Oncology, the First Affiliated Hospital of Nanjing Medical University, Nanjing, PR China

Peng Liu
Department of Hematology, the First Affiliated Hospital of Nanjing Medical University, Nanjing, PR China

Irene Amigo-Jiménez, Elvira Bailón, Estefanía Ugarte-Berzal, Noemí Aguilera-Montilla and Angeles García-Pardo
Cellular and Molecular Medicine Department, Centro de Investigaciones Biológicas, Consejo Superior de Investigaciones Científicas (CSIC), Madrid, Spain

José A. García-Marco
Hematology Unit, Hospital Universitario Puerta de Hierro, Madrid, Spain

Alessandro Pastore
Department of Internal Medicine III, University Hospital Munich, Ludwig-Maximilians-University Munich - Campus Grobhadern, Munich, Germany

Friederike Pastore, Wolfgang Hiddemann and Karsten Spiekermann
Department of Internal Medicine III, University Hospital Munich, Ludwig-Maximilians-University Munich - Campus Grobhadern, Munich, Germany
German Cancer Consortium (DKTK), Heidelberg, Germany
German Cancer Research Center (DKFZ), Heidelberg, Germany

Georg Wittmann
Department of Transfusion Medicine, University Hospital Munich, Ludwig-Maximilians-University Munich - Campus Grobhadern, Munich, Germany

Carol Lozano-Santos, Belen Fernandez-Cuevas, Natividad Polo, Belen Navarro and Jose Antonio Garcia-Marco
Department of Hematology, Hospital Universitario Puerta de Hierro Majadahonda and Instituto de Investigación Puerta de Hierro Majadahonda (IDIPHIM), Madrid, Spain

Isabel Millan
Department of Statistics, Hospital Universitario Puerta de Hierro Majadahonda and Instituto de Investigación Puerta de Hierro Majadahonda (IDIPHIM), Madrid, Spain

Jimena Martinez-Velasquez and Natalia Gomez-Lozano
Group of Immunogenetics, Hospital Universitario Puerta de Hierro Majadahonda and Instituto de Investigación Puerta de Hierro Majadahonda (IDIPHIM), Madrid, Spain

Jose Miguel Garcia
Group of Oncology, Hospital Universitario Puerta de Hierro Majadahonda and Instituto de Investigación Puerta de Hierro Majadahonda (IDIPHIM), Madrid, Spain

Rosa Collado and Felix Carbonell
Department of Hematology, Consorcio Hospital General Universitario de Valencia, Valencia, Spain

Pedro Sanchez-Godoy
Department of Hematology, Hospital Severo Ochoa de Madrid, Madrid, Spain

Jose Antonio Garcia-Vela
Department of Hematology, Hospital Universitario Ramón y Cajal de Madrid, Madrid, Spain

Xiao-Na Pan, Jia-Jie Chen, Le-Xun Wang, Ruo-Zhi Xiao, Ling-Ling Liu, Zhi-Gang Fang, Quentin Liu, Zi-Jie Long and Dong-Jun Lin
Department of Hematology, Third Affiliated Hospital, Sun Yat-sen University, Guangzhou, China
Sun Yat-sen Institute of Hematology, Sun Yat-sen University, Guangzhou, China

Minjie Gao, Guang Yang, Lu Gao, Xiaosong Wu, Yi Tao, Xiaojing Hu, Jun Hou, Ying Han and Jumei Shi
Department of Hematology, Shanghai Tenth People's Hospital, Tongji University School of Medicine, Shanghai, China

Van S. Tompkins
Department of Pathology, University of Iowa Carver College of Medicine, Iowa City, Iowa, United States of America

Hongwei Xu and Fenghuang Zhan
Department of Internal Medicine, University of Iowa Carver College of Medicine, Iowa City, Iowa, United States of America

Camilla Pedersen, Vanna Albieri and Ole Raaschou-Nielsen
Danish Cancer Society Research Center, Copenhagen Ø, Denmark

Elvira V. Bräuner
Danish Cancer Society Research Center, Copenhagen Ø, Denmark
Danish Building Research Institute, Aalborg University, Construction and Health, Copenhagen SV, Denmark

Christoffer Johansen
Danish Cancer Society Research Center, Copenhagen Ø, Denmark
Oncology Clinic, Finsen Centre, Rigshospitalet 5073, University of Copenhagen, Copenhagen Ø, Denmark

Naja H. Rod
Social Medicine Section, Department of Public Health, University of Copenhagen, Copenhagen K, Denmark

Claus E. Andersen
Risø National Laboratory for Sustainable Energy, Radiation Research Division, Technical University of Denmark, Roskilde, Denmark

Kaare Ulbak
National Institute of Radiation Protection, Herlev, Denmark

Ole Hertel
Department of Environmental Science, Aarhus University, Roskilde, Denmark
Department for Environmental, Social and Spatial Change (ENSPAC), Roskilde University, Roskilde, Denmark

Joachim Schüz
International Agency for Research on Cancer (IARC), Section of Environment and Radiation, Lyon, France

Natalia Ruiz-Lafuente, María-José Alcaraz-García, Silvia Sebastián-Ruiz, Natividad Montes-Barqueros and Antonio Parrado
Servicio de Inmunología, Hospital Clínico Universitario Virgen de la Arrixaca, Murcia, Spain
Instituto Murciano de Investigación Biosanitaria Virgen de la Arrixaca (IMIB-Arrixaca), Murcia, Spain

Alfredo Minguela and María-Rocío Álvarez-López
Servicio de Inmunología, Hospital Clı́nico Universitario Virgen de la Arrixaca, Murcia, Spain
Centro de Investigación Biomédica en Red de enfermedades hepáticas y digestivas, Murcia, Spain
Instituto Murciano de Investigación Biosanitaria Virgen de la Arrixaca (IMIB-Arrixaca), Murcia, Spain

Joaquín Gómez-Espuch and Consuelo Funes
Servicio de Hematología y Hemoterapia, Hospital Clínico Universitario Virgen de la Arrixaca, Murcia, Spain
Instituto Murciano de Investigación Biosanitaria Virgen de la Arrixaca (IMIB-Arrixaca), Murcia, Spain

José-María Moraleda
Servicio de Hematología y Hemoterapia, Hospital Clínico Universitario Virgen de la Arrixaca, Murcia, Spain
Universidad de Murcia, Murcia, Spain,
Instituto Murciano de Investigación Biosanitaria Virgen de la Arrixaca (IMIB-Arrixaca), Murcia, Spain

María-Carmen García-Garay
Servicio de Hematología y Hemoterapia, Hospital General Universitario Santa Lucía, Cartagena, Spain

Devaraj Jayachandran and Doraiswami Ramkrishna
School of Chemical Engineering, Purdue University, West Lafayette, Indiana, United States of America

Robert E. Hannemann
School of Chemical Engineering, Purdue University, West Lafayette, Indiana, United States of America
Weldon School of Biomedical Engineering, Purdue University, West Lafayette, Indiana, United States of America

Ann E. Rundell
Weldon School of Biomedical Engineering, Purdue University, West Lafayette, Indiana, United States of America

Terry A. Vik
Riley Hospital for Children, Indianapolis, Indiana, United States of America

Ling Wang and Shunbin Ning
Center for Inflammation, Infectious Diseases and Immunity, Quillen College of Medicine, East Tennessee State University, Johnson City, Tennessee, United States of America

Zhi Q. Yao and Jonathan P. Moorman
Center for Inflammation, Infectious Diseases and Immunity, Quillen College of Medicine, East Tennessee State University, Johnson City, Tennessee, United States of America
HIV/HCV Program, James H. Quillen VA Medical Center, Johnson City, Tennessee, United States of America

Yanji Xu
Shaun and Lilly International, LLC, Collierville, Tennessee, United States of America

Jaebok Choi, Matthew L. Cooper, Bader Alahmari, Julie Ritchey, Matthew Holt and John F. DiPersio
Division of Oncology, Department of Medicine, Washington University School of Medicine, St. Louis, Missouri, United States of America

Lynne Collins
BRIGHT Institute, and Molecular Imaging Center, Mallinckrodt Institute of Radiology, and Department of Cell Biology and Physiology, Washington University School of Medicine, St. Louis, Missouri, United States of America

Alenka Smid, Natasa Karas-Kuzelicki, Miha Milek and Irena Mlinaric-Rascan
Faculty of Pharmacy, University of Ljubljana, Ljubljana, Slovenia

Janez Jazbec
University Children's Hospital, University Medical Centre Ljubljana, Ljubljana, Slovenia

Jussara Hagen and Sebastian Sciegienka
Department of Pharmacology, University of Iowa, Iowa City, Iowa, United States of America

Sara M. Reed
Department of Pharmacology, University of Iowa, Iowa City, Iowa, United States of America
Medical Scientist Training Program, University of Iowa, Iowa City, Iowa, United States of America

Viviane P. Muniz
Department of Pharmacology, University of Iowa, Iowa City, Iowa, United States of America
Molecular and Cellular Biology Program, University of Iowa, Iowa City, Iowa, United States of America

Dawn E. Quelle
Department of Pharmacology, University of Iowa, Iowa City, Iowa, United States of America
Medical Scientist Training Program, University of Iowa, Iowa City, Iowa, United States of America
Molecular and Cellular Biology Program, University of Iowa, Iowa City, Iowa, United States of America
Department of Pathology, University of Iowa, Iowa City, Iowa, United States of America

Timothy R. Rosean
Interdisciplinary Program in Immunology, University of Iowa, Iowa City, Iowa, United States of America

Weizhou Zhang and Siegfried Janz
Interdisciplinary Program in Immunology, University of Iowa, Iowa City, Iowa, United States of America
Department of Pathology, University of Iowa, Iowa City, Iowa, United States of America

Nick Borcherding, J. Adam Goeken, Paul W. Naumann, Van S. Tompkins and David K. Meyerholz
Department of Pathology, University of Iowa, Iowa City, Iowa, United States of America

Isabelle Tigaud, Sophie Gazzo and Denis Souche
Laboratoire d'hématologie, Centre de Biologie Sud, Centre Hospitalier Lyon Sud, Pierre-Benite, France

Sarah Huet, Jean-Pierre Magaud and Sandrine Hayette
Laboratoire d'hématologie, Centre de Biologie Sud, Centre Hospitalier Lyon Sud, Pierre-Benite, France
Unité Mixte de Recherche 5239 Centre National de la Recherche Scientifique, Faculté de médecine Lyon Sud, Oullins, France

Pascale Cony-Makhoul
Service clinique d'he´matologie, Centre Hospitalier d'Annecy, Pringy, France

Maël Heiblig, Mauricette Michallet and Franck Nicolini
Service Clinique d'hématologie 1G, Centre Hospitalier Lyon Sud, Pierre-Benite, France

Amine Belhabri
Service clinique d'hématologie, Centre Régional de Lutte Contre le Cancer Léon Bérard, Lyon, France

Yuichiro Hasegawa, Hikaru Uchida and Makoto Makishima
Division of Biochemistry, Department of Biomedical Sciences, Nihon University School of Medicine, Tokyo, Japan

Hiromichi Takahashi and Masaru Nakagawa
Division of Biochemistry, Department of Biomedical Sciences, Nihon University School of Medicine, Tokyo, Japan

Division of Hematology and Rheumatology, Department of Medicine, Nihon University School of Medicine, Tokyo, Japan

Yoshihiro Hatta, Noriyoshi Iriyama, Jin Takeuchi and Masami Takei
Division of Hematology and Rheumatology, Department of Medicine, Nihon University School of Medicine, Tokyo, Japan

Index